W9-BLB-999

THE
NATIONAL WOMEN'S HEALTH
RESOURCE CENTER

BOOK OF WOMEN'S HEALTH

THE
NATIONAL WOMEN'S HEALTH RESOURCE CENTER

BOOK OF WOMEN'S HEALTH

Your Comprehensive Guide to Health and Well-being

ANTHONY R. SCIALLI, M.D.
EDITOR IN CHIEF

ILLUSTRATIONS BY MARK M. MILLER, MA, AMI

William Morrow and Company, Inc.
New York

Library of Congress Cataloging-in-Publication Data

National Women's Health Resource Center book of women's health : your comprehensive guide to health and
    well-being / Anthony R. Scialli, M.D., editor in chief.
        p.   cm.
    Includes index.
    ISBN 0-688-12434-8
    1. Women—Health and hygiene. 2. Gynecology—Popular works. 3. Obstetrics—Popular works.
    I. Scialli, Anthony R., 1952– . II. National Women's Health Resource Center (U.S.) III. Title: Book of
women's health.
    RG121.N35   1999
    613'.04243—dc21   98–43590
                                                                                                          CIP

The National Women's Health Resource Center Book of Women's Health provides comprehensive women's health information in an easy-to-use home medical reference. As the authoritative source on women's health, the book offers discussions about major health concerns confronting women today, based on the Center's extensive experience as the national clearinghouse for women's health information, as well as the experience of the book's medical and health editors.

The National Women's Health Resource Center's award-winning publication, the *National Women's Health Report*, also offers comprehensive information, translating complex medical and scientific information into easy-to-understand language for the consumer. To subscribe to the *National Women's Health Report*, contact the National Women's Health Resource Center toll free at (877) 986-9472. To learn about the Center, and to obtain additional women's health information, visit its web site — the one-stop shop for women's health information — at *www.healthywomen.org*

The National Women's Health Resource Center Book of Women's Health supplements the information and medical advice of your personal physician or health provider. It should not be used as a substitute for medical care. The National Women's Health Resource Center cannot accept responsibility for the application of the information herein to individual medical concerns.

The National Women's Health Resource Center does not endorse any company or products.

Printed in the United States of America

First Edition

1 2 3 4 5 6 7 8 9 10

BOOK DESIGN BY RENATO STANISIC

www.williammorrow.com

This book is dedicated to all women who want to improve their health and the health of their families.

We hope that you will use this book as your reference on women's health, and that it encourages you to embrace healthy life-styles.

Contents

❦

Foreword

The staff and Board of Directors of the National Women's Health Resource Center, Inc. (NWHRC), the national clearinghouse for women's health information, are pleased to recommend this book. *The National Women's Health Resource Center Book of Women's Health* is a medical reference that addresses the health issues that concern women most.

Written for women, largely by women, this practical, accessible home reference offers comprehensive discussions of women's health concerns, as identified by the NWHRC and its medical advisers.

The book addresses a broad range of common and not-so-common health conditions and diseases. Our contributing editors and staff have attempted to translate complex medical and scientific information into easily understandable language. Throughout, we have provided a focus on disease prevention, and steps you can take to maintain a healthy life.

Many medical and health professionals contributed to the book, and to them we are grateful.

On behalf of the NWHRC and our medical advisers and contributors, thank you for choosing *The National Women's Health Resource Center Book of Women's Health* as your medical reference.

—Amy R. Niles, M.B.A.
Executive Director
National Women's Health Resource Center, Inc.
The National Clearinghouse for Women's Health Information

Preface and Acknowledgments

❧

Several years ago, the National Women's Health Resource Center, Inc. (NWHRC), decided to undertake an effort to publish a comprehensive medical reference pertaining to women's health. The result is *The National Women's Health Resource Center Book of Women's Health*. Through this book, the National Women's Health Resource Center hopes to bring you information about the latest advances in women's health and to encourage you to seek the information you need to make informed health decisions.

There are many individuals I would personally like to thank. First and foremost, I would like to thank the Board of Directors of the National Women's Health Resource Center, Inc., for having the insight and initiative to create and publish this women's medical health reference. Two individuals deserve an enormous thank-you—Amy R. Niles, Executive Director of the NWHRC, who served as Executive Editor, overseeing the entire project and the work of our contributing editors, and Trish Reynolds, R.N., M.S., who served as Managing Editor, collaborating on a day-to-day basis with the Center's contributing editors.

I am extremely grateful as well to Constance J. Bohon, M.D., F.A.C.O.G., and to Stephen J. Horwitz, M.D., F.A.C.O.G., both of whom served as Associate Medical Editors. From the outset, they helped identify the women's health issues to be addressed and personally reviewed many of the chapters.

Of course, a special thanks goes to all of the medical and health contributing editors. These editors spent many hours reviewing several iterations of each of the chapters before going to print, and I am appreciative of their time and support. Our editors are all women's health specialists and represent a broad range of disciplines, including obstetrics and gynecology, breast health, cardiology, critical care, dermatology, hematology and oncology, infectious diseases, internal medicine, mental health, neonatology, nurse midwifery, nutrition and exercise, oral health, pathology, pediatrics, perinatology, radiology, reproductive genetics, sexual health, surgery, and urology.

It was a particular pleasure working with Hugh G. Howard of Red Rock Publishing, Inc., on this project. As Editorial Director, Hugh had an excellent understanding of the goals of the book and how it should be written. He was always timely with draft manuscripts and was instrumental in making sure "things kept moving."

We were fortunate to have the services of Mark M. Miller as medical illustrator. Mr. Miller came to us with a wealth of experience, and we believe his artwork has added a great deal to this medical reference.

Our publisher is William Morrow and Company of New York City. All of us are grateful to William Morrow for recognizing the importance of women's health and agreeing to publish this book. We also appreciate the ongoing support of Bill Adler Books, Inc. A special thank-you goes to Senior Editor Toni Sciarra of William Morrow. Toni supported the publishing of this book from its beginning days and was absolutely instrumental in helping to identify the "tone" for the book, not to mention the countless hours Toni spent reviewing and editing text.

As Editor in Chief, I have enjoyed working on this project and having the opportunity to collaborate with its editors and publishers. I hope that you, the reader, will use it as a reference when necessary, and, as a result, will become more informed about your health.

—*Anthony R. Scialli, M.D.*
Editor in Chief

The Contributors

EDITOR IN CHIEF
Anthony R. Scialli, M.D.
Director, Residency Training Program
Department of Obstetrics and Gynecology
Georgetown University Medical Center
Washington, D.C.

ASSOCIATE MEDICAL EDITORS
Constance J. Bohon, M.D., F.A.C.O.G.
Senior Attending, Obstetrics and Gynecology
Columbia Hospital for Women
Washington, D.C.

Stephen J. Horwitz, M.D., F.A.C.O.G.
Associate Clinical Professor, Obstetrics and Gynecology
George Washington University School of Medicine
Washington, D.C.

CONTRIBUTING MEDICAL AND
HEALTH EDITORS

Obstetrics and Gynecology
Alan B. Birnkrant, M.D.
Senior Attending
Columbia Hospital for Women
Washington, D.C.

Kenneth A. Blank, M.D., F.A.C.O.G.
Clinical Instructor, Obstetrics and
Gynecology
Georgetown University School of
Medicine
Washington, D.C.

Bruce G. Bonn, M.D.
Assistant Clinical Professor, Obstetrics and
Gynecology
George Washington University School of
Medicine
Washington, D.C.

R. Russell Bridges, M.D., F.A.C.O.G.
Senior Attending
Columbia Hospital for Women
Washington, D.C.

Rebecca A. Douglas, M.D., F.A.C.O.G.
Associate Attending
Columbia Hospital for Women
Washington, D.C.

Martin W. Dukes, Jr., M.D.
Senior Attending
Columbia Hospital for Women
Washington, D.C.

Conrad J. Duncan, M.D., J.D.
Chief, Obstetrics and Gynecology
W. W. Hastings Hospital
Indian Health Service
Tahlequah, Okla.

Michael A. Farrell, M.D., F.A.C.O.G.
Assistant Clinical Professor
State University of New York
Health Science Center at Syracuse
Medical Director
Department of Obstetrics and Gynecology
Our Lady of Lourdes Hospital
Binghamton, N.Y.

John A. Gschwend, M.D.
Assistant Clinical Professor
F. Edward Hebert School of Medicine
Uniformed Services University of the
Health Sciences
Bethesda, Md.

Sara L. Imershein, M.D., F.A.C.O.G.
Assistant Clinical Professor, Obstetrics and
Gynecology
George Washington University School of
Medicine
Washington, D.C.

Heather Lee Mitchell Johnson, M.D.
Senior Attending
Columbia Hospital for Women
Washington, D.C.

Douglas G. Kalesh, M.D.
Senior Attending
Columbia Hospital for Women
Washington, D.C.

Deena Adrian Kleinerman, M.D.
Assistant Clinical Professor, Obstetrics and Gynecology
George Washington University School of Medicine
Washington, D.C.

Edward G. Koch, M.D., F.A.C.O.G.
Assistant Clinical Professor
Georgetown University School of Medicine
Washington, D.C.

Stanley C. Marinoff, M.D., M.P.H., F.A.C.O.G.
Clinical Professor, Obstetrics and Gynecology
George Washington University School of Medicine and Health Sciences
Washington, D.C.

John H. Niles, M.D., F.A.C.O.G.
Senior Attending
Washington Hospital Center
Washington, D.C.

Joan Redfearn, B.S.N., M.D.
Medical Director
Regional Health Care Alliance, Inc.
Washington, D.C.

Morton J. Roberts, M.D.
Chief of Obstetrics
Columbia Hospital for Women
Washington, D.C.

April Rubin, M.D., F.A.C.O.G.
Senior Attending
Columbia Hospital for Women
Washington, D.C.

George Samman, M.D., F.A.C.O.G.
Director, Columbia Physician Group
Columbia Hospital for Women
Washington, D.C.

Janet A. Schaffel, M.D.
Senior Attending
Columbia Hospital for Women
Washington, D.C.

Marciana W. Wilkerson, M.D.
Senior Attending
Columbia Hospital for Women
Washington, D.C.

Breast Health

Katherine Alley, M.D., F.A.C.S.
Director of Breast Services
Suburban Hospital Healthcare System
An Affiliate of Johns Hopkins Medicine
Bethesda, Md.

Judith Macon, R.N., M.A.
Program Manager, Breast Center
Suburban Hospital Healthcare System
An Affiliate of Johns Hopkins Medicine
Bethesda, Md.

Cardiovascular Health

Marilyn Winterton Edmunds, Ph.D., N.P.,
Adult and Geriatrics Nurse Practitioner
President, Nurse Practitioner Associates, Ltd.
Ellicott City, Md.

Alan A. Oboler, M.D.
Cardiovascular Interventionist
Washington Hospital Center
Washington, D.C.

Elizabeth Ross, M.D.
Cardiologist
Washington, D.C.

Dermatology
Elizabeth A. Liotta, M.D.
Dermatologist
Bethesda, Md.

Douglas N. Robins, M.D.
Assistant Clinical Professor of
Dermatology
George Washington University School of
Medicine
Washington, D.C.

Family Practice
J. Ricker Polsdorfer, M.D.
Diplomate of the American Board of
Family Practice
Freelance Editor and Writer
Phoenix, Az.

General Women's Health
Trish Reynolds, R.N., M.S.
Health Education Coordinator
National Osteoporosis Foundation
Washington, D.C.

Heidi Rosvold-Brenholtz
Editor, *National Women's Health Report*
National Women's Health Resource
Center, Inc.
Washington, D.C.

Gynecology
Bruce L. Ames, M.D., F.A.C.O.G.,
F.A.C.S., F.I.C.S.
Senior Attending
Columbia Hospital for Women
Washington, D.C.

Violet Bowen-Hugh, M.D., F.A.C.O.G.
Associate Clinical Professor, Obstetrics
and Gynecology
George Washington University School of
Medicine
Washington, D.C.

John L. Marlow, M.D.
Clinical Professor, Obstetrics and
Gynecology
George Washington University School of
Medicine
Washington, D.C.

Steele F. Stewart, Jr., M.D.
Clinical Associate Professor, Obstetrics
and Gynecology
George Washington University School of
Medicine
Washington, D.C.

Hematology and Oncology
Henry B. Fox, M.D.
Assistant Clinical Professor of Medicine
George Washingon University School of
Medicine
Vice Chief of Medicine
Columbia Hospital for Women
Washington, D.C.

Infectious Diseases
Lewis Marshall, M.D., F.A.C.P.
Senior Attending
Columbia Hospital for Women
Washington, D.C.

Intensivists, Critical Care
Serena Joan Fox, M.D.
Medical Director
Adult Intensive Care Unit
Columbia Hospital for Women
Washington, D.C.

Elena Marie Tilly, M.D.
Medical Director
Adult Intensive Care Unit
Columbia Hospital for Women
Washington, D.C.

Internal Medicine
Marc I. Cinnamon, M.D.
Assistant Clinical Professor of Medicine
George Washington University School of
Medicine
Washington, D.C.

Mental Health
Rosemary Tofalo Bowes, Ph.D.
Psychologist
Washington, D.C.

Constance E. Dunlap, M.D.
Psychiatrist and Psychoanalyst
George Washington University Medical
Center
Washington, D.C.

Jerilyn Ross, M.A., L.I.C.S.W.
Director
The Ross Center for Anxiety and Related
Disorders
Washington, D.C.

Neonatology
Parveen Chowdry, M.D.
Neonatologist
Columbia Hospital for Women
Washington, D.C.

Kenneth L Harkavy, M.D., F.A.A.P.
Director of Neonatology
Columbia Hospital for Women
Washington, D.C.

Dorothy S. Hsiao, M.D., F.A.A.P.
Neonatologist
Columbia Hospital for Women
Washington, D.C.

Nurse Midwifery
Barbara Good, R.N., M.S.N., C.N.M.
Columbia Hospital for Women
Washington, D.C.

Carolyn Dutcher, M.S., C.N.M.
Columbia Hospital for Women
Washington, D.C.

Nutrition/Exercise
Stephanie Harris Jackman
Independent Fitness Consultant and
Founder, Bodies After Babies Indeed
Silver Spring, Md.

Janet Zalman, M.S., L.N.
Director, Zalman Nutrition Group
Washington, D.C.

Oral Health
Hazel Harper, D.D.S., M.P.H., F.A.C.D.
Assistant Professor
Department of Community Dentistry
Howard University College of Dentistry
Washington, D.C.
Past President,
National Dental Association

Pathology
William J. Jaffurs, M.D., C.P., A.P.
Director of Pathology
Columbia Hospital for Women
Washington, D.C.

Pediatrics
Janet L. Adams, M.D., F.A.A.P.
Attending
Children's Hospital National Medical
Center
Washington, D.C.

Dennis Reginald Wirt, M.D.
Vice Chair, Department of Pediatrics
Columbia Hospital for Women
Washington, D.C.

Perinatology
Jean C. Bolan, M.D.
Co-Director, Division of Maternal–Fetal
Medicine
Columbia Hospital for Women
Washington, D.C.

George F. Bronsky, M.D.
Co-Director, Division of Maternal–Fetal
Medicine
Columbia Hospital for Women
Washington, D.C.

Jon M. Katz, M.D.
Director, Division of Maternal–Fetal
Medicine
Franklin Square Hospital Center
Baltimore, Md.

Radiology
Leonard M. Glassman, M.D.
Chief of Radiology
Columbia Hospital for Women
Washington, D.C.

Kirsten A. Hanson, M.D.
Diagnostic Radiologist
Columbia Hospital for Women
Washington, D.C.

Reproductive Genetics
Evelyn M. Karsen, Ph.D., M.D.
Director, Division of Reproductive
Genetics
Columbia Hospital for Women
Washington, D.C.

Sexual Health
Julius Fogel, M.D.
Medical Director, The Fogel Foundation
Washington, D.C.

Surgery
Joseph D. Afram, M.D., F.A.C.S.
Chairman, Department of Surgery
Columbia Hospital for Women
Washington, D.C.

Richard L. Flax, M.D., F.A.C.S.
Senior Attending Surgeon
Columbia Hospital for Women
Washington, D.C.

Joseph E. Gutierrez, A.B., M.A., M.D.,
F.A.C.S., F.I.C.S., F.R.S.M.
Senior Attending
Columbia Hospital for Women
Washington, D.C.

Urology
John E. Bresette, M.D.
Chief of Urology
Columbia Hospital for Women
Washington, D.C.

Mary C. Dupont, M.D., F.A.C.S.
Director, Dupont Urogynecology Center
Bethesda, Md.

Editorial Director
Hugh G. Howard
Red Rock Publishing, Inc.
East Chatham, N.Y.

Executive Editor
Amy R. Niles, M.B.A.
Executive Director
National Women's Health Resource
Center, Inc.
120 Albany Street
Suite 820
New Brunswick, N.J. 08901

Managing Editor
Trish Reynolds, R.N., M.S.
Health Education Coordinator
National Osteoporosis Foundation
Washington, D.C.

Contributors
Richard Atcheson
Washington, D.C.

Jean Grasso Fitzpatrick
Ossining, N.Y

Dale Gelfand
Spencertown, N.Y.

Elizabeth Lawrence
East Chatham, N.Y.

Susan Lawrence Volkmar
Raleigh, N.C.

Dawn Micklethwaite Peterson
Maplewood, N.J.

Lyn Yonack
Great Barrington, Mass.

Elizabeth Tinsley
Chatham, N.Y.

Medical Illustrator
Mark M. Miller, M.A., A.M.I.
Liberty, Mo.

Introduction

✌

As the title suggests, *The National Women's Health Resource Center Book of Women's Health* is about taking good care of yourself to promote good health. This book is about life, specifically about the life of a woman. It's about any woman and about a specific woman—namely, you—whether you see yourself as a daughter, a wife, a mother, a grandmother, a friend, or simply a woman trying to improve her own health.

In the pages that follow, we will visit all of the key biological, emotional, social, and medical events and processes in a woman's life. We will address a vast range of opportunities for improved health. At the same time, you will encounter in these pages—just as you will in your life—challenges, too, health challenges to which you may need to accommodate yourself.

We have attempted to make this journey through the health-care landscape more personal by incorporating a great many stories. These stories are real; they feature women who have had to confront specific health challenges, and how they dealt with them. We hope you feel the presence of these women as they consider and cope and question just as you may be doing.

In today's world, a woman makes more decisions about her life than ever before. This book is intended to help you think about some of those decisions as they relate to your health and well-being. Today's woman has important choices to make about how she lives her life—and making the right ones can help her stay healthy and happy. Wise choices about what you eat, how much you exercise, and whether you avoid risky sexual behaviors and substance abuse: All of these can help you find a sensible and healthful road to take. This book will help you choose your road—*and* will help you identify avenues to avoid.

Every woman is ever-evolving, moving through the stages of her life in her own unique way. This book will not dictate which ways to turn at the multitude of crossroads you will encounter. On the other hand, you may find it helpful in addressing many questions and in putting your life into a broader perspective.

THE SEASONS OF LIFE

You began as an infant dependent upon your mother and father for virtually everything and later became an independent adolescent, poised on the brink of puberty and capable of amazingly complex and creative thought. A decade in an adult's life is relatively inconsequential—but in a child, that first decade is a time of almost unfathomable change.

Think about it. A girl comes into the world a wailing bundle of reflexes. Within a month, she is recognizing family members. By four months, the newborn—a miniature sleeping and eating machine—has already evolved into a little person, able to control her head movements and sit up with little support. At a year she's walking and making noises that adults around her vaguely recognize as words. At three, she is proudly using the toilet, just like "big" people. At five she's become a social butterfly, going off to kindergarten, maybe not even looking back when her mother says good-bye at the door.

Soon she's reading, writing stories, and learning math. By the end of elementary school, she may be bringing home spelling words that her parents have to look up in the dictionary. One day she may blush at the mention of a boy's name, and the next declare that she's never going to have anything to do with men. In a class photograph, you notice that she and some other girls tower over the boys. Her breasts begin to develop, and she may even have started menstruating.

If the preadolescent years are a developmental fast track, the teenage years can be an emotional and physical roller-coaster ride. Whoever said *Life isn't easy* might well have been a teenager—or the parent of one. These can be difficult years: wonderful, certainly exciting, but nevertheless trying. One moment the young teenager is seen sporting a face on which not one centimeter has been spared a coat of makeup; the next she scrubs her skin until the freckles shine through, and she looks ten again.

As a parent, you may feel that your little girl has been taken over by an alien being. As an adolescent, you are simultaneously thrilled and scared. Not long ago the little girl came home eager to share her day with her parents; as a teen, she bristles when her mother *dares* to inquire into the state of her life. Suddenly, friends seem to matter more than family, and the house may be overrun by an assortment of kids trying to act older than they really are.

(Conversely, if you're a teenager reading this, like many of your contemporaries you may feel you're without a friend in the world. For many girls and boys, the teenage years have less to do with proms and football games than with a sense that you just don't belong. This can be a lonely, heartbreaking time for those who, for whatever reason, don't seem to fit in.)

Even under the best of circumstances, the teenage years—for daughter and parents alike—are fraught with conflict. Unfortunately, the changes that turn girls into women (and boys into men) physically sometimes outpace emotional and psychological development.

A teenager, a girl about to become one, or the parent of one—each treads in uncharted territory. Everyone's adolescence is unique, and there are no hard and fast rules that work in every situation. But remember this: Teens graduate to adulthood and many of those difficult moments fade into memory for child and parent alike.

Sometimes high school graduation is a springboard to college; soon enough, the work world, serious relationships, or marriage will beckon, too—and, as anyone over thirty will tell you, the pace of life in young adulthood seems to quicken. Young adulthood for most women (and men) is the time when paths are chosen. The college student tries out various directions and decides that one feels better than the other; she may proceed to graduate school. Other women have already begun permanent jobs. Whether it's through work or more schooling, the woman poised at the opening of her third decade finds herself aiming at goals and opportunities that will shape her adult life.

If you are at the brink of adulthood, you may feel free to follow your career path for the first time in your life, even if it takes you three thousand miles from those you love. You may inaugurate a relationship or life-style that would raise your parents' eyebrows. It's your choice: You are, in short, an independent adult.

It is during this period, particularly in its early years, that a person, to a large degree, invents herself. True, your personality was formed long ago. But it is during adulthood that it is honed, its rough edges rounded out and polished. Even if you've always known who you wanted to be, these are the years when you discover who you actually are, and that person may be entirely different from the person you expected. Moreover, it is during this time that most people discover the types of personalities they want to be with, both friends and lovers. Many young adults have their first serious sexual relationship during their twenties. For some, these years may be a time of risky experiments with various sexual partners, alcohol, or drugs.

From a physical standpoint, the young adult years are relatively carefree. Your body probably will not change much during the third and fourth decades of your life. But if you haven't already done so, these are the years to develop good habits. Those who treat their body well early in life should find the transition to middle age and beyond smoother.

These years are the principal reproductive years, too. Most life choices can be made almost anytime: You can go back to school, shift careers every five years, move from one exotic place to another, or change partners at virtually any point in your adult life. But women have a finite number of years in which to bear children; past a certain point, nature grows less and less cooperative and eventually childbirth becomes impossible.

Thus, it is little wonder that reproduction and the many issues it encompasses play a major role for women during this stage of life. When it comes to reproduction, you will undoubtedly find that your priorities change over the years to fit your circumstances. Perhaps in your adolescence and your twenties, your main reproductive concern will be to avoid pregnancy, whereas a few years later you may embrace the prospect of bringing forth a new life. Or, if you are at the point where your reproductive days are numbered, you may be pouring all your efforts, emotional and financial, into trying to have a baby. As usual, there are decisions and challenges to be made and to be met.

As you age, you approach the time when estrogen production begins to fall and the time when no estrogen is produced. The medical name for these years is the *climacteric*; the menopause follows, with the actual cessation of menses.

This means more than simply the close of the childbearing years. As the amount of estrogen produced by your ovaries decreases, your body undergoes many changes. Your vaginal tissues begin to change, the ligaments that support your reproductive organs and bladder lose their elasticity, the amount of collagen in your skin progressively diminishes, and you lose bone mass and face an increased risk of heart disease. Moreover, women's bodies take on more fat as well as a gain in overall weight during this time.

Yet late midlife is often an intensely happy and productive time for a woman. Her obligations to her family are likely to be on the decrease; her marriage (new or old) has the opportunity to bloom and grow on its own terms. Career and life changes seem somehow less traumatic: it's the wisdom of age, tempered by the good health and energy of late midlife, that make it all work better.

The older years are next. Dreading them, are you? Well, if you had been born in a previous century, you need not have worried about these older years. In fact, the odds were that you would have died long before you were even well into what we now consider middle age; a woman born in 1841 lived, on average, only forty-two years.

Over the years things have changed. Diseases that once wiped out entire families and whole villages are no longer a threat. Better health care and improved access to that care, an explosion of medical technology, sophisticated medicines, and improved nutrition all have helped both men and women live longer and, more importantly, better lives.

Naturally, as a result of such improvements there are more people living past the age of sixty-five than ever before. If you are a sixty-five-year-old woman living today, statistics show us that you can expect to live another eighteen years, and if you are already seventy-five, you probably have another twelve years of life ahead of you.

How will these years be lived? It wasn't long ago that society's narrow view was of an older woman happy to sit by the fire rocking as she knitted a blanket for the next generation. This generation's older women have broken that mold. Today's older woman may be running a business or involved in a satisfying career, be politically active or a tireless volunteer. She may be pursuing a degree, learning French or art appreciation, or traveling the world. In short, these are the years when many women are free to make real what yesterday could only be dreams.

Any organism's aging begins the moment it is born. Yet even though the body is constantly evolving, the change is gradual. You don't go from the smooth face of your twenties to an eighty-year-old's complexion crosshatched with wrinkles in the blink of an eye. The rate at which the human body ages is highly variable, dependent upon a host of factors including genetics, health, environment, nutrition, stress, the amount of exercise you have done, and whether you are a smoker. Some women, in fact, may look sixty when they're eighty.

When you find yourself approaching seventy or even eighty, in many ways you will still feel the same as you did when you were twenty. You may hear yourself asking, *Where did the time go?* Everything has happened so fast.

HOW TO USE THIS BOOK

This book cannot, of course, offer a magic formula for successfully navigating through the often turbulent waters of adolescence, of young adulthood or midadulthood, and living to enjoy healthy later years. What it can do, however, is discuss some of the major issues you should consider, as they will determine much about the health, happiness, and duration of your life.

Part I: Maintaining Your Health offers a five-step approach to the preventive measures you can take to enhance your life now and later. There's good advice on eating and exercising, on healthy sexual practices, and on how best to use your health-care practitioner. Although no regimen can guarantee good health and longevity, living a healthy life increases your odds immensely.

Part II: Special Health Concerns is issue-oriented. In these chapters you'll find sound guidance about the questions you may face as you consider which birth control method to use or whether to have cosmetic surgery. Tobacco, drug, and alcohol abuse are also discussed, as are physical and sexual abuse. Feeling depressed? Considering cosmetic surgery? These are major considerations described in detail in Part II.

Part III: Pregnancy and Childbirth considers having a child, for many women the ultimate challenge and yet a process fraught with worries. In the four chapters of Part III—*Planning the Pregnancy, Being Pregnant, Labor and Delivery,* and *The Postpartum Period*—you will find discussions of the critical concerns, the physical and emotional issues, and the decisions relevant to the wonderful challenge of pregnancy and childbirth.

Part IV: Medical Disorders and Diseases of Women describes and discusses hundreds of ailments that a woman may encounter in her life. Breast disorders, menstrual problems, sexually transmitted diseases, muscle and bone disorders, vaginal problems, and a range of other issues are discussed. The book closes with discussions of the common medical tests and procedures you may encounter in dealing with the health-care system, which are referred to throughout this book, and with a Glossary of common medical and anatomical terms.

This book was written for women, largely by women. It isn't a universal health-care reference—the subjects discussed in it were carefully selected because each is of special interest and concern to women. In creating this volume, the goal was to offer clear explanations, sound information and accessible guidance to the crucial health-care and life-style issues that confront women today. It is the hope of all of us who have written, edited, and assembled this book that the words and pages that follow will help you maintain and enhance your health.

Part I

❧

MAINTAINING
YOUR HEALTH

Women today have come to understand that good health care consists of more than regular visits to appropriate health-care professionals. The consumer must assume personal responsibility for her behavior; she must be a participant in the pursuit of good health, in partnership with dedicated professionals and on her own.

If you are in search of advice on preventive strategies to minimize the risks of such ailments as osteoporosis, heart disease, and a wide array of disorders that can be prevented or minimized by an intelligent life-style, the following chapters can often be your guide. A combination of appropriate medical care, safe sexual activity, good eating, regular exercise, and an understanding of your body and how it changes—that is a healthy strategy for a healthy life.

CHAPTER 1

✺

The Healthy Life

CONTENTS

An ounce of prevention is worth a pound of cure." Just another tired cliché? Not when the subject is health and longevity. Although some medical disorders may be genetically determined—diabetes mellitus, cystic fibrosis, some breast cancers—many others are not only avoidable but preventable. If your goal is to attend your grandson's wedding or see your granddaughter through law school, there are habits of body and mind that can help get you there.

Whatever your state of health, one very useful thing you can do for yourself and for your health-care provider is keep a record of your family's medical history. Certain diseases and conditions tend to run in families. Cancers of the breast, ovaries, and colon are one example, as are cystic fibrosis, high blood pressure, even alcoholism. Knowing what you may be vulnerable to will help you and your health-care practitioner develop a preventive plan that may decrease the risk of your having the disorder and, in the event you do, ensure that it is detected early.

Some preventive measures you can take on your own; others you take under a health-care practitioner's supervision. The most important of them prevent a disease or physical impairment from occurring in the first place. Not smoking is a prime example of primary prevention; another is always wearing your seat belt when you travel in the car. Secondary prevention is aimed at detecting disease in its early stages, before symptoms appear, and includes annual physical exams, Papanicolaou (Pap) smears for cervical cancer, and bone density tests for osteoporosis. Once a disease has been diagnosed, tertiary prevention may keep it under control or slow its progression. Someone with heart disease, for instance, may minimize further damage by cholesterol reduction and exercise.

Primary Prevention. If adopting a healthy life-style strikes you as just too much work, keep in mind that disease-preventive habits can make you *feel* great, too. Maintaining your optimal weight through exercise and a low-fat diet means you can move more quickly, play softball with the kids, look good in your clothes, and be a star at your twenty-fifth high school reunion. Not smoking isn't just good for your heart and lungs; it allows you to climb stairs and walk a quick couple of miles without gasping, and your partner will thank you for not tasting like an ashtray.

As you might have guessed, the single most important preventive measure you can take is not to smoke. Lung cancer is the leading cause of cancer deaths in women, and *75 percent* or more of lung cancers are caused by smoking. The disease is not easy to detect in its early stages, and by the time it has spread to other organs, the five-year survival rate is about 2 percent. If you're already a smoker, *stop.* People who quit—regardless of age and how long they've been smoking—live longer than people who don't. Avoid exposure to secondhand smoke, too—and if it comes from family or friends, by all means try to convince them to quit. You'll be helping them *and* yourself.

Substance abuse of any kind—whether it be cigarettes, prescription drugs, illegal drugs, or alcohol—means bodily abuse and has no place in a healthy life-style. Chapter 8,

Substance Abuse, discusses the particular hazards of substance abuse to teens and pregnant women, the genetic and environmental factors that may contribute to substance abuse, and some strategies for quitting (see page 160).

Alcoholism, which takes a toll on the individual, the family, and the community, is associated with liver disease, ulcers, osteoporosis, some cancers, birth defects, and other disorders. Fortunately, alcohol dependency is no longer a taboo subject in our society, and as research continues to suggest a genetic basis or predisposition in many cases, more resources have become available to the alcoholic who wants to get on—and stay on—the wagon.

This is not to say that alcohol in any quantity is necessarily bad for you; on the contrary, researchers have discovered that a moderate amount of wine may actually be good for your heart and arteries. The key word is *moderate*, of course, and if you're trying to get your weight down, don't forget that four ounces of table wine contains about one hundred calories.

Speaking of weight, there's no avoiding it in this context. The only sensible ways to lose weight permanently are to take in fewer calories than you expend and to exercise regularly. To maintain your optimal weight, you need to balance caloric intake and output, and that is most efficiently done on a low-fat diet and regular exercise. If you don't do these things already, it's not too late to start. Nor should it be too difficult, particularly if you introduce changes gradually and experiment with what works for you and your family.

Low-fat eating and cooking means a shift in emphasis: occasionally replacing beef and pork with fish and chicken, for instance, or even with a meatless entrée; substituting low-fat or skim milk products for whole milk; serving more salads or steamed vegetables and fewer french fries (potatoes by themselves are a great food, but not when they're fried in deep fat or drenched in gravy, butter, or sour cream); offering fresh fruit for snacks or desserts instead of cookies and pastries. Chapter 3, *Nutrition* (see page 45), suggests many strategies for switching to a low-fat, high-nutrient regimen, including tips for post-menopausal women, seniors, and those hard-to-please eaters, children.

Exercise is a tougher challenge for many people than cutting back on cake and milkshakes. How many of us have begun an exercise program, kept it up for a few weeks, then started finding all sorts of good excuses for not doing it today, or tomorrow, or at all? How many of us madly start walking three miles a day a month or two before bathing-suit season, then put away the Nikes in September? Exercise needn't be an onerous chore—it should be something you enjoy, like swimming, or walking around the neighborhood after work, or joining an aerobics class with a friend—but it should also be done regularly and consistently. Twenty to thirty minutes at least three times a week can do wonders for your body and your psyche. For some suggestions on how to start, see Chapter 4, *Exercise* (page 72).

When you make a lifetime habit of low-fat eating and exercise you're accomplishing two very important goals: staying trim and staying healthy. Both habits benefit your heart, your bones, your cholesterol level, and your immune system, and they may help prevent certain kinds of cancer. What's more, you can feel and see the benefits—in your skin, your eyes, your energy level, even your outlook. Your ability to deal with stress, which more and more is being recognized as crucial to good health, is greatly enhanced both by vigorous exercise and by more relaxed regimens like yoga.

Okay, you've incorporated the basics of good health into your life—you eat well, you exercise, you don't smoke, you don't drink to excess or take drugs you shouldn't, you stay out of the sun between ten and three o'clock, you wear a helmet whenever you ride your bike. You make time for yourself and the things you enjoy doing. What other measures of primary prevention can you take?

If you're sexually active, safe sex is one. Careful, responsible sexual behavior can save your life, and maybe someone else's. The fundamentals include using devices that prevent not only pregnancy but also the spread of acquired immunodeficiency syndrome (AIDS) and other sexually transmitted diseases (STDs). The condom—which, legend has it, has been around since Roman soldiers used oiled animal bladders and intestines—is still your best protection against STDs. So-called natural condoms are fine if you're in a monogamous relationship with someone you know isn't infected, but in all other cases use only latex condoms, which inhibit the passage of microbes. Other safe sexual practices are described in Chapter 19, *Sexually Transmitted Diseases and Other Infections* (see page 440).

Secondary Prevention. Preventive measures that constitute the second line of defense against disease include the various tests that detect disease in the early stages, before symptoms appear—Pap smears, mammograms and breast self-exams, glaucoma tests, blood pressure screening, and others. Many otherwise fatal or debilitating diseases can be halted or even reversed if they are caught early and treated appropriately, either with medication or with dietary changes, stress management, or exercise.

If you're one of the many women who just haven't gotten around to making monthly breast self-examination a part of your routine, think about this: The majority of breast lumps are discovered by women themselves, either accidentally or during systematic self-examination. While 80 percent of all lumps are found to be noncancerous, malignancies discovered at this stage are more responsive to treatment, and the chances of saving both the breast and the woman's life are higher. *The smaller the cancer at diagnosis, the better the prognosis.* Breast examination by both you (monthly) and your health-care practitioner (yearly), coupled with mammograms at the frequency recommended for your age, can significantly reduce your risk of breast cancer. To learn how to examine your breasts and how often to get a mammogram, see Chapter 17, *Breast Disorders* (page 367).

Tertiary Prevention. If you have been diagnosed with a chronic or acute disease, there are ways to keep it under control and prevent complications from developing. Your health-care provider will determine the best course of treatment, but it's up to you to adhere to his or her recommendations, monitor your progress, and report any problems or concerns. To the extent that it's possible, it makes sense to continue the habits of healthy living described earlier and at greater length throughout this book. As we get older it becomes particularly important to combat what used to be considered the inevitable ravages of old age—osteoporosis, heart disease, stroke, arthritis, even overweight—which, though not always preventable, can at least be delayed or lessened in severity. Some of the health issues that face women in midlife are discussed in Chapter 5, *Menopause and the Climacteric* (page 87), and in Chapter 3, *Nutrition* (page 45).

Getting Started. If you haven't yet jumped on the health bandwagon, it's never too late—but the earlier you do so, the better. Get your spouse or partner to join you. It's easier and a lot more fun when you can set goals and work toward them together. And if you can start your children on a lifetime of health awareness, you'll be giving them one of the best gifts anyone can give to the people she cares about most.

TALKING TO YOUR DAUGHTER, TALKING TO YOUR MOTHER

A woman's biological life may be seen in three stages: the years leading to menarche, or the beginning of menstruation; the childbearing years; and menopause, the cessation of menses. In adolescence, a girl's body undergoes changes that prepare it for pregnancy; in midlife, a woman's body gradually loses its childbearing function. Both transitions often entail emotional as well as physiological upheaval.

If you're the mother of a teenage daughter, there are things you can tell her—if she'll listen—about what to expect as her body changes and she grows into a sexual being, about how to take care of herself, about the lure of sex and smoking and drinking and other "adult" behaviors. Although teenagers tend to get much of their information and outlook from their peers or the media, you can teach by communication and by example.

Nutrition is one of the areas in which you can try to exert some influence. A nutritious breakfast containing protein and carbohydrates is a good way to help your daughter keep her energy and concentration high during the school day; lots of vegetables and whole grains at other meals and fresh fruit snacks and desserts help with weight control and skin care. Calcium is particularly important for future bone health; she should be getting 1,000 milligrams (mg) a day (see Chapter 3, Nutrition, *page 45).*

Encourage your daughter to exercise, either in organized sports or by walking, dancing, or some other form of vigorous physical activity. Weight-bearing exercise builds bone density and helps in maintaining healthy weight. If sound nutrition and regular exercise become enjoyable habits for your daughter during these years, she's more likely to stick to them for the rest of her life (see How Can I Get My Child to Eat Properly? *page 66, and Chapter 4,* Exercise, *page 72).*

Teen sexuality is a topic many parents would rather tiptoe around, but it's crucial that you keep the channels of communication open as your daughter makes the transition to womanhood. Whatever your beliefs about premarital sex, she needs to know she can come to you for guidance and help. Although most schools include sex education in their curriculum, you should reinforce the message that unprotected sex and sex with multiple partners carry the risk not only of pregnancy but of several sexually transmitted diseases (see Teenage Sexuality, *page 19).*

Talking to your mother about the health issues relevant to her generation is different in the specifics from talking to your adolescent daughter, but many of the basics are similar. A balanced diet and regular exercise still form the foundation of good health in the years after menopause. One difference is that most older women need to cut back on their caloric intake as their metabolism slows, in order to maintain their optimal weight. Another is that, to counter the risk of osteoporosis, older women should make sure they're getting enough calcium—1,000 mg a day for women who take estrogen, 1,500 mg for women who do not. Calcium is important for younger women also, as 98 percent of a woman's peak bone density is achieved by age twenty. Exercise, too, will help your mother keep her bones healthy and is good for just about everything else, including her state of mind (see Nutrition and Exercise in Midlife, *page 96).*

If your mother has taken good care of herself over the years and is conscientious about annual checkups, she knows how important it is to see her doctor regularly for Pap smears, pelvic exams (including the rectal exam), mammograms, bone density tests, and whatever else may be recommended for her. Don't let her forget the dentist, either!

Midlife may be a time of great change for your mother, but you can assure her that it can also be a time of great opportunity. Many women have found that, free of the responsibilities of child rearing, they have time to do all those things they put off for years, time for themselves, and time, perhaps, to reconnect with a spouse or partner. The renowned anthropologist Margaret Mead spoke of postmenopausal zest. *With a positive attitude, a continuing awareness of her health needs, and the determination to stay active and engaged, any woman can make the last phase of her life truly golden years.*

IMMUNIZATIONS

Immunization is the process by which a person is made resistant or immune to a particular disease. One way to develop immunity is to have a disease, at which time your body produces antibodies that destroy the invading organism and make you immune to further infection by that organism. The other, safer way to immunity is to ingest by mouth or through an injection a vaccine made of dead or harmless microbes. Thanks to advances in immunology, many childhood illnesses that once killed countless children are now rarely seen in the industrialized world.

Children in the United States must receive various immunizations before they can enter school. The following is an immunization schedule for normal, healthy infants and children:

Two months: diphtheria/tetanus/pertussis (DTP) and oral polio virus

Four months: DTP and oral polio

Six months: DTP

Fifteen months: measles, mumps, rubella (MMR)

Eighteen months: DTP and oral polio

Two years: Hemophilus B (Hib) conjugate vaccine

Four to six years: DTP and oral polio before entering school

While the majority of immunizations are given during the first years of life, don't assume that when you are an adult your vaccination days are over. Both teenagers and adults can benefit from certain immunizations:

Td. *A tetanus and diphtheria (Td) booster should be given every ten years to everyone over twelve, the first between the ages of fourteen and sixteen.*

Hepatitis B Vaccine. *Hepatitis B is a potentially dangerous form of hepatitis that can result in liver damage and even cancer. Those at highest risk include recreational drug users and sexually active people. Because many teenagers begin experimenting sexually at an early age and may have multiple partners over the years, many physicians recommend a series of three shots to protect them against this disease, to be started even as early as the preteen years. Ask your health-care provider for his or her recommendation.*

Viral Influenza. *If you are in good health, there is no reason to have an annual flu shot. However, if you are at high risk for lower respiratory infections or have a chronic condition such as asthma, cystic fibrosis, diabetes, or heart disease, yearly immunization may be advisable. Many physicians recommend flu shots for all people over age sixty-five to reduce the risk not only of infection but of possible complications and hospitalization.*

HOW OFTEN SHOULD I SEE MY HEALTH-CARE PRACTITIONER?

Both women and men routinely put off medical checkups because they feel just fine and believe that nothing is wrong with them. But because many diseases in their early stages have no symptoms, the main goal of periodic medical examinations is to detect problems when they are still treatable.

How often you see your health-care provider depends on many factors. If you have a family history of breast cancer, for example, more frequent mammograms may be recommended for you than would normally be indicated at your age. Thus the following should be used as a guideline only if you are in good health; if, however, you have pain or other worrisome symptoms, see your clinician.

Regular Physical Examination. If you are younger than thirty, you should have a routine physical examination every five to six years; between thirty and forty, every three years; and after forty, every year.

What can you expect during your checkup? First you will be weighed and your blood pressure taken. After questioning you about your family history, general health, and any medications you may be taking, your clinician will take your pulse and temperature, listen to your heart; examine your eyes, ears, nose, throat, and skin; and feel your abdomen for enlargement or other abnormalities. If you have a gynecologist, he or she should perform your annual pelvic examination and feel your breasts for lumps; if not, your regular physician will do it during your checkup. Depending on your family history and the results of your checkup, the physician may recommend further tests, such as a cholesterol count, tuberculosis (TB) screening, a stress test, or perhaps a glaucoma test.

Pelvic Examination. The American College of Obstetricians and Gynecologists recommends that women have a yearly examination of the pelvic organs. An important part of the pelvic exam, particularly for older women, is the rectal examination, during which the doctor inserts a finger into the rectum to check for colorectal cancer. Many health-care advocates recommend a yearly digital rectal exam for all women over forty, earlier if family history dictates the need.

Pap Smears. During your routine pelvic examination, your doctor will scrape some cells from your cervix onto a slide to test for cervical cancer. Once a woman becomes sexually active, most doctors recommend an annual Papanicolaou (Pap) smear.

Mammograms. If you have no symptoms and no family history of breast cancer and are between the ages of forty and forty-nine, your health-care provider will recommend a baseline mammogram with which to compare future X rays. The test should be repeated every one or two years and then annually after you reach fifty. If, however, breast cancer runs in your family, you may be told to start mammograms at an earlier age.

Proctosigmoidoscopy. If you do not have a family history of colon cancer, this test, which involves the insertion of a lighted tube into the large intestine via the rectum, is recommended at the age of fifty and every other year thereafter. More frequent tests may be in order if colon cancer has occurred in your family.

Bone Density Test. After menopause, if you elect not to take hormone replacement therapy (HRT), your health-care practitioner may recommend bone densitometry to estimate the density of calcium in your bones, which is compared to the average for women your age. Repeating the test after a year or two may help predict how rapidly you are losing bone mass. Some women find such predictions helpful in deciding whether HRT is right for them.

THE GYNECOLOGICAL EXAMINATION

When was the last time *you* had a pelvic exam? According to the American College of Obstetricians and Gynecologists, all women should have annual pelvic examinations after the age of eighteen and earlier if they're sexually active. But many women forget to make that yearly appointment or just keep putting it off; others find the examination of their most private body parts embarrassing or unpleasant.

For any woman—but especially one who is nervous about being examined—the first step is feeling comfortable with her health-care practitioner. For that reason many women go to their family physician or internist, a person with whom they have an ongoing professional relationship, for their pelvic exam. Some women prefer a woman doctor, in the belief that a woman will be gentler and more sensitive; for others gender is less important than a relaxed, helpful, nonjudgmental attitude. Because the gynecologist is the primary care physician for many women, these specialists today are trained to treat not only problems of the reproductive organs but also bronchitis, rashes, depression, and other nongynecological afflictions.

No matter whom you choose to do the exam, most routine pelvic examinations begin with questions about the date of your last menstrual period, past pregnancies, current contraceptive method, and date of last general physical. You will be weighed and have your blood pressure taken. Sometimes a urine sample is required, especially if you have not recently had a physical examination. The clinician may ask you about your sexual history and ask whether you have a problem with drug or alcohol abuse. If the doctor is not familiar with your general state of health, he or she may delve into your family's health history.

Then comes the pelvic exam, a relatively simple procedure. You will be asked to disrobe and be given a gown to wear. Then you will be instructed to lie on an examining table, with your knees bent and your heels in metal supports or stirrups.

Some health-care providers begin the examination with a general physical, including a breast exam. (If you don't know how to do self-examination, this is a good time to ask to be taught the proper technique.) Physicians can often detect lumps as small as one centimeter that even a diligent self-examiner has missed. A clinician's examination resembles the one you perform at home (see *Breast Self-examination*, page 373).

The genital exam follows. First, the external genitals are inspected for sores, swelling, or discoloration that could indicate an infection or other problem. Then, with an instrument called a speculum inserted into your vagina to hold the vaginal walls apart, your doctor inspects the vagina and cervix for lesions, inflammation, or suspicious discharge. The next step is a Pap smear, a painless procedure in which the cervix is gently rubbed with a cotton swab, brush, or small spatula. The cervical cells picked up by the instruments are then sent to a laboratory and analyzed for the presence of cancer or precancerous changes (see *The Pap Test*, page 531).

Some women are curious about how their reproductive organs look. If at any time during the exam you have the urge to see what's going on, ask for a mirror and take a look (you can do this on your own at home, too). Don't be afraid to ask questions.

After the Pap smear you will be examined internally. Although your uterus and ovaries are not visible, your practitioner has been trained to detect abnormalities by touch. He or she inserts one or two lubricated, gloved fingers into your vagina and, by pressing down on your abdomen with the other hand, can locate and feel the uterus and ovaries. This simple examination will reveal whether these organs are normal in size, shape, and consistency. If you have a tumor or cyst, it may be detected during the exam.

To feel ("palpate") your organs from a different angle—and to check for colorectal cancer—the clinician may insert one finger into your rectum and another finger into your vagina at the same time. Any stool deposited on the glove may be tested for blood, a sign of a possible colon cancer. The digital rectal exam is recommended for women over forty as part of their annual pelvic checkup.

Most healthy women find the exam uncomfortable but not painful. Relaxation is the key: the more you can relax those muscles, the less uncomfortable you'll be. If you do feel pain, tell your examiner immediately, as this could indicate a problem.

BREAST SELF-EXAMINATION

A woman's best hope for early detection of breast cancer—and therefore survival—is regular breast self-examination.

Regardless of your age, it's never too late to begin regular breast examination. Try to make it as much a part of your routine as exercise. It costs nothing, it can be done in the privacy of your home, and it's easy to perform once you understand the basics. It can save your life.

The procedure for breast self-examination is described in detail on page 373. Follow the procedure and any additional advice your health-care practitioner offers regarding breast self-exam.

Should you discern a lump when you're examining your breasts, consult your provider immediately. Don't panic; though it's natural to be frightened by the prospect of cancer, remember that 80 percent of all breast lumps are noncancerous.

THE MAMMOGRAM

Like any cancer, breast cancer is most successfully treated in its earliest stages. And nothing—not even diligent monthly self-examination—can detect a breast tumor as early as a mammogram. This special breast X ray can detect small tumors that are often years away from being large enough for even an experienced health professional to feel.

Two important studies have addressed just how effective mammography is at detecting minute cancers in women with no overt symptoms. In the first study, conducted by the Health Insurance Plan of New York in the 1960s, women were given an annual physical exam and mammogram for five years and then followed for ten to fourteen years. The study found a 30 percent decrease in breast cancer deaths among these women when compared with a control group of women who did not have mammograms. A larger study, the Breast Cancer Detection Demonstration Project, was conducted by the National Institutes of Health and involved the screening of 275,000 women over a five-year period. During this time, 3,557 breast cancers were found, 42 percent of which were discovered only with the help of mammography.

The question, then, is not whether a woman should have a mammogram but when and how frequently. In the 1970s many doctors were reluctant to prescribe mammograms for patients under the age of fifty, questioning the benefits to these relatively low-risk women when weighed against the possible harm of radiation. Today, improved diagnostic techniques and equipment have reduced the risks of radiation to a negligible level. Furthermore, we now know that women under the age of fifty are at higher risk of development of breast cancer than was previously thought: One third of breast cancers occur in this age group.

Even so, the National Cancer Institute (NCI), in a major policy shift, recently dropped its recommendation for women under fifty, citing inconclusive evidence that mammograms save lives in this group. The reason? The density of breast tissue in premenopausal woman makes detection less exact. (The recommendation still applies to women under fifty who are at greatest risk—those whose close female relatives have had breast cancer.)

Despite the NCI shift, the debate over the efficacy of mammograms for younger women is by no means concluded. The American Cancer Society recommends a baseline mammogram by the age of forty, a mammogram every one to two years between the ages of forty and forty-nine, and an annual mammogram after fifty. Many health-care providers and professional organizations still recommend periodic mammograms for women under fifty. The decision about how often to have mammograms is best made on an individual basis, taking into account family history and other risk factors.

Although a mammogram takes only a few moments, the tight compression of the breast can be uncomfortable. To minimize discomfort, schedule the X ray for a time other than just before or during your period, when your breasts are generally more tender. After the procedure, the X-ray result is examined by a specially trained radiologist and compared to any previous mammograms to identify changes that could indicate a developing problem.

Keep in mind that no test is foolproof. In some cases mammography has failed to spot an early tumor or has mistakenly identified a problem where none existed. So, effective as they are, mammograms should not take the place of either monthly breast self-examination or annual exams by a health professional. Nor is mammography the only radiological technique used in the diagnosis of breast diseases, although to date it is the procedure that combines the highest effectiveness with the least risk. Some other methods are *ultrasonography*, a painless procedure in which high-frequency sound waves are employed to examine body tissue; *computed tomography (CT)*, which has greatly enhanced physicians' ability to diagnose many diseases but is more problematic in diagnosing breast cancer than mammography; and *magnetic resonance imaging (MRI)*, which is capable of differentiating between benign and malignant tumors and could ultimately reduce the need for breast biopsies.

CHAPTER 2

❦

Female Sexuality

Contents

Writing about female sexuality for today's woman presents an especially complicated and sometimes daunting challenge. On the one hand, many contemporary women in midlife—accomplished, vigorous, satisfied women—grew up at a time when female sexuality at best was shrouded in mystery and sometimes shame, and at worst, assumed to be appropriate only in service of a man and a marriage. On the other hand, a good many somewhat younger women—vital, energetic women—grew up believing themselves to be fully entitled to rich sexual lives, and any suggestion to the contrary would strike them as surprising.

These two groups of women have been exposed to the controversies stirred by the sexual revolution, a period of history in which readily available and effective birth control, reliable research, therapy and counseling, legal and safe abortions, work, money, and greater independence came together to bring empowerment to women. Contemporary women, young and old, are consequently more likely to be open and more demanding in their sexuality than were their predecessors a generation ago. It is this willingness to be openly sexual and responsible for their own sexuality that forms a bridge for women of all ages as they explore their sexual selves and seek sexual expression.

In the late 1950s, sexual experimentation certainly was not unheard of. However, most women waited until their early adult years actually to engage in intercourse. Research now tells us that for the vast majority of women, sexual intimacy was viewed as a step toward marriage, and intercourse was reserved for the men they intended to marry. In contrast, today an estimated 75 percent of women in the United States have enjoyed sexual relations by the time they are twenty. Sex is often viewed as an end in itself—something a woman does for the sheer pleasure of it. By the time a woman marries—the average age now is twenty-four—she is likely to have had several sex partners. What is more, while American women still head for the altar, many do so two, even three times: An estimated 50 percent of marriages now end in divorce, twice the number of thirty years ago. To add to this complex mix, more than two million American couples live together without marriage.

In recent years, two topics, acquired immunodeficiency syndrome (AIDS) and menopause, have informed discussions of sexuality in new and important ways. As a greater percentage of women have economic and political impact, the subject of menopause has gained greater attention. This stage in a woman's reproductive life no longer carries the same stigma it did just a decade ago. Menopause represents an inevitable end to a woman's fertility and ushers in considerable physical and emotional change. Yet, far from being a "deficiency disease," as one feminist critic, Frances B. McCrea, has characterized its traditional perception, menopause presents an opportunity for renewed sexual richness and pleasure.

AIDS, on the other hand, is not an inevitability. Still, it will touch every woman's life in some way. This frightening, deadly, but mostly preventable sexually transmitted disease emerged in the eighties, as did the birth control pill in the 1960s, as a major influence in shaping sexual mores and behavior.

The sexual lives of women have clearly changed over the last few decades. Few women today feel the same embarrassment about expressing sexual needs. Women no longer have to be afraid to admit when something isn't right, whether it be a loss of sexual desire or the inability to experience orgasm. Lesbian life-styles, too, are more accepted, even as the courts and the general public grapple with issues such as homosexual parenting and discrimination against homosexuals in the workplace.

Despite what sometimes seems to be greater candor around and interest in sex—as well as the media's seeming willingness to sensationalize and exploit this candor—there are clearly gaps in our understanding of sexuality. A recent report by Indiana University's Kinsey Institute found that 55 percent of the two thousand adults surveyed could not answer adequately basic questions on such topics as contraception, AIDS, sexual stereotypes, and general sexuality. Of women respondents between the ages of thirty and forty-four, only 55 percent performed well on the questionnaire.

Given the tremendous changes in sexual attitudes, behavior, and complexity, it is not surprising that American women find this highly charged area confusing. Even in our enlightened age, most women, whatever their stage of life or personal experience, need to have questions answered and want to understand their options. In this chapter we will explore various elements of female (and, to a lesser degree, male) sexuality as it manifests itself and evolves through adolescence, adulthood, the menopause years, and beyond. We will also discuss such personal concerns as lack of desire and difficulty in reaching orgasm. To begin, we will talk about female sexual arousal and the steps that normally lead to orgasm.

SEXUAL AROUSAL AND ORGASM

Susannah can recall a time when no matter how hard she tried, she just couldn't become sufficiently aroused to have an orgasm. It wasn't exactly that her husband didn't touch her in the right places, but he seemed impatient. Beyond that there were the children sleeping in the next room, likely to wake and call her at any time. And she kept remembering that argument she had had with her assistant at work. Thoughts of her mother's ailing health and pending need for a nursing home in the near future also distracted her. It just didn't seem quite right that she should be enjoying sex now. But she missed it.

Jessica had been suffering from a slight depression and hadn't really been interested in making love for some time. The depression quickly lifted after her doctor prescribed fluoxetine hydrochloride (Prozac), but the medication did nothing to restore her interest in sex. She began to worry that it would affect her relationship.

Yvonne was crazy about her new partner, yet sex was not exactly thrilling. She did not want to hurt her partner's feelings by telling him that she wanted to be touched in a different way. After a while, she began to think that maybe this was not such a promising relationship.

Susannah and her husband found a sex therapist who helped them make room in their stressful lives for each other and for sex. Jessica told her doctor about her decreased libido, and her doctor helped her understand the problem: Though Prozac had alleviated her symptoms of depression, it had interfered with her sex drive. And Yvonne decided to check her embarrassment and talk openly with her lover about what kinds of touch felt good and what satisfied her.

The list of reasons why women may have less than satisfactory sexual experiences is long and complicated. For some women, physical or emotional problems stand in the way of becoming aroused and achieving orgasm (see *Sexual Difficulties and Dysfunction*, page 34). For these women, therapy—medical, psychological, or a combination of both—can help them move closer to a satisfying sex life. For other women, the difficulty lies in their situations: a new and unfamiliar partner, outside pressures and preoccupations, other health problems. Nevertheless, most women *can* become sexually aroused and *do* have the capability of reaching orgasm, especially when they know how their body works and what they need to reach sexual fulfillment.

The Stages of Sexual Response. Much of what we know about female sexual response comes from the 1966 Masters and Johnson book *Human Sexual Response*. Through their research, the authors identified four phases of sexual response: excitement, plateau, orgasm, and resolution.

EXCITEMENT. The excitement or seduction phase is characterized by deep breathing, increased heart rate and blood pressure, a feeling of warmth throughout a woman's body as well as in her genitals, and increased sexual tension. A woman's breasts become engorged with blood and some women develop a rash on the breast, known as sex flush. A woman's labia may become swollen and the clitoris erect. As she becomes more excited, her vagina secretes more fluid and her breathing deepens.

PLATEAU. During this stage of sexual excitement, parts of a woman's body become further engorged with blood. Her breasts and nipples continue to swell, as do her labia and the lower third of the vagina. Her vagina contracts by about 50 percent, enabling her to enjoy greater friction. The clitoris retracts.

ORGASM. This phase occurs when the sexual tension that has built up is released. During orgasm, muscles throughout a woman's body contract, especially those of the vagina, uterus, and anus. The contractions repeat every second. Both the number of contractions and their intensity vary among individuals. Some women studied by Masters and Johnson didn't realize they were experiencing orgasm. Other women had multiple orgasms that left them pleasurably drained. The researchers found that an orgasmic response could be heightened when the excitement phase was prolonged through masturbation or the use of a vibrator.

RESOLUTION. When the orgasm has passed, a woman's body returns to its usual state. Typically, a woman who has had an orgasm experiences a feeling of well-being. Unlike a man, whose resolution phase includes a period during which restimulation to orgasm is not possible, a woman is capable of enjoying an immediate repetition of lovemaking and orgasm without pause or recovery.

Research conducted by Masters and Johnson further concluded that the clitoris was the main focus of a woman's sexual satisfaction. For most women, regardless of their age, penile thrusting alone is not enough to bring on orgasm; clitoral stimulation before or during lovemaking is necessary. But like most other experiences in a woman's life, orgasm is a unique and complex phenomenon, one that brings together sensations from the skin, breasts, clitoris, labia, and possibly points within the pelvis.

FOREPLAY

Most women want and need foreplay before they are ready to have intercourse. During foreplay, both partners become increasingly excited. A woman's vagina feels wet as it secretes a lubricant that makes it easier for the male's erect penis to enter. Her nipples also may become erect. The amount and duration of foreplay vary with each relationship. For some couples, a special look may be all it takes to prepare both for sex. Others may take pleasure in more extended physical contact.

Foreplay takes many forms. Seductive whispers; sharing graphic fantasies; watching or reading erotic materials together; using vibrators and sex toys; gentle kissing, touching, and stroking of each other's bodies, breasts, and genitals; anal stimulation; and oral sex—stimulation of the male and female organs, fellatio and cunnilingus, respectively—have all been known to incite passion in women. The more familiar a woman is with the pleasures and responses of her own body, the more individualized, varied, and pleasurable foreplay becomes.

For most women, foreplay forms an integral part of lovemaking. To consider it a mere introduction or addendum to the sex act is clearly out of date.

THE G-SPOT

In the 1980s, the question of whether the female orgasm originated in the vagina or clitoris became a subject of heated debate among gynecologists and feminists alike. Unquestionably, the clitoris is key to female sexual response; at the same time, some researchers suggested that there was an area on the vaginal wall that, when stimulated, became engorged and, during orgasm, actually produced a fluid from the urethra, the tube through which urine passes from the bladder. The scientists labeled this area the G-spot (G being the last initial of the first researcher to write about it). In studies the researchers noted that when this area was stimulated, the female subjects became sexually excited. If the stimulation continued to the point of orgasm, liquid with qualities similar to those of a male's prostate fluid was ejaculated from the urethra.

    However, the existence of the G-spot remains unproved. Some research suggests that the cervix with its rich bed of nerves may be involved in sexual response, although this too has not been proved. What does this all mean in terms of sexual response? It is another indication of the somewhat mysterious quality of a woman's sexual experience.

TEENAGE SEXUALITY

Most girls have distinct sexual feelings in early childhood. A three- or four-year-old girl may enjoy openly and freely masturbating, depending, of course, on parental response. These early sexual feelings, though, blend into a girl's emerging awareness of herself and her body, as she struggles at this developmental stage with the understanding that she exists separately from her mother.

As girls enter adolescence, they become better able to isolate and identify these sexual urges and attractions, and to anticipate and understand the implications of these feelings. They feel some anxiety and confusion as well. Suddenly, a girl finds herself more interested in sexual matters. She may think about a boy she likes in school and imagine what it would be like to touch him or have him touch her. She and her girlfriends may laugh at dirty jokes or look at books or magazines that they wouldn't necessarily want their parents to see. What feels like forbidden, almost naughty enjoyment that girls often share at this phase in their development creates a bond between them; in fact, it is not uncommon for young teenage girls to kiss, fondle, and explore sexual feelings with each other. This kind of natural behavior does not predict, one way or the other, lesbian interest later in life.

As a girl's body changes, she may actively explore—both visually and through touch—her breasts and vagina in the privacy of her bedroom or bathroom. Some girls masturbate to the point of climax. Though for some the pleasure of masturbation is mixed with fear and shame, exploration is a perfectly natural part of discovery and development—just as an adolescent actively experiments with many aspects of identity as she strives to develop and consolidate a maturing sense of self.

Because teenagers are by nature so highly invested in their peers, young men and women feel strong pressure from outside to engage in increasingly intense sexual activities, whether or not they feel emotionally prepared to do so. After intercourse, some girls may feel guilty, scared, embarrassed, and confused, and these feelings may overshadow any pleasure they experience during their first sexual encounters.

There is a prevailing sense that today's children are growing up faster than ever before. Indeed, a girl today will begin to menstruate on average three years earlier—the average age at menarche is thirteen—than her great grandmother did at the turn of this century. This difference is attributed to better nutrition and general health habits.

But the rate at which a girl or boy moves through childhood toward adulthood is not limited to physical development. Other aspects of growing up have changed, too. Relaxed sexual mores, the availability of contraceptive devices, a loosening of parental supervision and authority, single-parent households (which often mean more open parental sexuality), the instability that divorce frequently brings, media that bombard us with provocative and glorifying images of sexual activity—these and many other factors make the teenage years a riskier, more confused time than it was a generation or two ago.

Consider these facts:

- Today more teenagers are sexually active—and often at a younger age—than ever before. Most will have had intercourse before they enter their twenties, and one in ten will have had multiple partners.
- More than one million American teenage girls become pregnant each year. Of this number, one third will have more than one pregnancy by the age of nineteen. The majority of these girls go on to give birth; 90 percent of them opt to raise the child themselves.
- Before AIDS reached into every layer of our society, an unwanted pregnancy or a sexually transmitted disease—troublesome but in most cases curable—was the most serious physical consequence of sexual behavior. Today, casual, careless sexual activity threatens a young woman's health and future. Thus far, there is no cure for AIDS, which spreads to women primarily through sexual contact or sharing of needles with someone infected with the virus.

What, then, does a teen need to know about sex? How can a parent or trusted friend communicate the wonders and the risks, the pleasures and the encumbrances of responsible sex?

For a parent of a teen, the need to forge open discussion about sexuality becomes a particularly tricky business. One of the tasks of adolescence is to separate and form an identity apart from her parents, so a teen's budding sexuality may well become a primary vehicle by which she may react against parental authority and assert her independent identity. The goal should be to find a way to talk about sex without prompting the exact kind of behavior—irresponsible sexual acting out—one wishes to prevent.

ROMANCE AND REALITY IN TEENAGE SEXUALITY

For many teenagers, sexual feelings in early adolescence are romanticized. As they move through their adolescent years, they typically add sexual behavior and experimentation to their imaginings. Let's look, for example, at Lucy.

At thirteen, Lucy dreamed about an older boy from a distance. She didn't fantasize about his touch or his lips or his genitals. Instead, she wondered what it would be like to hold hands at school, go to the movies with him, and talk on the phone. She spent time with her girlfriends talking about him, focusing on a desire for romantic tenderness. She was giddy as she carried on love affairs from afar.

As she got older, Lucy began to develop a greater awareness of herself as a sexual female. Now, at sixteen, she has a boyfriend. She spends more time with him and less with her girlfriends. He reciprocates her feelings, and they have begun to engage in sexual experimentation. Lucy feels aroused when he touches her. For Lucy, later adolescence is at once an exciting and a frightening time.

Late adolescence is also a trying time for Lucy's parents. Her boyfriend is unlike anyone in the family, and her parents don't like him very much. It seems to them that, by her choice, Lucy is actively rejecting them and their value system. In fact, although she is not aware of it, Lucy has chosen this boy as a way both to explore her evolving sexuality and to forge an identity that is distinct from her mother's. Yet, partly because her parents remain patient and available and resist criticizing, Lucy is able to move through the confusing transformations of adolescence and toward adulthood with an increasing understanding of herself as well as a greater sense of her own responsibility as a sexual being.

TALKING ABOUT SEX WITH YOUR TEENAGE DAUGHTER

Despite the advent of sex education and health programs in most schools, it remains the parents' responsibility to educate their children about sexuality and the consequences of sexual activity. How, then, does a parent go about it?

• Begin talking about sex early. *If a parent calls the parts of the body— vagina, breast, penis, anus—by their correct names (just as a leg is called a leg, and an eye is called an eye); if she describes accurately the process by which babies are conceived before the child is old enough to be embarrassed or self-conscious—perhaps as early as age three or four—talking about sex will always seem natural. Then, when it becomes important to talk about it, it won't seem to be such a big deal.*

• Don't assume that information is all your daughter needs to make the right choices. *No matter how much information she receives from her peers and teachers, her parent needs to be the primary source of information. That way parents can include discussions of their own value systems as well as listen to what their children think, believe, and want. Although you may feel uncomfortable talking about intercourse and imagining the child you once diapered as a sexual being, your approach should be honest and straightforward.*

• Emphasize that she can talk to you about sex anytime. *Share your own feelings about sex. If you think she should wait to engage in sexual intercourse, say so. But try to avoid being negative or critical of her choices, friends, boyfriends, and behavior. If a parent's opinion sounds like an order, a teen may feel pushed around or criticized. Few teens have been dissuaded by a dictatorial parent. Furthermore, an adolescent who feels that her parents are overbearing and judgmental is likely to turn away from them and toward friends for information, or worse, to act out in sexually irresponsible ways just to prove that she can't be pushed around.*

• Explain the relationship between sexual activity and AIDS and other sexually transmitted diseases. *Emphasize that should she decide to become sexually active, she is entitled to safe, responsible experiences. Therefore, she should protect herself. One way is to insist her partner wear a condom not only during intercourse, but in sexual play and anal stimulation as well (see* Birth Control, *page 101).*

• Be clear and explicit about birth control, and the reality and consequences of unwanted pregnancy. *When your daughter makes the decision to become sexually active, she should be in a position to make responsible choices and take appropriate precautions. In a time when so many young people are having sex, more than 50 percent of teenagers who get pregnant have neglected to use any means of birth control.*

Above all, let your daughter know that she can trust you: that you are there for her, no matter what happens.

MASTURBATION

The stimulation of one's own genitals for sexual pleasure is a normal and healthy practice. Masturbation offers a very personal way for a woman to release sexual tension, give herself pleasure, indulge in sexual fantasy, and develop a fuller sense of herself as a sexual being. Mutual masturbation and self-masturbation during lovemaking can heighten the experience. Some women find that more intense orgasms are brought on by masturbation than through intercourse.

The process of masturbation varies. Some women gently massage the clitoris itself; others rub a larger area around the clitoris. Still others insert a finger or other object into the vagina. Some use vibrators or running water (in the tub, for example) to bring on orgasm. This kind of stimulation leads to orgasm, in which involuntary muscular contractions produce a pleasurable sensation. The sensations are described differently from woman to woman; the methods of achieving them also differ. Whatever the method, however, masturbation enables a person to enjoy sexual activity without a partner.

Regardless of marital status, most women masturbate. This is true even when they are involved in sexually satisfying marriages or relationships. According to one recent study of female sexuality, 82 percent of women surveyed said they masturbated. Of that number, 95 percent said they were always able to have an orgasm during masturbation.

WHAT DO WOMEN REALLY WANT?

With all the attention female orgasm has received in the media, in movies, and on television, it would appear that, just as with men, sexual pleasure for women is in danger of being reduced to a simple process of genital stimulation and release. Moving the focus in sex to a localized, goal-oriented activity overlooks the richness and variety that are possible in a woman's sexual life. There is no question that, when they are asked, a more textured picture emerges: Different women enjoy different types of sexual pleasure, just as the same woman will enjoy and indeed feel deeply satisfied with different sexual experiences at different times in her life.

- Jackie: *"I really enjoy sex, being held, being close, feeling sexy and warm. There's just nothing like it. But—and I'm a little embarrassed to admit it—I've never orgasmed. I guess, though, that if it doesn't bother me or my husband, it's not really that important. I've been married almost twenty years, and I think we have a good sex life."*

- Kathy: *"It's okay if I don't orgasm every time. But, most of the time, I do feel sort of entitled to it. My husband wouldn't think that sex was over before he orgasms. Why should I be satisfied with less?"*

- Gwen: *"I love the energy of orgasm, the feeling of moving outward toward my lover and inward toward myself at the same time. I wouldn't consider sex completely satisfying if I didn't orgasm. I feel it in my ovaries, my uterus, my breasts, the back of my neck—everywhere. Sometimes when I just think about sex, I shiver at the thought of orgasm."*

- Sunny: *"When I was young, I thought that if I didn't have an orgasm, there was something wrong with me. Or I thought that my partner would feel somehow inadequate. So I sometimes faked it. Now that I'm older, I just like having sex. To tell you the truth, I don't have to have it all that often. But I'm satisfied because it's just part of my really full life."*

- Gerriann: *"I orgasm only through masturbation, so actually, I hardly bother with it during intercourse. I feel pressured when there's someone else around, like I have to hurry up and come. There have been times when I was with a man who seemed patient and caring, in which case I felt okay about letting him masturbate me to orgasm or doing it myself. That's rare, but when it happens, it's great."*

- Martha: *"I was in my late thirties when I first orgasmed, and I couldn't believe I'd lived that long without it. Suddenly, I felt this intense hunger, an ache, and the blood throbbing throughout my body, not just around my clitoris. It was like sparks. And then—it was as though I fell right into my lover. I'd always liked making love, but I must say, orgasm was just an added bonus to the whole wonderful experience."*

LESBIANISM AND BISEXUALITY

While the majority of men and women are involved in heterosexual relationships, a substantial and increasingly active segment of the population live openly as homosexuals. Many others are bisexual, that is, sexually attracted to members of both sexes.

According to a survey by Indiana University's Kinsey Institute, the pioneer in the study of sex, an estimated 4 percent of men and 2 percent of women are exclusively homosexual throughout their life. Currently, there are an estimated two to three million women living openly as lesbians in the United States, though experts believe there are many more lesbian women who are not open about their sexual practices. Many more are bisexual or have experimented sexually with members of the same sex on occasion. This practice is relatively common among girls and boys during their early years; such adolescent experimentation, however, is not necessarily a predictor of later sexual orientation.

What causes a woman to prefer another woman to a man for sexual relations? Until 1974 the American Psychiatric Association listed homosexuality as a mental disorder; today, after long and serious debate, homosexuality has been redefined by the medical establishment as a life-style, not a disease. Rather than a choice that one makes, sexual orientation is more often conceptualized as an aspect of identity that is likely to be inherent and later nurtured by environment and circumstance.

Just what accounts for gender identity—what makes a person heterosexual or homosexual—may never be fully understood. No doubt, the determinants of sexual orientation are complex and varied. However, myths, such as those that hold that women become lesbians as a result of aloof, distant, and rejecting fathers and smothering, overinvolved mothers, are clearly oversimplified and unfounded. It would be a mistake to attribute sexual orientation to parents' shortcomings. Further, such simplistic explanations imply and endorse the belief that homosexuality is a developmental deviation.

A recent study offers compelling evidence that homosexual orientation may be, at least in part, genetic. At the National Cancer Institute's Laboratory of Biochemistry, researchers found a significantly higher proportion of homosexual male relatives among the families of seventy-six gay men. Most of the gay relatives were on the mother's side of the family. This interesting observation prompted researchers to examine the X and Y chromosomes, which determine gender. Men receive the X chromosome from their mother and the Y chromosome from their father. When the deoxyribonucleic acid (DNA) from forty pairs of homosexual brothers was studied, researchers found that thirty-three pairs of brothers shared five different patches of genetic material grouped around a particular area on the X chromosome.

The significance of this finding to our understanding of homosexuality in general and to lesbianism in particular has to do with the fact that gene combinations are highly variable even among siblings. The degree of similarity between brothers who share the same sexual orientation cannot be dismissed as mere coincidence. The only trait, in fact, that any of these brother pairs shared was their homosexuality, leading scientists to believe they had discovered a genetic component.

Homosexuality's link to the maternal chromosome may help explain what has long puzzled scientists. Gay men are less likely than heterosexuals to have children. If homosexuality is indeed genetic, it would be difficult to explain why the trait hasn't disappeared over time. This new research suggests that the genes for male homosexuality can be carried and passed by heterosexual women to their children.

A similar study of lesbians is being conducted but is not yet complete because the genes responsible for sexual orientation are taking longer to identify. In another study that suggests a genetic link, researchers compared the sexual orientation of pairs of female identical twins and found that they have a higher incidence of lesbianism than pairs of fraternal twins or adopted sisters. (Identical twins share all the same genes, whereas fraternal twins have both genetic similarities and differences.) Researchers interviewed more than one hundred pairs of women about their sexual orientation. They recruited lesbians with an identical or fraternal twin or adoptive sister. Nearly half the identical twins were both either lesbian or bisexual, whereas one quarter of the fraternal twins and one in six of the adopted-sister pairs were both homosexual.

Regardless of homosexuality's genesis, it is important to understand that physically a lesbian is no different from a heterosexual woman. She reaches puberty, menstruates, can bear children if she chooses, and goes through menopause.

What is different, of course, is that lesbians have loving relationships with other women that go beyond friendship. Many of the sexual activities between two lesbians are similar to those between a man and woman. The lovers kiss and caress each other. Whereas in a heterosexual relationship, foreplay often acts as a prelude to penile penetration, this does not happen in lesbian sex. Some lesbian couples use dildos to add the feeling of penetration. Most lovemaking between women centers around clitoral stimulation. Lesbian lovers use mutual masturbation and cunnilingus (oral stimulation) to bring each other to orgasm. Vibrators are often used for enhanced clitoral stimulation. Tribadism, a practice in which one woman lies on top of the other and moves in a way that stimulates each partner's clitoris, is another way two women make love.

Many lesbians, having dealt with health-care providers who have been intolerant or insensitive, do not feel comfortable in health-care settings and as a result avoid seeking medical attention. Lesbians have gynecological examinations and Pap smears less often than heterosexual women. They may not seek help in the early stages of an illness when the problem is most effectively addressed.

Although a lesbian is just as susceptible to such common vaginal infections as trichomonas or yeast infections, and is at least as likely to contract human immunodeficiency virus (HIV) infection and therefore needs to follow the same preventative measures and seek the same treatment as heterosexual women, she is less likely to contract syphilis or gonorrhea. On the other hand, for those involved exclusively in lesbian relationships, there is no need for birth control or obstetrical care (unless a woman decides to be artificially impregnated).

As with heterosexuals, lesbian relationships assume different forms. Some women are basically on their own. They may have a wide circle of friends, date, and have relationships with different lovers. Others are involved with only one person at a time. Increasingly, many lesbian lovers are involved in and open about long-term monogamous relationships.

Motherhood is a natural part of the lesbian world. Many women were mothers before they acknowledged they were lesbians or before they assumed openly gay life-styles. Some publicly avowed their lesbianism and promptly lost custody of their children. On the other hand, it is becoming more common to find families headed by two mothers, families in which one or both women have children from prior heterosexual relationships, or into which children are adopted or conceived through artificial insemination with the sperm of a male friend or anonymous donor. In relationships in which one partner bears the child, the other parent, though not biologically related, may legally assume parental responsibilities and rights through adoption.

SEXUALITY AND SUBSTANCE USE AND ABUSE

Despite myths about sex under the influence, drugs and alcohol seldom enhance sexual performance or sexual experience. On the contrary, the use of excessive amounts of alcohol or drugs is likely to suppress a woman's sex drive and interfere with a man's ability to perform. Alcohol and drug use can also depress a person's ability to make reasonable and responsible choices in terms of partners and judgments about protection.

Alcohol is the most commonly abused substance. The National Institute on Alcohol Abuse and Alcoholism estimates that ten million Americans abuse alcohol with enough regularity to characterize them as alcoholics. Another seven million use alcohol in such a manner as to warrant some kind of intervention—either professional treatment or a twelve-step Alcoholics Anonymous–type program. Two thirds of all Americans over the age of fourteen drink alcohol from time to time.

Alcohol, even in modest amounts, affects libido. Consuming too many beers or glasses of wine will depress brain function, altering thought processes, emotions, and judgment. Driving and operating machinery after even moderate drinking pose an alarming danger to the drinker and to those around her. But even when alcohol consumption isn't particularly irresponsible, it can, when coupled with sex, result in awkwardness and regret.

A case in point: Although Mara and her husband, Adam, would deny that they abuse alcohol and certainly would not consider themselves alcoholics, Mara has found that too much drink interferes with her plans to make love and, over the long run, with their marriage. When Adam indulges, he is unable to perform in bed—either to maintain an erection or to bring himself to ejaculate. Despite his best intentions, once alcohol's sedative effect kicks in, he ends up snoring instead. As for Mara, while she is physically capable of making love, after she's had too much to drink, she too falls asleep, despite faint stirrings of desire. This happened only on occasion early in their marriage and Mara thought it was nothing to worry about. But as the years went on and parties became more regular and the few drinks imbibed to deal with stress became many, Mara's husband became impotent, and she became uninterested.

Drugs, too—both illegal drugs and prescribed medications—can alter sexual feelings. Heavy use of the opioid drugs, which include heroin, methadone, morphine, and opium, will depress a person's sex drive. Other street drugs such as Ecstasy, Ice, MDA, Crystal, and

Special K impair sexual functioning. Valium can hinder a woman's ability to have an orgasm; in males, it can impede ejaculation. Other prescription medications such as lithium, phenytoin sodium (Dilantin), alprazolam (Xanax), clomipramine hydrochloride (Anafranil), anabolic steroids, and amphetamines produce similar sexual impairment. However, it is important that any side effect of prescribed medications be discussed with the health-care practitioner, and that the woman taking these medications continue at the recommended dosage until she is able to consult her clinician.

Perhaps even more worrisome than the impairment of sexual function are the effects that alcohol and drugs have on reasoning and judgment. Inhibitions are compromised, and it becomes difficult to anticipate consequences. Not infrequently, people who are high have sexual encounters without the protection of condoms. This can result in pregnancy and/or a sexually transmitted disease.

Although most drugs that have an impact on sexual function inhibit lovemaking, in some cases a drug may be used by a couple to enhance orgasm. One such drug is amyl nitrite. This drug is a vasodilator, similar to medications prescribed for angina pectoris (a type of chest pain), which causes small blood vessels to expand. When taken prior to sex, amyl nitrite (also called "poppers") produces intense orgasm. Another substance sometimes used to intensify sex is butyl nitrite, an inhalant found in room deodorizers. Although these substances are not addictive, they can have serious side effects—there is a risk of lung, brain, and heart tissue damage—that may endanger a user's health.

A TIMETABLE FOR CHANGE

At what age do girls develop? Although that may seem to be a simple question, there really isn't a simple answer except to say that pubertal development is highly variable. One girl's breasts may begin to bud—the first sign of breast development—when she is only eight, while her sister may not notice any changes much before her twelfth birthday. Nonetheless, both are within the normal range.

So the age at which a given girl will begin puberty is difficult to predict. Not so, however, for the sequence of development, which, in most cases, proceeds in a fairly predictable manner.

The increase in height ("growth spurt") will be the first change a girl is likely to notice as her body begins to mature. Breast development is next, followed a few months later by pubic hair. Some degree of breast development generally occurs between the ages of eight and twelve; fewer than 1 percent of American girls have not had developed breast buds by the time they reach their teens. Pubic hair generally occurs between the ages of eight and thirteen. At the same time that this is happening, a girl notices a change in the distribution of fat on her body, especially around the hips. The average girl undergoes these changes between the ages of ten and eleven.

As the next stage of pubertal development unfolds, many internal changes occur. The vagina lengthens and the outer genitals become more pendulous. A white vaginal discharge may appear. The reproductive organs enlarge. You may notice you perspire under your arms, and an increase in activity of sebaceous glands in your face may lead to an eruption of acne. During this time—on average between the ages of eleven and twelve—you continue to grow rapidly.

In the next year or two, expect your breasts to grow larger and the areola, the darker tissue around the nipple, to form a mound that is separate from the rest of your breast. Your pubic hair will continue to spread and your reproductive organs will further enlarge. You are still growing but at a less rapid pace than before. Probably the most noticeable change in this stage is the onset of menstruation, which occurs in the majority of girls between the ages of twelve and thirteen.

Most girls between the ages of thirteen and a half and fifteen now have breasts and genitals that appear adultlike. Periods gradually become more regular. The growth spurt by this time is generally over.

MENARCHE

The day a girl begins to menstruate is usually a memorable one. After all, menstruation is, in many ways, a turning point in the adolescent girl's life—and as such isn't something you're likely to forget. Only yesterday you were in so many ways a child. Now, in the space of one day, things are suddenly changed forever. You are no longer a child, yet you are only really grown up in a reproductive sense.

Menstruation is the signal that a teenager is becoming capable of pregnancy. Every month from menarche to menopause, one of the hundreds of thousands of eggs your ovaries have contained since well before your birth begins to ripen within a tiny sac called a *follicle*. During the process, called *ovulation*, the ovaries secrete a high level of estrogen, which causes the lining of the uterus (endometrium) to grow and thicken. A day or so prior to ovulation (when the egg is released), estrogen levels fall and the hormone progesterone is produced. The egg is then released to begin its six-day journey to the uterus.

If an egg traveling down the fallopian tube en route to the uterus is fertilized by sperm, it burrows into the blood- and nutrient-rich bed of the uterus and begins to grow into an embryo. If fertilization does not take place, however, upon reaching the uterus the egg either disintegrates or is expelled in vaginal secretions. Dropping hormonal levels trigger the uterus to shed its lining—twice its usual thickness—because it isn't needed to nourish a growing embryo. The menstrual flow is made up of the blood, secretions, and tissues of this lining.

The average menstrual cycle is twenty-eight days, although some women may have a period every three weeks, and others may go as long as thirty-five days between periods. Each monthly period normally will last between three and seven days. Initially, many girls have irregular periods and even those whose periods are usually like clockwork can occasionally be irregular without cause for concern, unless, of course, there is a chance of pregnancy (see *The Menstrual Cycle*, page 404, for more details).

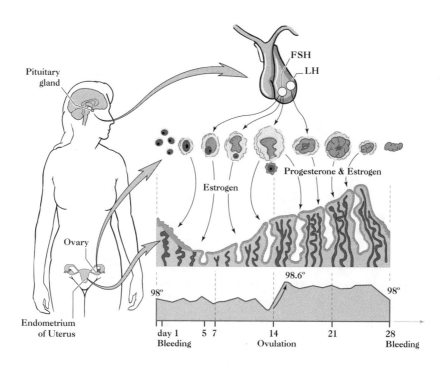

FSH
LH
Pituitary gland
Progesterone & Estrogen
Estrogen
Ovary
Endometrium of Uterus

98.6°
98°   98°

day 1   5 7   14   21   28
Bleeding   Ovulation   Bleeding

During the twenty-eight-day menstrual cycle, the pituitary gland at the base of the brain secretes follicle-stimulating hormone (FSH) and luteinizing hormone (LH). The result is an increase in estrogen production and a thickening of the uterine lining. At the midpoint in the cycle, ovulation occurs. An egg is released, and it travels through the fallopian tubes to the uterus. If the egg is fertilized, it implants itself in the uterus and pregnancy begins. If not, the egg will pass out of the body along with the menstrual flow, which consists of the blood, secretions, and tissues of this lining.

Although menstruation is a perfectly normal physical process, many girls and women have some uncomfortable symptoms prior to or during their period. The hormonal changes in your body may cause your skin to break out with acne a few days before your period. Some women have bloating and even a slight weight increase. Some women find themselves becoming depressed, irritable, or moody around the time of their period. Many devise strategies involving exercise (a regular program may minimize menstrual discomforts), nutrition (avoidance of coffee and alcohol, for example), and even an over-the-counter pain medication such as ibuprofen that helps them feel better. An estimated 2 to 5 percent of women, however, have such severe premenstrual syndrome (PMS) that they require additional therapy, but PMS is more common in women in their twenties and thirties than in teenagers (see *Premenstrual Syndrome*, page 410).

Adolescents who have recently started menstruating often worry about keeping themselves and their clothes clean during their period. The answer certainly isn't douching, which, rather than being healthful, can change the pH balance of the vagina and may irri-

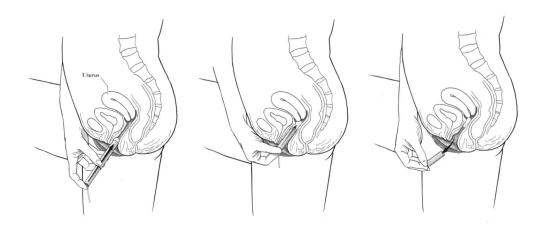

Uterus

*Standing with one leg raised or sitting on the toilet, gently hold open the skin surrounding
the vaginal opening and position the tampon applicator, if any (left), or the tampon itself
at the entrance to the vagina (center). Using the injector or your index finger, ease the tampon inside
your body, aiming it toward the small of your back. When the tampon is placed within
the vagina, remove the applicator (right).*

tate the delicate tissues. Most girls start out using disposable external pads to absorb the
flow. These are especially effective today because the belts that women once had to use to
hold the pads in place have been replaced by pads that adhere directly to the panty.

Although many girls are nervous about using tampons, even a girl who has never had
intercourse should be able to use one with practice because the hymenal membrane normally does not cover the vaginal opening completely. If you do opt to use a tampon, though,
be sure you change it every three to four hours because of the risk of toxic shock syndrome,
a rare but sometimes fatal condition associated with tampon use. Instead of using a tampon,
you may also want to use a pad at night to minimize the risk of toxic shock (see *Toxic Shock
Syndrome*, page 428).

SEXUALITY AND THE CLIMACTERIC

Until very recently, menopause was associated exclusively with endings: the ending of a
woman's fertility, the ending of her sex drive and her sexuality, the ending of her femininity. But these associations were a product of an era in which a woman's value was defined in
terms of her childbearing capabilities, so that once her reproductive years were over, so was
her usefulness.

Luckily, the greater presence of women in the work force, feminism, and sexual awareness have changed this perception. Although it is true that menopause marks the end of a
woman's reproductive capabilities, it is also true that women's attitudes toward and experience of menopause have changed, thanks largely to better health habits, greater awareness,
and new therapies. Certainly, a woman's need to express herself sexually does not end just

because she reaches a certain age. For most women, the years during and after menopause present the opportunity to reexamine their lives and, often, to rediscover the sexuality of their youth. With family responsibilities shifting and the threat of unwelcome pregnancies eliminated, many couples in midlife have time and attention to devote to one another. Sexual options broaden. Now that the kids are out of the house, sex can be as spontaneous as it was when a woman first fell in love.

For some women, however, the climacteric—the period during which the ovaries begin to reduce their production of estrogen, leading to what is called menopause—is not so kind to their sex life. Various health problems that go hand in hand with aging can interfere with sexual activity. Then, too, for many women, midlife presents not only physical changes but life-style alterations as well. Some find that with children off at college or established in lives of their own, their love relationships lack the flexibility or richness to weather the changes; there seems little reason to stay together. Divorced or widowed, many women are without permanent sex partners for the first time in their adult life and find dating and renewing intimacy awkward and, at times, just plain difficult.

Because many contemporary women have waited longer to start families, some women approach menopause at a time when they are still caring for young children. Many have busy and exacting jobs that yield various degrees of personal satisfaction. In some cases,

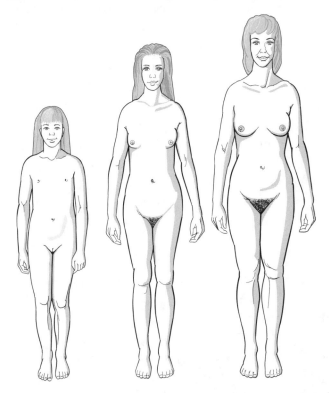

The female form of a young girl (left); *an adolescent* (center); *and a mature woman* (right).

these very same women are called on to care for elderly parents, so that the stress that internal changes can bring is, at times, magnified by external demands.

As a woman nears midlife, however, especially if she has a history of sexual problems or dissatisfaction, it may be tempting to dismiss sex as something, like a wrinkle-free complexion, belonging to a different era. But it is not necessary to do so. Women in their seventies and eighties have active sexual feelings. Considering that women generally outlive men, the opportunities for sex late in life may be limited. Nevertheless, desire does not die out, and, given the opportunity, most women are capable of having satisfying sexual experiences.

Let's look at some of the sexual obstacles in midlife that may stand between you and a rich and rewarding sex life.

Lack of Desire. Some women notice that once they reach menopause their interest in sex has diminished. In many cases this lack of interest points to a larger problem in the marriage or relationship. If lack of desire stems from relational problems, professional counseling for both partners is the recommended approach.

Moodiness, resulting from reduced estrogen levels at menopause, may diminish sexual desire. On the other hand, progestins, which are commonly prescribed together with estrogen during menopause to guard against the increased incidence of endometrial cancer associated with long-term estrogen replacement, can induce or exacerbate emotional volatility. Other medications, such as diuretics, antidepressants, and antianxiety drugs, can interfere with a woman's sex drive.

Some women who have undergone hysterectomy report that, even with estrogen therapy, their pleasure during sexual intercourse has been significantly lessened. Hormone therapy does not compensate for the lack of androgens, which were once secreted by functioning ovaries and which contribute to a woman's sexual desire and responsiveness. Moreover, the loss of the cervix may alter the intensity and quality of a woman's sexual experience.

However, most women can address diminished libido in consultation with their health-care provider. Treatment may include having therapy for depression, changing or discontinuing medication, or beginning estrogen replacement therapy (see *Hormone Replacement Therapy*, page 90). In cases in which a woman is on hormone replacement therapy and still experiences a marked decline in her sex drive, the health-care practitioner may recommend a small dose of an androgen such as testosterone. Usually given orally in addition to estrogen, testosterone can recharge the sex drive of women who have lost it and induce desire in women who have never felt it. As with any therapy, the risks and benefits of hormone therapy must be thoughtfully weighed.

Vaginal Changes That Make Sex Difficult. Once a woman goes through menopause, her body no longer produces the large amounts of estrogen it once did. This is a radical change that affects many parts of the body. A woman may feel that her vagina is uncomfortably dry, making sex difficult or painful (dyspareunia). Along with a decrease in vaginal secretion comes a thinning of vaginal tissue, making it vulnerable to irritation. During intercourse, a woman may feel itching or burning or have bleeding from these delicate tissues.

In some instances, the inner pelvic structures may lose their usual shape as a result of estrogen deprivation and as the ligaments that hold them give way (see *Uterine Prolapse*, page 496). When this happens, the bladder, rectum, or small bowel may protrude into the vagina. These conditions may necessitate vaginal strengthening exercises; the use of a pessary or rubber device, which, placed in the vagina, supports the uterus; or surgical correction.

Postmenopausal women frequently cite vaginal discomfort as a reason for avoiding sex. When vaginal tone and lubrication decrease, intercourse is less comfortable, and, in many cases, less than satisfying. When a woman has these problems, she should see her health professional. A lubrication problem can be eliminated with the use of a water-soluble lubricant. The most effective treatment for the vaginal and pelvic changes that occur in menopause is hormone replacement therapy. Studies have shown that by taking estrogen, women can prevent many troubling physical changes as well as guard against heart problems and osteoporosis. Even after a woman's vaginal tissues have thinned, the condition can be treated with hormones (see *Hormone Replacement Therapy*, page 90).

Depression. Someone who is severely depressed generally has no interest in sex. Health providers observe severe depression in many of their patients, menopausal or not. One of the symptoms of clinical depression is a loss of interest in sex.

Although it is natural to feel sad sometimes, a depression that persists for any length of time and that interferes with the ability to enjoy any of life's pleasures (such as family, food, and sex) should not be dismissed as inconsequential. See your health practitioner for help.

Your Partner Isn't Interested. Clarissa found the years around menopause particularly gratifying. She was energized by her career, pleased with the paths her children had taken, and freed up to enjoy sex with her partner. Unfortunately, her husband, Edward, didn't feel the same way. Although men don't undergo the physical changes that women do during midlife, Edward, like so many men during these years, felt the change on a deep and disturbing emotional level. As he looked at his life, he experienced regret at what he had never achieved and boredom with what he had accomplished. He feared aging and losing his virility. He was unable, therefore, to match Clarissa's renewed passion.

It isn't unusual—especially after the age of sixty—for a man to want sex less often than in his younger years. For Clarissa and Edward, their sexual relationship had always added zest to their marriage. With the help of a couples therapist, Edward was able to express, manage, and accept many of these feelings, and he and Clarissa were able to renew their sexual intimacy (see *Male Sexual Problems and Dysfunction*, page 40).

Communication about sex is a continuous process. Women who have learned to be open, curious, and expressive about their needs will find that most changes and problems can be addressed as they surface.

SYMPTOMS OF DEPRESSION

According to the American Psychiatric Association, depression is characterized by at least three of the following symptoms, experienced over an extended period and with considerable severity:

- *Insomnia or hypersomnia (oversleeping)*
- *Low energy level or chronic tiredness*
- *Feelings of inadequacy, loss of self-esteem, or self-deprecation*
- *Decreased effectiveness or productivity at school, work, or home*
- *Social withdrawal*
- *Loss of interest in or enjoyment of pleasurable activities such as sex*
- *Irritability or excessive anger*
- *Inability to respond with apparent pleasure to praise or rewards*
- *Less activity or talkativeness than usual or feeling slowed down or restless*
- *Pessimistic attitude toward the future, brooding about past events, or feeling sorry for oneself*
- *Tearfulness or crying*
- *Recurrent thoughts about death or suicide*

SEXUAL DIFFICULTIES AND DYSFUNCTION

Sexual problems and dysfunction that stand in the way of a person's having or enjoying sex affect almost half of all married couples. Although for many couples sexual difficulties are reflections of unhappiness in other parts of their marriage, a surprising number who experience problems claim to be otherwise happily married. In one study of married couples, 83 percent rated their marriage as happy or very happy, yet 63 percent of these women and 40 percent of the men said they had some degree of sexual dysfunction.

Sexual dysfunction occurs in both men and women, and when one person has sexual difficulties, the other does as well. Hence, the woman involved in a sexual relationship with a man who ejaculates even before he enters her will likely not be sexually satisfied, nor will the man whose partner, despite his best efforts, cannot reach climax.

The most common male sexual dysfunction problems are impotence and premature ejaculation (see *Male Sexual Problems and Dysfunction,* page 40). Women most commonly manifest sexual difficulties in lack of sexual desire, sensation disorders, or the inability to achieve an orgasm. In this section, we will discuss female sexual dysfunction, its causes, and its treatment.

Inhibited Sexual Desire. Many couples seek counseling for a problem when one partner wants to make love more often than the other. However, a more modest sexual appetite does not necessarily signal a desire disorder. Often, counseling will focus on negotiating a middle ground as well as exploring and identifying ways in which both partners can feel safely sexual. Every person's sexual needs are individual and variable. There has to be room in relationships for differences.

Most people experience diminished or negligible desire at one time or another. Women with young children, for example, often feel too tired for sex. Demands from jobs, the community, and family responsibilities will distract a woman from her sexual life, as will health problems. Disagreements and anger, which are inevitable parts of relationships, will at times affect a woman's amorous feelings. An ebb and flow of sexual desire is normal.

If, however, a woman finds that her aversion to sex is severe or persistent, she may indeed have a problem. Consultation with her health-care provider is advisable.

There are many factors that affect sexual desire. As couples mature, it is natural that sexual desire changes. Many who maintain a satisfying sexual relationship after many years together say that sex with a trusted and beloved partner continues to be rewarding, both physically and emotionally. Sometimes, though, one partner no longer finds the other sexually attractive.

Isabel, for example, looks at her partner, Howard, after forty years of marriage and instead of a trim and taut-bodied youth, sees a flabby, overweight old man. She truly loves her husband, yet she finds it difficult to imagine him in a sexual role. With the help of short-term therapy, Isabel was able to examine some of her feelings about the aging body, including her own, and come to a more realistic view of Howard.

Marital discord, an uncaring partner, and a history of emotional or physical abuse are other reasons that a woman might be reluctant to have sex with her mate. If her partner is selfish, caring only about satisfying himself, with little regard for her feelings or needs, it is understandable that she would shrink from sex with him.

Thus, before a woman assumes that something is lacking in her, it is wise to examine the relationship and work to open it up. If establishing a dialogue with her mate proves frustrating, a therapist may be able to help.

If you are happy with your partner in the other areas of your relationship but still have no desire to make love, it is possible that the cause is physical. For some women, for example, there is a decrease in pleasure and desire following tubal ligation. Health professionals speculate that because tubal ligation affects blood flow to the ovaries, a woman's hormonal balance is thrown off and vaginal dryness may result.

Some disorders actually make it painful for a woman to have sex (see *Painful Intercourse*, page 37). Naturally, a woman who experiences pain every time she makes love won't be eager for sex. Hormonal changes, such as a drop after menopause in a woman's level of estrogen, the physical and emotional adjustments during and after pregnancy, or medications that treat such conditions as high blood pressure, depression, and anxiety also can put sex on the bottom of a woman's priority list.

Identifying the problem underlying the dysfunction will usually point to a solution. In the majority of women, however, a lack of sexual desire has no physical cause but is instead a symptom of an emotional problem. Some women consciously or unconsciously associate sex with shame, fear, or guilt. Depression commonly reduces sex drive, as will stress, alcohol, and/or drug abuse (see *Sexuality and Substance Use and Abuse*, page 26). If a health professional determines that nothing is wrong physically, he or she may recommend counseling for a woman and her partner. Treatment combining psychotherapy with sex therapy is often successful in breaking through the psychological barriers to achieving sexual satisfaction.

Before you lose any sleep over your sudden lack of desire, however, ask yourself whether the problem could be related to a conflict in schedules. For many couples, simply setting aside time to be alone together is the first step toward recharging desire.

How Much Sex Is Enough?

Ever since the sexual revolution of the sixties, women have been told that it is "normal" to want sex often. Today, there is still a lot of pressure on women to desire and engage in sex regularly. But as with many activities in life, most women find that their appetite and their opportunities for sex fluctuate—according to their attraction to certain partners, other demands in their lives, their health, their menstrual cycle, and their stage and circumstances in life.

Melanie feels lucky that she's in such a happy relationship because she finds that having sex three or so times a week is just about right for both her and her partner. For Estelle, once or twice a month is more than enough. Diane finds that if she goes too long without sex, her desire drops to such a degree that she hardly misses it. Then she worries that there is something wrong with her. Yet when she makes love again, her desire and pleasure return readily.

Carol goes for extended periods without sex, and she wants it only when she is in a relationship with someone for whom she has special feelings. In Amy and Bob's fourteen-year marriage, there have been long periods when they didn't make love. The longest period lasted for almost two years; at that time, although they didn't have intercourse, there were other expressions of physical closeness.

The answer to the question, How much sex is enough? is as often as you and your partner want it. There cannot be too much sex if the frequency suits both partners. Two or three times a week is common for people in stable relationships. Many people have sex more often, and some are satisfied with less. And quite normally, there are periods in most people's lives that are celibate. Before the age of fifteen or twenty or twenty-five people usually go without sex, and other developmental stages, such as pregnancy, widowhood, old age, and divorce, are often periods of celibacy.

Frequency normally declines with age, but many couples maintain a high rate of sexual intimacy well into their later years.

It is important, though, not to become compulsive or worried about frequency. There naturally will be times when you or your partner want sex less often, and times when you want it more. Don't hold yourself up to a timetable or scoreboard.

Sensation Disorders. A woman with a sensation disorder experiences desire, but her body doesn't cooperate. Despite stimulation, she can't seem to get excited. Because she isn't excited, her vagina does not secrete adequate lubricant, often resulting in painful intercourse (below).

Many women think they have a sensation disorder when what they really have is an inadequate lover. Most women respond to patient and attentive foreplay. Without this kind of stimulation, the female body is less than cooperative.

The most common cause of sensation disorders lies in a woman's feelings about her partner. If she feels hostility or anger, her body probably will not respond to sexual cues. Or perhaps her lover isn't sensitive to her needs or doesn't know how to touch her. Creating open communication should be the initial tactic for improving libido. Try showing him where and how you want to be touched.

Although a sensation disorder is not immediately harmful to a woman's health, it can impair a relationship if it persists over too long a time. It certainly affects a woman's feelings about herself and her circumstances. Treatment often involves sex therapy to help partners learn how to best make love with one another. If there are unspoken resentments or disappointments in the relationship, couples counseling, not just sex therapy, may be recommended.

Painful Intercourse. Understandably, a woman who experiences pain during intercourse may give up on sex. But painful intercourse (dyspareunia) can usually be treated once the cause is determined.

The first step is to consult a health professional, who will take a careful history. In an attempt to get to the root of the problem, he or she will want specific descriptions of the discomfort. Does pain occur only when the penis penetrates the vagina? Or is it most painful when penile thrusting deepens? Although discussing sexual matters can be embarrassing, it is important to be frank and specific in order to arrive together with a health-care professional at an accurate diagnosis.

Dyspareunia is rooted in either physical or psychological problems or a combination of both. In many cases, lack of lubrication makes penetration difficult. Women who are breastfeeding and those past menopause are prone to dryness because the body's estrogen production is low. As a result, vaginal tissue often becomes drier, thinner, and more vulnerable to irritation. Allergic reactions to laundry detergents, vaginal deodorant sprays, condom rubber, and spermicides can irritate the vulva, making sex uncomfortable. So can such infections as herpes, genital warts, or yeast (see pages 454, 457, and 505). A woman who has a bladder infection (page 484), pelvic inflammatory disease (page 449), an ectopic pregnancy (page 286), endometriosis (page 545), or a pelvic mass such as a large ovarian cyst or fibroid may find intercourse uncomfortable, especially when her partner thrusts.

Once the physical source of the pain is found, appropriate treatment can start. Some infections are treatable with antibiotics. Dryness problems may be addressed with the application of a lubricant (K-Y Jelly, saliva, or birth-control foam, cream, or jelly) to the vaginal area prior to intercourse. (Do not, however, use Vaseline, since a petroleum-based lubricant will cause the rubber of a diaphragm or condom to deteriorate.) In the case of a woman past menopause, her provider may recommend hormone replacement therapy (see page 90).

When a woman has painful intercourse due to a severe case of endometriosis (see page 545), in which bits of tissue lining the uterus are implanted in other areas, surgery or medication may be recommended. Some women who have painful intercourse may get some relief simply by changing positions during sex. For example, by sitting on top (the female superior position), a woman better controls rhythm and depth of penetration. Thus, it's a good idea to experiment with various ways of making love.

In rare cases, painful intercourse is caused by vaginismus, the involuntary spasm of muscles around the vagina. This problem is often rooted in confusion around sexual identity or such sexual trauma as childhood sexual abuse. The thought of inserting even a tampon or vaginal suppository can cause a woman with vaginismus such anxiety that her vagina stops producing lubricant and essentially closes up (see page 506).

Treatment for this problem usually combines counseling (individual and/or couples counseling) with a technique in which progressive vaginal dilation is accomplished by the use of medically prescribed tubes or dilators. Beginning with the smallest, the woman gently inserts a tube into her vagina. Once she can tolerate that without pain, she progresses to the next size, and so on, until she is able to insert a penis-size dilator without pain.

Orgasm Difficulties. There are many ways for a woman to enjoy her body and express herself sexually. It's too simplistic to describe the route to sexual pleasure as a step-by-step progress from foreplay to intercourse to orgasm. However, if a woman wishes to reach orgasm, through either masturbation or lovemaking, and habitually fails to do so, doubts and anxiety about her own sexuality and about her sexual relationships can disrupt her sense of well-being.

Every orgasm is different. Some are barely noticeable; others are explosive. And women achieve orgasms at different rates and through various means. Some women never have orgasms but have satisfying sex lives. An estimated 10 to 15 percent of all women have never had an orgasm, while another 25 to 35 percent will have difficulty reaching a sexual climax on any given occasion. Others have orgasm every time they have intercourse.

For many women who have trouble reaching orgasm, the most important step is to consider what would make sex more satisfying for them and to communicate this to their partners. Perhaps more or different kinds of foreplay would help. Sometimes novel positions or sex toys and vibrators would enhance lovemaking. Too often shame and guilt prevent women from touching and exploring their own body, then sharing such sexual understanding with their partner. As with so many problems around sexuality, understanding and communication provide the best avenue to solutions.

If better self-knowledge and communication fail to address the problem, a couple should look to other factors. Dyspareunia (painful intercourse; see page 506) stemming from infection, allergic reactions, abrasions, or a lack of lubrication can inhibit a woman's ability to relax and enjoy sex to the point of climax. Depression, a lifeless relationship, anger, stress, or other factors all can interfere with a woman's ability to focus on pleasurable sexual sensations and reach orgasm. Some women have an intense fear of letting go with another or are reluctant to appear vulnerable.

SEEKING THERAPY FOR A SEXUAL PROBLEM

While there are counselors and therapists specially trained to treat sexual disorders, it may not be easy to locate adequate help. If you and/or your partner needs to talk to someone, call your local women's health center, free clinic, medical center, or teaching hospital, or ask your health-care provider. Since it is possible for anyone to assume the title "sex therapist" regardless of education, credentials, and training, it is best to contact the American Association of Sex Educators, Counselors and Therapists (AASECT), 11 Dupont Circle NW, Suite 220, Washington, D.C. 20036 for names of licensed counselors in your area.

When a couple have sexual problems it is usually the woman who actively seeks help. Perhaps this is because traditionally it is easier for women to admit to and talk about relationship concerns. It may also be that when there are problems in relationships, women are all too ready to assume responsibility. Yet sexual problems, by their very nature, reflect and express problems created by two people. It is therefore most helpful if both partners are committed to working on and working out a solution to the difficulties.

Single and homosexual women may find that they have even fewer resources than heterosexual couples. It may be necessary to ask around among friends, acquaintances, and advocacy groups in addition to relying on traditional resources. Other organizations that can help people navigate this area include the following:

Impotence Anonymous
South Ruth St.
Maryville, Tenn. 37801
(615) 983-6064

Sex Information and Education Council of the United States (SIECUS)
130 West 42nd St.
New York, N.Y. 10019
(212) 819-9770

SEX THERAPY: A SOLUTION FOR MANY

When the problem in achieving orgasm is not the result of a medical problem, treatment often aims at helping both partners become more sexually sensitive to each other. Take, for example, the relationship between Lianna and her boyfriend, Jack. Lianna had read about orgasm, had talked with her friends about it, but had never actually climaxed. In fact, she had never masturbated, at least not in her adult life, nor was she familiar with her own body. She felt a vague dissatisfaction that something was missing in her sexual life. Then she met Jack, who also wished her to have a fully gratifying sexual experience. Together they sought professional help.

As is typical in sex therapy, their therapist gave them homework: She instructed Lianna to explore her body, to look at her vagina using a mirror, to touch and enter her vagina with her fingers, to manipulate her clitoris. Then she was to use a vibrator. All the while, she and Jack were to restrict their lovemaking to tender and sensual play and to postpone intercourse for a period of weeks. With the vibrator, Lianna discovered that she was not, as she had feared, incapable of experiencing orgasm; the ease with which she climaxed reassured her. With greater confidence, she was able to take fuller pleasure from her time with Jack, and in fact could have an orgasm as Jack stimulated her clitoris through both masturbation and cunnilingus.

However, once the therapist suggested that they try intercourse again, Lianna tensed up. She found herself distracted with worries about penetration, anticipating her own failure. The therapist encouraged them to cuddle, and to experiment with positions and touching exercises. She suggested that Jack delay penetration and that Lianna concentrate on her own sensations, not her thoughts. She also recommended simple Kegel exercises, in which Lianna was to contract her pelvic-floor muscles for a second, then release them completely. By repeating this ten to twenty times per daily session, women can prevent sagging of the pelvic muscles and reduce incontinence, as well as strengthen orgasms. Thanks to her own commitment to her sexuality, a patient and considerate partner, open communication, and a good therapist, Lianna soon reached orgasm, not only in masturbation but in intercourse, and was able to develop a rich and satisfying sexual life. Their experience in therapy lasted about six months, which is the usual length of time in relatively uncomplicated cases.

MALE SEXUAL PROBLEMS AND DYSFUNCTION

Male sexual problems manifest themselves primarily in premature ejaculation and the inability to achieve or maintain erection. While there may be a physical cause of male dysfunction that will respond, to a greater or lesser degree, to treatment, often a man with a sexual problem suffers from stress, depression, or other emotional factors.

Impotence. When a man has difficulty attaining or maintaining an erection, he is said to be impotent. In ordinary circumstances, a man who is sexually aroused gets an erection. This happens because nerve impulses cause obstruction of blood flow out of the penis. Continued sexual arousal maintains the obstruction to blood drainage, maintaining the erection. After ejaculation, or when the excitation passes, excess blood drains out and the penis returns to its nonerect size and shape. If something interferes with any of the steps in this process—which entail communication between the nervous system and the vascular system—impotence can result.

Most men at some time experience impotence. Excessive amounts of alcohol and nicotine, inadequate sleep, work-related stress, and relationship problems can sabotage many a man's sexual plans. If this happens occasionally it is nothing to be concerned about. But if it persists, impotence needs to be taken seriously.

An estimated ten million American men are impotent. The older the man, the greater the chance of impotence; almost 20 percent of men at age sixty are unable to have an erection, while 70 percent are impotent by the time they reach eighty.

The cause of impotence can be either physical or psychological. The most common physical causes include diabetic neuropathy (nerve damage consequent to diabetes), cardiovascular disorders, use of prescription drugs, surgery for prostate cancer, injury to the spinal cord, multiple sclerosis, hormone disorders, and alcoholism or drug abuse. Many cases of impotence are due to emotional factors. Depression, negative feelings toward the partner, fatigue, and anxiety can each render a man impotent. Moreover, each time a man experiences impotence, he will likely worry about his sexual performance and what it says about his virility and find it difficult to perform at all.

Treatment for impotence depends upon cause. If it is not caused by a physical problem, a health professional may recommend treatment by a psychiatrist, psychologist, social worker, or sex therapist. Some forms of impotence respond to hormone treatment. Eliminating or adjusting the dosage of some medications, when advised to do so by a doctor, may also eliminate a sexual problem. Medications such as beta-blockers prescribed for hypertension, antidepressants, estrogen used for prostate conditions, and chemotherapy will interfere with a man's sexual functioning. When impotence is caused by hardened arteries that obstruct blood flow to the penis, surgery to reconstruct the vascular system in that area of the body can be performed.

Even in the event that impotence cannot be cured, a man can still have a satisfying sex life. Surgically implanted devices can enable a man to experience intercourse. Among the varieties used today are malleable implants that maintain firmness at all times but allow the penis to be tucked close to the body when not in use for intercourse, and an inflatable device that uses fluid reservoirs and a hand pump to produce an erection mechanically.

Other Erection Abnormalities. While impotence is the most common erection disorder, some men suffer from a condition called *Peyronie's disease*, in which curvature of the penis makes intercourse difficult, even impossible, in extreme cases. This disorder most commonly occurs in men between the ages of forty and sixty and is caused by scar tissue that forms inside the penis for no apparent reason. Fortunately, most cases of Peyronie's disease resolve on their own without treatment, typically within one to three years. When the disease is so severe that intercourse is impossible, the deformity can be corrected with surgery.

The other erection disorder is priapism. This condition is the opposite of impotence. A man who is not sexually excited nevertheless has a prolonged and often painful erection. This rare condition, often resulting from a spinal cord disorder, leukemia, reaction to some drugs, or an inflammation of the urethra, requires immediate medical attention if the ability to have a normal erection is to be restored.

Ejaculation Disorders. Premature ejaculation, the most common ejaculation disorder, occurs when a man ejaculates too early in the sexual process. This happens most commonly after the penis enters the vagina, but in some instances, mere touching, kissing, or holding a woman can trigger ejaculation. In almost every case, the man feels that he lacks control over the timing of his ejaculation and experiences frustration—as does the woman. Often, premature ejaculation disrupts foreplay and preempts a woman's ability to become sufficiently aroused, as well as preventing full sexual enjoyment for the man. Premature ejaculation probably happens to every man at least once in a while. Young men just embarking on a sexual relationship are especially prone. But men who chronically experience premature ejaculation frequently become preoccupied with and anxious about the difficulty.

The cause of the problem is rarely physical. While not a health risk, chronic premature ejaculation can interfere with a relationship. Moreover, a man who consistently ejaculates prematurely may grow so frustrated that he becomes impotent.

For men who have problems with premature ejaculation, help may be as close as their partner. The "squeeze" technique is a common remedy—a collaborative method wherein a patient partner squeezes the end of the man's penis when he indicates that he's about to ejaculate, usually at the point where the glans joins the shaft. After the penis is squeezed, the couple waits thirty seconds or so and then returns to foreplay. Squeezing causes the penis to shrink, but it soon regains its firmness with adequate stimulation. The squeeze can be repeated as often as necessary. After a few sessions, many men can stop themselves from having premature ejaculation without direct assistance.

The other ejaculation disorder is retrograde ejaculation, a condition in which little or no semen emerges during intercourse. In this unusual and harmless condition, the semen doesn't exit through the end of the penis but instead enters the bladder.

Retrograde ejaculation is most likely to occur in diabetics but also is seen in men after prostate surgery or urethral surgery and in those taking mood-altering or antihypertension drugs. Because the semen is expelled in the urine, this condition poses no physical threat to a man, but it may prevent him from fathering a child through any method other than artificial insemination.

Treatment of retrograde ejaculation depends upon the cause. If a doctor suspects that a particular drug is behind the problem, she may recommend the drug be eliminated or the dosage be adjusted.

THE MALE SEXUAL ANATOMY

The primary function of the male sexual organs is to produce sperm and deliver it to the female's reproductive system, where millions of these minute cells strive to fertilize an egg. The major male sexual organs are the penis, the testicles, the vas deferens, the seminal vesicles, and the prostate gland. The male sexual organs also are linked to the body's urinary system.

The penis is the most visible sexual organ during intercourse; at other times, it is used to discharge urine. The urethra, a narrow tube that runs the length of the penis, is used to carry both semen, the fluid containing sperm, and urine. The penis is rich in blood vessels and when a man is sexually aroused these vessels fill three cylindrical, spongelike structures that run parallel to the urethra. As blood continues to flow into these structures, the penis becomes larger, straightens, and stiffens in preparation for intercourse, when it will enter the vagina.

The testicles, or testes, are the site of sperm production as well as the secretion of the male hormone testosterone, which promotes masculinity. Produced in different degrees in both men and women, testosterone creates libido and regulates sexual desire, responsiveness, and performance.

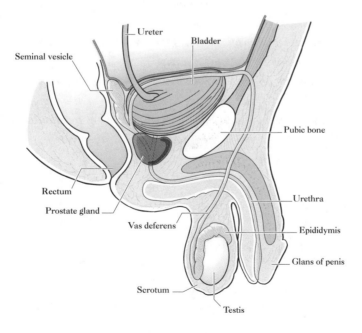

The two oval-shaped testes are housed in a skin pouch known as the scrotum. *Although a female is born with all the eggs she will ever have, a male doesn't begin to produce sperm until puberty, a process that continues throughout his life. In order for sperm to be produced, the temperature within the testes must be lower than the body's temperature. Hence, the scrotum hangs below the abdomen and behind the penis, enabling it to maintain a cooler temperature than the rest of the body. Cords that suspend the testes within the scrotum help to maintain the optimal temperature. If it is cold outside, the cords draw the testes upward, where they stay warmer. Similarly, when the outside temperature is increased, the cords lower the testes away from the body to keep them cool.*

As sperm are produced, they pass into the epididymis, a long, tightly coiled tube behind each testis. It is here that the sperm cells are allowed to mature for two or three weeks before they enter a duct known as the vas deferens, *a sperm storage system. In addition to containing sperm, semen is composed of fluids secreted by the seminal vesicles and the prostate gland. These secretions mobilize and nourish the sperm and increase their ability to withstand the acidic environment of the vagina.*

When everything is working well, a man is able to have and maintain an erection and impregnate a woman. A variety of problems, however, can stand in the way of both (see Male Sexual Problems and Dysfunction, *page 40).*

ELENA AND JOHN

Elena was bothered by her husband's sudden inability to make love to her; John had always been such an eager and responsive lover. She assumed his new difficulties resulted from his anxiety about his health. It never occurred to her to ask about the effects of his hypertension medications. Nor did it occur to John to ask his doctor about his impotence even though he saw him regularly.

The doctor never inquired about John's sex life. Rather than the source of joy it had always been, John and Elena's sex life became a source of disappointment. Had they known to ask, the problem could have been easily resolved by substituting a diuretic for the beta-blockers used to treat John's high blood pressure.

Nutrition

CONTENTS

Healthy eating ought to be simple—but in recent times American consumers, especially women, have been bombarded with advice. It comes from sources as diverse as the tabloids at the grocery checkout and official-sounding governmental bodies. First one study get lots of television publicity. Then a few months later somebody else's research is reported and it directly contradicts the first. Should we eat eggs or not? What about red meat? Do we dare allow our children to eat sweets? Should we be struggling to reduce our calorie intake as we get older, or should we accept some weight gain as an inevitable part of aging? In short, how are we to go about eating in a way that will keep us healthy throughout our life span?

Many women bear the primary responsibility not only for feeding themselves but for purchasing food for entire households, storing it properly, preparing and serving it safely and appealingly, and organizing the eating habits of those with whom they live. These women—all women, in fact—must become nutritionists in the interest of good eating and good health.

Thus, it's no surprise that we eagerly seek out the newest news about diet and nutrition. Perhaps the best way to wade through the masses of available information on food, vitamins, minerals, and other supplements—some of it correct and useful; some of it confusing, misleading, or even false—is to begin with the basics. Even though the experts' opinions on diet and nutrition seem to change every few months, certain guidelines can serve as building blocks with which we can develop sensible and nutritious eating habits. With a little experimentation we can demonstrate even for younger eaters the radical notion that food that's good for you can taste good, too.

THE BASICS OF HEALTHY EATING

The foods we eat are made up of carbohydrates, proteins, and fats, with small amounts of vitamins and minerals. Combined appropriately, these substances provide us with the nutrients our bodies need to function effectively throughout our life. The challenge, of course, lies in combining them properly, in the appropriate amounts. Some basic definitions of the kinds of food may be helpful.

Carbohydrates. Carbohydrates are compounds made up of carbon, hydrogen, and oxygen. They are classified as complex or simple, depending on how their chemical elements are arranged. Carbohydrates take the form of starches or sugars, which are digestible, or the form of fiber or roughage, which passes through the digestive tract undigested. Complex carbohydrates, which include starches, are found in breads, cereals, grains, beans, fruits, and vegetables. Simple carbohydrates, or sugars, are found in fruits, syrups, honey, and white and brown sugar.

Nutrition experts now urge us to consume at least 35 percent of our calories in the form of carbohydrates. This means six or more daily servings of bread, cereals, and legumes and five or more daily servings of fruits and vegetables. These complex carbohydrates are good substitutes for fatty foods and also help to protect us from heart disease, hardening of the arteries, and other diseases. They also provide fiber, which, although it has no nutritive value, helps the large intestine function optimally. Fruit skins, seeds, berries, and oat and wheat bran are the richest sources of fiber; other sources are whole-grain breads and cereals, fruits, vegetables, beans, peas, and nuts.

Protein. Proteins are essential to our diets because, unlike fats or carbohydrates, they provide us with the amino acids our bodies need to produce energy and to make the thousands of different kinds of proteins in muscle, bone, skin, hair, and organs. Our bodies cannot manufacture some of the amino acids that are essential to health; those must come from the food we eat.

Meat and dairy products are the richest sources of complete protein, but they also contain fat—which most of us get too much of in our diet. Nutrition experts now emphasize the importance of sticking to lean meat (up to six ounces a day), fish, chicken without the skin, and low-fat dairy products. Beans, nuts, and cereal grains supply *incomplete* proteins—so called because they are missing one or more essential amino acids—but these foods can be combined to provide a complete protein. Beans and rice (or tortillas), for instance, supply a high-quality protein.

Fats. The fat compounds provide us with energy, and some fat is essential for good health. Like carbohydrates, fats free protein to perform its principal job in the body, which is building and repairing tissue. Fats also facilitate absorption of vitamins A, D, E, and K. Foods that contain significant amounts of fat include meat, dairy products, chocolate, pastries, nuts, and a few fruits and vegetables such as coconuts and avocados.

Fats are made up of fatty acids, which exist in different forms. Those with the largest numbers of hydrogen atoms are known as saturated fatty acids and are found mostly in foods of animal origin. Those with fewer hydrogen atoms are monounsaturated (found in olives and peanuts), and those with the least are polyunsaturated (fish and some seed oils). Some fatty acids, such as linoleic acid, are termed essential because the body cannot make them and must obtain them from foods.

These nutritional building blocks—protein, carbohydrates, and fat—do not contain the same amount of calories per unit. One gram of protein provides four calories of energy, as does one gram of carbohydrate. However, one gram of fat provides over twice as many calories, about nine calories per gram. That's one major reason to limit fats and eat more carbohydrates.

Cholesterol. While not exactly a fat, cholesterol is similar to fat in some ways. It is an important component of many body tissues but is not an essential nutrient because the body manufactures as much as it needs. Cholesterol is found in many foods, such as egg yolks, liver, some shellfish, and whole-milk dairy products, so people whose blood cholesterol level is too high must limit their intake of these foods. Cholesterol is found only in animal products.

Vitamins and Minerals. Vitamins and minerals are critical to our health. Women have special needs for some of these nutrients, in particular, calcium and iron, throughout life—infancy, early childhood, puberty, pregnancy, menopause, and later.

Calcium is considered especially important in preventing osteoporosis, or thinning of the bones. The National Institutes of Health recommends that women consume 1,200 milligrams (mg) of calcium per day from age eleven to twenty-four, 1,000 mg as adult women, 1,200 mg when pregnant or lactating, 1,500 mg when postmenopausal and not taking estrogen, and after age sixty-five.

Many women take in less than half that amount. Dairy products are a good calcium source, as are canned salmon and sardines; dark green vegetables like broccoli, kale, spinach, and bok choy; and beans. Some foods, like yogurt and orange juice, are now calcium-enriched.

Other necessary minerals include iron, magnesium, phosphorus, potassium, sodium, and sulfur. Magnesium and phosphorus, along with calcium, are important for the development and health of bones and teeth. Sodium regulates body fluids, and sulfur is important in protein tissues. Women tend to be particularly prone to iron deficiency, in part because of the monthly blood loss that occurs with menstruation. Good food sources for iron are red meat, organ meat, brewer's yeast, wheat germ, and whole grains.

Other minerals known as trace elements are needed in very small amounts. These include iodine, zinc, copper, fluoride, selenium, and manganese.

Vitamins are organic substances found in plant and animal tissue. They are essential to good health, but only in small amounts. They help in the processing of proteins, carbohydrates, and fats, and they also contribute to the production of blood cells, hormones, genetic material, and the chemicals of the central nervous system. Some vitamins, such as A, D, E, and K, dissolve in fat; others, like vitamin C and the B vitamins, are soluble in water. Our bodies cannot synthesize most vitamins, and nutritionists recommend getting our daily requirements through the food we eat, to the greatest extent possible, rather than relying on vitamin supplements, because we are less likely to get too much of them that way.

Excessive amounts of vitamins or minerals may damage the body; thus, self-medicating with megadoses of vitamins is not a wise idea. In general, it is safe to take a daily multivitamin and mineral supplement that provides 100 percent of the recommended dietary allowances (RDAs), particularly for those whose diet is very limited. However, it is even better to make sure that you eat at least five servings of fruits and vegetables every day, four or more servings of breads and cereals, two or more servings of low-fat milk and other dairy products, and two servings of lean meat, fish, chicken without the skin, low-fat dairy products, or beans, nuts, and cereal grains.

Pregnant women are usually given vitamin and mineral supplements because their need for iron, folic acid, and calcium is greatly increased. Women who menstruate heavily may need iron supplements. Vegetarians who eat no animal products may have trouble getting enough vitamin B_{12}, vitamin D, calcium, and iron in their diet. A dietary shortage of vitamin D (which is found in milk) can cause softening of the bones (osteomalacia).

A deficiency of folic acid, a member of the B-vitamin group, can cause anemia. Folic acid is found in a wide variety of foods, especially raw fruits and vegetables, dry beans, liver, and kidney, but can be destroyed by excessive cooking. Supplemental folic acid, when taken by pregnant women shortly after conception, decreases the risk of neural tube defects. Thus, all women who might become pregnant should take such supplements.

Recommended Dietary Allowances. The term *recommended dietary allowances*, usually abbreviated RDAs, refers to the amounts of vitamins and minerals thought necessary to prevent nutritional deficiencies. RDAs are determined by the Food and Nutrition Board of the National Research Council, which is a part of the National Academy of Sciences. The RDAs identify cover intake levels for a number of vitamins and minerals by age and sex groupings. A simplified version of RDAs, known as the United States Recommended Dietary Allowances, or USRDAs, recommend the highest RDA of each nutrient. They are listed on vitamin and mineral supplements and on some packaged foods.

Reading Labels. In recent years, the government has made efforts to improve the standards for labeling packaged foods. The intent of this reform is to give consumers more nutritional information about the food they buy. However, the new guidelines apply only to packaged foods, not to fresh meat, poultry, fish, produce, or restaurant food.

In essence, the labeling guidelines require food manufacturers to put nutrition labels on their products listing the total number of calories per serving, the percentage of calories derived from fat, total fat content, and percentage of saturated fat content, cholesterol, carbohydrates, complex carbohydrates, sugars, fiber, protein, sodium, calcium, iron, and vitamins A and C. The guidelines also establish uniform serving sizes for thousands of foods in order to prevent manufacturers from offering information based on unrealistically small portions to suggest that their products are low in fat and salt, for instance. Uniform standards are also set for such terms as *high fiber, low fat, organic,* and *natural.*

The information on amounts is given in terms of both mass per serving and percentage of the daily recommended minimum or maximum intake. The percentages of daily values are based on a diet of 2,000 calories per day, which is considered the appropriate food intake for most women and children. The guidelines also specify that for a food to be termed *light, healthy,* or *low-fat,* it must contain 25 percent or less of a particular nutrient than does the original product.

Food Additives and Contaminants. Substances may be added to foods intentionally, to preserve or flavor them, or incidentally as a by-product of food processing, storage, or handling. For the most part food additives are necessary and pose no risks to consumers. In addition to preserving processed food, additives may be used to enhance flavor or nutritional value: vitamin D in milk, vitamin A in margarine, B vitamins in breads and cereals, and iodine in table salt. These additives have helped virtually eliminate nutritional deficiency diseases that were once common, such as rickets, beriberi, pellagra, and goiter. Even nitrates and nitrites are added to bacon and other cured meats for a very specific reason: to inhibit the growth of the toxin that causes botulism, a form of food poisoning that can be fatal. Sulfites are added to fresh fruits and vegetables to keep them fresh and prevent spoilage. Some people are sensitive to sulfites and should avoid foods containing them, but by and large they are harmless and useful in preventing mold and decay.

Food contaminants, on the other hand, can cause problems. Some are naturally occurring substances, such as molds. Others, like pesticides or drug residues, may contaminate foods before they reach our tables. The food supply is routinely and periodically tested to keep these occurrences to a minimum. When preparing foods at home, it is important to wash fruits and vegetables carefully, since pesticide residues, if present, remain on the surface.

A Basic Dietary Approach. With the help of food-labeling guidelines and the information discussed here, making your way through the nutrition information forest to find a path to healthy eating is actually fairly simple. The National Academy of Sciences' Committee on Diet and Health has established a set of dietary guidelines that the U.S. Department of Agriculture has used to develop a food guide. The feature of the guide that has received the most attention in recent times is the Food Guide Pyramid, an illustration of the guide's most basic components (see page 53). But before examining the pyramid, let's look at the guidelines from which it was developed.

NINE DIETARY GUIDELINES

These guidelines were developed by the National Academy of Sciences' Food and Nutrition Board to help people stay healthy and reduce their risk of many chronic diseases. Think of them as the nutritional commandments—nine rules to eat by.

The first guideline *advises us to limit total fat intake to 30 percent or less of total calorie consumption, to lower saturated fatty acid intake to less than 10 percent of calories, and to reduce cholesterol intake to less than 300 mg daily.*

Diets with more fat, especially saturated fatty acids and cholesterol, cause cholesterol to build up in the bloodstream. Fatty plaque then accumulates in the blood vessels, causing the arteries to become narrower, less elastic, and obstructed (see Atherosclerosis, *page 563). Heart attacks and strokes can result.*

Since dairy and meat products are the biggest sources of saturated fat, the best way to lower fat consumption is to limit intake of fatty meats, whole-milk dairy products, and egg yolks as well as oils and fried foods. Substitute fish, poultry without the skin, lean meats, and low-fat or nonfat dairy products. Keep the size of meat portions to three ounces (six ounces per day) and eat more vegetables, fruits, cereals, and legumes.

The second guideline *recommends eating five or more servings of fruits and vegetables (especially dark green and yellow vegetables and citrus fruits) each day and six or more servings of breads, cereals, and legumes, which provide potassium, a mineral that may help lower your risk of stroke. Eating fruits and vegetables also is thought to lower susceptibility to cancer of the lung, stomach, and colon.*

Starches and other complex carbohydrates found in whole-grain breads, cereals, and legumes are good sources of vitamins, minerals, and fiber and good substitutes for fatty foods. They may also lower the risk of cardiovascular disease.

The third guideline *recognizes that protein-containing foods are primary sources of amino acids.*

The fourth guideline *stresses the importance of getting regular, moderate exercise to maintain appropriate body weight and prevent obesity. Obesity is linked to such chronic disorders as non-insulin-dependent diabetes, high blood pressure, heart disease, gallbladder disease, osteoarthritis, and endometrial cancer.*

The fifth guideline *advises against the regular use of alcohol, even though some studies have shown that drinking moderately can offer some benefits. If you do drink alcohol, limit the amount to no more than two cans of beer, two small glasses of wine, or two average cocktails per day. If you are pregnant, avoid alcohol. Alcohol has no nutritional value but is high in calories and, in excess, is linked to heart disease, high blood pressure, chronic liver disease, some forms of cancer, neurological diseases, nutritional deficiencies, and many other diseases as well as patterns of abuse and addiction in susceptible individuals.*

The sixth guideline *recommends limiting salt intake to six grams per day (a little more than a teaspoonful) and avoiding or minimizing consumption of salty foods. Higher levels of dietary salt are linked to high blood pressure, and excessive consumption of salt-preserved or pickled foods has been linked to stomach cancer.*

The seventh guideline *recommends maintaining adequate calcium intake by consuming low-fat or nonfat milk and milk products and dark-green vegetables. Women and teenagers must be especially careful to get enough calcium in their diet.*

The eighth guideline *cautions against taking dietary supplements that provide more vitamins or minerals than are recommended in the USRDAs. Some groups of people may need supplements, including women with excessive menstrual bleeding, pregnant women or women who may become pregnant, some vegetarians, and people taking medications that may interfere with the intake, digestion, absorption, metabolism, or excretion of nutrients. However, high-potency vitamin, mineral, or protein supplements have not been proved to be effective and can be harmful to your health.*

The ninth dietary guideline *recommends maintaining an appropriate level of fluoride in the diet, especially for children. In most areas this is provided through fluoridation of drinking water supplies, but in many rural areas supplements may be prescribed by dentists.*

THE FOOD GUIDE PYRAMID

The guidelines discussed here served as the basis for a recent effort by the U.S. Department of Agriculture (USDA) and the Department of Health and Human Services (HHS) to improve people's understanding of healthy eating through the distribution of dietary guidelines and the Food Guide Pyramid, a graphic representation of food groups and the optimal amounts people should consume.

In brief, the USDA–HHS guidelines are as follows:

1. *Eat a variety of foods.*
2. *Maintain a healthy weight.*
3. *Choose a diet low in fat, saturated fat, and cholesterol.*
4. *Choose a diet with plenty of vegetables, fruits, and grain products.*
5. *Use sugars only in moderation.*
6. *Use salt and sodium only in moderation.*
7. *If you drink alcoholic beverages, do so only in moderation.*

The Food Guide Pyramid was designed to replace traditional food charts that urged people to select foods from four basic food groups—meat, dairy, grains, and fruits and vegetables. In the new graphic, foods to be consumed in the greatest quantities are at the base of the pyramid, with those to be eaten in smaller quantities placed above them. At the top of the pyramid are fats, oils, and sweets, which are not classified as a food group and are to be eaten only sparingly.

Key to the pyramid approach is the USDA's emphasis on three essential elements of a healthy diet: proportion, moderation, and variety. Proportion relates to the relative amounts of food to be chosen from each major food group. Moderation relates to eating fats, oils, and sugars sparingly and using them as accents for other foods rather than as primary sources of calories. Variety emphasizes the importance of selecting different foods from each food group rather than relying on a few favorite items.

As the newest in a long line of food guides, the pyramid has received its share of attention. The design was intended to meet several goals, chief among them the promotion of overall health and well-being in a way that is easily understandable. Foods are grouped in familiar categories by nutrient content. No foods are banned completely— instead, the idea is to balance selections so that high-fat choices can be balanced by lower-fat options. Variations in age, sex, and activity levels are addressed by the range of suggested servings from each food group. For example, six to eleven servings from the bread group is recommended. A very active young person would opt for the higher end of the range, while older adults and relatively inactive people would go for the lower end.

At the pyramid's base is the bread, cereal, rice, and pasta group, which should provide most of our daily calories. Although many of us have been trained to think of starchy foods as fattening, they aren't. It is the high-fat toppings like butter, sour cream, and cheese that put on the pounds.

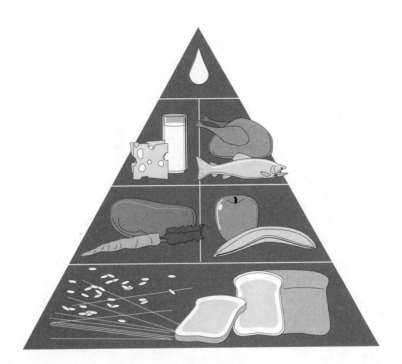

On the bottom layer are starchy foods, which include grains, bread, rice, and pasta. Next are vegetables and fruits. On the third layer are dairy products, as well as meat, poultry, and fish. At the top, fats, oils, and sweets are represented. This deceptively simple image actually conveys a great deal about good dietary practices.

Above the bread group are the vegetable group, from which we should select three to five servings a day, and the fruit group, two to four servings. In earlier diet guides, fruits and vegetables were often lumped together. Both are good sources of fiber and are naturally low in salt and fat, but they offer different kinds of nutrients. Green, leafy vegetables are good sources of beta-carotene, vitamin C, calcium, iron, and potassium. Squash is a good source of beta-carotene and vitamin A.

The third layer of the pyramid, the milk, cheese, and yogurt group, is especially important as a source of calcium. Dairy products also provide protein, riboflavin, vitamins A and B$_{12}$, thiamine, and often vitamin D. Yogurt is particularly recommended because it provides substantial amounts of complete protein with relatively few calories. Having two to three servings a day of these foods is recommended—three for pregnant women, breast-feeding mothers, and young people up to age twenty-four.

Low-fat or nonfat dairy products are recommended over whole-milk varieties. People who have trouble digesting milk may want to use products that contain lactase, the enzyme that breaks down lactose.

The next layer of the pyramid comprises meat, poultry, fish, dry beans, eggs, and nuts; two to three servings a day from this group is recommended These foods are primary sources of protein. Meat, poultry, and fish also provide iron, zinc, and B vita-mins. Eggs, despite their recent bad press as a source of cholesterol, are recommended in moderation because they provide complete protein. Comsuming up to three eggs per week should cause no problems.

At the very tip of the pyramid are fats, oils, and sweets. These substances should be used as condiments rather than as primary sources of calories. A little fat in a meal can help you feel satisfied, but rich desserts, chocolate, salad dressings, cream, butter, and margarine should be occasional treats, not dietary staples, because they offer little nutritional value but a wagonload of calories. Sugary sweets like soft drinks and can-dies should be limited for the same reason.

By following these guidelines and the Food Group Pyramid, it should not be too difficult to plan healthy menus. Most important is making sure that you eat at least five servings a day of fruits and vegetables and six servings of complex carbohydrates. Although this may sound like a lot of food, keep in mind that one serving is equivalent to one piece of raw fruit or a cup of raw leafy vegetables; a half cup of raw or cooked vegetables or fruit; a half cup of cereal, pasta, or rice; a cup of milk or yogurt; or one roll, muffin, or slice of bread. A three-ounce serving of meat is about the size of a deck of playing cards.

Learn to avoid visible sources of fat—oil, butter, marbled meat, cream sauces, and soups—and less visible sources such as whole milk and cheese, avocados, and nuts. Limit your consumption of meat, poultry, salty foods, and sauces. Snacks and desserts need not be eliminated as long as you steer clear of those that are high in fat, added sugar, and salt. Serve fruit, raw or minimally cooked, for dessert. Small quan-tities of such sweets as cake, cookies, and ice cream can be worked into menus without wreaking dietary havoc.

A growing number of cookbooks reflect the recent dietary initiatives discussed here. Rather than offering high-calorie recipes, they provide information on such low-fat cooking techniques as microwaving and suggestions on how to enhance food flavor with a minimum of salt, fat, and sugar.

CONTROLLING YOUR WEIGHT

If you haven't already, now is the time to begin eating a healthier diet, as a way of both main-taining your health and avoiding the weight gain that so commonly settles in as midlife approaches.

As a teenager perhaps you went from one junk food meal to the next and still managed to look and feel great. Unfortunately, your adult metabolism (the rate at which your body burns energy) may not be so forgiving. Many women who were thin as teens begin to gain weight during their twenties and thirties. When they start families, each pregnancy adds a few pounds, and after the birth of several children a woman may be left with a serious weight problem. Other women may become overweight simply by eating too much of the wrong things and exercising too little.

As you age, expect your body to change. Between the ages of thirty and thirty-five your muscle mass slowly begins to decrease. What does that mean in terms of the way you look? If at forty you weigh ten pounds more than you did at twenty, you may actually be fifteen to twenty pounds "fatter." The distribution of that fat changes with age. In the older body, the subcutaneous fat in the face, arms, legs, and neck tends to shift to the center of the body, namely, the trunk and abdomen. You have probably noticed older people with thin faces and limbs but bellies that even the most tightly cinched belts can barely contain.

At the same time that your body is changing, your metabolism begins to slow down. As a result, the same diet you ate at twenty may end up making you fat at forty.

While thus far no one has stumbled upon a magic potion that will keep the body forever young, there are things you can do to help your body stay healthier and more youthful longer.

A healthy diet—high in fiber and low in fat—can do wonders for the way you feel, but it alone isn't enough. If you want to lose weight, keep your joints flexible, tone your muscles, and strengthen your heart, you must include exercise in your daily routine. A good exercise program incorporates aerobic exercise, as distinguished from endurance training. Walking, bicycling, jogging, aerobic dancing, cycling, and swimming are good aerobic exercises. Weight training, yoga, and stretching exercises help make your body stronger and more flexible.

In designing your exercise program, be sure to choose an activity that is easily accessible and that you enjoy, so that you will be less likely to make excuses to avoid exercising. For maximum gain, you should exercise twenty to thirty minutes about every other day of the week.

If you have a chronic health problem, are over the age of forty, smoke, are obese, or have never exercised, see your health professional before embarking on an exercise program (see *Exercise*, page 72).

TAKING A LOOK AT VEGETARIANISM

Vegetarianism has been practiced for centuries in many cultures, notably among the Hindus in India. In the United States it is considerably less common, and until fairly recently most people believed a healthy diet had to include meat. Some are still convinced that meat should be the cornerstone of any serious athlete's diet.

Wendy, who's been a vegetarian for over half of her thirty-two years, would vehemently protest this view. She renounced meat when she was twelve. Her mother, though dismayed, was certain she would get over it—lots of kids, when they're old enough to make the connection between cute barnyard animals and the meat on their plates, go through a phase of refusing to touch it. But Wendy's convictions were no passing phase. She has not eaten meat in twenty years.

What began as a purely moral stand has since been reinforced in other respects.

Wendy agrees with those who believe that beef production is an inefficient use of resources, that the land on which cows graze would feed many more people if it were planted with food crops. Then there's the health angle. Red meat is high in fat and cholesterol; there is also a concern (among some) about the chemicals and antibiotics fed to the animals before slaughter. While the meat industry and the USDA have assured the public that these are perfectly safe for humans, Wendy would just as soon not worry about it at all. Besides, she says, her diet gives her all the nutrients she needs anyway. The USDA agrees: Vegetarian diets meet the nutritional requirements set by its 1995 Dietary Guidelines for Americans (with the recommendation that vegans, who eat no animal products, supplement their diets with vitamin B_{12}).

There's tantalizing evidence that vegetarians may be at lower risk than meat eaters for certain diseases—heart disease, high cholesterol level, high blood pressure, and others. In fact, some studies suggest that vegetarians live longer. Of course, most vegetarians are very health-conscious overall—they tend to drink less alcohol and not smoke, are less likely to be overweight, and with all those grains and fruits and vegetables their diets are full of fiber—so it's probably misleading to point to the meatless diet as the sole explanation for their good health.

Still, the evidence provides food for thought. For the rest of us who can't bear the thought of life without medium-rare steak, less extreme measures can be very beneficial. Replacing meat dishes with grains and vegetables at least a couple of times a week is a good start. Serving more fish and chicken and less beef and pork is another. Offering fresh fruit as a snack and a dessert is good for everyone's heart and waistline. You don't have to give up meat to be healthy, but a few servings of the vegetarian life-style wouldn't hurt. Actually, paying more attention to nutrition generally—using the guidelines described in this chapter (see The Food Guide Pyramid, *page 52, and* Nine Dietary Guidelines, *page 50, along with regular exercise, make a huge difference in anyone's health picture.*

NUTRITION AND EXERCISE DURING MIDLIFE

At forty-seven, Betsy didn't look bad for her age, although it was getting harder and harder to pull the zipper on her jeans all the way up, she hadn't worn a sleeveless dress in years, and she wouldn't have been caught dead in a sweater that didn't cover her hips and bottom. Shopping for a bathing suit was torture akin to root canal. She'd gained twenty pounds in twenty years but until recently refused to take them seriously. "I can get rid of those pounds like that," she'd say, snapping her fingers. "I'll give up cream cheese on my bagels. I've done it before and I can do it again."

Six months ago, having finally had it with circulation-impairing waistbands, she started a low-fat diet and a walking program—three miles, three times a week. What she was shocked to discover was how much harder it is at forty-seven to lose weight—and keep it lost—than it was at twenty-five. She's now lost eight pounds and feels terrific, but she realizes that the diet and exercise are habits she can't give up unless she's willing to wear sweat pants for the rest of her life.

In your younger years, like Betsy, you might have been able to coast on a junk food diet and minimal exercise. Well, with the advent of midlife those days are over. More than ever, sound nutrition and a regular exercise program are essential to continued good health.

Most men and women are at their heaviest weight around the age of fifty. A combination of a sedentary life-style, overeating, and consumption of too much alcohol is the most common culprit. Add that to an overall slowing of your metabolism and you have the basic ingredients for obesity and the host of health problems that often accompany it, such as heart attack, high blood pressure, and diabetes. In fact, recent research suggests that a weight gain of eleven to eighteen pounds after age eighteen puts women at 25 percent greater risk of heart attack; with a weight gain above twenty-five pounds, the risk is a sobering 200 to 300 percent higher.

If you are among the many Americans with weight to spare, perhaps the first step to midlife fitness is losing it. Consult a weight table if you are in doubt about whether you need to lose weight, or try this test: Pinch a fold of skin from your abdomen while you are standing. If you can pinch more than an inch, don't just think about dieting. Do it.

Get Some Exercise. Of course, even if you eat a healthy diet, you will never be truly fit if you never do anything more strenuous than operate the remote control on the television. Your body was designed for use. Your heart was meant to beat strong and hard, pushing your blood throughout your body. And your muscles, bones, and joints were intended for movement more vigorous than lifting fork to mouth.

No one has found a panacea for the aging body. But you can minimize the effects of aging by combining a healthy diet with an exercise program. A good half-hour aerobic workout three or more times a week will strengthen your heart by increasing its capacity to pump blood, perhaps even slowing or preventing the progression of atherosclerosis. Joints that are exercised regularly remain supple and healthy, and muscles stay strong, toned, and defined. Moreover, it is a fact that women who exercise regularly prior to menopause have a better chance of avoiding osteoporosis than their less physically fit counterparts.

What kind of exercise is best for you? It is important to find something that you enjoy doing and that can be done conveniently. Brisk walking, lap swimming, cross-country skiing, bicycling, aerobics, and jogging are a few of the ways in which countless American women stay fit. If you have or are at high risk for osteoporosis, weight-bearing exercises such as walking, riding a stationary bicycle, or working out on a rowing machine may be your best bet (for exercise programs and other advice on physical activity, see *Exercise*, page 72).

Remember, before you embark on any exercise program—especially if you have been sedentary, are a heavy smoker, have health problems, and/or are overweight—consult your health-care practitioner.

NUTRITION AND EXERCISE IN THE OLDER YEARS

Long before you reached this stage in your life, you undoubtedly learned that your body was past the point where you could eat whatever you wanted, whenever you wanted it. Try that now and you will probably put on unwelcome pounds and may even aggravate one of the chronic diseases that are more likely to strike during the golden years.

Everyone—young, old, and in the middle—benefits from a nutritionally balanced diet. In recent years, however, our ideas about what constitutes such a diet have changed as we've learned more about the body and what nourishes it. We now know that most Americans eat too much and that their diets tend to be high in fat and low in complex carbohydrates. The reverse would be healthier.

For an older person, however, it may not be as simple as following the standard nutritional guidelines (see *Nine Dietary Guidelines*, page 50, and *The Food Guide Pyramid*, page 52). Your nutritional plan may be complicated by a chronic disease that restricts your food choices. A woman with hypertension, for example, may be advised to go out of her way to avoid salt. For a woman with adult-onset diabetes, sugar, not salt, may be the enemy. Or perhaps because of heart disease it may be necessary for you to limit your intake of fat and cholesterol stringently.

In the absence of disease, most of your nutritional requirements remain unchanged from earlier years. Your vitamin needs, for example, are virtually the same as at any other time in your adult life. As always, the key for most people is eating a wide variety of healthy foods. Eat less red meat and more chicken and fish or, even better, replace meat at some meals with beans, pasta dishes, or other high-energy, low-fat foods.

A concern for all women should be osteoporosis, the often crippling bone disease that strikes one in four women, typically after menopause. A diet rich in calcium helps prevent the bone loss that occurs with osteoporosis (see *Osteoporosis*, page 598).

No matter what you eat or drink, practice moderation. As you age, your body's energy requirements are diminished, and you require less food. Unfortunately, we tend to be creatures of habit, and many of us continue to eat the way we've always eaten, and the result is the intake of more calories than are needed to keep the body going. When that happens, the pounds tend to accumulate. Aside from interfering with your self-image, obesity is bad for your health and can put you at risk for serious diseases such as diabetes and hypertension.

Many senior citizens drink alcohol. There is nothing wrong with having a drink before dinner. In fact, some evidence suggests that a small amount of alcohol every day is beneficial; it makes a person feel good and may help keep the cardiovascular system healthy. Like most food and drink, however, alcohol is safe when used in moderation. The problems come with excess indulgence. People who are depressed may self-medicate with alcohol; alcohol also tends to worsen depression. And, since alcohol is high in calories, weight gain is a potential problem.

Something you almost can't drink too much of, though, is water. People who don't drink enough water may have constipation problems, so make an effort to drink eight glasses a day.

All the nutritional strategies in the world won't amount to much if you don't make an effort to eat. All too often, older people skip meals. Sometimes it's a matter of not having the money to buy enough food. In other cases a person may no longer feel capable of coping in the kitchen or may simply opt for the ease of opening a can of soup instead of preparing a more nutritious dinner. Then, too, depression can kill the appetite. If you do not have access to enough food or are no longer able to prepare food for yourself, there are meal delivery programs such as Meals on Wheels that help many thousands of senior citizens eat better than they otherwise would. If you feel depressed, talk to your health-care practitioner.

No matter what your age, one thing that generally will make you feel better is activity. Today, more older Americans than in any previous generation are exercising on a regular basis. Not only does vigorous exercise—when combined with a healthy diet—help keep the extra inches at bay, but it enables your heart and lungs to operate more efficiently and helps your joints maintain their flexibility. If you are already exercising, keep it up; most clinicians suggest at least three vigorous twenty- to thirty-minute workouts a week. If you haven't yet joined the exercise bandwagon, it's not too late. Be sure to check with your health-care practitioner before beginning, however. And no matter how enthusiastic you feel, begin your exercise program slowly, gradually lengthening your workout as your body becomes stronger.

Controlling weight is not easy for many people, especially as they age. The newest federal dietary guidelines recommend maintaining one's body weight within ten pounds of that attained at the time of reaching full adult height (assuming that weight was within the healthy range). Unfortunately, after age thirty our metabolism slows by about 5 percent every ten years, so people must learn to decrease their food intake by about that much to avoid gaining weight.

Aside from limiting calorie intake, the other key element in weight control is exercise. Basically, weight control is quite simple: if you burn more calories than you take in, you will lose weight; conversely, if you take in more than you burn, you will gain weight. The body burns calories in the normal processes of breathing, moving around, and performing other functions, but the rate at which calories are burned changes, depending on the level of exertion as well as body size.

If you sit quietly, you burn between 50 and 100 calories in one hour. If you are walking at 2 miles an hour (mph), you will burn roughly 125 calories in an hour. At 4 miles an hour, you burn between 260 and 360 calories per hour. If you jog at 5 mph, you burn between 460 and 640 calories per hour. Running at 10 mph burns between 860 and 1,200 calories per hour. Calorie expenditure varies widely, depending on type of activity, from aerobic dancing to chopping wood, and also on body weight: Lean people expend fewer calories than do heavy people engaged in the same form of exercise.

How *Not* to Lose Weight: Fad Diets and Bad Habits

The American obsession with weight loss and gimmickry is evident to anyone who peruses the nutrition and health shelves—or magazine racks—of her local bookstore, library, drugstore, or supermarket. New diets proliferate, each touted as a surefire program with no hunger pangs or other discomfort. Hucksters peddle the wonders of a bewildering variety of vitamin and mineral combinations, all "guaranteed" to melt off excess poundage.

Unfortunately, the vast majority of such claims are worthless. Most fad diets lighten pocketbooks rather than waistlines. With their intriguing but faulty rationales, many quick-fix diets enjoy short-lived popularity.

Fad diets can be dangerous as well as ineffective. Most so-called crash diets cause abnormal losses of water and protein from the body. Since over half the human body is composed of water, fad diets that promote water loss can produce a dramatic weight plunge. However, loss of body fat occurs much more slowly.

One perennial favorite among fad diets is the low-carbohydrate diet. This program generates a carbohydrate deficiency that slows the production and storage of fat while accelerating the rate of fat release into the bloodstream. It also limits the metabolism of fat, producing compounds called ketones *that inhibit appetite. It may cause tissue protein to break down and be converted to carbohydrates in order to maintain blood sugar levels and increase the loss of water and minerals in the urine. Most such diets are high in fat and can cause the body's metabolism to adapt in a way that leads to rapid weight gain whenever normal consumption of carbohydrates is resumed.*

Another currently popular fad diet relies on fasting to avoid the consumption of protein or the use of liquid protein preparations instead of food. Although this approach does produce results, weight is generally lost from lean tissue; such a loss can weaken the body and may damage the vital organs. Furthermore, studies of liquid protein preparations have indicated that the protein is of extremely poor quality.

One danger of many fad diets is that they are likely to cause imbalances in vital processes such as the acid–base balance, waste excretion, metabolism of carbohydrates, and fluid distribution within the blood and body tissues. Electrolyte imbalances, gout, or metabolic disturbances can result.

Even trying to lose weight by carefully counting calories can have its pitfalls. To lose weight, one must take in fewer calories than one expends, but calorie restriction can cause nutritional deficiencies if one is not careful to select foods from all the important food groups.

Those not trying to curb their weight through the newest and trendiest fad diets often find their efforts to be healthy frustrated by bad eating habits. Most of us must eat under less than optimal circumstances and do not have the time to sit down at home to three carefully balanced and prepared meals each day. Those who must eat at the office or elsewhere may put on weight because they eat what is offered in restaurants, cafeterias, fast-food emporia, or vending machines. Breaded and deep-fat–fried foods; pastries; high-calorie snacks such as french fries, fatty meats, and other delicatessen items; rich dishes like casseroles and lasagna; and ice cream, sodas, and the like can all add unwanted pounds. Socializing, too, can lead people to eat more food, and higher-calorie food, than they really want.

Nutritionists recommend identifying bad eating habits and changing them. Many people eat when they are not really hungry but are emotionally overwrought, bored, or frustrated. If emotional problems appear to trigger overeating, finding a way to address those problems more directly may be beneficial. Other people tend to eat snacks while engaging in certain activities, like watching television. Identifying settings one associates with eating can help the dieter avoid temptation. Joining a weight-loss group is another step many experts recommend. It is important to learn beforehand how the group is organized and how it operates, to make sure that whatever diet is being promoted is safe and healthy and that the group's approach fits well with the dieter's personality.

THE LINK BETWEEN NUTRITION AND DISEASE

Nutritional problems can occur as a result of nutrient deficiencies or nutrient excess. According to many surveys, nutrient deficiencies are quite common in women (as well as in the general population). Women from adolescence on, especially those who diet for prolonged periods and those in low-income groups, tend to be at risk for iron, calcium, vitamin B_6, and magnesium deficiencies. Iron deficiency is often observed in pregnant women as well as in women between the ages of twenty and forty-four. Long-standing calcium deficiencies and decreased vitamin D intake and metabolism increase the risk of osteoporosis (weakening of the bones) in postmenopausal women. Excess consumption of alcohol and lack of exercise are also linked to osteoporosis.

Nutritional Deficiencies. Careful attention to diet can ensure that adequate levels of these nutrients are maintained, and supplements may help prevent deficiencies. The most common deficiencies are the following:

IRON DEFICIENCY ANEMIA. Iron deficiency anemia occurs when the body does not have enough iron to make hemoglobin, the protein in red blood cells that carries oxygen to body tissues and removes carbon dioxide from them. Up to 20 percent of women in this country are thought to suffer from this condition, which usually results from insufficient consumption of iron-containing foods, loss of blood, or poor iron absorption. The cause in most women of childbearing age is menstruation. Iron deficiency anemia develops in many pregnant women if they do not take iron supplements because blood volume increases during pregnancy, and the existing stores of iron in their bodies must provide the fetus with a source of hemoglobin.

Iron deficiency anemia is a particular problem because it does not cause any initial symptoms. People may feel tired and eventually become pale, but the best diagnostic test is a blood test. The key preventive strategy is proper nutrition. The iron in vegetables and grains is not in a form that is easily absorbed by the body, so it is important to eat other iron-rich foods such as meat, fish, shellfish, poultry, eggs, legumes, potatoes, and rice. In particular, people on weight-reducing diets, infants, and strict vegetarians require an adequate supply of iron. Pregnant and lactating women are usually given iron supplements, and infants are sometimes placed on supplemental iron or iron-enriched cereal after about four months of age.

FOLIC ACID DEFICIENCY. Another form of anemia that sometimes develops in pregnant women is caused by a deficiency of folic acid. Alcoholics may also have this problem if they are malnourished and their digestive tract is less efficient at absorbing nutrients than it used to be.

Folic acid, one of the B vitamins, is important in the production of red blood cells.

Diet is important in preventing this problem and in correcting it. Raw fruits and vegetables, orange juice, dry beans, wheat germ, liver, and kidneys are good sources of folic acid, which can be destroyed by extensive cooking. Eating a balanced diet, minimizing alcohol consumption, and taking folic acid supplements when not actively using contraception are good ways both to avoid deficiency and to reduce the risk of a certain type of birth defect.

OSTEOPOROSIS. Osteoporosis involves low bone mass. It naturally occurs as a consequence of diminishing estrogen at the time of the climacteric and after. As a result, women are particularly prone to osteoporosis.

Thus, consuming quantities of calcium before menopause is a healthy strategy. Good dietary sources of calcium include such dairy products as milk, cheese, and yogurt. Skim-milk products can provide this essential nutrient without contributing large amounts of fat to the diet. Other recommended foods include canned salmon and sardines, and dark green vegetables like bok choy, broccoli, kale, and spinach. Kidney, navy, and pinto beans and soybeans as well as black-eyed peas are good sources.

Calcium supplements may be needed by those who can't meet their daily requirement through diet alone. A dosage of 1,200 to 1,500 mg a day is often recommended. Some foods, such as orange juice, yogurt, and milk, are now sold in calcium-enriched form. Note, however, that after menopause calcium alone may not be sufficient to prevent bone loss.

Getting regular weight-bearing exercise (but avoiding high-impact exercise), eating adequate amounts of dairy foods and dark-green vegetables, keeping protein intake down to recommended daily amounts, and getting enough vitamin D through exposure to sunlight and proper diet can all be helpful in minimizing the risk of osteoporosis (see also *Osteoporosis*, page 598).

Nutritional Excesses. Excessive nutrient consumption has been implicated in obesity, hypertension, and cardiovascular diseases. Women are more likely than men to be obese, especially between the ages of forty-five and fifty-four. The consumption of fat has been linked with breast and colon cancer, while salt-cured and smoked foods are linked to stomach cancer.

CARDIOVASCULAR DISEASE. Some factors for cardiovascular disease are hereditary, but one major factor that can be controlled relatively easily is cholesterol intake. Blood cholesterol concentrations play a large part in such problems as coronary artery disease, atherosclerosis, and stroke. Experts recommend that those with high blood fat levels make dietary changes to bring the levels down. These may include avoiding simple sugars and alcohol as well as foods that are high in cholesterol and saturated fat, and increasing intake of complex carbohydrates such as cereals and vegetables. Polyunsaturated or monounsaturated fats such as peanut, olive, canola, or safflower oil are healthier than saturated fats like butter. In recent years, fish oils have been recommended as an easy way of lowering one's risk of a heart attack; however, most nutritionists recommend eating fish rather than taking fish oil supplements.

HYPERTENSION. High blood pressure is a major risk factor for heart disease and other problems. If left untreated, it can damage the walls of the arteries. Because it does not cause immediately recognizable symptoms, many people do not realize they have the condition until it is detected during routine physical examinations.

Many people with hypertension are sensitive to salt. For those, eliminating or restricting salt intake can lower blood pressure substantially. Although we all need some salt for our bodies to function normally, most people routinely ingest up to *sixteen* times as much salt as they need. Strategies for lowering salt intake include using other spices to season food; avoiding highly salted foods like potato chips and pretzels or pickles; and minimizing consumption of processed foods like canned soups, cheese, lunch meats, bacon, and ham. Condiments like ketchup, mustard, and soy sauce are also very high in salt content.

Caffeine can increase blood pressure over the short term, so limiting caffeine intake is probably a good health measure.

OBESITY Obesity is defined as weighing at least 20 percent more than the recommended weight for one's body type and height. Obesity is the result of consuming more calories than the body can use, and they are then stored in the form of fat. Theoretically, all one needs to do to prevent obesity is not to take in more calories than are needed; however, dealing with obesity is rarely quite so easy. For one thing, fatty tissues may not always release fats when the body needs calories. Some people also appear to retain water when they metabolize body fat, while others seem to have extremely efficient metabolism. To lose one pound a week, most people must create a calorie deficit of 500 calories a day. To lose two pounds a week, they must create a deficit of 1,000 calories a day.

Some of the strategies for dealing with obesity have already been addressed (see *Controlling Your Weight*, page 54, and *How* Not *to Lose Weight*, page 60). Anyone with a tendency toward obesity must strive to eat a balanced diet that provides adequate amounts of nutrients without excess calories. Crash diets are not helpful. What is helpful is devising a dietary plan in conjunction with exercise that one can stick to over a prolonged period.

The Food Guide Pyramid discussed earlier (see page 52) is a good guide for selecting an adequate variety of foods, helps the dieter stave off the impulse to binge on one favorite high-calorie treat, and also ensures that caloric restriction does not result in nutrient deficiency. Paying attention to which foods in each group are more filling but less fattening than others allows the dieter to eat more without gaining unwanted weight. For example, within the bread group, pasta, crackers, bread, and cereal have fewer calories than do biscuits, stuffing, muffins, donuts, cakes, or cookies.

Fish and seafood offer the same complete protein found in red meat and poultry but at a considerably lower caloric cost and with less fat. A serving of a fish like flounder, for example, has about half the calories and 3 percent of the fat of an equivalent amount of beef rib roast. When eating meat, stick to lean varieties like chuck and round cuts, which contain only about 55 calories per ounce compared to the 100 or so calories per ounce in meats like ham, porterhouse steak, prime rib, rib lamb chops, and spareribs.

When it comes to milk products, skim milk has substantially fewer calories per ounce than whole milk. Even 1 percent or 2 percent milk offers savings in calories to the dieter. Cheeses can be very high in both fat and calories. One ounce of American cheddar cheese or cream cheese contains over 100 calories. A yogurt spread may offer just as much taste for far fewer calories.

Raw vegetables, of course, are the dieter's mainstay. With their high fiber content they provide a sense of fullness but only negligible amounts of calories. Fruits are especially valuable because they provide sweetness without added sugar, a source of empty calories.

Dieters must develop strategies that allow them to stick to their planned caloric intake regardless of the circumstances in which they find themselves. Eating lunches packed at home can help the office worker avoid high-calorie entrées in restaurants or cafeterias. Eating out is possible if the dieter is vigilant. At restaurants featuring buffets, concentrating on fruits and vegetables, avoiding sauces and desserts, and sticking with only one main dish or starchy side dish is a good idea.

The dieter should do the grocery shopping when he or she is not hungry and shop from a prepared list to minimize impulse buying. Confining eating to specific times and circumstances can help the dieter restrain the impulse to snack. Dieters must learn not to eat just because others around them are eating. Chewing more slowly and savoring each bite are good habits to cultivate; they are beneficial to the digestion, too. Preparing only enough food for a meal and serving appropriately sized servings remove the temptation to eat too much at mealtime. Storing leftover food as soon as the meal is over can prevent the dieter from feeling the need to finish it up so it won't go to waste (a common "Mom syndrome").

Weight control groups may be very helpful to those who need support in their efforts to reduce and may offer opportunities for socializing that are not organized around food.

Exercise is a significant component of most weight reduction programs, although it cannot be expected to produce weight loss unless combined with reduction of caloric intake. Not only does regular exercise expend calories, but it can also clear fats from the bloodstream, increase the flow of blood to organs and tissues, lower blood pressure and blood sugar level, slow the heart rate, reduce the rate of calcium loss from bones, firm up muscles and improve appearance, and reduce tension from emotional stress. Exercise also makes you feel good—and that can be a powerful motivating force in any weight reduction program.

CONSTIPATION AND DIARRHEA. Despite what many people think, constipation is not the inability to have a bowel movement every day. Normal bowel function varies from person to person; some people may move their bowels once a week, while for others bowel movements are part of their daily routine.

Constipation occurs because the colon removes water from the waste products in your body. Alterations in the speed at which waste passes through the colon or in the amount of water removed from it can produce dry, hard stools that are difficult to pass.

Take Sandra. Her lifelong struggle with constipation began when, as an adolescent, she became supersensitive about all her bodily functions. She had a bowel movement perhaps twice a week, sometimes less, and she had to strain to pass it. The time she spent in the bathroom was a source of hilarity for her siblings, which only aggravated the problem. It wasn't until she was in her late thirties that she finally decided to do something about what had become an unpleasant part of her life.

After talking to her doctor, she started exercising regularly, added more fiber to her diet (in the form of bran cereals, unprocessed wheat bran, and lots of raw fruits and vegetables), and drank at least eight glasses of water a day. She avoided laxatives and enemas, which her doctor warned her might aggravate her constipation if she used them too often. She noticed an improvement within a couple of weeks. She doesn't move her bowels every day, but when she does, the stools are larger and softer and easier to pass than before. The chronic bloated feeling in her stomach is gone, too. She's amazed that being regular can make such a difference in her disposition and sense of well-being.

Diarrhea can be caused by any number of disorders, so an effort should be made to find out what the underlying problem might be. Food poisoning, bacterial or viral infection, and medications can cause this symptom. Another common cause is carbohydrate malabsorption due to a deficiency of lactase, the enzyme the body needs to break down lactose. Lactase deficiency occurs in up to 75 percent of adults in all ethnic groups except those of northwest European origin, affecting up to 90 percent of Asians and 75 percent of American blacks and Native Americans. Avoiding milk is one solution; adding the lactase enzyme to milk or buying reduced-lactose milk (available in most supermarkets) is another. Calcium supplements should be taken by those who forgo milk products altogether.

Excessive intake of some of the sugar substitutes used in dietetic food, such as sorbitol and mannitol, can also cause diarrhea. Discontinuing consumption of these products clears up the problem. Some foods may also exacerbate diarrhea—apple juice, pear juice, grapes, honey, dates, nuts, figs, and fruit-flavored soft drinks, for example—because they are high in fructose. The caffeine in coffee, tea, colas, and some headache remedies can also worsen the problem, as can antacids containing magnesium.

How Can I Get My Child to Eat Properly?

Nancy's first child, Kate, was a delight when it came to eating. She had a good appetite and ate anything her mother put in front of her: broccoli, bean sprouts, yogurt, even tofu. In contrast, Nancy's second child, Ross, decided before his first birthday that green and yellow foods were not meant for human consumption.

Nancy had to learn a subversive form of cooking familiar to many mothers, in which extra ingredients like pureed carrots and spinach are secretly added to spaghetti sauce, hamburgers, lasagna, muffins—in short, to just about everything. Ross eventually allowed two or three shreds of lettuce and a raw carrot on his plate next to his grilled-cheese sandwich, but at the age of eleven that's as far as he'll go. Meanwhile, his sister asks for sushi and arugula and stir-fried Chinese vegetables. Their mother sighs resignedly as she prepares two separate meals every evening, but she knows better than to force Ross to eat what he doesn't want to. That method backfires every time.

Worries about their children's nutritional habits are among the most common concerns that plague parents of small children. Paradoxically, most experts agree that the single most important factor in ensuring that children receive adequate and appropriate nutrition is maintaining a relaxed, low-stress attitude toward food and meals. Eating should be a pleasant experience for a child, not an ordeal during which he or she is quizzed about school performance or lectured sternly about proper table manners.

It is important for parents to remember that children have a small stomach and need snacks as well as regular meals. A child under age twelve should eat, on average, three servings from the milk group each day, two servings from the meat group, four servings of vegetables or fruits, and four servings from the bread and cereal group. However, growing children have unpredictable appetites. They may, especially if they have been very physically active, seem like bottomless pits one day and then barely pick at their food the next.

Children also tend to find the flavors of many foods to be very strong, especially those of some vegetables. Most go through phases when they are passionately attached to a few foods and vehemently opposed to others. The wise parent will try to provide as broad a variety as possible and attempt to substitute foods of roughly the same nutritional value as those the child expressly rejects.

Children need to be allowed to eat at their own pace, even if they seem to be dawdling or playing with their food. Most children need more time to eat than do adults. And bear in mind that some aspects of childhood, such as tooth loss or braces, can have a substantial impact on a child's food preferences and eating habits. Becoming obsessively concerned with every detail of a child's daily food intake is likely to have a negative effect on the child's ability to develop healthy eating habits. Although some children, particularly in the United States, struggle with obesity in childhood, trying to restrict caloric intake for a growing child can be risky and should not be undertaken without consulting a pediatrician or dietitian. And banning whole categories of food, like cookies, can have the undesirable effect of causing a child to focus excessively on the forbidden treat.

One big problem for parents, of course, is the influence of television advertising on childhood food preferences. Most children's programming is surrounded by commercials for high-sugar items like candy, cookies, and breakfast cereals.

School lunch programs can cause problems, too, since many depend on government surplus items such as cheese, butter, and fatty ground beef. Many schools have opted for selling fast foods rather than staff and operate full in-house cooking operations. Since institutional cooking—food prepared in large quantities and left to languish on steam tables—often does not appeal to children, parents can pack nutritious lunches for them instead. Again, it is important to pay attention to fat and salt content; many lunch meats are high in both and low in nutritional value. Most children, however, will eat raw vegetables such as carrots, celery, or broccoli florets, and many, given the choice, actually prefer a snack like yogurt to cookies and crackers. Outside school, parents can exert some low-key control over their children's eating habits by minimizing trips to hamburger stands and other fast-food outlets.

Children are influenced by those around them, so one of the best strategies for parents is to follow a healthy, varied eating regimen themselves. Making sure the family eats at least one meal a day together is not only beneficial to family life, but also allows you to introduce your children to new foods in a relaxed, convivial setting.

There's no getting around the fact that many children are picky eaters. However, when offered a wide array of healthy food, most children will eat a nutritionally balanced diet. Remember too that your child's energy requirements vary at different stages of her development. So there will be times when she does not need or want the large quantities of food she required at an earlier time. Don't force your child to eat when she isn't hungry; that may only serve to promote a weight problem later.

What are the foods your daughter should be eating during the first twelve years of life?

The First Year. In her first few months of life, your daughter needs only breast milk or formula, a combination of processed cow's milk or soy proteins mixed with vitamins and minerals. Some practitioners also prescribe a vitamin supplement. Eating schedules during this stage vary. Some breast-fed babies may need to eat every two or three hours; others are content to feed every four hours or go even longer between feedings.

As some point during the first year you will want to start your baby on solids. Some pediatricians recommend that formula-fed babies begin on rice cereal after the fourth month. Others wait until the sixth month. A lot depends upon how hungry your baby seems. If she is drinking a quart of formula a day or nursing more rather than less often yet still seems ravenous, it is probably time to introduce solids.

You have two options with solids—buy commercially prepared baby food or use a blender or food grinder to prepare your own. In addition to cereal, good initial choices include mashed banana and fresh fruits and vegetables that have been cooked (without salt!) and then pureed. Later you can introduce pureed meat. After about eight months, most babies delight in bits of table food that they can eat with their fingers. Small pieces of cheese, toast, scrambled egg, and pasta are good choices (again, unsalted and unsugared).

The Preschool Years. Whereas it may seem that your infant never stops eating, the parent of a preschooler often has the opposite problem. Children this age do not grow at the same rapid pace as infants, and their slackened appetite often reflects this lower energy expenditure. Thus you may find that your preschooler rarely sits down to eat a full meal, instead getting the bulk of her nutrition from small healthy snacks that you provide throughout the day.

While you may be tempted to argue with your child about her eating habits, it is best not to make an issue of them. Instead, make sure that all the choices you offer provide good nutrition, then let her make her own decisions. She may, for example, turn up her nose at cooked carrots at dinner, yet happily munch on carrot sticks in midafternoon.

We used to think that dietary fat was something that only adults had to be concerned about. Today, however, we know that even the diet of young children could benefit from a reduction in fat. Not only does an early fat-rich diet promote obesity and possible cardiovascular disease, but it establishes a lifelong eating pattern that is often difficult to break.

You need not be a fat-free zealot; children do, in fact, need fat, although not as much as most of them eat. The following are a few relatively painless steps you can take to reduce some of your child's fat intake:

- After your child turns two, buy 2 percent rather than whole milk.
- Trim the fat off meats.
- Serve more fish and poultry and less red meat. Avoid lunch meats and other highly processed foods.
- Buy low-fat cheeses and yogurt and replace ice cream with frozen yogurt.
- Limit the number of eggs you serve your child to no more than three a week.
- Bake or broil foods instead of frying.
- Serve cookies that are lower in fat such as oatmeal cookies, animal crackers,

ginger snaps, vanilla wafers, or fig bars. Don't leave salty, high-calorie snacks like chips where children can easily get at them—better yet, rarely keep them in the house.

The School-Age Child. School-age children need between 1,650 and 3,000 calories a day for normal development. Children involved in vigorous sports need more. Like adults, children should get the bulk of these calories from the basic food groups: milk products, meat, fruits, vegetables, and breads and cereals. An after-school snack is fine as long as it is something nutritious like a piece of fruit and does not make the child too full to eat dinner.

As with the preschooler, you should attempt to reduce fat intake whenever possible, but don't overdo it. Children need some fat in their diet to grow.

Many children of this age skip breakfast. Even if your child has to get up earlier in order to eat in the morning, stress the importance of starting the day with a nutritious meal. Avoid instant cereals, which typically have added salt and sugar; regular or quick-cooking cereals take only marginally longer to prepare. A bowl of hot oatmeal or Cream of Wheat with sliced fruit or nuts on top appeals to many children. If dry cereals are preferred, stick to those that are not overly sweetened. Yogurt, whole-grain toast, cheese, or an egg is also a good choice, with milk or unsweetened fruit juice on the side.

In addition to eating a healthy diet, children should be encouraged to exercise. Not only is a physically active child less likely to become overweight, he or she is more likely to continue the fitness habit as an adult. While most schools require that children take physical education, that alone is not enough exercise; they should be encouraged to be active at home. Most children would probably have a difficult time scheduling a regular workout, so it might make more sense to get them involved in an organized sport or activity they enjoy. You can help your child learn to like exercise by letting her see you involved in your own regimen. Encourage her to spend her after-homework hours not in front of the television set but riding her bicycle or taking a walk with you.

Adolescence. Adolescence is a particularly trying time when it comes to nutrition. Many teenagers seem to subsist entirely on huge quantities of burgers, potato chips, and soda. Others, especially girls, are obsessed with a fear of fat. Visions of unrealistically thin fashion models or movie and television stars can cause adolescents of perfectly normal proportions to worry excessively about their weight. In extreme situations this obsession may lead to the development of anorexia nervosa or bulimia, which must be addressed with the help of a doctor or therapist (see *Eating Disorders*, page 70).

Again, the experts advise parents to take a relaxed attitude toward their adolescents' eating habits. Teenagers are experiencing many profound physiological changes and may find reassurance in familiar and comfortable foods. As long as these are not too fatty, salty, or sugary, they are not a problem. However, most adolescents are not aware of the impact the foods they eat can have on their body either in the short term or later in life, so parents must make sure that healthy alternatives to junk food are readily and plentifully available.

EATING DISORDERS

If you've ever watched your body transformed into a massive blob through the distorted glass of the trick mirrors often seen at carnivals, you can visualize how the girl with anorexia nervosa, an eating disorder, sees herself.

She may, in fact, be so thin that her ribs protrude and her legs resemble matchsticks. Yet when she looks in the mirror, all she sees is fat.

Anorexia nervosa and another disorder called bulimia (binge eating and purging) are eating disorders that generally affect adolescents and young adults.

Anorexia Nervosa. An estimated one in one hundred adolescent girls suffers from this eating disorder, which is nine times more common in females than males. The typical girl with anorexia nervosa is in the middle to upper socioeconomic group. The condition is especially common among girls who are involved in ballet, modeling, sports, and any other fields in which appearance is particularly important.

Anorexia is a disease and is often a symptom of a psychological problem related to the girl's family. Many girls, for instance, are from families that frequently think and talk about the "proper" amounts or kinds of foods to eat. These girls may use their refusal to eat as a way of manipulating their parents. Other girls may stop eating as a way of halting their sexual maturation, since a poorly nourished adolescent is not likely to develop breasts or to menstruate. In some cases, the disease may be triggered by a sexual experience. In one study, researchers found that two thirds of the anorectic girls interviewed had been sexually abused during childhood or early adolescence, usually by an older man whom the girl knew.

A girl with this disorder sees herself as obese. Typically, the illness starts as a simple diet to lose weight and then snowballs. Over time, the girl eats less and less and her stomach shrinks so that her desire for food is diminished. At times, she may go on food binges, eating everything in the refrigerator and then inducing herself to vomit (see also *Bulimia*, page 71). She may also take heavy doses of laxatives to speed what little food she does eat through the digestive system.

Even while the anorectic is becoming skeletally thin, she may be bursting with energy. Although she won't touch food, she may spend a lot of time in the kitchen preparing elaborate meals for the family. She'll insist she's feeling great but her skin eventually will look like paper and become sallow. After her weight drops to about twenty-six pounds below normal, she stops menstruating.

If your daughter shows any of the signs of this eating disorder, it is imperative that you get help quickly. Consult your family's primary care provider, doctor, school nurse or counselor, or community mental health clinic. If untreated or if treated too late, anorexia nervosa can be fatal. An estimated 15 percent of anorectics die of starvation or of infections caused by undernourishment or dehydration or commit suicide.

Treatment for this condition may require hospitalization. In severe cases, the anorectic may have to be fed intravenously. Cognitive behavior therapy is aimed at changing the girl's body image.

Bulimia. An estimated 50 percent of girls with anorexia nervosa also have bulimia, also known as binge eating and purging. Many bulimics, however, are not underweight; that makes identifying the problem much more difficult.

The girl with bulimia typically goes on eating binges where she becomes obsessed with food, devouring an extraordinary amount and then inducing herself to vomit. Bulimics also are known to use excessive amounts of laxatives to purge the digestive system after an eating binge.

Unlike anorexia, which eventually becomes impossible to ignore, bulimia may escape diagnosis because many bulimics maintain their normal weight or even gain weight. One telltale sign of the disorder is wildly fluctuating weight.

The treatment of bulimia is similar to that of anorexia but may not require hospitalization or forced feeding. Consultation with a health-care professional is recommended to be sure the treatment thoroughly addresses the problem, both psychologically and physically.

CHAPTER 4

❧

Exercise

CONTENTS

Ask any exercise aficionado and she will probably be all too happy to recite the numerous advantages of a regular workout. Many are readily apparent a few weeks or months after beginning a program. Improved muscle tone, strong and supple joints, better physical stamina, reduced tension, extra energy, a healthy glow to the skin, and even weight loss (provided you also decrease your caloric intake) are all benefits of regular exercise that are visible soon after you begin a program.

For many exercisers, these reasons alone would be sufficient to keep them pumping iron or logging more miles on already well-worn jogging shoes. But exercise has hidden benefits that, while not apparent to the eye, have major consequences for the body's health and longevity.

No doubt you know by now that vigorous exercise is good for your heart and lungs. When you exercise hard, your muscles require more oxygen. As a result, you are forced to breathe more deeply to fill your lungs. Your heart must beat harder and faster to meet the muscles' increased demand for blood. As a result, your heart becomes stronger and your lungs more efficient. That is why you may notice after several months of a vigorous exercise program that you don't get winded as easily when climbing stairs or performing some other strenuous task. In addition to these benefits, exercise may widen the arteries, making it less likely that a fat deposit or clot could block blood flow.

Women should also know that some types of exercise may reduce the risk of osteoporosis, a degenerative bone disease that poses a major health risk to a large segment of postmenopausal women. Studies have shown that weight-bearing exercise such as walking will strengthen the bones and may help lessen the risk of this often crippling disease.

So if you haven't already begun to exercise regularly, think about starting today. All it takes is three twenty-minute sessions per week to benefit your entire body. But what type of exercise is best for you?

To learn about different types of exercise, how to match particular exercises to specific health problems, and how to force yourself from the couch to the gym, pool, or track, read on.

AN EXERCISE PROGRAM FOR YOU

Martha walks for enjoyment and for keeping herself in shape. Three or four times a week, rain or shine, she treks up and down the hills of the small town in which she lives.

The idea of traipsing through the town holds no appeal for Martha's sister, Natalie. Her exercise of choice is an assortment of barbells and dumbbells. Natalie's body, with more peaks and valleys than most mountain ranges, is testament to the zeal with which she trains.

These activities illustrate the two basic types of exercise—aerobic being the former and anaerobic the latter. They're certainly different—but are they equally good for you?

According to exercise experts, no. Although weight training and floor exercises can help increase muscle size and shape and tone your body, they do not push the limits of your cardiovascular system the way aerobic exercise does. So if we were able to peek inside the cardiovascular systems of these women, Martha's would probably be stronger and more efficient.

What is *aerobic* exercise? This form of fitness involves continuous motion, the kind of motion that causes your heart to pound and your body to sweat. When you perform aerobic exercise, you breathe deeply to fill your lungs in order to supply your moving muscles with the extra oxygen that this level of activity demands. Your heart must work harder and faster to pump blood throughout your body and you feel it pounding in your chest. Your breath comes out in puffs, you begin to feel warm, and, even though you don't physically feel it happening, your body burns extra calories.

Anaerobic exercise, on the other hand, does little to promote a stronger and healthier cardiovascular system. Anaerobic exercise usually is of such short duration that the heart and lungs are not taxed. This is not to say that anaerobic exercise has no place in your fitness program. Lifting weights or performing certain exercises will increase your muscle strength and tone your body. In short, you will have a better figure.

Just remember that a good exercise program must include aerobic activity. Activities that can help keep your heart and lungs healthy include walking, running, bicycling, swimming, cross-country skiing, and aerobic dancing. One way to incorporate both methods might be to use light weights when you walk. Or, consider doing aerobic exercise three times a week and anaerobic on two or three of the off days, but be sure to warm up before you start pumping iron.

Once you make the decision to begin your fitness program, aim for at least three twenty- to thirty-minute sessions of aerobic activity each week. Remember, though, the old adage "Rome was not built in a day" applies to physical fitness as well as ancient architecture. If you are just leaving the exercise starting blocks, don't expect to be capable of a full workout immediately. The key to success is to start with a realistic goal and gradually increase the intensity and duration. Most people notice improved fitness within two to three months of starting an exercise regimen.

FITNESS TESTING

You've been thinking about changing your life-style. Last night you choked down the last Twinkie in the house, unplugged the TV, and started searching the newspaper for sales on running shoes. But before you purchase new equipment to embark on your goal of physical fitness, it might be prudent to get your existing equipment—namely, your body—checked out.

If you are a relatively healthy adult, the chances are that however long it has been, you can probably start exercising, as long as you begin gradually. However, if you are over forty, are overweight, or are a smoker, or if you have had a heart attack or are diabetic, see your health-care provider before you embark on your new exercise regimen. A pregnant woman who has not been regularly exercising should also check with her clinician, though, in the absence of potential complications, most practitioners will probably enthusiastically endorse the plan.

Your health-care provider may ask you to undergo an exercise tolerance or stress test. This test may be given if you have a history of heart disease, if you have symptoms that suggest possible coronary artery disease, or if you are over forty and have other heart risks. Other risk factors that could make this test worthwhile for you include high blood pressure, high cholesterol level, smoking, and a family history of stroke.

During the test, which is done on a treadmill or stationary bike, electrodes are placed on your chest and a blood pressure cuff on your arm. Then you begin the test on the machinery. As the workout commences, your provider monitors your heart rate, your blood pressure, and your heart's electrical impulses and then watches how your heart tolerates the workout as it becomes increasingly more strenuous.

The test takes about thirty minutes. It correctly identifies the presence of coronary artery disease in nearly three fourths of those who have the disease and take the test.

If your heart's function is normal throughout the test, you probably will not encounter any cardiovascular problems during a workout, provided you start slowly and gradually increase your activity. When the practitioner detects a problem, he or she may not advise against exercise but may help design a program that works within the limits of your cardiovascular capabilities. For example, rather than endorsing your plan to jog, the clinician may recommend walking instead.

In considering an exercise program, look for something that will give your cardio-vascular system the workout it needs. To do this, find your "target heart rate." Begin by subtracting your age from 220 and then take 70 percent of this number. If, for example, you are 40 years old, 220 minus 40 is 180; 70 percent of 180 is 126. This means that your target heart rate during exercise should be 125 beats per minute. If during the duration of your workout your heart does not achieve that target rate, it means you are not exercising hard enough. Keep in mind, however, that this formula is for healthy adults; if you have a health problem, your health-care provider may recommend that you start with a lower target heart rate and gradually work your way up.

THE RISKS-VERSUS-BENEFITS EQUATION

After years of sitting in front of a computer developing the software that would put her fledgling company on the corporate map, Lily decided it was time to ease up. She would start exercising, she decided, get her body back in shape. So when a friend suggested a ski trip, Lily jumped at the chance to resume the sport at which she had excelled in high school.

One day into the trip, Lily took a hard fall—and a ligament in her right knee ripped like paper.

Lily was right in thinking that an exercise program would be a worthwhile addition to her life. Her mistake was not finding the right program. The lean seventeen-year-old body that had negotiated with ease the tricky path down a slope filled with moguls was a far cry from the softening form of the thirty-five-year-old executive whose joints hadn't in years attempted anything more strenuous than bending to sit down.

An unexercised body eventually bears the signs of neglect. The pounds may pile up and the muscles weaken; the result can be extra strain on the joints and ligaments. The heart and lungs grow lazy with untapped potential. At the same time, a body exercised improperly is an accident waiting to happen. We all have heard stories of people with heart problems who have massive coronaries while out for the morning jog around the park, or people who sustained serious joint injuries on their "weekend athlete" regimen.

Once you decide to incorporate exercise into your life, the next step is choosing the program that best fits not only your fitness goals but your body itself. This involves weighing the benefits of a potential exercise program against the risks.

Remember to take into consideration your stage of life. Although you may have been a good long-distance runner in your twenties, that form of exercise isn't appropriate if you have been diagnosed with osteoporosis. An exercise that places weight on the joints but does not jolt the body (walking and bicycling are excellent choices) would be more suited to you now.

Perhaps you've always desired the definition that weight lifting gives to the muscles, but you have a bad back and are wary of damaging it further. In fact, a proper weight program might well benefit both your muscle definition and your back—but care must taken to select the right equipment and an appropriate regimen to prevent further damage of your already vulnerable back. Some people combine using weight machines with another exercise program. An aerobic activity such as swimming, bicycling, or walking will also strengthen the cardiovascular system and joints, firm muscles, and generally tone the body.

Let's look at some of the most common health problems and the exercises that are both effective and safe for those with such concerns.

Obesity. If you are overweight, a combined diet and fitness program can help you lose those extra pounds. However, this extra weight places additional stress not only on your heart and lungs but on your joints and ligaments. In evaluating types of exercise, opt for one that will not place further stress on your joints, that will gradually strengthen your cardiovascular system, and that will expend a good number of calories to help you move closer to your weight-loss goal.

Walking is an excellent choice and is often recommended for inactive or overweight people who want to become more fit. If walking has no appeal for you, other aerobic exercises that would be safe are swimming and bicycling.

Osteoporosis. Studies have shown that one weapon in the battle against the development of the often crippling bone disease osteoporosis is exercise to help prevent bone loss. Doctors believe that women who begin exercising before they have the disease may decrease their risk. If osteoporosis develops after menopause—the time of life when this disease typically develops most rapidly—exercise will not cure the problem but can help improve overall health. Again, the key is the correct exercise.

Exercises that generate a high force on the bones (so-called weight-bearing exercise) help maintain the bone density. But think in terms of gentle stress. Walking is an excellent choice; running, on the other hand, is not the best option for some people. Jogging stresses the vulnerable bones and joints, and, in women who run great distances, estrogen production is often decreased, and that decrease may make the ardent runner prone to this disease in her later years. Other good weight-bearing exercises for both younger women and older women who already have the disease are riding a stationary bicycle and working out on a rowing machine.

Heart Problems. The days when survivors of heart attack were treated as invalids are long past. We now know that exercise is an important component in maintaining cardiovascular health. It is also important in helping the damaged heart recover its strength after a heart attack.

Your health-care provider or a member of the cardiac rehabilitation team at your local hospital will help you plan a fitness program that works for you. Walking is often recommended for heart patients. You will be instructed to start slowly and gradually increase the duration and pace of your workout. For example, the first two weeks of your program, your practitioner may recommend you walk about one mile per exercise session. As that becomes easier, you can increase it to two miles, and so on. Walking on a treadmill, riding a stationary bicycle, and swimming are also good exercises to help strengthen the damaged heart.

Remember, though, whatever exercise you choose—you must listen to your body. It will tell you if you are overdoing. If you experience pain, nausea, or dizziness during exercise, stop immediately and rest. Call your clinician if the symptoms persist.

Back Problems. The good news is that most back problems will not prevent you from exercising. However, you must choose your fitness program with care to prevent further damage to your back. Forget sports that involve sudden twists and turns or that put you at a high risk for falls. Tennis, downhill skiing, football, soccer, horseback riding, and aerobic dancing are not good choices if your back hurts; walking, swimming, and bicycling are excellent exercises that not only strengthen your heart and lungs but help tone your back muscles, making them less prone to injury.

If your back continues to be a problem, consult a physical therapist, who will teach you various exercises to stretch and strengthen your back muscles.

ALICIA'S STORY

When Alicia was coming of age in the early 1950s, exercise was something most women did only as a last resort when a waistband became too tight.

As Alicia puts it, "I never had to worry about that. I was thin, probably too thin. Besides, who needed to do a hundred sit-ups a day or run around the block to stay in shape? I got all the exercise I needed chasing two toddlers and doing housework."

Forty years later, Alicia still has little fat on her body. And even though for years she'd been reading about the overall health benefits of a regular exercise program, to Alicia, the words exercise *and* overweight *were synonymous. That was until a lifetime of poor health habits caught up with her.*

A heavy smoker, Alicia was recently diagnosed with emphysema, a chronic lung disease that compromises air flow to the lungs, making breathing difficult. A few months later, she began having chest pains and her doctor ordered tests that revealed blocked coronary arteries, the vessels that feed the heart. If something wasn't done, Alicia would probably have a heart attack.

Six months ago Alicia had surgery to correct the blockage. Following her doctor's orders, she threw away her last pack of cigarettes and resolved to eat more fruits, vegetables, and grains and fewer high-fat foods. But those measures alone, while important, would not be adequate, her doctor explained. To strengthen her heart and to help her reduced lung capacity become more efficient, she would need to begin to exercise.

So Alicia enrolled in a cardiac conditioning course at her local hospital. It was slow going at first. A sedentary person can no more take on a full exercise load than a baby can run before it walks. Alicia's instructor suggested she start with two minutes on the treadmill and slowly work her way up. Within a few months, she was up to twenty minutes of exercise three times a week.

One year after starting her exercise program, Alicia says she has more energy, looks better in her clothes, and, more importantly, feels stronger and healthier.

Although it took a long time, Alicia finally discovered what many people have known for years: Exercise not only is good for you, it makes you feel good.

LOOSENING UP, BEFORE AND AFTER

On a frigid morning, chances are you wouldn't think of driving your car without first warming it up for a moment or two. Experience has taught you that not doing so is to risk stalling on the way to the freeway. Yet many people, in an attempt to race through their exercise regimen, may be tempted to skip the critical warm-up period. True, you may save a few minutes—but at the risk of stiffness, sore muscles, and even injury.

No matter what the nature of your exercise program is, you should always allow a few minutes to warm up. A good warm-up will ease you gently into your workout, stretching and loosening your inactive muscles and gradually increasing your heart rate, body temperature,

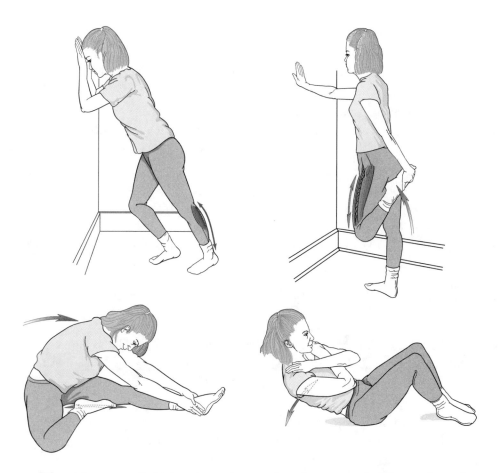

When doing your calf, thigh, or hamstring stretch, make sure you don't bounce. Instead, hold the position steadily for ten seconds before relaxing and moving on to another repetition of the same stretch or to another exercise.

and blood flow to the muscles. Once you have loosened your muscles, they become more flexible and as such are less prone to injury.

How long you warm up is up to you, but most experts recommend at least five to ten minutes of exercise prior to starting your primary workout. Remember when performing stretching warm-up exercises to hold each position for thirty seconds—but do not bounce. The goal is to stretch gently, not pull the muscle. Although you will feel a pulling sensation, you should not feel pain. If you do, your body is telling you to ease up. There are many good stretching exercises that will do the job, but here are a few basic ones that suit a range of exercise regimens.

Calf Stretch. To perform this stretch, stand an arm's length away from a wall. Lean forward, resting your forearms against the wall, and bring your forehead to rest against the backs of your hands. Bend one leg at the knee, bringing it toward the wall, while keeping the other leg straight with the heel on the floor.

Keep your back straight while you move your hips toward the wall. When this stretch is done correctly, you should feel a pull in the calf muscle of the straightened leg. Hold the position for ten seconds and repeat with the other leg. Do six repetitions with each leg.

Thigh Stretch. Placing your left hand on the wall for balance, reach behind you and hold your right foot or ankle with your right hand. Then pull the foot gently toward your buttock. You should feel a stretch in your thigh. Again, hold this position for ten seconds. Again, do six repetitions with each leg.

Hamstring Stretch. While sitting on the floor, extend your left leg straight ahead of your body. Bend your right leg so that the bottom of the right foot touches the inner thigh of the left leg. Bending forward from your waist, slowly move both hands down your left leg. If you are doing the movement correctly, you will feel a pull down your hamstring, the long muscle that runs along the back of your thigh. After holding the stretch for ten seconds, repeat the movement with the other leg. Do six repetitions.

Bent-leg Sit-ups. Another excellent candidate for the warm-up period is bent-leg sit-ups. Lie on your back, with your knees bent. Holding the palms of your hand on opposite shoulders, bring yourself partway up to a sitting position (at roughly a forty-five-degree angle to the floor). Start with ten sit-ups before a workout, and increase gradually to thirty.

After you have warmed up for ten minutes or so, you are ready to move on to the main exercise course, whatever that may be. To achieve the full benefits from your aerobic workout, you should exercise at least twenty minutes three times a week on nonconsecutive days. Longer and more frequent workouts will result in faster physical conditioning and weight loss if that is a primary goal.

At the end of your workout, your heart will be beating fast in your chest. Now is not the time to quit cold turkey and run off to take a nap. Instead, your body needs a cool-down period to allow your heart rate to return to normal and to prevent blood from collecting in your legs, which may make you feel dizzy.

Allow three to five minutes to bring your heart and respiration levels back to normal. Some runners use this time for slow walking. If you use a stationary bicycle, you might pedal slowly for a few minutes. Once you have begun to cool down, you should end the workout with a few minutes of stretching exercises—the ones described here are fine—to keep your muscles supple and to prevent stiffness and soreness. Check your heart rate after the cool-down period to ensure it is normal.

KINDS OF EXERCISE

It doesn't matter how beneficial an exercise is for your cardiovascular system or how well it tones the muscles in your body—if you *hate* doing it, all the benefits in the world probably are not enough to make you incorporate it into your life.

This isn't to say that everyone who has made the decision to work out on a regular basis loves every lap she swims or every mile she walks. For many of us, exercise is simply a means to an end. We like the results that a thrice-weekly workout reaps, the way it tones and strengthens the body, inside and out, and makes us feel wonderful. Lots of us like exercise best *after* we've finished doing it.

That's why it's so important to find the exercise program that's right for your needs and stage of life. You may not love spending twenty minutes three times a week pumping your legs up and down on your stationary bicycle, but is it something that you are willing to do? If not, then it isn't the exercise program for you.

The first step to finding your best exercise regimen is to identify your goals. Sheryl, for example, has decided she wants to redefine or sculpt her body. The walking program that has kept her friend Jodi's body trim and toned and her cardiovascular system healthy will do little to give Sheryl the muscle definition she desires. Sheryl needs a weight-training course to sculpt her muscles—a program that is supplemented by an aerobics program that will keep her heart and lungs healthy.

In designing your exercise program, be sure to take both your general physical health and your life-style into consideration. If you are overweight and have never exercised, initiating a strenuous running program would be for you like an elementary school student's trying to learn calculus before she has mastered basic math. Walk before you run.

Swimming laps may appeal to you. That was the workout that Terri initially chose. But with the closest pool a twenty-minute ride away and with two toddlers at home and only sporadic baby-sitters, Terri soon found that her visits to the pool were few and far between. Instead she bought an exercise bike and installed it in her home office, and now she happily pedals away on a regular basis while her children nap.

Whatever variety of exercise you choose, you control the intensity during your workout. A workout should not be so strenuous that you are ready to collapse at the end, but it must be hard enough to get your heart and lungs working hard. You need to find your target heart rate. If, for example, your target heart rate is 125 beats per minute, your heart should reach that target rate and remain there for twenty minutes or more during the workout. To test whether this is happening, use your pulse as your guide. During the workout, use the tips of your index and third fingers to locate your pulse between the wrist bone and thumb side of either wrist. Press gently. Then, using the sweep hand of a clock or watch, count your pulse for ten seconds. Multiple this number by 6 to determine whether you are achieving your target heart rate.

You say you still don't know what exercise would be best for you? Perhaps after reading the following section, you will have a better idea of what various exercises have to offer you.

WALKING

The most popular exercise today requires no special skills or instruction and little in the way of equipment other than a good pair of shoes. Maybe that's part of the reason why thirty million Americans have taken to the streets in an effort to walk their way to better health.

Walking is a wonderful way to improve your cardiovascular fitness, reduce the stress of a difficult day, strengthen bones and ligaments, and tone muscles in your legs, hips, buttocks, and abdomen. For dieters, it has the additional benefit of burning calories. The amount of calories burned in an hour's walk depends on your weight and the distance you walk. If, for instance, you weigh 150 pounds, you will burn roughly 240 calories by walking two miles.

Walking is frequently recommended by doctors as the best way to start safely exercising, particularly for those who have heart problems, are overweight, or have simply been sedentary. Regular walking also may lower your risk of development of osteoporosis by helping prevent the loss of bone density (see *Osteoporosis*, page 598).

As with any exercise, a beginning walker is advised to ease into the program. Plan to walk three times a week on alternating days, for twenty minutes or more, to achieve aerobic benefit. Prior to and after the walk, do stretching exercises to warm up and cool down your muscles (see *Loosening Up, Before and After*, page 78). Initially, set a modest goal for yourself, perhaps a rate of one mile every fifteen minutes, then gradually work up to two twelve-minute miles, and so on. By your third month of walking, you may find yourself walking four or five miles during the workout.

Equip yourself with good shoes for your walk. The best walking shoes are lightweight, fit well, and have a slightly elevated heel. The shoes should have good arch support, plenty of width in the toe, a well-cushioned heel that absorbs shock, and good traction.

And remember, keep your body well hydrated, especially if you walk in warm weather. Drink water before and after your workout.

JOGGING

When you jog, your heart pumps hard and you huff and puff as your lungs work harder to meet the muscles' greater demand for oxygen. The muscles in your legs, hips, buttocks, abdomen, and arms gain strength and tone. If you are in overall good health, jogging may be just the exercise you are looking for. Like walking, it is inexpensive (all you need is a good pair of shoes and a good bra), can be easily adapted to most schedules, and is done virtually anywhere.

Jogging also is an excellent way to burn calories. If you weigh 120 to 130 pounds, for example, and jog at the rate of five miles per hour, you will expend 460 calories per hour.

Unlike walking, however, jogging is not recommended for everyone. If you have a heart or lung problem, are substantially overweight, or have joint problems, jogging may be too strenuous. Jogging, with its constant pounding of feet against asphalt, is physically stressful to the bones and joints. So if you have osteoporosis or have back or knee problems, this is probably not the exercise for you.

If you decide that you would like to try jogging, start gradually; otherwise you substantially increase your risk of injury and muscle and joint discomfort. If you haven't exercised in a while, consider starting with walking. After you can comfortably walk two miles in thirty minutes, try alternating jogging with walking.

In beginning your jogging program, run at a comfortable pace, aiming at perhaps 50 percent of your target heart rate (see *Fitness Testing*, page 74). Your first time out, jog one minute and then walk for one minute, repeating each sequence twelve times for a total workout of twenty-four minutes. Your next workout, increase your jog to two minutes and walk one minute, and so forth. Each subsequent workout, increase each jogging sequence by one minute, while the walking sequence remains stable at one minute. By your tenth workout session, you may want to try jogging for twenty straight minutes. If you can do that comfortably, gradually increase your jog to thirty minutes.

As with walking and other forms of aerobic exercise, to achieve full cardiovascular benefit, plan on jogging at least three times a week on alternating days for a minimum of twenty minutes each time. Remember to begin and end your workout with stretching exercises.

BICYCLING

An estimated twenty million American adults hop on a bike in their quest for physical fitness, pedaling around town, on country roads, or even without setting foot from their home.

There is no question that bicycling—whether you opt for the stationary kind or a fancy racing model—is good aerobic exercise when done three times a week in minimum twenty-minute sessions. When done correctly, bicycling exercises the leg, thigh, and abdominal muscles. Some stationary bicycles also exercise the arm and chest muscles with handlebars that are pulled and pushed.

The key to using bicycling as an aerobic exercise is intensity. A leisurely little ride three times a week will not give you the exercise you need. In order for you to achieve full aerobic benefit, you must be pedaling your bicycle twice as fast as you would move your legs during a brisk walk. You should be able to maintain your target heart rate for the duration of your workout. Your workout should not be so intense that you cannot carry on a conversation during the exercise, but you should have to time your words to your breathing pattern. Finally, if you come to the end of your workout without having perspired, you need to challenge yourself more.

Some beginning bikers make the mistake of setting the gears in such a way that pedaling is especially hard. This is not an effective way to work the heart. From an aerobic standpoint, you'd be much better off maintaining a rapid rate of pedaling.

The calories burned during bicycling vary tremendously, according to how hard you are working. On an outdoor bicycle, a 120-pound woman may burn anywhere from 170 to 800 calories over the course of an hour; on a stationary bike the range is 85 to 800 calories.

Bicycling is an excellent weight-bearing exercise, the type recommended by health-care practitioners to help strengthen bones against the risk of osteoporosis. However, if you have heart disease, high blood pressure, diabetes, or a high cholesterol level or smoke, consult your health-care provider before you begin bicycling for exercise.

If you decide on this form of exercise, your most important decision is selecting the right bike. Some people prefer a stationary bike because they can exercise any time of day or night in any weather. The workout, however, may not be as challenging.

In selecting a road bicycle, you will have to choose among racing, mountain, and touring bikes. Racing bikes are lightweight and have narrow tires, low-slung handlebars, and typically between ten and eighteen gears. When you ride a racing bike, your upper body is parallel to the ground.

A mountain bike is sturdier, with wider tires. Designed for off-the-road riding, this bike has upright handlebars and often more gears than a racing bike. Your posture on this type of bike is more nearly erect.

Finally, the touring bike is a cross between the mountain and racing bikes, typically with ten or twelve gear settings and an upright posture.

When shopping for a bike, sit on the bike, with your foot on the pedal lower to the ground. Your leg should be not quite fully extended in this position and you should be able to reach the handlebars to brake and shift gears without taking your eyes off the road. When you straddle a racing bike with your feet on the ground, there should be one to three inches of clearance above the crossbar; a mountain or touring bike should have three to six inches of clearance.

SWIMMING

If you like the water and have access to a pool, swimming may be tailor-made for you.

Although swimmers exercise virtually every muscle in the body, there is no stress placed on the joints and bones, making this an ideal exercise for people with back or joint problems. Moreover, swimming is an excellent exercise during pregnancy. And this sport is often high on the list of activities for people with various disabilities. For all its advantages, however, swimming should not be your exercise of choice if you are at high risk for osteoporosis because this is not a so-called weight-bearing activity and as a result does not help strengthen bones.

When done correctly, swimming provides an excellent aerobic workout, helps slim you down, and tones and strengthens your muscles. If you are carrying around extra pounds, a combination of swimming and a sensible diet will help you lose that weight. A 120-pound person, for example, expends anywhere between 230 and 690 calories during an hour-long swim session.

Of course, in order to reap the physical rewards swimming can offer, you have to be serious about your workout. Those who derive aerobic benefits from this sport do not simply "play" in the pool but swim continuous laps for at least twenty minutes, three times a week. To exercise different muscles and to help prevent boredom, you can alternate strokes. For example, you might want to do a few laps of the crawl stroke, which is excellent in trimming your torso, followed by several laps of breast stroke, a stroke that uses the chest muscles.

Like any of the exercises we've discussed, swimming should be preceded and followed by stretching exercises to warm up and cool down the muscles.

WEIGHT TRAINING

Weight training used to be the domain of oiled-skinned behemoths whose muscles bulged as they affected poses designed to show off the rippled musculature that resulted from their considerable labors.

Those days, though, are long gone. Now the person pumping iron is just as likely to be your neighbor, working feverishly in a last-ditch effort to wear a bikini this summer, or your elderly aunt, who has decided she's had it with flab. Untold numbers of men and women are flocking to gyms or establishing their own home exercise rooms to lift barbells, hoist dumbbells, and work out on machines designed to resist the efforts of targeted muscle groups.

The name of the game is body sculpting, the act of chiseling body fat to expose "abs," "biceps," "quads," and "glutes." For many exercisers these days, it is not enough to be trim and relatively bulge-free. Instead, they want a defined look, a rib cage that resembles a washboard, the muscles rippling like gentle water underneath a cover devoid of fat.

For the most part, the men and women who train with weights have no illusions of becoming Arnold Schwarzenegger look-alikes. Rather, the goal is to become stronger, tone and tighten muscles, and burn body fat. Although weight training can help you do just that, one thing it will not do is give you the aerobic workout your cardiovascular system needs. So those who train with weights are encouraged to engage in an aerobic activity in addition. At some gyms, trainers often combine aerobic activity with weight training. For example, one way to combine the two might be to do a weight routine and then exercise for twenty minutes on a rowing machine or a cross-country ski machine, either of which would provide an aerobic workout. Many exercise experts also recommend weight training as a supplement for people devoted to aerobic sports. Studies have shown that bicyclists who lift weights can substantially improve their cycling performance, as can swimmers and runners.

Before you contemplate weight training, be sure you do not have physical problems that would be exacerbated by this type of activity. If you have high blood pressure, for example, lifting weights could make your pressure soar. People with heart disease or back or joint problems should consult their health-care practitioner before taking up this sport.

Once you have decided to begin weight training, you must choose the type of weights to use. Unless you have Olympic aspirations, the five-hundred-pound barbells previously associated with this sport are not a good choice. Instead, most people today use resistance training, which works on the principle of muscle overload. You exercise a targeted group of muscles to the point of exhaustion, rest, and then exercise again, gradually increasing the amount of weight.

There are several types of weights commonly used. So-called free weights are what people most often associate with body building. Dumbbells are weights held in one hand, whereas barbells require a two-handed grip. To exercise, you simply lift the weight, the direction determined by the muscles you are trying to increase. Though inexpensive, easy to use at home, and effective, these weights have been known to cause injury. To minimize your risk of injury, always exercise with a partner.

One of the most popular ways to weight-train is at a gym using machines that isolate specific muscle groups, providing resistance. Although the machines may seem intimidating, they are usually safer than free weights.

No matter where you train, make sure you use the weights properly. Never bounce the weight or bend your body during lifting, as this can cause an injury. Do not hold your breath when you lift weights.

CHAPTER 5

❧

Menopause and the Climacteric

CONTENTS

An you become older, your ovaries gradually decrease their production of estrogen. When the amount of estrogen is so low that it is no longer capable of stimulating the uterine lining to grow, your periods stop and you are said to have reached menopause. While the literal definition of menopause is the cessation of the menses, generally the word is used to describe the years between the time when estrogen production begins to fall and the time when no estrogen is produced. The medical name for these years is the *climacteric*, with the word *menopause* reserved for the actual cessation of menses.

CLIMACTERIC: THE DECLINE OF OVARIAN FUNCTION

As the amount of estrogen produced by your ovaries decreases, your body undergoes many changes, perhaps the most noticeable of which is the loss of menstruation and the ability to get pregnant. Your vaginal tissues begin to change, becoming thinner and less well lubricated. The ligaments that support your reproductive organs and bladder may lose their elasticity. A deficiency of estrogen also can cause urinary problems such as urgency, increased frequency, and even incontinence. The amount of collagen in your skin progressively diminishes, producing thinning of the skin and increased wrinkling. As we've discussed previously, you will lose bone mass and the risk of heart disease is markedly increased after menopause. Moreover, in many women the body takes on more fat and there is a gain in overall weight during this time.

For most American women today, menopause occurs during midlife. Ninety-five percent of American women reach menopause between the ages of forty-five and fifty-five, with the average age being fifty-one.

Predicting when a particular woman will reach menopause is difficult. Neither race, socioeconomic factors, education, height, weight, the age at which your first period occurs, or your age at your last pregnancy appears to be related to menopause. The only external factor that appears to influence the onset of menopause is cigarette smoking. Studies have shown that smokers on average experience menopause as much as four years earlier than do nonsmokers.

No matter what a woman's age, the time from menarche to menopause is variable. Some women—as many as one third of the female population—have no inkling that menopause is imminent. Others begin to notice changes in their periods. Perhaps your cycles will begin to get shorter or longer. Some women skip periods as they draw closer to menopause or notice a marked change in the amount of the menstrual flow.

Although an estimated 25 percent of all women have no side effects other than a gradual cessation of menstruation, most women are not quite so lucky. Fifty percent of all women have mild side effects, and for 25 percent of the population, menopause symptoms can be severe. The following are the most common symptoms of menopause, and the ways in which they are treated.

Hot Flushes. If you are going through menopause, you may find yourself awakened in the night, drenched in sweat. You throw off the covers, even though it is the dead of winter and the room is cold enough to preserve food. You feel as though you have run a marathon in the tropics. Your face is red, your heart is pounding, and try as you may, you can't get back to sleep. While the majority of hot flushes occur at night, they can also occur at other times of day, even at work.

Hot flushes are associated with a decrease in the amount of estrogen circulating in your system and last anywhere from thirty seconds to five minutes. Although as many as 75 percent of women going through menopause will have a hot flush once in a while, thin women are more likely to be bothered by them than their heavier counterparts because fat tissue produces its own estrogen. Half of the women who have hot flushes report at least one every day, while 20 percent have more than one a day.

While hot flushes are uncomfortable and bothersome and can be embarrassing when they happen to occur in the middle of an important meeting, rest assured that they cease, usually within two or three years. If you are among the one third of hot flush sufferers with symptoms severe enough to seek medical attention, your health-care provider may prescribe estrogen. Alternative drug therapies that are effective in some women are hormones called *progestins* and an antihypertension drug called clonidine (Catapres). The latter is usually prescribed as a skin patch.

Vaginal and Urinary Discomfort. During the menopause years you may notice disconcerting changes in your vagina. Because your vaginal tissues have become thinner, you may find yourself more prone to vaginal and urinary infections. Your vagina may itch or burn and the tissue may sometimes bleed. Intercourse may be painful because of a decrease in lubrication. And you may suddenly find that when you exercise or sneeze, urine leaks out (stress incontinence).

If you have these symptoms, see your health-care provider. He or she may want to prescribe estrogen, which can alleviate or even prevent these changes.

Depression. Many women during this stage of life feel depressed and anxious, easily fatigued, and sometimes irritable. Are these side effects of the hormonal changes that occur during menopause or simply a function of midlife and the life-style changes it usually brings? The answer is probably a little of both.

There is no question that midlife is a time of change for most women, often radical change. Children leave; many marriages fail. The loss of a job and the diminished prospects of finding another, poor health, the responsibility for aging parents, the push to pay for college and still save for retirement—all of these pressures can result in feelings of depression. When you add to the equation the hormonal changes that are taking place in your body during menopause, it comes as no surprise that some women have a hard time emotionally during these years.

Everyone feels sad or depressed at times. For most people, the feeling passes and in a day or two they are feeling more positive about life. Sometimes, however, the depression doesn't automatically give way to happier feelings. In some instances, the cause even may be biological, as a shortfall of a brain messenger called *serotonin* is more common in older people, a disorder termed *endogenous depression*.

Some of the symptoms of a more serious depression include generalized sad or numb feelings that prevent you from enjoying your normal activities, difficulty in sleeping, loss of appetite, irritability, crying for no reason, difficulty in making decisions, withdrawal from others, and a decreased interest in sex. If you have these symptoms, you need to see your health-care provider or seek the counsel of a mental health professional (see *Mood Disorders*, page 190).

PREMATURE AND SURGICALLY INDUCED MENOPAUSE

While the vast majority of women go through menopause spontaneously at some time during midlife, some women's ovaries either stop producing estrogen prematurely or are removed surgically before natural menopause.

If you stop menstruating spontaneously before the age of thirty-five, you have gone through premature menopause, also known as *premature ovarian failure* when it occurs at such an early age. Studies have shown that as many as 1 percent of all women stop menstruating before their fortieth birthday.

Upon examination, the ovaries of a forty-year-old woman who stops menstruating are similar to those of a postmenopausal woman. Premature menopause can occur as a result of autoimmune diseases, conditions in which the body's immune responses are directed against itself. These include diseases such as hypoparathyroidism, Hashimoto's thyroiditis, and Addison's disease (see pages 474, 470, and 474, respectively). Genetic abnormalities, chemotherapy, radiation of the ovaries, and infection also may be responsible for premature menopause.

The surgical removal of the ovaries is sometimes done during a hysterectomy, an operation to remove the uterus. Naturally, a woman whose uterus has been removed cannot get pregnant, nor does she still have periods, but if her ovaries remain intact, her body is still getting the estrogen it needs, so she won't suffer any of the other symptoms associated with premature menopause. Sometimes, however, the ovaries are also removed.

To help prevent osteoporosis and heart disease, many clinicians recommend that women with premature or early surgical menopause use hormone replacement (see *Hormone Replacement Therapy*, below).

HORMONE REPLACEMENT THERAPY

Should you or shouldn't you? If you have already entered the ranks of postmenopausal women or are likely to do so soon, no doubt you've heard of hormone replacement therapy (HRT). On one hand, there are those who tout its virtues enthusiastically. They point to studies that show that as a result of replacing nature's depleted hormones with those contained in a pill or patch, your skin will be less wrinkly, intercourse will be better, you'll be less likely to have a heart attack, and your bones will escape the crippling fractures so common among older postmenopausal women. It all sounds too good to be true—until, that is, you hear the other side of the debate, those who cite possible increased risks of breast cancer in women who take hormone replacement therapy.

Despite widespread evidence that replacing hormones after menopause clearly benefits most women, only between 10 and 15 percent of postmenopausal American women are currently having estrogen replacement. While many clinicians appear to be writing prescriptions for HRT, an estimated one quarter of women who get prescriptions never have them filled, while another quarter discontinue therapy within the first year.

Only you—with your health-care provider's guidance—can decide whether you want HRT. It is the purpose of this section to give you the facts, as we now know them, so that you can make the decision that is best for you.

What Is HRT? Simply put, HRT is an artificial way of replacing the hormones your ovaries no longer produce now that you have reached menopause. Such replacement became popular in the 1960s, only to lose much of its appeal when researchers discovered a link between estrogen replacement and cancer of the endometrial lining of the uterus. As a result, many women were afraid to use HRT.

You should know, however, that today's HRT differs markedly from that of earlier decades. For one thing, the estrogen dose has been reduced to its lowest effective level. Moreover, progestins (hormones similar to the body's natural progesterone) were added to the regimen after studies showed that this would reduce the risk of uterine cancer.

If you decide to try HRT, your health-care provider will prescribe a low-dose estrogen in combination with a progestin if you still have your uterus. If your uterus has been removed, you will take only estrogen because you don't need the endometrium-protecting properties of a progestin. If you have not undergone a hysterectomy, you also may elect, upon consultation with your clinician, to use estrogen only. This option may be particularly appropriate when progestin-related side effects, such as headache, bloating, and mood changes, occur.

There are various treatment regimens that can be prescribed. Some so-called cyclic therapies require that you take estrogen tablets fifteen days of the month, followed by estrogen and progestin for ten days. Then you stop for several days, during which time you may have vaginal bleeding for a few days, similar to a period, and a major reason why many women opt not to take HRT.

An alternative treatment approach is for your health-care provider to prescribe a continuous combination of estrogen and progestin. In such regimens, both the estrogen and progestin may be taken every day; or the estrogen may be taken daily, accompanied by progestin during the first ten to fourteen days of the month. Women who opt for this combined continuous therapy don't have the end-of-the-cycle bleeding common to those who follow a sequential therapy, but they do sometimes have some breakthrough bleeding, particularly in the first six months of therapy. After that time bleeding usually isn't a problem, but any bleeding that does occur should be reported to your health professional.

The Benefits of Hormone Replacement Therapy. A multitude of studies have shown that taking estrogen by mouth, vaginally, or as a patch, both during and after menopause, can ease some of the symptoms associated with the climacteric. Even more importantly, HRT has been demonstrated to prevent some life-threatening diseases that strike once a woman's ovaries cease production.

The following are some ways in which estrogen therapy has been shown to be of benefit:

GENITOURINARY SYSTEM. The decrease in estrogen during menopause leads to atrophy of the vagina, a painful condition with symptoms that include dryness, itching, burning, and bleeding. The vagina becomes less capable of lubricating itself, making intercourse unpleasant and even painful. To make matters worse, the tissues that provide support for your vagina, bladder, and urethra may lose their ability to hold the organs in position, causing a loss in vaginal tone and uncomfortable urinary symptoms such as incontinence, and an increase in both the urgency and frequency of urination.

We now know that these conditions can be alleviated or prevented altogether with HRT.

HOT FLUSHES. While an estimated 75 percent of all women going through menopause experience hot flushes, only about one third of them have symptoms severe enough to require medical treatment. If you are within this group, your health-care provider may prescribe estrogen, which has been shown to be effective in reducing the number of hot flushes (see page 88).

CHANGES IN THE SKIN. Upon reaching menopause, perhaps you noticed that the rate at which your wrinkles are appearing has increased. That's because once you no longer produce adequate amounts of estrogen, your skin's collagen, a protein that helps skin maintain its strength and elasticity, becomes thinner. When that happens, the wrinkles happen faster.

Studies have shown, however, that HRT reduces skin thinning. Women who use estrogen after menopause have significantly thicker skin and fewer wrinkles than those who take no medication.

ATHEROSCLEROSIS. There is little doubt that women who use estrogen replacement after menopause are less likely to have atherosclerosis, the dangerous narrowing of the blood vessels that can lead to heart attack and stroke.

Once thought to be primarily an affliction of aging men, atherosclerosis is now known to pose a very real threat to women, but only after they reach menopause. Then, however, coronary artery disease becomes the leading cause of death in this age group.

Various studies have found a 50 percent reduction in heart attacks among post-menopausal women who take HRT in comparison to those who have not. Even if a woman does have atherosclerosis, she may be able to retard its progression by taking estrogen. In a study of 345 women who underwent a diagnostic test for suspected heart disease, estrogen users were only half as likely to have severe disease as women who didn't take HRT.

Survival rates for estrogen users with heart disease also were higher: 97 percent ten years after diagnosis, compared to only 60 percent for nonusers. Estrogen use also has been found to reduce significantly the risk of death from stroke in women between the ages of seventy-five and eighty-five (see also *Cardiovascular Disease*, page 561).

OSTEOPOROSIS. As a result of the high risk in postmenopausal women of development of osteoporosis, a disease in which bone density is low, and can result in an increased likelihood of bone fractures, your health-care provider may recommend HRT.

Numerous studies have shown that HRT significantly reduces both the amount of postmenopausal bone loss and the number of fractures. In one study, for example, of young Scottish women whose ovaries had been removed, half were treated with estrogen, the other half with a placebo. Ten years later, the estrogen users' bones had no decrease in density, whereas the other group had shown a steady decline in bone mass. Some of the latter group had even lost height, indicating the presence of small fractures in the vertebrae.

For estrogen to be its most effective in the fight against osteoporosis, it may need to be taken indefinitely once you reach menopause. One group of women who took estrogen for four years and had no bone loss began losing bone mass at the same rate as the group that took a placebo once they discontinued HRT.

Estrogen is best started before you have suffered any bone loss. Once your bones have started to deteriorate, HRT will not greatly reverse the damage. However, it can halt the progression of osteoporosis in women who already have the disease (see also *Osteoporosis*, page 598).

THE RISK OF CANCER WITH HRT

In recent years many women have refused to consider hormone replacement therapy because they fear an increased risk of cancers of the breast and endometrium. By taking HRT do you indeed increase your chances of development of these malignancies?

Breast Cancer. There is disagreement among scientists as to whether estrogen will cause a cancer to grow in your breast. However, it is possible that if you already have the beginnings of a malignancy that thus far is too small to detect, it might accelerate its growth.

A plethora of studies have been published on the relationship between estrogen replacement and breast cancer, most of which have concluded that estrogen use after menopause does not significantly increase risk of development this disease. Some stud-

ies, however, have shown a slightly increased risk in women who take estrogen for fifteen years or more. Some scientists predict a breast cancer epidemic if massive numbers of baby boomers decide to use HRT.

The addition of progestin to a hormone replacement regimen does not appear to have an impact either way on your risk of breast cancer.

Endometrial Cancer. *There is no doubt that women who take high doses of estrogen over a period of several years significantly increase their chance of cancer of the endometrial lining of the uterus. Depending upon the dosage and length of therapy, the risk of disease is three to seven times that of women who do not use estrogen.*

In the early 1970s, the incidence of uterine cancer in the United States reached an all-time high when estrogen replacement therapy was introduced as a way to make women "forever feminine." Most health-care providers now know to prescribe smaller doses of estrogen, along with low doses of progestin, in order to eliminate the dangers to the uterine lining.

While no one wants to think about the possibility of development of cancer, if you are an HRT user and eventually do have cancer of the endometrium, you should know that this form of cancer is usually detected early enough to cure it by removing the uterus.

In deciding whether or not to use HRT after menopause, you must weigh the potential benefits against your own concerns about cancer. For example, if heart disease runs in your family, HRT might be of great benefit to you, whereas a woman whose mother and sister have had breast cancer might not consider the possible increased risk worth taking. Consider, too, that the lives saved by estrogen use to prevent the occurrence of osteoporosis and cardiovascular disease are estimated to be ten times *the number lost from the increase in breast cancer.*

Your health-care practitioner can help you determine what is best for your long-term health.

SEXUALITY

Sex after menopause can be better than ever. Finally, the fear of pregnancy is behind you. No more fumbling at the last minute for your diaphragm or trying to remember whether you took your pill.

All too often, though, sex after menopause may be less than satisfying. Some postmenopausal women complain that they simply have no sexual desire anymore. Others may have the desire but say that intercourse is painful. Some women—particularly those who have been recently divorced or widowed—for the first time in their life don't have a sexual partner and are finding a dearth of interesting and interested men. To complicate the picture, many men at this stage of life are having their own sexual problems. It isn't uncommon for men in this age group to suffer from chronic health problems that require daily medications, some of which can adversely affect a man's ability to become aroused or maintain an erection.

Yet those couples who successfully scale the sexual hurdles of midlife often say that making love has never been so rich or fulfilling as it is in the middle years.

If you are one of the many women who after menopause just seemed to lose interest in sex, you shouldn't simply assume this is a normal function of age. On the contrary, it is very normal for even very old women to want sex. First, take a look at your relationship. Is your partner still loving and considerate? Do you find him physically attractive? Does he want to make love? Is he interested in your sexual and emotional needs, not just his own? If the answer to these questions is yes and yet you still don't want to have sex, there may be a physical cause of your lack of libido. Disease, chronic fatigue, and some medications have been known to suppress sexual desire.

As we discussed earlier in this chapter, as the ovaries produce less and less estrogen, many physiological changes occur in the vagina, as well as in other parts of the body. Along with the thinning of vaginal tissues comes a loss of lubrication and general vaginal muscle tone. For many women, a marked decrease in the vagina's natural lubricants makes for painful intercourse. This can usually be remedied by the application of a water-soluble lubrication jelly prior to sex or by the use of a vaginal cream containing estrogen.

If you are having any sexual problems, do not hesitate to see your health-care provider. Your symptoms may warrant estrogen therapy, which has been proved effective in alleviating and even preventing postmenopausal changes in the vagina.

MALE MENOPAUSE

Women aren't the only ones whose sexual and reproductive capabilities change with age. Men, too, go through a version of menopause.

Unlike a woman, a man remains fertile well into old age. Although the production of the male hormone testosterone gradually decreases, it does not come to a halt, so a healthy man, however elderly, continues to produce sperm.

Midlife, however, is a time of sexual changes for many men. A lessening of sexual desire, an increase in the time it takes to become sexually aroused, and a decrease in the force and contents of the ejaculate are common.

Impotence can strike at any time during a man's life, but it frequently occurs during this middle period, when other emotional issues such as job dissatisfaction, health problems, marriage upsets, and a sense of mortality can shake anyone's emotional foundation. If a man is impotent once in a while, that does not mean he has a sexual problem. If a man frets over a period of poor sexual performance, he can create a cycle that becomes difficult to break. If the man in your life has a long-term impotence problem, consult a health-care provider. It may be that a medication he takes is causing the problem.

Another factor may be alcohol consumption: Men who already have some decrease in performance may treat themselves with alcohol under the mistaken impression that it will relax them and improve their function. While alcohol can contribute to sexual desire, it also can inhibit ejaculation.

NUTRITION AND EXERCISE IN MIDLIFE

In earlier years you might have been able to consume junk food and exercise sporadically. In midlife, however, sound nutrition and a regular exercise program are essential to your continued good health.

Around the age of fifty, most men and women are at their heaviest. A sedentary life-style, overeating, and excessive use of alcohol can combine with an overall slowing of your metabolism—the rate at which your body burns energy—to set the stage for obesity *and* the host of health problems that often come with it such as heart attack, high blood pressure, and diabetes.

The first step to midlife fitness may be losing weight if you are among the many Americans with some to spare. Consult the weight table on page 97 if you are in doubt about whether you need to lose weight. Or try this test: Pinch a fold of skin from your abdomen while you are standing. If you can pinch more than an inch, it's time to do more than just think about losing weight.

Eat Sensibly. Everyone—no matter his or her weight—needs a balanced diet to keep the body in good health. As a woman approaching or already through menopause, you are now more vulnerable to atherosclerosis than ever before. To help prevent fatty deposits from narrowing your blood vessels, you should reduce the amounts of fats and cholesterol you eat. A diet high in fiber will help reduce your risk of colon cancer. And an increase in foods containing calcium (or a calcium supplement) will help make you less vulnerable to osteoporosis, especially if your diet has always been rich in calcium.

The following are a few basic rules of good nutrition:

- Eat meat less often and in smaller portions. Substitute fish and poultry for red meat. Remove the skin from chicken.
- Bake or broil instead of frying. When you do fry, use polyunsaturated oils such as corn oil instead of butter or margarine.
- Reduce your salt intake.
- Increase the amount of complex carbohydrates and fiber in your diet. Try to eat five or more one-half-cup servings of fiber-rich fruits and vegetables every day, and six or more complex carbohydrates such as bread, pasta, cereals, and legumes.
- If you drink alcohol, limit yourself to one drink a day.
- Try to eat foods containing at least one thousand milligrams of calcium

each day. Many women avoid calcium-rich dairy products because they are high in fat and calories. However, you can substitute skim for whole milk and cottage cheese for the higher-calorie hard cheeses. Other calcium-rich foods include dark green vegetables, such as broccoli and spinach, and beans. However, the calcium in these foods is less accessible to your body, so you must combine them with other calcium sources. Some brands of yogurt and orange juice are also enhanced with calcium. For a more detailed discussion of dietary considerations, see *Nutrition*, page 45.

USDA SUGGESTED WEIGHTS FOR ADULTS

Height	Weight in Pounds	
	19–34 years	>35 years
5'0"	97–128	108–138
5'1"	101–132	111–143
5'2"	104–137	115–148
5'3"	107–141	119–152
5'4"	111–146	122–157
5'5"	114–150	126–162
5'6"	118–155	130–167
5'7"	121–160	134–172
5'8"	125–164	138–178
5'9"	129–169	142–183
5'10"	132–174	146–188
5'11"	136–179	151–194
6'0"	140–184	155–199

Get Some Exercise. Of course, eating a healthy diet will not result in true fitness if you never do anything more strenuous than punch buttons on the television remote control.

Your body was designed for use. Your heart was meant to beat strong and hard, pushing blood throughout your body. Your muscles, bones, and joints were meant for movement.

No one can stop the aging process. But you can minimize the effects of aging by combining a healthy diet with an exercise program. A good aerobic workout for at least twenty minutes three times a week will increase your heart's capacity to pump blood, perhaps even slowing or preventing the progression of atherosclerosis. Joints that are exercised regularly remain supple and healthy, and muscles stay strong, toned, and defined. Women who exercise regularly prior to menopause have a better chance of avoiding osteoporosis than their less physically fit counterparts.

What kind of exercise is best for you? It is important to find an exercise activity you enjoy doing and can do conveniently. For example, if you live in a cold climate and the nearest indoor swimming pool is an hour away, an exercise program that revolves around swimming probably won't work for you. Brisk walking, lap swimming, cross-country skiing, bicycling, aerobics, and jogging are a few of the ways in which countless American women stay fit. Weight-bearing exercises such as walking, riding a stationary bicycle, or working out on a rowing machine may be your best bet if you have or are at high risk for osteoporosis. For exercise programs and other advice on physical activity, see *Exercise*, page 72.

Be sure to consult your health-care provider before you embark on an exercise program—especially if you have been sedentary, are a heavy smoker, have health problems, and/or are overweight.

Part II

❧

SPECIAL
HEALTH CONCERNS

The pages that follow will address a variety of issues of particular importance to many, though not all, women. These include birth control, substance abuse, mental health matters, violence in the home, abortion, cosmetic surgery, and occupational and environmental concerns.

The guidance in these pages is less specific than in Part I. Here, the emphasis is on discussion, though, where possible, the topics are viewed in a prescriptive way. More often, rather than concrete solutions and options, the various perspectives and viewpoints are presented in an even-handed fashion. These chapters are designed to help you learn about issues of concern so that you can shape your own opinions and make your own choices.

CHAPTER 6

Birth Control

CONTENTS

Consider this: A healthy and fertile woman who begins having unprotected sexual intercourse at the age of seventeen and who continues the practice throughout her childbearing years can expect to bear thirteen children. Needless to say, the prospect of delivering and rearing thirteen children would be daunting to most women, even those wanting a large family. But thanks to the advent of contraceptive devices, couples don't have to sacrifice their sex life to prevent pregnancy. Today's wide range of effective birth control options gives a woman and her partner the ability to determine whether they will become parents, how many children they will bear, and when.

This isn't to say that our current contraceptive methods are perfect. Odds are you have at least one friend who had an unplanned pregnancy, despite every precaution. Or perhaps you can count yourself among those whose family planning efforts went awry. Still, though any birth control method has a margin of error, women who use contraception seize a large degree of control over their reproductive life—a relatively new concept and one that would amaze our ancestors (and even some modern-day cultures).

The harshness of life in ancient times meant that most children didn't live to adulthood, making it vital that a couple have more offspring than they wanted simply to ensure that one or two would live to support them in their old age. Yet some four millennia ago women were apparently trying to gain some control over their body, as is evidenced in the Babylonian Code of Hammurabi, which, to discourage abortion, imposed death by crucifixion as its penalty. Three hundred years later, Genesis, the first book of the Old Testament, carried many references to coitus interruptus, apparently a widespread contraceptive practice among the early Hebrews. And, in A.D. 130, Soranus, a gynecologist, discussed the merits of contraception versus abortion as a means of limiting family size, concluding it was safer to prevent conception than to destroy its results.

And so the quest to prevent pregnancy began.

Following the advice of the Talmud fifteen hundred years ago, couples drank a brew of roots to reduce their fecundity, while Native Americans sipped a specially concocted tea. Sixteenth-century Arabs seeking to prevent their camel herds from growing in size may have been the most ingenious in their contraceptive efforts, fitting their beasts with stones—crude versions of our modern-day intrauterine devices (IUDs).

Some methods of preventing pregnancy that can only be termed bizarre continue even today. The women of an isolated Russian enclave practice a contraceptive ritual in which a young girl puts a few drops of her menstrual blood into a hole in a hen's egg, which she then buries for nine days and nights; when the egg is dug up, the number of worms inside represents the number of children she will bear. If she wishes to have them, she throws the egg into water; if she chooses not to have them, she hurls the egg into fire, thereby destroying her ability to bear children. A tribe in New Guinea believes the power to induce sterility can be passed from mother to daughter. To render a young woman sterile, an older woman in control of the power sits behind her while uttering incantations and making passes over her abdomen, at the same time burning roots and herbs for the young woman to inhale.

Neither method has been proved workable.

While it may not surprise you that our ancient ancestors didn't have foolproof means to prevent pregnancy, what hits closer to home is that until 1936 women in this country weren't much better off when it came to family planning. In fact, it was illegal in the United States to use or dispense birth control devices. This changed through the tireless efforts of Margaret Sanger, a nurse who saw firsthand the effects of unwanted pregnancy on the poor immigrant women she nursed in the slums of Lower Manhattan. Appalled, she opened the first birth control clinic in the United States in 1916—for which she was sent to prison. After organizing the first World Population Conference in Geneva in 1927, Sanger helped obtain passage of laws allowing doctors to dispense contraceptive devices to their patients.

Today, the use of some form of contraception is the rule rather than the exception. Data from a recent National Survey of Family Growth showed that all but 3.8 percent of women at risk for pregnancy (those who were sexually active, had not had a hysterectomy, and were not infertile, pregnant, or trying to conceive) used some form of birth control. Married women were twice as likely as single women to use a contraceptive device.

If you're considering using a contraceptive method, this chapter gives you a look at all the options, to help you decide which one may be best for you.

Three methods rely mainly on the male's compliance. A *condom* is a rubber sheath that the man places over his erect penis before intercourse. When used correctly and with a spermicide, the condom is fairly effective in preventing pregnancy. It will also help protect both partners from acquired immunodeficiency syndrome (AIDS) and other sexually transmitted diseases (STDs). *Coitus interruptus* is the age-old practice in which the man withdraws his penis before he ejaculates, but is not only frustrating for both partners, but ineffective in preventing pregnancy. *Vasectomy*, male sterilization, is highly effective but should not be undertaken unless a man is sure he doesn't want to father any more children because it isn't reversible in all instances.

The remaining methods of contraception depend primarily on the woman. *Natural family planning* (a.k.a. *periodic abstinence*) involves closely monitoring the menstrual cycle and abstaining from intercourse during the days when ovulation—and therefore pregnancy—is most likely to occur. Its success depends on the predictability of your ovulation, accuracy of your assessments, and diligence of your efforts to avoid intercourse on the most-fertile days. An *intrauterine device* (IUD) is a specially designed piece of plastic that a doctor inserts into your uterus and that prevents pregnancy by making it difficult for a fertilized egg to implant in the uterine lining. So-called barrier methods such as the *diaphragm* and *cervical cap* are under a woman's control, as are the *spermicidal creams and jellies* used in conjunction with these methods. A relatively new form of birth control developed in 1985, *injectable steroids*, is currently being used by millions of women. *Contraceptive implants* are highly effective (they involve the insertion of capsules containing small amounts of synthetic progestin hormone just under the skin of the upper arm). Of all the nonpermanent methods of birth control, *oral contraceptives* are still the most popular. Introduced in 1960, "the pill" is often credited with helping to change our society's sexual mores by taking much of the worry out of sex. The final method of birth control that we will examine in this chapter is *female sterilization*. Like a vasectomy, a tubal ligation should be viewed as permanent, even though it's sometimes possible to reverse the procedure.

Which method is right for you? The best contraceptive is the one that fits your lifestyle. If, for example, any loss of sexual spontaneity would greatly diminish your enjoyment of sex, a diaphragm or a condom probably isn't a good choice. On the other hand, if you don't have intercourse on a regular basis, a diaphragm may be preferable to taking the pill every day or having an IUD inserted.

Remember, too, that fertility declines as we age. An estimated 7 percent of women between the ages of twenty and twenty-four are infertile. That number increases to almost 15 percent in the early thirties, and by the time a women enters her forties, almost 30 percent of her peers are unable to conceive. In terms of choosing a contraceptive device, this means that the same high level of birth control you used in your twenties may not be necessary later in life, although you still must use some form of contraception if you want to prevent pregnancy.

In this chapter, we'll explore in detail your contraceptive options and the pros and cons of the various methods.

NATURAL FAMILY PLANNING

Perhaps because of a wish to avoid any of the adverse side effects that can result from use of chemical or mechanical birth control methods or perhaps because of religious restrictions, a relatively small percentage of couples prefer to rely on "natural family planning" (periodic abstinence) as their means of birth control. This depends on a woman's ability to judge the fertile and infertile days of her cycle and to refrain from sexual intercourse on those days when pregnancy is most likely to occur.

There are four main methods of periodic abstinence:

1. Calendar Rhythm Method. The calender rhythm method, the oldest of the natural family planning methods, requires figuring out your ovulation days, on the basis of observations over several months, and abstaining from intercourse on those days when fertilization could occur.

This method relies on the following assumptions: (1) The female egg can only be fertilized for about forty-eight hours after it enters the fallopian tube; (2) sperm remain capable of fertilization for only seventy-two hours after intercourse; (3) ovulation generally occurs fourteen to sixteen days prior to the start of the next period. However, in young women ovulation may occur much closer to menses, so instead of ovulation's occurring fourteen days before menstruation, ten days might be more accurate.

Once you have recorded the length of several menstrual cycles, you can establish your fertile period by subtracting eighteen days from the longest cycle and eleven from the shortest. Having determined that, you and your partner must not have sex during the days when your egg could be fertilized—which means that couples who practice this method must abstain for about one third of the days of every menstrual cycle.

This method will obviously work less well if your periods are irregular, but even in women who menstruate regularly, pregnancy rates range from 14 to 47 percent. This high pregnancy rate is attributed in part to the fact that many couples end up having unprotected intercourse on fertile days.

Few health-care practitioners recommend this method, which is no longer considered effective by itself.

2. Temperature Method. Most women have a slight rise in body temperature just after ovulation, and it remains elevated until just prior to menstruation, when it drops. If you opt for this method of natural family planning, which is also referred to as the *basal body temperature method*, you must take your basal body temperature every day, first thing in the morning, using a special ovulation thermometer. A sustained temperature rise for at least three consecutive days means that ovulation has taken place and it is "safe" to resume intercourse. Note, though, that the temperature method is not an aid in calculating "safe" days *before* ovulation. Because intercourse should take place only after the sustained elevation in temperature, this can mean abstinence for more than half of a standard twenty-eight-day cycle.

This method, too, usually isn't used alone to prevent pregnancy.

3. Vaginal Secretion Method. Perhaps you've noticed that a few days before you ovulate, your vaginal secretion becomes thin and profuse. With this method, which is sometimes referred to as the Billings method, you gauge your ovulation by feeling the changes in the amount and consistency of your vaginal secretion. Immediately after menstruation there is no noticeable discharge, and your vagina feels relatively dry. As ovulation approaches, the secretions become thin, elastic, and slippery, similar in consistency to raw egg whites, and can be stretched between two fingers. A woman using this method must not have intercourse from the onset of this sign until four days after her secretion has peaked and this slippery mucus dries up again. Intercourse can then be resumed until the next menstrual period. For most women, this method would require about seventeen days a month of abstinence.

The efficacy of this method is poor. Studies of couples who have used it after three to five months of training found pregnancy rates of 20 to 24 percent. As many as 75 percent of practitioners discontinued the method during the first year, with fewer than 10 percent continuing after one year.

4. Symptothermal Method. The symptothermal method combines the temperature and vaginal secretion methods with the calendar rhythm method to determine peak fertility days. More effective than any one natural family planning method, it's also more difficult to learn: A woman figures out her first fertile "unsafe" day with the calendar method, then confirms her calculation by monitoring her vaginal secretions. At the same time, she takes her basal body temperature to determine the beginning of her "safe" days after ovulation.

One study found that couples who conscientiously used the symptothermal method had pregnancy rates of roughly 11 to 20 percent.

Hormonal Tests. A primary problem with natural family planning is the lengthy period when couples must not have intercourse during each cycle. Several tests that detect hormonal changes have been developed recently and may make complying with natural family planning easier in the near future. These self-administered tests may perhaps be used to reduce significantly the number of days a couple who practice natural contraception must abstain during each cycle, from as many as seventeen to as few as seven. These hormonal tests are still being studied since their effectiveness has not yet been established.

Natural family planning has become one of the least popular contraceptive methods mainly because people don't want restrictions placed on when they can make love—and those who succumb to an urge to do so often find themselves expecting an unplanned child. Some couples practicing this method overcome the frustration of too many unsafe days by using a barrier contraceptive—a diaphragm or a condom—during times when intercourse is desired during highly fertile days in the cycle. This combination of natural family planning and barrier contraception constitutes *fertility awareness methods* (FAMs). Studies have shown that women using the symptothermal method plus a barrier method during the fertile period reduce their chance of becoming pregnant to about 10 percent.

INTRAUTERINE DEVICES

It has been more than twenty-five years since the first intrauterine devices (IUDs) were introduced into the marketplace after doctors found that placing such a foreign body into the uterus created an inflammatory reaction in the uterine lining, thereby inhibiting the implantation and growth of a fertilized egg. Clinical studies also suggest that the devices interfere with sperm transport and fertilization or may affect the number and viability of sperm.

However it works, an IUD—a small piece of flexible plastic, usually covered with copper, inserted into the uterus—not only is a highly effective way to prevent pregnancy, but also has the highest continuation rate (that is, when used for extended periods) of all reversible methods of contraception.

Several features make the IUD an attractive birth-control method. First, its pregnancy rate is low—between 1 and 3 percent, depending on the type of IUD used. Also, unlike methods such as the pill or diaphragm that require patient compliance, once her IUD is inserted, a woman can basically forget about it for years. Unlike the pill, injections, or implants, this method of contraception produces no systemic effects.

This isn't to say that the IUD is perfect. It must be inserted by a health professional, a procedure that is often uncomfortable. More importantly, some women—about 15 percent in the first year of use—have problems, mainly increased menstrual pain, backaches, and bleeding between periods. Heavier or prolonged periods, even after years of IUD use, are common. IUD users are more likely than other women to have serious complications such as pelvic inflammatory disease (see page 449) or perforation of the uterus.

In fact, though the risk of such serious side effects is low, many American health-care providers no longer recommend IUDs, especially for women who haven't completed their family, unless a woman has already been using one and has had no problems with it. Moreover, many former manufacturers of these devices discontinued production because a proliferation of lawsuits against them made it too expensive to continue (in the case of only one IUD, however, the Dalkon Shield, was the manufacturer found liable). At this time, only a Copper T 380A and a progesterone-releasing IUD are available in this country, though others are marketed in other parts of the world.

In the early years of the IUD, concerns that the devices would increase the incidence of pelvic inflammatory disease (PID)—a sexually transmitted disease that can cause sterility—appeared ill founded. But with the introduction of the Dalkon Shield years later, a high incidence of young single women who had never had children experienced severe infections while using this type of IUD. Today, though the connection is not well understood, the incidence of PID among wearers is about 1 percent for the two IUDs now being sold in the United States, with most infections occurring within four months of insertion.

In considering whether an IUD should be your contraceptive choice, you should know that most American clinicians don't recommend IUDs for women who might want to have more children and, because of the increased risk of pelvic infection, recommend against their use by women with multiple sex partners. They also aren't recommended for anyone who has had unexplained abnormal vaginal bleeding, a recent history of pelvic infection, a history of tubal pregnancy, a recent abnormal Papanicolaou (Pap) smear result, or a lowered immune response caused by diseases such as leukemia or human immunodeficiency virus (HIV), or for someone with an artificial heart valve (because of the risk of infection). A good candidate for an IUD might be a woman wanting no more children yet not wanting to be permanently sterilized and in a monogamous sexual relationship.

If you decide to have an IUD, you'll need to consult your health-care professional.

An IUD can be inserted safely at any time in the menstrual cycle, but it's usually done during menstruation. To insert the device, your clinician will use a speculum to expose your cervix. An instrument shaped like a large drinking straw is loaded with the IUD and threaded through the cervical canal into the uterine cavity, where the IUD is deposited. A small string hangs down from the IUD into the vagina; it will not interfere with intercourse, but does make it easy for a professional to remove the device and allows you to check whether it's still in place. The most commonly used IUD needs to be removed and a new one reinserted every ten years.

Expect some cramping both during the insertion and for a brief period afterward. Be aware that during the first year about 10 percent of IUDs are expelled and another 15 percent are removed, mainly as the result of heavy bleeding and pain. As an IUD wearer, you may find your periods unusually heavy and lasting longer than usual. Since heavy blood loss can lead to severe iron deficiency, you should have a periodic blood test for anemia. If your bleeding is severe and doesn't abate within a few months after insertion, your IUD may have to be removed.

Rarely, the IUD may puncture the wall of the uterus, a problem usually associated with faulty insertion, and surgery may be required to remove the device. The incidence of uterine perforation ranges from about one in six hundred to one in one thousand insertions.

What if you should become pregnant while wearing an IUD? While it's a very effective birth control method, between 1 and 3 percent of IUD wearers do become pregnant. There is no evidence that a fetus conceived in spite of an IUD has a higher incidence of congenital abnormalities, but the IUD should be removed immediately if pregnancy occurs. Removal reduces chances of miscarriage, although in some cases it may trigger miscarriage. However, when removal can't be performed, a woman is three times more likely to have a miscarriage than she would be without an IUD in place. Further, in the rare case when an IUD fails, there is a chance the pregnancy will be ectopic (tubal)—that is, the egg will be implanted in the fallopian tube.

If you wish to get pregnant, and assuming you haven't had an untreated pelvic infection while using an IUD, once the device is removed, your fertility returns immediately. Because of the slight risk of infection from an IUD, many doctors suggest that women who want to maintain their childbearing capabilities use a different contraceptive method.

FEMALE BARRIER METHODS

Barrier methods of contraception help prevent pregnancy by blocking the merging of egg and sperm. Some methods, like the condom, accomplish this by putting up a physical barrier. Others are chemical barriers in the form of creams, jellies, foams, or suppositories. The effectiveness of barrier methods is enhanced when physical and chemical barriers are used simultaneously, as with the diaphragm. Note, however, that none of the female barrier methods of contraception provides significant protection against acquired immunodeficiency syndrome (AIDS) or other sexually transmitted diseases (see *What Is Safe Sex?*, page 442).

Failure rates with these methods range considerably. For example, some studies have shown that diaphragm users in their thirties have only a 1.1 percent pregnancy rate when they use the device correctly and consistently, and other studies found failure rates as high as 21 percent among first-year diaphragm users. It appears that the most important factors relating to these methods' effectiveness as birth control devices are proper use of the device or product, a good fit, and assurance that the diaphragm, cervical cap, or condom—male or female—isn't damaged or worn.

Barrier techniques are most effective in women over the age of thirty, with failure rates highest among women under twenty-five. Perhaps older women fare better with these forms of birth control because they've already completed their family and are more highly motivated to avoid pregnancy than their younger counterparts. Moreover, fertility decreases with age.

Barrier methods also have been shown to reduce the rate of some sexually transmitted diseases.

Diaphragm. A diaphragm is a dome-shaped soft rubber cap about three inches in diameter with a flexible rim that you slip into your vagina to cover the cervix; it stays in place by means of spring tension. Developed more than one hundred years ago, the diaphragm is the most effective barrier method for women, with a success rate of 98.5 percent when used properly and consistently. If you decide to use a diaphragm, you'll need to see your healthcare provider to be fitted; fit is crucial to preventing the device from being dislodged during intercourse. During a pelvic examination, your practitioner will fit you with the largest size that's comfortable. If you gain or lose ten or more pounds, have abdominal or pelvic surgery, or become pregnant, the diaphragm needs to be refitted.

A diaphragm must be used with a spermicidal cream or jelly placed along the rim and inside the center of the device. If you insert your diaphragm more than four hours prior to intercourse, another application of spermicide will be necessary. After intercourse, the device should be left in place at least six hours. If you make love again during that time, insert more spermicide but don't remove the diaphragm. When properly fitted, the

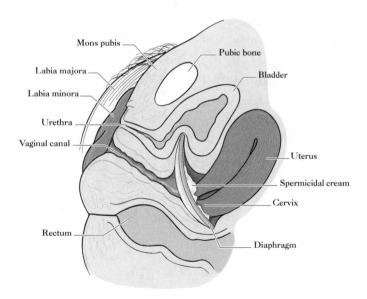

When properly positioned, a vaginal diaphragm rests at the top of the vaginal canal, holding the spermicide against the cervix.

diaphragm should be completely comfortable, with neither partner aware of its presence, and it won't interfere with a woman's coital sensations.

To prevent the risk of damage to vaginal tissues, never wear your diaphragm for more than twenty-four hours at a time. Wash the device with mild soap and water, and inspect it periodically for pinholes, cracks, or thinning, indicators that you need a new one. Never use Vaseline or other petroleum-based products since they tend to damage the rubber.

The downside of using a diaphragm is an increased risk of bladder or urinary tract infection, possibly caused by the slight pressure the diaphragm exerts against the bladder, which may obstruct the flow of urine. On the other hand, studies have shown that diaphragm use helps protect the cervix from being infected with gonorrhea and human papillomavirus (HPV). The only other physical problem associated with a diaphragm is the rare instance of an allergic reaction to the spermicide or the latex.

To maximize sexual spontaneity while using this method, perhaps the most satisfactory tactic is to insert the diaphragm routinely every night (with spermicide, of course) before going to bed, remove it and clean it the next morning, and reinsert it the following evening. That way it's always in place, and its use is separated from the sex act, enhancing the aesthetic aspects of this form of birth control.

Medically speaking, the diaphragm remains the most acceptable form of contraception from the standpoint of absence of complications and rate of effectiveness.

Cervical Cap. Although the cervical cap has been used for decades in Europe, it was only approved in this country in 1988. Unlike the much larger diaphragm, this soft rubber (or sometimes hard plastic) thimble-shaped device fits deeper into the vagina directly over the cervix; it remains in place by suction. Cervical caps are often used by women who can't use diaphragms because of anatomical disorders (such as a prolapsed uterus), and because it covers only the cervix, it doesn't require refitting if pelvic muscle tone changes as a result of weight loss, aging, or childbirth. Like the diaphragm, the cervical cap is used with a spermicide. Many women find it more comfortable than a diaphragm; also, it can be left in place longer—up to forty-eight hours—and using additional spermicide for each sexual act isn't necessary, a feature that can add to spontaneity.

Proper fitting is critical and must be done by your health-care professional. The degree of suction depends on how good the fit is; inadequate suction may allow the cap to slip off, resulting in pregnancy. Also, since a cervical cap needs to go onto the cervix and not just into the vaginal canal, some women may find it more difficult than a diaphragm to insert and there may be a tendency to leave the device in place longer than the recommended forty-eight hours. Women with very short fingers may have difficulty inserting or removing a cervical cap.

There is some concern about the possibility that the cervical cap may adversely affect cervical tissue. Many clinicians recommend that any woman using this method of birth control have a Pap smear three months after being fitted, and if you've had an abnormal Pap

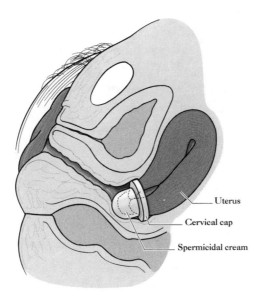

The thimble-shaped cervical cap fits directly over the cervix, acting both as a barrier to sperm and to contain the spermicide.

smear finding, your health-care provider may advise against this method. Also, the cap has caused some degree of irritation and abrasion of the cervix. Unlike the diaphragm, the cervical cap won't cause bladder infections.

The cervical cap's effectiveness in preventing pregnancy is virtually the same as that of the diaphragm: 98.5 percent. Its disadvantage is that some women complain of odor within a day or so of insertion, and because of a tendency to leave the cap in place for longer than is recommended, a malodorous secretion may collect inside. If you find this to be the case, the cap should be removed and washed, then filled with fresh spermicide.

Over-the-Counter Spermicides. The over-the-counter spermicides—in the form of cream, vaginal foam, jelly, film, and vaginal suppositories—contain a substance (generally nonoxynol-9) that kills or immobilizes sperm. About ten minutes prior to intercourse, you insert these spermicides into your upper vagina. These methods aren't effective for more than an hour after insertion, and additional spermicide should be inserted if you have repeated sex. Do not douche for six to eight hours after lovemaking.

One of the newest forms of spermicide is vaginal contraceptive film (VCF), a small square of material only slightly thicker than plastic wrap that, after being inserted with the finger high in the vagina, dissolves quickly into a gel that immobilizes sperm. Its effectiveness is the same as that of other spermicides, it's very inconspicuous to carry and use, and only minor vaginal irritation has been reported.

A spermicide alone is not the most foolproof way to avoid pregnancy. Failure rates vary from about 10 to 18 percent and are considerably higher—up to 40 percent—in those who don't use the products correctly, though spermicides seem to be more effective in older age groups. But if your partner wears a condom, a spermicide may be an excellent contraceptive choice for you. In fact, according to Planned Parenthood, VCF and condom used together have virtually the same effectiveness rate as the pill: 98 to 99 percent. Moreover, studies have shown that these preparations decrease your risk of being infected with gonorrhea by 50 percent, and proper condom use is regarded as a safeguard against HIV infections as well (see *What Is Safe Sex?*, page 442).

Disadvantages depend on the specific method. The spermicides in the foams, jellies, creams, suppositories, and film may irritate the penis or vagina, although switching brands may solve this problem. Some women experience a sensation of "heat" when the suppository is foaming, and allergic reactions to some products have been reported.

ZANDRA'S DILEMMA

It seemed to Zandra that her diaphragm—the method of contraception she had chosen several years earlier and had been using with satisfaction and without any problems whatsoever—had suddenly turned against her and was now her mortal enemy.

Every time she tried to insert the new diaphragm her health-care provider had given her, she felt as if she were in a slapstick comedy—or that, without warning, she had grown thumbs where her fingers used to be. Instead of ending with her diaphragm properly inserted, the process seemed usually to conclude with her fingers smeared with contraceptive jelly. The final straw for her was one particularly memorable occasion when she had the diaphragm folded in half and was attempting to insert it into her vagina when the spring in the rim popped back open and the diaphragm flew out of her hand and stuck to the tiled bathroom wall. Zandra washed it off, put it back in its plastic case, and didn't have sex with her partner that night.

The next day she made an appointment to see her gynecologist. When she finally saw the physician, she whipped the diaphragm out of its case and held it up for inspection. "I don't know what's going on," she told her doctor. "I've been using a diaphragm for years and never had any trouble before. Now I feel completely inept. But this one doesn't behave at all like my old one. It doesn't fold the way the old one did. I can't control it at all. Is it me or it?"

It turned out that the diaphragm had a different rim spring, which gave it a different action. It was a learning experience for Zandra, and she raised her gynecologist's consciousness, too. The doctor promptly wrote a prescription for the old brand of diaphragm, and Zandra was once again a satisfied diaphragm user.

CONDOMS

Condoms have long been used by couples to prevent pregnancy. These days, however, these thin latex rubber sheaths, which are worn over the penis to entrap semen, are just as likely to be used to help prevent sexually transmitted diseases such as AIDS, genital herpes, gonorrhea, and hepatitis B.

An estimated 10 to 15 percent of couples use condoms. Probably one reason for their popularity is their ready availability, without a prescription, in any drug store and even in vending machines. Condoms are made of various materials, although those of latex rubber offer protection against sexually transmitted viruses, whereas those made of animal skin don't. Some are lubricated; others are not. They are available in various colors and textures. You can buy single condoms or packages of large quantities. Just be aware that the shelf life of packaged condoms is two years. And don't use a condom that's been sitting in a wallet getting nice and warm for any length of time; heat breaks down the latex, causing it to tear.

To be effective, the condom must be placed on a man's erect penis before it enters the vagina. Using a condom with a receptacle tip (for the ejaculate), your partner—or you, if you want to make this part of your foreplay—should place the rolled condom on the end of the erect penis, leaving a half inch of space at the tip. If your partner is uncircumcised, he should pull back his foreskin before putting on the condom. The tip of the condom should be squeezed as it is rolled on so that no air is trapped in the end; this will prevent it from bursting when ejaculation occurs and leave room for the ejaculate. Roll the condom down over the penis, smoothing out any air bubbles. If you use a lubricant, use only water-based ones like K-Y Jelly (or saliva) or a spermicide. Don't use oil-based lubricants like mineral or vegetable oils or petroleum jellies (Vaseline), which cause the latex to deteriorate. After your partner climaxes and before his penis becomes flaccid, he must withdraw from your vagina while holding the rim of the condom against his penis. This should prevent the condom from slipping and spilling semen into the vagina. The used condom is then discarded.

Most condom failures are the result of rupture or leakage around the base. Leaving room at the tip and lubricating the condom can help reduce this risk.

How effective are condoms? One large study on condom use found a 3.6 percent failure rate during the first year of condom use—but the longer a couple used condoms, the higher the rate; at two years the pregnancy rate was between 8.4 and 10 percent. Using a spermicide in conjunction with the condom reduces the risk of failure. Like those of other barrier methods, condom failure rates are lowest in women over thirty.

Aside from the chance of pregnancy, there are no ill effects associated with condoms and, particularly for women who have multiple partners, latex condom use is the best protection against sexually transmitted diseases. The main complaint is that condoms dull sexual sensation for the man and interrupt spontaneity.

THE FEMALE CONDOM

The newest contraceptive is the female condom—also known as the vaginal pouch *and marketed under the name Reality—a polyurethane sheath that lines the vagina during intercourse. Approved for use by the U.S. Food and Drug Administration, these condoms are available over the counter in drugstores and discount outlets.*

The female condom consists of a soft, loose-fitting polyurethane sheath with flexible rings at each end. The pouch is inserted deep into the vagina like a diaphragm. The ring at the closed end of this prelubricated condom serves as an insertion mechanism

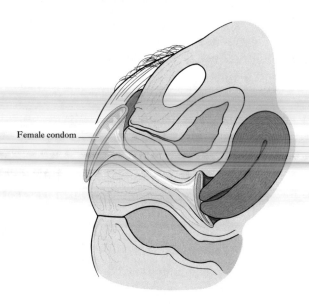

Female condom

The sheathlike female condom, made of polyurethane, is inserted into the vagina to surround the male penis during intercourse and contain the ejaculation.

and holds the pouch inside the vagina, while the outer ring hangs about an inch outside the vagina, resting between the woman's labia and the base of the man's penis during intercourse. Unlike a male condom, the female condom can be inserted prior to sexual activity.

As for its effectiveness, studies have shown a pregnancy rate of between 21 and 26 percent, although its manufacturer claims that when properly used, the female condom is even more effective in preventing pregnancy. Preliminary studies have shown that the condom is effective against the transmission of sexually transmitted diseases, but more research is necessary to confirm these findings.

A common complaint among men who have had intercourse with women using the female condom is that it interferes with sensation. However, women who have used it report that sensation during the sex act is similar to that of unprotected intercourse. The main complaint among both men and women is the unnatural presence of the anchoring ring hanging outside the labia.

Who is expected to use the female condom? Its manufacturer predicts women who want to exert more control over their sexual activity will be interested in trying this product, as well as women who are allergic to latex but want to use a barrier device or those who have been on the pill but now want to try different barrier methods.

As with diaphragms and cervical caps, women who aren't comfortable about touching their genitals probably won't like using the female condom.

IMPLANTS

Hormonal implants that prevent pregnancy have been used by more than 500,000 women worldwide. But it wasn't until 1991 that the U.S. Food and Drug Administration approved the product known as Norplant for use in this country.

This method, consisting of six match-shaped flexible capsules that release a small amount of a synthetic progestin hormone over five years, is one of the most effective methods of reversible contraception. Studies have shown that the annual pregnancy rate in the first year of use is only about 0.2 percent and is comparable with that of sterilization.

The implants prevent pregnancy by suppressing ovulation and by acting on the cervical mucus to make it thick and impenetrable to sperm. They also cause thinning of the lining of the uterus, preventing attachment of a fertilized egg.

The Norplant capsules are inserted just under the skin on the inner surface of your upper arm in a simple outpatient procedure performed by your gynecologist. After using a local anesthetic to numb the area, your doctor will make a small incision (about one eighth inch long) in which to insert the implants. If at any time you decide you want them removed, another small incision is made by which to do so. If after five years you still don't want to get pregnant and want to remain on Norplant, the implants must be replaced.

The potential side effects of Norplant are irregular periods, irregular bleeding between periods, cessation of periods (amenorrhea), and heavy, prolonged menstrual bleeding, all the consequence of the hormones in the preparations. About half the women using Norplant have bleeding about every twenty-one to thirty-five days; an estimated 40 percent have irregular bleeding, although in most cases the blood loss is minimal; and 10 percent don't bleed for three or more months at a time. Bleeding usually becomes more regular after nine to twelve months, although a small number of women experience irregular bleeding throughout the five years. Also, some Norplant users have had difficulty in having the implants removed, and it isn't yet known how often difficult removal can be expected to occur. Like those using the IUD, a sizable percentage of women who use Norplant continue with this method for several years—perhaps because to discontinue their use, the implants have to be removed in a procedure much like the one done to insert them. According to a study done between 1991 and 1993 by the *Journal of Family Practice*, 63 percent of patients surveyed would use Norplant again and 74 percent would recommend the method to a friend.

Other possible side effects include infection, irritation around the area of the implant, headaches—30 percent of implants are removed for this reason—nervousness, nausea, dizziness, weight gain or loss, change in appetite, acne, dermatitis, breast tenderness, increased facial or body hair, hair loss, and mood changes. Other conditions that have been reported are breast discharge, cervicitis, muscle and skeletal pain, abdominal discomfort, vaginal discharge, and vaginitis.

The package labeling says that a woman who has had breast cancer should not use Norplant, nor should anyone with blood clots, unexplained vaginal bleeding, or serious liver disease. However, information on whether Norplant increases complications in women with such medical conditions is scarce. Norplant works much as the birth control pill does but contains no estrogen. Since smoking while using the pill greatly increases the risk of blood clots, heart attack, and stroke in women over thirty-five, and since it isn't known yet whether this happens with Norplant, women using it are advised to stop smoking.

Will Norplant affect your future fertility? In a word, no. If you decide the time is right to have a child, simply have your implants removed. You should begin ovulating shortly afterward.

INJECTABLES

Long-acting injectable steroids are extremely effective at preventing pregnancy. They work by inhibiting ovulation and by thickening the cervical mucus, making it a hostile environment for sperm. Millions of women around the world have three injectable formulations available to them, but only one has been approved for birth control in the United States by the Food and Drug Administration.

The injectable contraceptives currently available are depo-medroxyprogesterone acetate, or DMPA (the formulation available in the United States); norethindrone enanthate (NET-EN); and various progestin–estrogen combinations.

DMPA. The injectable DMPA, the most widely used, is the contraceptive of choice for millions of women worldwide. In this country, DMPA has been approved by the FDA for the treatment of endometrial cancer as well as for contraception. Manufactured by Pharmacia Upjohn, DMPA's trade name is Depo-Provera. It is administered in an intramuscular injection; the shots are required at regular three-month intervals.

The pregnancy rate among DMPA users is very low, with studies showing a rate from 0.0 percent to 1.2 percent, lower than that of the birth control pill and on a par with the rate for sterilization or Norplant. Injected every three months, DMPA prevents pregnancy by suppressing ovulation and altering the cervical mucus. Even after you stop using DMPA, it

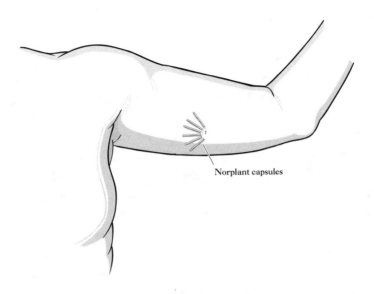

Norplant capsules

Norplant capsules are inserted beneath the skin through a small incision. The tiny "sticks" of the Norplant are virtually invisible.

may take months to resume normal menstruation. An estimated 50 percent of DMPA users begin to have periods (although not always regularly) within six months after discontinuing the injections; 75 percent have regular menstruation by the end of the first year. Although DMPA does not cause sterility, it can take an average of ten months for a woman to get pregnant after discontinuing the drug.

Most women adjust to DMPA with few or no problems, but as with all medicines, some women may experience some side effects. The major side effect experienced by DMPA users is the disruption of the menstrual cycle. These changes are variable from one woman to another. After the first injection, about 30 percent of women stop bleeding, while another 30 percent have irregular bleeding for more than eleven days each month. Other women may continue to have regular periods but with breakthrough bleeding in between. The longer a woman uses DMPA, the more likely she is to stop menstruating. More than half of DMPA users have no periods after one year of use; this rises to 70 percent after two years of treatment. Periods return within six to eighteen months after the injections are stopped.

Other side effects may include change in appetite, some weight gain, headache, sore breasts, nausea, abdominal discomfort, nervousness, dizziness, depression, skin rashes or spotty darkening of the skin, hair loss, increased facial or body hair, and an increased or decreased sex drive. Remember: There is no way to stop immediately the effects of DMPA—and that means that any side effects may continue until the shot wears off in three months' time.

You will be advised not to take DMPA if you have liver disease or jaundice, blood clots in your legs or lungs, abnormal vaginal bleeding, a history of breast cancer, or an allergy to the chemicals in the drug.

If you're willing to risk the side effects and fit the patient profile, the primary advantage of this injectable is pregnancy prevention for three months at a time. With nothing to be taken daily or put in place before intercourse, spontaneous sex is pretty much yours if you want it.

Net-En. The injectable contraceptive NET-EN, currently not available in the United States, is given every two months. The pregnancy rate with this drug is comparable to that of DMPA, rising slightly when the time between injections is increased by a week or two. The risk of side effects is much the same as with DMPA.

Progestin–Estrogen Injectables. Various combinations of estrogen and progestin are widely used in Mexico and some Latin American countries. Irregular bleeding is less of a problem with these formulations than with DMPA and NET-EN.

Like those of the other injectables, failure rates are extremely low. But because of concern regarding the side effects of high doses of estrogen, these monthly injectables aren't available in most countries, including the United States.

ORAL CONTRACEPTIVES

The groundwork for oral contraception was laid as far back as 1940, when researchers found that estrogen inhibited ovulation—and without eggs there could be no pregnancy. The original birth control pills dispensed in the early 1960s had higher amounts of estrogen than necessary, and these caused severe side effects such as blood clots, high blood pressure, and heart attacks. Further research showing that lower estrogen doses were equally effective led to the widespread use of the combination estrogen–progestin contraceptives marketed today. In addition, the progestin-only "minipill," though not as effective as combination formulas, is useful for women who can't take estrogen.

When used correctly, oral contraceptives are a very effective form of reversible contraception. Of one hundred women using the combined pill as directed during a given year, fewer than one will get pregnant; the figure is slightly higher for the progestin-only mini-pill. The combined pills suppress ovulation and prevent implantation of a fertilized egg, while the progestin-only pills work mainly by thickening the cervical mucus, preventing sperm from joining with an egg; they also prevent fertilized eggs from implanting in the uterus. Women on the combined pill don't release a monthly egg, but they do continue to menstruate, usually just a light flow and in some cases limited to spotting. Pill users typically have little menstrual cramping before and during the period.

Given the effectiveness and ease of use of birth control pills, it's not surprising that today one in four women under forty-five uses the pill to prevent pregnancy. If you're interested in taking an oral contraceptive, consult your health professional. Birth control pills are dispensed by prescription, though over-the-counter availability is currently being debated. Like any contraceptive, the pill is effective only when used correctly, so you must take it exactly as directed. The combined pills are taken at the same time each day for twenty-one days and then stopped for seven days. (To remove the risk that a woman might forget to start the pills again after the seven days off, some packages contain seven inert tablets to continue the daily habit of taking a pill.) Most women begin to bleed about three days after their last hormone-containing birth control pill. But if your period doesn't begin, just start taking the pills again one week after you've taken the last hormone-containing pill. If after this second cycle you miss a second period, consult your clinician. By contrast, the minipill is taken every day with no off time. Women using this method usually but not always have a period.

While the pill's side effects are not as severe as they were in the days of higher doses, some women still have problems, most of them minor. These include fluid retention, nausea, weight gain, breast tenderness, spotting, mood changes, and acne.

A small percentage of pill users do experience serious health problems. In rare instances some can be fatal, especially blood clots in the lung or brain. The chance of development of these complications increases with age, and the risks are greatly multiplied by smoking more than fifteen cigarettes a day and when other conditions such as poorly controlled diabetes, high blood pressure, obesity, or high cholesterol level are present. Women who are often advised not to use oral contraceptives include those with cerebrovascular or coronary artery disease, high blood pressure, or a history of breast or endometrial cancer or malignant melanoma, and those over thirty-five who smoke more than fifteen cigarettes a day.

Concerns have been voiced over the impact of prolonged pill use on a woman's risk of breast cancer, but studies have not found an increase in risk. Long-term pill use is, however, associated with an increased risk of development of precancerous cervical dysplasia (see *Cervical Dysplasia*, page 529).

Yet the pill offers some protection against ovarian and endometrial cancers as well as fibrocystic breast and ovarian cysts. Pill use also reduces anemia (because women bleed less during menstruation) and the incidence of pelvic infections.

Is the pill a safe choice for you? Part of making an informed decision about which contraceptive is right for you is learning the pros and cons of the method. If you don't smoke and fit the medical guidelines given, your health-care provider may recommend the pill.

If you decide you want to get pregnant, you can attempt to do so right after you stop taking the pill. Calculating your due date, however, will be more accurate if at least two normal periods have occurred before conception. As for your fertility prospects, it isn't uncommon for a few months to pass before a normal menstrual cycle resumes while your body adjusts to the changes. It may take several months before you conceive, but the percentage of users of oral contraceptives who stop and then conceive is no different from that of women who have conceived after stopping other methods of contraception.

TALKING WITH YOUR PARTNER

Talking about birth control with your partner isn't the easiest thing in the world to do. Just about everyone feels embarrassed when discussing something as personal as sex— especially when you're discussing it with someone you're attracted to and may not know very well yet. But you owe it to yourself and to your partner to communicate clearly about contraception—and you owe it to yourselves as a couple to make this decision together.

To be able to talk about the subject intelligently, first read about the different methods available and which one(s) might be best for you and why. If you have a clear picture of your needs, it'll be easier to discuss them with your partner.

Are you in a monogamous relationship? The answer to that question will help you to determine whether you need to use a barrier method or not, to prevent the transmission of sexually transmitted diseases (STDs).

Pick a good moment to bring up the subject—and don't wait until you're about to have sex to do so. Good sense can fly right out the window when you're in the throes of passion. If you're worried that your partner will think you're being unromantic by making sure you're protected, think how not protecting yourself could change your life forever—and not necessarily for the better.

Remember that using birth control makes good sense for both of you. Not only can couples make their contraceptive choice a part of their lovemaking—you can put on your partner's condom, for example, or he can insert your diaphragm—but eliminating worry about pregnancy also will make you more relaxed and may make sex more enjoyable.

If at some point in your relationship you decide to stop using condoms, either to become pregnant or to switch to another birth control method, you may want to consider having an HIV test before you discontinue condom use. Such a precaution makes particular sense when either of you has had a number of previous partners or has other risk factors for HIV infection.

If you don't agree on a choice of method right off the bat, don't worry about it. Maybe the next time you talk about it, you will. But don't have sex until you talk.

If your partner is unwilling to talk about birth control or refuses to use it, then perhaps knowing this will save you from a lot of grief down the road. Anyone who would be willing to risk your health or risk unplanned pregnancy is not someone who has your best interest at heart.

POSTCOITAL CONTRACEPTION

Sometimes birth control is needed *after* sex: Your partner's condom broke or slipped off or you neglected to use your diaphragm or you had sex when you didn't expect to. If you had unprotected sex and are certain you don't want to be pregnant, there may be a solution. But you must act fast! If your need for postcoital contraception is a result of rape, go immediately to a hospital emergency room or rape crisis center.

Postcoital contraception is the medical term for what is commonly called the morning-after pill, which is actually a misnomer, since this hormonal contraceptive protection can, in fact, be started up to seventy-two hours after intercourse—but no more than seventy-two hours.

The method of treatment currently used is a short course of medium-dose combined oral contraceptives. This method has a failure rate of two to four pregnancies for every one hundred women treated. The regimen consists of two doses of two pills combining a progestin and estrogen. The first dose should be taken as soon as possible after unprotected sex; the second dose, twelve hours later.

This treatment probably works by disrupting the function of the fallopian tubes and disturbing the development of the uterine lining, thereby either preventing the egg from being fertilized or preventing a fertilized egg from being implanted. The disruptions last only a few days.

Temporary side effects, consisting primarily of nausea and vomiting, are fairly common. (If you vomit, call your physician as soon as possible because you may need to take another dose.) Other short-term side effects that may be experienced are headaches, breast tenderness, dizziness, and fluid retention.

Make sure your clinician knows your medical history before you take this treatment. Since this form of postcoital contraception contains the same hormones found in birth control pills, if you are unable to take oral contraceptives, you might not be able to use the morning-after pill.

Since the treatment is not 100 percent effective, you should have a pregnancy test one month after treatment to ensure that you aren't pregnant. In the rare incidence of failure, the pregnancy need not be terminated because there is no evidence that treatment can be detrimental to the developing fetus.

FEMALE STERILIZATION

If you can say unequivocally that no matter what happens to any children you have or to your relationship, you want no more children, then sterilization may be an appropriate birth control option for you.

Female sterilization is accomplished by means of a *tubal ligation* ("tying the tubes"), which blocks off the fallopian tubes so that eggs can't travel down the tubes and sperm can't journey upward. The result, of course, is that the two don't make contact, making fertilization virtually impossible. Unlike a vasectomy, the male counterpart to this operation, the surgery immediately makes the woman incapable of pregnancy.

About 650,000 women a year opt for tubal ligation in the United States. (In developing countries, where it's often the most common form of birth control, tubal ligation is even

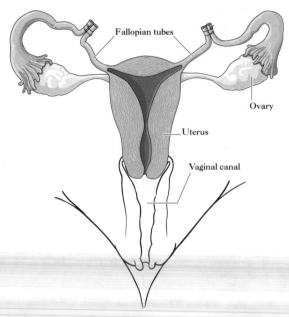

Fallopian tubes

Ovary

Uterus

Vaginal canal

The female sterilization procedure called a tubal ligation *is a minor surgery during which the fallopian tubes are divided, preventing the release of eggs from the ovary to the uterus during ovulation.*

more popular.) The procedure, which takes about fifteen minutes, is done on an outpatient basis. The surgery is done through the abdomen by making a small incision just below—or perhaps inside—the navel, using local, regional, or general anesthesia.

The most widely used method of sterilization involves the use of laparoscopy. After making the incision and pumping a harmless gas into your abdomen to distend the abdominal wall away from your other organs, your gynecologist then inserts a laparoscope, a fiber-optic instrument that gives your doctor direct visual examination of your reproductive organs. Another instrument—an abdominal forceps—is then inserted through either the original incision or a nearby opening. The doctor uses this to pick up a portion of the tube and uses one of two methods to close the passage and make it nonfunctional: either electrocautery or use of a ring or a clip. The incision is then closed with a few stitches.

Allow yourself a few days to rest after sterilization. Many women feel weak and tired for the first couple of days and may experience dizziness, nausea, and bloating. Only about one in one thousand has a serious problem after the surgery. These include injury to the bowel, bleeding, infection, and complications from the anesthesia.

The failure rate for all tubal ligation procedures is extremely low (pregnancy rate following female sterilization is around 0.3 percent). A failed sterilization doesn't usually become apparent until the woman becomes pregnant, and that may be years later.

Although you can decide at any time during your reproductive life to be sterilized, some women choose to do so just after childbirth. At this time the uterus is near the navel, where the doctor will make the incision. In the case of a cesarean birth, a tubal ligation can be performed immediately after delivery, while the abdomen is still open. The length of your postpartum hospital stay won't be affected by this additional procedure. But you should be aware that postpartum sterilization fails about three times as often as laparoscopic sterilization.

If you decide that sterilization is right for you, your physician will advise you of the risks and benefits of the procedure. If you are young or don't have children, you should consider using another method for a while before undergoing the procedure. Above all, in considering sterilization, you should view it as a permanent choice. Doctors can sometimes reconnect the tubes, but this surgery is difficult. Success depends on how much of the tube has been blocked off, the surgical technique used, and the length of tube remaining. If your circumstances change and you decide you want to have a child, the possibility of reversing a procedure done with a ring or a clip is much greater than the possibility of reversing one done by cauterization. Fewer than half of the women who have reversal procedures bear a child, and there is an increased risk of ectopic pregnancy. In some instances, women have reported a decrease in pleasure and desire after tubal ligation.

VASECTOMY

The male counterpart of a tubal ligation is a vasectomy, a procedure that involves cutting and sealing each of the two tubes that carry the sperm from the testes to the penis, the vas deferens, from which comes the term vasectomy. *Many couples choose male sterilization over the female procedure because it's less physically difficult, is less costly, and necessitates less lost work time.*

A vasectomy is a minor procedure often done in a urologist's office. After local anesthetic is injected into the skin of the scrotum, a pair of small incisions is made in the scrotal skin to locate the vasa deferentia. The physician cuts, ties, cauterizes, or clips the tubes and stitches them closed. Then the incision is closed with absorbable stitches that generally dissolve in a week or so. After the twenty-minute procedure, a man usually is asked to minimize the risk of swelling by resting for a day with ice packs on the scrotal area. Most men can return to work the next day.

It should be emphasized that a vasectomy should in no way physically interfere with a man's ability to maintain an erection or reach orgasm, although some men may have an adverse psychological reaction to the surgery, which causes sexual problems. After a vasectomy, men continue to produce male hormones, and they ejaculate the same amount of semen with no change in its appearance. The only difference is that the semen contains no sperm.

Swelling and pain in the scrotum are usually mild after surgery. In the event of persistent or severe pain or fever, your partner should call his doctor.

The failure rate for vasectomy is less than one per one thousand procedures. Generally, if a vas deferens is going to reattach, it does so within the first few months after surgery.

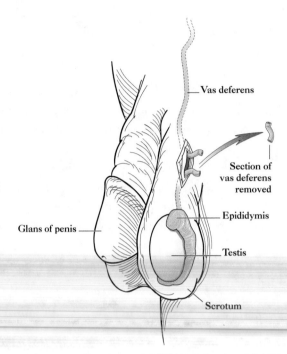

Vas deferens

*Section of
vas deferens
removed*

Epididymis

Glans of penis

Testis

Scrotum

Conducted as outpatient surgery, a vasectomy *is a male sterilization procedure.
The physician will make two small scrotal incisions in order to reach the vas
deferens, which are then cut, tied off, cauterized, or clipped closed. This prevents
the release of sperm in the ejaculate.*

Unlike women who are sterilized, men are not immediately rendered sterile by
the procedure because sperm are stored above the point where the vasa deferentia
were tied. Usually it takes between fifteen and twenty ejaculations before the ejaculate is sperm-free. A man is not considered sterile until a semen analysis finds no
evidence of sperm. Until that time, continue to use a contraceptive.

A vasectomy, like a tubal ligation, should be considered permanent. However,
an estimated 6 to 7 percent of men who have had vasectomies change their mind for
a variety of reasons. The reversal of a vasectomy is a more major procedure than the
vasectomy itself. And although the majority of men who have the procedure do then
ejaculate sperm, only about 30 to 40 percent can father children.

DISCUSSING BIRTH CONTROL
WITH YOUR TEENAGER

For many parents, discussing sex and its consequences with their teenage children is a daunting task. Yet, when you consider that as many as seven of ten teenage girls have had intercourse by the time they leave their teens, the necessity of this communication becomes apparent. Teenage pregnancy rates are skyrocketing: More than one third of all abortions are performed on teenage girls—most of whom admit afterward that they've never used any form of contraception. (Sometimes if a girl has sex but doesn't become pregnant, she assumes she's infertile and continues having unprotected sex— and often must suffer the consequences.) Either health education classes aren't comprehensive, parents aren't advising their children in matters of sex information, or teenagers just aren't listening.

Most of us want to believe that our children will be in no hurry to embark on a sexual relationship. If that's actually the situation in your family, you're very lucky. Even so, as a parent you owe it to your daughter to see that she has the information she needs to be adequately protected in the event she does decide to have sexual intercourse.

It's not easy talking about sexual issues with our kids. Probably most parents are uncomfortable discussing the subject. Even more so are kids, who, to cover their anxiety about the subject (this probably means—yikes!—their parents *have sex!), act as if they're bored to tears. Some parents think they don't know enough about sexuality to impart accurate information, so they avoid the subject altogether. And most kids either are too embarrassed to talk about sex with their parents, think they already know everything, or feel guilty just thinking about sex. But one of the most important things you can do for your kids is to be receptive to and open about their questions about sexuality. By doing so you can reinforce the positive aspects of a loving sexual relationship while advising on the consequences of risky behavior.*

Naturally, if you strongly oppose premarital sex, you should certainly communicate your feelings. Many teens succumb to early sexual experimentation as a result of peer pressure. Tell your daughter that there's nothing wrong with not *wanting to have sex. It doesn't make her abnormal. In fact, it's a very mature attitude. Be sure to let her know that.*

Equally important is to let her know that if she chooses to have a sexual relationship, she has a responsibility to protect her body, both from the risk of pregnancy and from disease. All too often teens plunge headfirst into sexual waters, as if having sex in the throes of passion makes them less responsible for their actions than if they had consciously made the decision and then planned for it.

As for birth control, if you both feel comfortable, you can provide your daughter with contraceptive information, discussing the pros and cons of each method and even helping her make the choice that's right for her. But for many parents and their teens such openness is out of the question. If you find yourself unable to discuss specifics with your daughter, you can offer to make an appointment for her at a reputable family planning clinic or with a health professional, either of whom can offer information and advice. Medical and family planning professionals want to reduce the pregnancy and abortion rates among teenagers, and they won't be judgmental toward a young woman—or a young man—who's taking steps to prevent unwanted pregnancy.

Remember, the question isn't whether *your children will have sex, but* when. *By openly discussing sexuality with them, you can help them mature into sexually healthy, caring, and responsible adults.*

If you're a teen reading this, be aware that a contraceptive is only effective when it's used correctly. The failure rate for the pill, for example, is extremely low, yet if you can't remember to take the pill consistently, it won't work for you. In making your contraceptive choice, choose a method that you feel comfortable using and then use it (see also Teenage Sexuality, *page 19).*

CHAPTER 7

Abortion

CONTENTS

Few issues in recent U.S. history have been as divisive and controversial as abortion. Although a woman's right to terminate her pregnancy was guaranteed by the Supreme Court in its 1973 landmark case *Roe v. Wade*, abortion opposition is as strong as ever, and the issue continues to be a political hot potato.

Yet abortion has been practiced throughout recorded civilization. Five thousand years ago Chinese herbalists recommended mercury to induce abortion. Abortion was common in ancient Greece—though not nearly so as infanticide—and the philosophers Plato and Aristotle advocated abortion as a means of controlling overcrowding. (Aristotle, incidentally, conjectured that life began forty days after conception for males and eighty days after conception for females.) Roman society believed the fetus wasn't a person until birth, and abortion was widely practiced.

Religious views on the subject waxed and waned over the centuries. According to Jewish tradition, induced abortions were only justified to save the life of the mother. In the early days of Christianity, the accepted position was that a fetus was not alive until sometime after conception. An ongoing debate was carried on over the centuries as to when such animation occurred. Somewhere around A.D. 400, St. Augustine theorized that a fetus wasn't fully formed until forty-five days after conception—though he agreed with Aristotle that the female was slower in development than a male. From A.D. 600 to 1100, with the distinction between unformed and formed fetuses widely accepted, an abortion was considered a sin only if a formed fetus was extracted. In the thirteenth century, Thomas Aquinas, recognizing St. Augustine's notion of fetal development, advocated that a fetus had no soul until it moved—"quickened." Thus abortion could be done during the first sixteen weeks of pregnancy. Three centuries later, the church amended that time frame back to the first forty days of pregnancy. Still, the policy of the Catholic church was that since a fetus didn't have a soul until animation, abortion wasn't a sin. Then in 1869, Pope Pius IX restored the sixteenth-century dictum that life begins at the moment of conception, making abortion a grievous sin.

In the United States, Connecticut was the first state to pass an antiabortion law: In 1821, the state forbade the use of poisons to induce postquickening abortions. In 1828, New York State banned postquickening abortions by all methods, except when it was necessary to preserve the life of the mother. Then in 1846 Massachusetts passed the nation's most restrictive law—one supported by physicians—and New York quickly followed suit. These laws disregarded quickening and stipulated punishments for both abortionists and their patients. By 1880, forty states had adopted similar statutes, and by 1900 induced abortion—with the exception of abortion to save the mother's life—was a criminal offense nationwide.

That these laws were seldom enforced is evident by estimates that from 1820 to 1830 one in every twenty-five or so pregnancies ended in induced abortion, between 1850 and 1860 roughly one in five pregnancies so ended, and during the first half of the twentieth century perhaps as many as every third pregnancy was aborted.

While abortion laws undoubtedly deterred some women from the procedure, those who were determined to terminate pregnancy often found the means to do so, either self-induced or performed by lay people under unsanitary conditions. Women died of hemorrhage, infection, or complications of uterine perforation; many survivors were rendered incapable of childbearing. In the early nineteenth century, the death rate from infections even when abortions were performed in hospitals was high; some estimates have it as high as *30 percent*. Given that the mortality rate from childbirth at that time was under *3 percent*, a great many women were clearly willing to risk their life to end unwanted pregnancies.

In later years, doctors often circumvented the laws by performing "therapeutic abortions." Poverty was a widely accepted reason during the 1930s depression, and psychiatric reasons were often cited during the 1940s and 1950s, although increasing scrutiny soon limited these practices. Yet it wasn't until the 1960s, when mothers were unable to get legal abortions in the United States, that proponents of legalization began to be heard. Ironically, the American Medical Association (AMA), which had been an outspoken opponent of abortion in the nineteenth century, began advocating legalizing abortion.

In 1970 Hawaii was the first state to repeal its criminal abortion law and legalize early abortions, and other state legislatures gradually authorized abortion for other than lifesaving reasons. Then came the 1973 Supreme Court ruling that recognized abortion as the private right of a woman.

Giving women access to legal abortions done by trained physicians in a medical environment made a profound difference. In 1955, 100 out of every 100,000 abortions resulted in the woman's death; thirty years later that figure was 0.4 death per 100,000 abortions—compared to 6.6 deaths per 100,000 *births* that same year.

After steadily increasing, the number of abortion procedures performed leveled out during the 1980s. In 1988, an estimated 1.6 million elective abortions were performed in the United States, about 29 percent of all pregnancies. Some 58 percent were done on women under twenty-five, including about 26 percent on teenagers; only 20 percent were performed on women thirty and older. About one fourth of all abortions are performed on married women.

Women have abortions for many reasons, and terminating a pregnancy is always a serious decision. Many unmarried women feel they are too young or are unable to support and nurture a child adequately. Some women, already burdened by the challenge of caring for other children, choose not to bring another one into the world. Couples often choose abortion after genetic testing reveals their baby will be severely handicapped or have a serious disease. Sometimes therapeutic abortions are done because the mother's life is jeopardized by the pregnancy.

Despite rational reasons for termination, opponents vehemently lobby against a woman's right to choose abortion. Some argue that abortion is legalized murder, believing life begins at conception, not months later, when the fetus is capable of living on its own. Others say abortion is simply immoral or severe psychiatric consequences await the woman who has one. No matter what their rationale, many antiabortion advocates are committed to stopping abortion—sometimes at any cost. Groups frequently picket abortion clinics, determined to dissuade women from entering the facilities or attempting to hinder or even at times to harm the physicians who perform the procedures.

Even the language of the debate has become highly politicized: Many religious leaders and politicians support the antiabortion movement under the banner of being "prolife"; other religious and political leaders have stood up for a woman's right to abortion, characterizing themselves as "prochoice" as they insist upon women's having the option to choose as a moral and legal imperative.

In recent years, antiabortion groups have also fought to keep the so-called abortion pill, RU-486, unavailable in the United States, but they finally lost that battle. On the other hand, antiabortion advocates have gradually eroded some abortion rights. For example, Medicaid no longer pays for abortions, effectively denying access to many poor women. Moreover, many states now legally require minors seeking an abortion to have parental permission or, in lieu of that, a court's consent.

While the opposing groups either battle against further government restrictions or lobby for tighter restrictions and ultimately for making the procedure illegal, in most states the decision of whether to have an abortion remains a woman's choice through the twelfth week of pregnancy. Ninety percent of all abortions are done during this time. Some states regulate second-trimester abortion services in the interest of preserving the health of the woman; however, some states' restrictions limiting second-trimester abortions to hospitals have been declared unconstitutional.

This chapter examines the various abortion methods. Some, such as dilation and extraction, have been used for years; one, the abortion pill RU-486, may be finally available in this country by the time this book goes to press; and other physicians are already using other, readily available medications to induce abortion. We also will discuss the emotional aspects of this very personal, often difficult choice.

ABORTION TECHNIQUES

Since its legalization in 1973, induced abortion has become one of the most common gynecological surgeries in the United States. When performed by a trained health-care provider in a medical setting, it's a very safe procedure with few complications and an overall mortality rate of less than 1 per 200,000 abortions.

There are several methods of abortion. The technique a clinician uses will depend primarily on how advanced the pregnancy is. Generally, abortions aren't performed before six weeks from the last menstrual period (LMP). The safest time to have an abortion—and the least physically and emotionally traumatic—is between seven and ten weeks after the LMP. (Some 90 percent of women who obtain abortions are in their first trimester of pregnancy, meaning that less than thirteen weeks has passed since the LMP.)

Before we describe the specific techniques used, let's first clarify some terminology. Most people regard abortion as a voluntary choice made about a pregnancy. However, in this and other health books, you'll see references to *spontaneous abortion, missed abortion*, or *threatened abortion*. All are medical terms for what most people think of as miscarriage or threatened miscarriage.

A *spontaneous abortion* or miscarriage occurs naturally, typically either before a woman even knows she's pregnant or during the early weeks of pregnancy. A *threatened abortion* is the term used when there are early symptoms of miscarriage—vaginal bleeding with or without cramping—but miscarriage has not yet occurred. A woman is said to have a *missed abortion* if the fetus or embryo dies in utero but neither it nor the placenta is expelled naturally.

If you now or in the future are pregnant and believe that an abortion is the best choice, chances are that one of the following methods will be used to terminate the pregnancy.

VACUUM ASPIRATION

The most common technique used today for first-trimester abortions is removal of the contents of the uterus by vacuum aspiration, called variously *vacuum aspiration, aspiration and curettage*, and *suction curettage*.

Performed between the sixth and twelfth weeks, this procedure is safest between seven and ten weeks after your last menstrual period (LMP). Prior to six weeks after the LMP, it's possible the abortion will be unsuccessful.

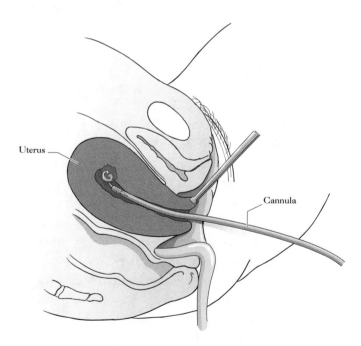

To perform an abortion by vacuum aspiration, your physician will insert a tube called a cannula *into the uterine cavity. It is attached to a suction machine that will enable the practitioner to suction out the embryo and placenta.*

Vacuum aspiration is generally done on an outpatient basis under a local anesthetic. For this and all other abortion procedures, you lie on your back with your thighs spread apart, as you do for your yearly gynecological exam. After your cervix is washed with an antiseptic solution, an anesthetic is injected into and around the cervix to minimize discomfort. Successively larger dilators are used to enlarge the cervical opening; then a strawlike tube called a *cannula* is inserted, the outer end of which is attached to a suction device similar to that used by dentists to clear the mouth of saliva. When everything is in place, the cannula is rotated and the embryo and the placenta are aspirated through the tube into a receptacle.

Though the cervix is anesthetized, the uterine cavity isn't, so during the suction procedure the patient will experience a cramping similar to moderate-to-severe menstrual pain as the uterus contracts in response to the suction.

After the tissue has been suctioned out, the clinician gently scrapes the walls of the uterus with a spoon-shaped metal instrument called a *curette* to ensure that no tissue remains. The entire procedure takes about ten minutes, after which you'll be instructed to rest until you feel well enough to go home. Most women resume normal activities within a day or so.

As with any medical procedure, the possibility of complications exists, though the chance of complications is only about 1 percent for a first-trimester abortion. The most common complication of this technique is infection. To reduce the risk of infection, some practitioners prescribe a short course of antibiotics, as well as medication to contract the uterus back to its normal size.

Perforation of the uterus is another potential risk. In very rare instances the fetal tissue isn't completely removed and a second procedure may be necessary.

DILATION AND EXTRACTION

Only one tenth of the abortions done in the United States are performed in the second trimester (between the thirteenth and twentieth weeks) because abortions become increasingly difficult as pregnancy progresses through this period, and the potential for serious complications grows week by week.

The usual method used for termination until the sixteenth week (though occasionally up to the twentieth week) is dilation and extraction (D & E), which is basically an expansion of the vacuum aspiration method used in first-trimester procedures (see page 131). Because this advanced stage of pregnancy means larger fetal tissue and a softer, more easily injured uterus, this procedure is complicated and requires considerable skill of practitioners. Still, D & E procedures are usually done on an outpatient basis.

First, the cervix is anesthetized, and then dilators are inserted to enlarge the cervical opening. To determine the correct size dilators to open the cervix sufficiently, your provider must know the exact size of the fetus, and that may require an ultrasound a few days prior to the procedure. Depending on the method used, initial dilation may take several hours to as long as overnight.

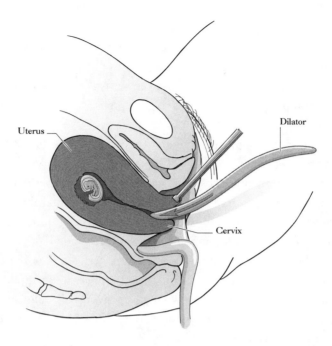

A dilator may be used to enlarge the opening to the cervix in order to perform a dilation and curettage.

The dilator absorbs fluids and gradually expands, widening the cervix. One such dilator is laminaria, a sterilized seaweed about the diameter of a pencil and three inches in length; another is a hydroscopic (moisture-attracting) gel. Sometimes only one dilator is inserted, although women who have previously given birth usually can tolerate several laminaria inserted side by side into the cervix.

Once the cervix is adequately dilated, the dilators are removed and a speculum is inserted into the vagina to expose the cervix. A tube is inserted into the uterus to suction out the amniotic sac, and forceps remove fetal parts too large for the suction tube. Finally a spoon-shaped curette is used to remove any remaining tissue from the walls of the uterus. The procedure itself takes from ten to thirty minutes, after which you'll be instructed to rest until you feel well enough to go home.

As in all abortions, if you are Rh-negative, you'll be given a dose of hyperimmune anti-D globulin (Rhogam). This prevents sensitization, in order to prevent your antibodies from attacking an Rh-positive fetus in subsequent pregnancies.

The risks of abortion complications increase with the length of gestation; after sixteen weeks they're comparable to those associated with childbirth. The most common complications of this procedure are infection, uterine hemorrhage, perforation of the uterus, cervical laceration, and retained pregnancy tissue. If you experience fever, excessive bleeding, or pain, consult your provider. Your health-care provider will likely prescribe an antibiotic to reduce the risk of infection and a medication to help the uterus contract, slowing the bleeding that normally occurs.

INDUCTION ABORTION

Sometimes second-trimester abortions even as late as the twenty-second week of pregnancy are done by dilation and evacuation. In many states this is illegal, but even where it is legal, many clinicians won't use D & E because the fetus is by now quite large and difficult to extract. Most abortions performed at this stage of pregnancy use techniques that induce early labor and expulsion of the fetus.

An induction abortion, given at sixteen to twenty-four weeks of pregnancy, is a more difficult procedure emotionally than a D & E, and fewer than 5 percent of abortions are performed beyond the sixteenth week of gestation. In many cases the decision to abort at this relatively late date is made after tests reveal a serious congenital abnormality in the fetus.

A late-stage abortion requires hospital admission. In an induction abortion, the usual method is to give prostaglandin compounds, by either a vaginal suppository or an injection, to induce labor. The drugs, often used in conjunction with a dilator to hasten the process, are administered every two to three hours until the fetus dies and is expelled. Prostaglandins create prolonged contractions, and most women are given pain-relieving drugs to help them through the labor. Other medications counter the prostaglandin-induced fever, nausea, vomiting, and diarrhea that can be expected.

Typically, uterine contractions begin within twelve to twenty-four hours after the first dose of the prostaglandin. The fetus is generally expelled within a few hours after the onset of labor; within an hour, the placenta follows. However, in about half of all induced-labor abortions, the placenta isn't expelled, and the health-care provider must use instruments to remove it.

Today's techniques to induce early labor are much safer than previous methods. Even so, side effects such as gastrointestinal distress, fever, and chills can result. Infection and hemorrhage are also risks.

After labor and delivery, most women can be discharged from the hospital. Expect to have some bleeding, often for longer than you would during a heavy period. Signs of more serious complications would be fever, excessive bleeding, or pain. If those symptoms occur, consult your provider.

RU-486

RU-486—the "abortion pill"—is a nonsurgical method of terminating a pregnancy during its earliest weeks. Though used in Europe since 1989 by approximately 200,000 women, RU-486 has been used so far in this country by only a few women involved in a clinical study in California. It may become more generally available.

Efforts to introduce the pill in the United States were, until recently, entirely stalled, mainly by threats from antiabortion groups to boycott other products made by the parent company of the pill's French manufacturer. But the company agreed to donate its product patent and technology to the Population Council, a nonprofit contraceptive research organization that will conduct research trials involving about two thousand American women and then choose an American company to manufacture the pill. By donating its patent, the French manufacturer isn't subject to product liability claims. The product will also be rigorously scrutinized by the Food and Drug Administration before becoming available to American women. Needless to say, antiabortion groups have declared their intent to boycott any American company that agrees to produce and market the pill.

RU-486 has been shown in Europe to be an effective method of terminating pregnancy up to about seven weeks after the last menstrual period (LMP) or three weeks after a missed period. The drug, whose chemical name is mifepristone, works by preventing the body from preparing the uterus for pregnancy. Normally after conception takes place, the hormone progesterone prevents the uterus from contracting or bleeding, creating an environment capable of sustaining a fetus for nine months. Mifepristone counters that action. Blood to the developing embryo is then cut off, bleeding and contractions begin, and eventually the embryo is flushed from the uterus.

While it may seem simple, RU-486 isn't a magic pill that transforms a woman from pregnant to nonpregnant in a matter of minutes. Women who use RU-486 need to make three or four trips to their health-care provider. The first will likely be to discuss the procedure and to receive the pill. In conjunction with RU-486, a prostaglandin, misoprostol, is given to increase contractions and therefore the likelihood of abortion. It generally takes several days for the embryo to be expelled. During that time cramping will occur. About two weeks later, a follow-up examination by the provider is appropriate to ensure that the abortion was complete.

Studies have shown that RU-486 in combination with prostaglandin is about 97 percent effective in selected patients. In the remaining cases, the abortion is incomplete and must be followed with a surgical procedure.

The main side effect associated with the pill is bleeding. About half of the women studied have bleeding more severe than that of a heavy period. About one in five hundred requires a blood transfusion to replace lost blood.

An abortion with the pill is initially expected to cost about as much as a surgical abortion, although the cost may go down in time. Some experts predict that if RU-486 becomes generally available, eventually 25 to 40 percent of this country's annual 1.6 million abortions will utilize the abortion pill instead of surgery.

Backers of RU-486 believe its biggest advantage is that it will make abortions available to any woman, as long as her health-care provider knows how to prescribe the drug properly. Today, 31 percent of all women and about 83 percent of those who live in rural areas have no easy access to abortion services. Moreover, taking the pill will be considerably more private than going to an abortion clinic, where many women, who may already be emotionally distraught, are forced by jeering protesters to view pictures of aborted fetuses and are subjected to other humiliations. Proponents hope that by broadening the access to abortions, health-care practitioners and clinics who perform the procedure will be less of a target for antiabortion violence.

THE ALREADY AVAILABLE ABORTION DRUG

A legal, well-established, and very safe drug that, like RU-486, allows for a nonsurgical abortion of early (eight weeks or less) pregnancies is already available by prescription at any pharmacy, and abortion opponents can't possibly outlaw it. The drug, methotrexate, is only now starting to be used for abortions by some doctors in the United States, but it's likely that its use for this purpose will soon become widespread and mainstream.

Classified chemically as a folic acid antagonist, methotrexate stops the normal cell division that folic acid, a B vitamin, promotes. This action is the reason that methotrexate is primarily used—and has been since 1948—to treat cancerous tumors, arthritis, lupus, and other conditions. Because its original therapeutic applications are so long established and beneficial, methotrexate can't be taken off the market, making it safe from attack by abortion foes.

As a drug that chemically induces miscarriage, methotrexate was first used successfully to terminate ectopic pregnancies. This successful application led to the obvious conclusion that it could be used to terminate any pregnancy, and this was first tried clinically in 1993. Methotrexate is now being used in clinical trials under the auspices of the FDA, which has classified it as experimental for pregnancy termination, and the researchers doing studies of the drug for this purpose are expected to work closely with the FDA and an overseeing review board. But since health-care providers frequently prescribe drugs for nonapproved purposes when they've proved beneficial in other applications, practitioners aren't limited to strict guidelines, and it's likely that many physicians in the United States will follow the lead of some of their peers and prescribe methotrexate to their patients who want to terminate pregnancy. However, as an experimental drug, is it probably not covered by insurance when used for abortion.

Using the drug is very similar in procedure to using RU-486 in that it involves administration first of the methotrexate (by injection) followed a week later with a prostaglandin, misoprostol (which is, in fact, a common ulcer medication), to cause uterine contractions to expel the embryo. In tests, the efficacy of the methotrexate/misoprostol combination was nearly identical to that of RU-486, with a success rate of 96 percent. As with RU-486, side effects were minor—basically just cramping and bleeding—and no major complications were reported. Methotrexate will, however, fail on some occasions to terminate the pregnancy. The surviving pregnancy will be at risk of birth defects as a side effect of its use.

The widespread availability of a safe, legal drug that permits safe, legal terminations gives women—and their health-care providers—a new option for those who are prochoice. It enables a decision about abortion to remain a private matter involving a woman, her conscience, and her practitioner, and not a drama that must be played out in the public arena.

THE EMOTIONAL ISSUES OF ABORTION

Abortion, especially when done in the earliest stages of pregnancy, is a commonplace procedure, and a woman's physical recovery afterward is usually swift, provided the procedures are carried out properly. But for the majority of women who opt to terminate a pregnancy, the physical ramifications are only a part of the overall abortion picture. There is also an emotional side.

While some abortions are done because a woman's health is threatened by her pregnancy or because a couple learns that their fetus has a congenital abnormality, the majority occur because a woman—sometimes married, more often not—wakes up one morning to the symptoms of an unplanned pregnancy. Perhaps she's a teenager, still in school and without the means, financial or otherwise, to make a good life for a child. Perhaps she's older with a promising career; she may find the prospect of rearing an infant without a loving partner too daunting. Or perhaps she's married but has economic problems, has a troubled marriage, or is already stretched thin by the demands of her existing family.

Facing an unplanned pregnancy is hard no matter what your age, but it may be especially terrifying for a young woman. Teens account for more than four hundred thousand abortions each year. *To whom do I turn?* a teen may ask herself as she struggles to decide what to do about her situation. The father of her baby may or may not be a source of support, depending on their relationship and his level of maturity. Many young women summon their courage, take a deep breath, and confide in one or both parents. An unplanned pregnancy may be difficult for parents to accept, but most will stand by their daughter, steering her to experts who can help. If you're a pregnant teen, a strong support system can get you through the difficult days ahead, so seriously consider telling your parent(s). No woman, no matter what her age, should have to shoulder this alone. Share your situation with someone—if not your husband or lover, then a friend or relative who, if nothing else, can just be there for you when you want to talk.

The first step once you know you're pregnant is to speak with someone knowledgeable about your options. Many unexpectedly pregnant women have at least an inkling of what they want to do, but they may need information. Some women are vehemently opposed to abortion, and if they're not in a position to keep their child, they'll go through with the pregnancy and give up the baby for adoption. Others feel the only way out of their situation is to terminate the pregnancy. An increasing number of women go through with their pregnancy and keep their babies.

Even if you lean in one direction, you should still examine all your options before you make a decision. If you have a health-care provider, he or she may be able to give you information or at least refer you to someone who can. Abortion clinics advertise in the Yellow Pages of the phone book, but not every clinic offers the same quality of services, so be careful. It's better to call your nearest Planned Parenthood facility for a referral to a reputable clinic.

Planned Parenthood has found that most women—some 98 percent—who have had an abortion have no regrets and would make the same choice again. The majority of women find the procedure to be a maturing experience, and they discover a sense of strength in having successfully coped with a personal crisis by having made and carried out an important decision.

The overwhelming emotional response to first-trimester abortions is relief. A mild, transient depression occurs immediately postoperatively for about 20 percent of women who have had an abortion, though this quickly passes. A smaller number, some 10 percent, experience lingering depression, though it may be the experience of an unwanted pregnancy, not the abortion itself, that's the actual cause of any depression. Shame and guilt sometimes come into play. You may be ashamed of having become pregnant and then feel guilty for having aborted your fetus. If you and your partner choose to abort a fetus that has severe congenital defects because raising the child would be beyond the scope of your abilities, you may be filled with sadness and regret even though you feel you made the right decision. Some women, especially those having second-trimester abortions, experience sadness and a sense of loss and go through a grieving process. Though the vast majority of partners either have unchanged feelings toward each other or feel closer as a result of their decision, for some couples problems in their relationship develop, especially when one partner was opposed to the abortion.

All these emotions are normal and there's no evidence that women who have abortions experience serious psychiatric disorders as a result. In fact, a panel of experts assembled by the American Psychological Association said in a report to Congress that legal abortion "does not create psychological hazards for most women undergoing the procedure," and further noted that since some 21 percent of American women have had an abortion, if severe emotional reactions were common, there would be an epidemic of women seeking psychological treatment—and there's no evidence of such an epidemic.

Some women may find counseling beneficial before or after an abortion. It may also be a comfort to know that having a properly performed abortion rarely affects a woman's ability to have children in the future.

TWO SIDES, TWO STORIES

Quite by chance, Catherine and Louisa found themselves sitting side by side in the waiting room of their counseling clinic. They first connected because each realized the other felt as bad physically as she did. Both were experiencing the nausea and discomfort of pregnancy for the first time and each recognized the other's queasiness almost instantly.

They fell into talking and soon realized they had more than their pregnancy in common. Both were married but neither had planned to become pregnant. "I don't even know when it could have happened," complained Catherine. "I know exactly when it did," Louisa commented dryly in response.

One woman waited for the other, and they had a cup of coffee after they'd seen the doctor and talked some more. Both had considered having abortions, although Louisa, as a Catholic, knew her faith forbade it. Catherine wanted children badly but was very concerned that the timing be right, and her husband had just lost his job. They talked for almost two hours and agreed to talk again after they'd made their decisions.

Both women had an abortion and a few days afterward they met again. Neither woman had had any complications; the procedure had been the least of the experience. But both were grappling with the emotional aftermath. Catherine was having the tougher time, with bouts of tearfulness that came on her with no warning. Louisa had told her mother, and, to her surprise, her mother hadn't become hysterical. She'd been upset, but, after they had talked, her mother had reinforced her daughter's decision. That had helped.

In the coming months, both Louisa and Catherine got on with their lives. A year later, Catherine became pregnant—intentionally—and she is happily expecting a boy. She feels it was the decision to get pregnant that lifted the cloud and still has doubts that she did the right thing in having the abortion. Louisa's happier with her decision, as she pursues her career with growing success. The two women haven't kept in touch, though. Even though their memories of their abortion are no longer fresh, neither wants to revisit that time.

BIRTH CONTROL AFTER ABORTION

Abortion is *not* a method of contraception and should never be viewed as such. As we have seen, a properly done early surgical abortion is a relatively simple procedure, but even relatively simple surgery poses more potential risk to a woman than does using an approved contraceptive device.

Although most women aren't cavalier about abortion, some are lax about using a contraceptive, often with the idea that one can always terminate a pregnancy should it occur. But most women who have had an abortion don't consider it a preferred or desired form of contraception. Studies of these women indicate that while 70 percent of them used no form of birth control before their first abortion, only 9 percent didn't use a contraceptive method *after* their abortion. Despite propaganda to the contrary, women clearly don't take abortion lightly and don't want to go through it again.

After an abortion, most providers or family planning clinics counsel the patient about effective contraception to avert additional unplanned pregnancies. If you want to prevent another pregnancy, you must use a contraceptive consistently and correctly (see *Birth Control*, page 101). Be aware that although you won't have a period until some four to eight weeks after your abortion, *you can get pregnant again immediately, even before your next period.* One thing's sure: If you didn't know before that you could get pregnant, you certainly know now.

POSTABORTION CARE

If you have a surgical abortion, you'll need to do several things postoperatively:

- *Abstain from vaginal sexual intercourse until given the OK by your health-care provider after a follow-up exam.*

- *Avoid strenuous exercise and activity for a week or so and use sanitary pads instead of tampons.*

- *Be alert for a high fever, pelvic pain, excessive bleeding, or unusual vaginal discharge—all signs of possible delayed complications.*

- *Pamper yourself—or, if it's an option, let someone else pamper you. You've just gone through a physically and emotionally difficult procedure, and you deserve some "tender, loving care."*

CHAPTER 8

Substance Abuse

Contents

For some people, the term *substance abuse* brings alcohol to mind—after all, alcohol is in almost universal use in American society as a recreational beverage and social lubricant. Every social class, from very rich to very poor, uses *and* abuses alcohol and has done so since the first casks of rum were brought over on the *Mayflower* and the first colonial tavern opened in Boston.

Over the years, substance abuse has come all too often to include drug use, too. Opium and opium derivatives found their way into some patent medicines and, in more recent years, a wide variety of powerful prescription and street drugs came to be abused. Yet the dominant substance abused has been, for most of our history, alcohol.

Beer was by far the most popular (and cheapest) drink; breweries were numerous in almost every sizable city and town, and men frequented taverns and saloons to imbibe beer from freshly tapped kegs. Drinking was deemed an unladylike thing to do, so officially, at least, only women of ill repute drank and visited saloons. Practically speaking, women of polite society might indulge a bit, but rarely more than an occasional glass of wine at dinner—except, perhaps, in secret.

Drink informed the American way of life, and nobody feared the hazards though everybody knew of them. If you drank to excess, you were inebriated or "drunk." The condition bore no stigma if it occurred only occasionally, and people paid little attention. But if you got drunk constantly, particularly in public, you were labeled a "drunkard," and the full force of moral disapproval descended upon you. The idea never occurred to anyone that a stumbling drunkard might be in need of help; compulsive drinking showed a man to be a moral degenerate, plain and simple. However, fashionable society rarely applied such labels. Drinking to excess wasn't what was done, certainly, but tippling was sometimes considered amusing or at least tolerable.

Among working-class men, however, excessive drinking created serious social problems. Some workers spent their wages on drink, and some lost their jobs and left their families destitute, situations that led to the Temperance movement. Assaults on saloons by its members became a celebrated theme of the period; the indefatigable Temperance leader Carry A. Nation achieved fame for her practice of charging into saloons and wielding her hatchet on a bar's elaborate inlaid woodwork. To Temperance leaders, drinking was a sin, and they were determined to stamp out "demon rum" by whatever means they could, even if such means were illegal. In the end, their most effective weapon was lobbying state and national legislators. Eventually, several states passed laws prohibiting the sale or consumption of alcoholic beverages, and in 1920 both the United States Senate and the House of Representatives voted for a constitutional amendment that stretched the ban from ocean to ocean.

Prohibition was hailed initially as "The Great Experiment," but its popularity soon soured. Transforming alcohol from something commonplace into something hard to get only made it more glamorous and more expensive. The law was effectively unenforceable, and Prohibition ushered in a period of defiance that united everyone from gin-running gangsters to factory workers to society swells. This was the roaring twenties, with its speakeasies (illegal bars), bootleg hooch (whiskey bought from gangsters), and bathtub gin (homemade liquor). The Great Experiment became a great social disaster, and when Franklin Delano Roosevelt took office as president in 1933, Prohibition was quickly repealed. The nation immediately celebrated with an orgy of legal drinking.

Hollywood movies are our best remaining evidence of the period immediately after Prohibition. William Powell and Myrna Loy in *The Thin Man* series epitomized the country's new idea of smart, sophisticated behavior: Their characters were always drinking and usually tipsy. The humorist Robert Benchley, one of the more cerebral wits of the thirties and forties routinely—and hilariously—portrayed himself as a gentleman who had taken "a tew foo many martinis." By contrast, W. C. Fields, playing a workingman's drunk, was irascible, confused, and often falling down. (A significant difference is that Fields often *was* drunk, even when working, tickling his fans but infuriating his colleagues.) In these and many other instances, typical on-screen drinking mirrored typical off-screen drinking and was regarded as perfectly normal.

Naturally, everybody knew that some people couldn't "handle their liquor" and couldn't limit their consumption to "social drinking"—which in polite society in those days might include a few cocktails before dinner, wine with dinner, and possibly cognac after. In barroom society the routine would be a lot simpler: an endless succession of shots and beers. The word *drunkard* had been retired with nineteenth-century melodrama, but people who couldn't *not* drink were still known as "drunks," and they cut across all class lines. Those who had money might eventually go to a sanitorium to "dry out." A few began to find their way to Alcoholics Anonymous, a self-help organization that got its start at this time. But the vast majority of "dipsomaniacs"—a name derived from their uncontrollable craving for alcohol—drank their way into the gutter and an early grave, and medical science found no certain way to help them to stop.

In that same period, a few people on both the bottom and top rungs of the social ladder were also using drugs—mainly cocaine, heroin, and hashish—but the numbers were too small to interest or alarm the general public. *Reefer Madness*, a lurid film released in 1936—and today a cherished camp classic—purported to show that marijuana was turning American kids (especially young women) into sex maniacs, so sensationalizing the effects of a single puff of marijuana that the movie was laughed out of movie houses.

By the mid-1940s, addiction—to alcohol or heroin—was being recognized as a serious problem, on the rise among the white middle class, and again Hollywood held the mirror to society. When Ray Milland played an alcoholic suffering with delirium tremens (DTs) in the 1945 film classic *Lost Weekend*, horrified audiences were forced to face the destructive emotional and physical effects that alcoholism can wreak. They were shocked again in 1956 when, in *The Man with the Golden Arm*, Frank Sinatra portrayed the trauma of trying to kick a heroin habit cold turkey.

By the 1960s, Americans were well aware that drinking could be dangerous and that people who regularly got drunk were in need of help. But aside from the occasional movie, the danger of drugs hadn't really penetrated public consciousness, mainly because Americans then had so little exposure to them. Yet we knew that drugs were out there—somewhere—and parents were beginning to fear their kids might run into them.

By 1968, the year of Woodstock—remembered as "the summer of love"—we were a changed people. The concert was a watershed in America's understanding of itself, and few people were surprised to learn from news stories that a haze of marijuana had wafted over the multitude of "hippies" who had gathered for that event. By then most Americans knew from press and television reports, if not firsthand, that immense numbers of young people all over the country were using drugs casually, socially, much as their parents used cocktails. Unlike alcohol, these newly popular substances—mainly marijuana but also psychedelics such as LSD and psilocybin mushrooms ("magic mushrooms"), cocaine, and, to a very limited extent, heroin—were illegal, and to use them was to break the law. Thus the term *substance abuse* came into being.

The generations of young Americans since Woodstock have all grown up around drugs and alcohol, and it's evident that over the past thirty years, drug substances particularly have powerfully influenced the music, art, and thinking of the entire culture. In the mid-1990s, American users of alcohol and/or drugs are numbered in the tens of millions. The vast majority of people currently over twenty-one have certainly had at least one drink and/or inhaled a little marijuana smoke.

As for addiction, many millions also tried cocaine or Ecstasy or other so-called boutique drugs without becoming addicted. Marijuana, the illegal substance most widely used, is not chemically addictive, and although government and law-enforcement agencies have railed against it and laws criminalize those who sell, buy, or use it, it continues to be popular. Not incidentally, marijuana has been subjected to many scientific studies. While none has proved it to be injurious to health, the illicit drug industry has managed to breed strains of cannabis that are many times more potent than the naturally occurring variety. The massive doses of THC (tetrahydrocannabinol—marijuana's active ingredient) now available may significantly magnify the danger of this substance. Time will surely tell; street users now provide a natural laboratory for studying many events that cannot ethically be generated in controlled experiments. However, abundant evidence proves that perfectly legal alcohol can be a dangerously addictive substance, as are illegal heroin, cocaine, crack cocaine, amphetamines, and barbiturates.

So how is it that some people can occasionally use potentially addictive substances and walk away unaffected while others are quickly hooked? Many members of Alcoholics Anonymous (AA) and Narcotics Anonymous (NA) subscribe to the idea of an "addictive personality," a predisposition to compulsive drinking or drug use that they believe is genetic. Many AA and NA members also see addiction as a "disease," an idea supported by the medical establishment, notably doctors who run "detoxification" clinics for alcoholics and addicts.

The American medical community wholeheartedly supports AA methods, including its

Twelve-Step program of recovery. When the program is closely followed or "worked," in AA parlance, alcoholics and addicts are able to maintain sobriety.

Substance Abuse and Sex and Violence. "A loaf of bread, a jug of wine, and thou," has long been the classic recipe for love. But don't go overboard on the wine. Too many jugs will certainly work against the sexual intentions of any couple. Excessive use of alcohol inhibits a man's ability to attain and sustain an erection. Sexual reaction in women is more complex: Alcohol may somewhat inhibit physiological response, but at the same time it tends to relax inhibitions. Men and women alike should also keep in mind that a relaxing of the important rules of safe sex can be dangerous.

Abuse of other drugs is also inimical to sex. People who come together for sex and first get stoned on marijuana may well become distracted and forget the original reason for meeting. Cocaine is often used to stimulate sexual sensation; cocaine addicts, though, find sex secondary to the need to maintain the habit. The same is true of heroin addiction; with junkies, most normal human activities are sublimated to the drive to get a fix, which produces in the addict a sense of being returned to normal, a feeling of physical well-being, and an irresistible drowsiness. Sexual activity among women addicted to heroin or to crack cocaine is high, but only because so many women addicts prostitute themselves to pay for their drugs.

Violence is virtually unknown in connection with the use of marijuana and is rarely associated with the *use* of cocaine, heroin, and the like. However, addicts who rob and burglarize to get the money to sustain their habit may well be violent in the commission of these crimes. And alcohol could be said to be the most violent of drugs: Violence often erupts at home or in public places when men (and, infrequently, women) fall into disputes while drinking. Alcohol is very often linked with domestic violence: Disturbances and conflicts range from verbal assault to spousal and child battery to spousal abuse and rape, and even murder (see *Violence Against Women*, page 205).

HOBBLED BY HABITS: MATERNAL SUBSTANCE USE AND ABUSE AND THE EFFECT ON CHILDREN

Roughly 300,000 children a year are born with physical and psychological impairments as a result of their mother's alcohol use. Some 500,000 infants yearly are harmed by drug abuse during pregnancy. And at least 250,000 children a year suffer low birth weight—which stunts far more than growth—as a result of nicotine exposure.

Grim statistics all—and all preventable if mothers put the needs of their unborn children above their own. Mothering, as well as fathering, must begin at conception, not at birth.

Fetal Alcohol Syndrome. *Even in antiquity the dangers of alcohol to the fetus were known. References to the connection between alcohol consumption and deformed and mentally impaired babies can be found in the Bible and in the writings of such ancient Greeks as Aristotle. Ancient Carthaginians were forbidden to drink wine on their wedding night lest it harm the resultant offspring. But the concept was generally ignored until the nineteenth century, when several British studies noted that alcoholic women showed dramatic rates of stillbirth, growth deficiencies, and malformations in their offspring.*

Widespread recognition of the risks of alcohol consumption during pregnancy didn't really occur until the early 1970s, with the publication of the findings on what the researchers called fetal alcohol syndrome, *or FAS, the severe and irreversible physiological and behavioral problems present in children born of chronically alcoholic women.*

Alcohol freely crosses the placental barrier, creating a blood alcohol level in the fetus similar to the mother's. The result can be damage to the embryonic cells and profound and permanent congenital anomalies. The impairment can be extensive: Central nervous system deficiency causes mental retardation, fine motor dysfunction, and behavioral problems, including hyperactivity, irritability, and attention-deficit disorder; growth deficiency causes retarded intrauterine growth and failure to thrive after birth; abnormalities occur in facial characteristics, including small eye openings, microcephaly (a small skull and brain), and internal and external bodily abnormalities, including heart defects.

If you're planning a pregnancy, it's preferable that you stop drinking before conceiving.

Fetal Drug Exposure. *Low-birth-weight babies are common among cocaine and crack users as well as marijuana users. In infancy, exposed babies can experience problems in sleeping and waking, resulting in exhaustion and poor development. Childhood problems range from vision and motor control; to learning, speech, and language disabilities; to difficulties with social interaction. A baby's exposure to drugs in utero can result in impaired ability to pay attention or sit still, and visual, auditory, and language skills may not develop fully.*

Maternal Smoking. *If, as a smoker, you think that you have nine months in which to quit before secondhand smoke creates a hazard for your baby, think again. Pregnant smokers put their unborn babies at great risk of complications. Smoking during pregnancy has long been known to be related to low birth weight. Moreover, children of smokers are smaller in stature and lag in cognitive development and educational achievement.*

The latest findings indicate that as few as five cigarettes smoked daily by the mother creates a risk of growth retardation in her baby. Compared to the offspring of nonsmokers, children of heavy smokers were nearly twice as likely to experience school failure by age seven and were particularly subject to hyperactivity and attention-deficit disorder.

ALCOHOL ABUSE

Alcoholism—the uncontrollable need to drink alcohol on a regular basis to feel calm and be able to function normally—is a chronic psychological and nutritional disorder that affects about fourteen million American adults. Almost 2 percent of all adults report becoming intoxicated weekly.

The *amount* of alcohol an addicted person requires for maintenance will vary widely from individual to individual; it's the essential dependence itself, in whatever amount, that characterizes the alcoholic.

Alcoholism may be identified by specific behavioral changes that are symptomatic of the disease. By this definition, symptoms include an inability to control alcohol consumption, a preoccupation with alcohol, continued use of alcohol despite adverse consequences, and distorted thinking, notably denial of alcohol abuse.

People who drink can have alcoholic symptoms at any age, from very young to very old, but the largest population of American alcoholics falls between the ages of thirty-five and fifty-five. For some people, the compulsion to drink begins with the first taste of alcohol, an urge likened to being, in the jargon of Alcoholics Anonymous, "off to the races," suggesting a heedless and headlong gallop from one drink to the next to the next, with no stopping and no turning back. But for most, alcoholism is a progressive process that begins with mild to moderate drinking and only gradually results in habitual and uncontrolled excess.

This process, which usually takes place in a largely social context, may initially be entirely unobserved by family and friends. Many alcoholics report having had a remarkable ability to "handle" their drinking from an early age; they could consume far more alcohol than their friends yet rarely if ever get drunk. A few drinks every day, or even less often—consumed to relax, to be social, to overcome pressures and fears—may have no apparent ill effect for years, apart, perhaps, from the hangovers, which prompt the traditional recipe for cure: "the hair of the dog that bit you" (another drink), which makes the drinker feel all right again—for a time.

At a certain point *some* drinkers move from social drinking to abusive, habitual drinking and from there to dependence on alcohol. To date, researchers cannot explain why this happens to some and not to others.

THE EFFECTS OF ALCOHOLISM

Sharon wasn't a drinker, but her husband was. She learned the hard way that when drinkers find they're compelled to drink, they keep very quiet about it. It's a disagreeable realization, and one that is often denied for a very long time. But when Roger lost his job, the dirty little secret came out.

She had been denying the truth of it, but when he came home drunk one night, she confronted him. And for the first time in their eight years together, he hit her. That hurt—but the fact he didn't seem to feel any remorse about it made her even more upset. And then he became increasingly cautious and surreptitious in his drinking behaviors, afraid the secret would be discovered by other family members or coworkers, especially his new employer. It was a dangerous cycle.

Only when Sharon left, taking the children with her, did Roger take action. He got himself on a program and his new boss even admitted that he himself had once had a problem. Over time, Roger and Sharon negotiated the terms of a new start. Without alcohol.

Alcoholism interferes with personal life and job performance, but some alcoholics are extremely good at covering up, even for long periods. However, a confirmed alcoholic will rarely be able to fool all of the people all of the time. Erratic and roller-coaster moods and emotionality at home, coupled with increasingly frequent absences from the workplace, are a tip-off. Most alcoholics can't hide the watery eyes, jittery nerves, and permanently flushed complexion that often come with the territory.

Nobody wants to be an alcoholic, of course, so the affected person is highly conflicted, both knowing and at the same time denying that he or she is in trouble. Most out-of-control drinkers use denial as a personal shield against the truth: "*I* don't have a problem" is the usual defense. Rather, the problem is blamed on *them* (family, friends, associates who express concern). Denial is why so few people in trouble with alcohol voluntarily ask for help. Doing so would be an admission that the problem exists. Most alcoholics must be prodded to face up to the situation.

When looking back at their alcoholic behavior, recovering alcoholics always speak of the helplessness their compulsive drinking engendered and the relief they eventually felt at not *needing* to drink again. Many experienced blackouts in their drinking years, periods about which they remember nothing, waking up in strange beds with strangers, for example, with no idea of how they got there. But even a series of such terrifying episodes is rarely enough to frighten alcoholics into stopping or moderating their drinking. Most simply see these blackouts as an inevitable, even acceptable, hazard of the drinking life, a life in which drinking itself becomes the single most important function of the day and night, at the cost of every other consideration.

Drinkers can become so physiologically dependent on alcohol that they can't behave "normally" without it. Attempts to stop drinking at this stage are doomed to failure; the body is so accustomed to regular doses of alcohol that without them, alcoholics experience rising panic and often fear impending death. These alcohol-induced terrors, accompanied as they usually are by violent and uncontrollable shaking, send drinkers quickly back to the bottle. Acutely aware that they can't stop drinking and can't afford to be seen as alcohol-dependent, alcoholics may resort to drinking as much on the sly as in public, hiding bottles in secret places even at work to ensure a supply.

Situations as desperate as this almost certainly require an intervention by family members or friends to force the alcoholic into treatment. When concerned family and friends do have to intervene, they should expect an angry and resentful drinker who will make the exercise a memorably painful process for all because alcoholics seldom go into treatment willingly. Not surprisingly, alcoholics don't want to admit that they have a problem, and they're frightened of surrendering their independence to the will of others, even if they're clearly ill to the point of incapacitation.

It's usually recommended that alcoholics undergoing withdrawal be managed with medical supervision. Drinkers this "toxic" may be in greater physical danger than they know. Aside from producing the shakes and profuse sweating, withdrawing from alcohol at this point can induce hallucinations (delirium tremens or DTs) and even shock, convulsions, and cardiac arrest.

The Bodily Effects. The toxic effects of alcohol on the liver, especially cirrhosis, in which scar tissue replaces live cells, are well known. Heavy drinking can also cause an alteration in fat metabolism by the liver, resulting in an accumulation of fatty acids. Bouts of heavy drinking can induce alcoholic hepatitis, a serious liver inflammation.

The cardiovascular system is also affected. Prolonged and immoderate consumption can cause arrhythmic heartbeat, enlargement of the heart, and thrombosis, along with high blood pressure. Heavy drinking can lead to angina pectoris, decreased cardiac efficiency, and cardiac arrest.

Prolonged heavy drinking can result in a chronic undersupply of the male sex hormone, which doesn't just cause a temporary loss of potency—it can actually shrink the testicles and cause the breasts to enlarge. There also seems to be a correlation between cancer and alcohol, which apparently acts either as a causative agent or as a promoter of cancerous cells that are initiated by other factors. Heavy drinkers are two to six times more likely to have cancer of the throat or mouth, and if heavy smoking is added to the heavy drinking, the risk increases by *fifteen* times compared to that of nondrinkers and nonsmokers.

The most radical effects of alcohol are, of course, witnessed in the central nervous system. Alcohol seems to destroy brain cells permanently. Irreversible brain damage seems to occur, as identified by intelligence tests taken over an extended period of excessive alcohol use.

Women are more sensitive to the effects of alcohol than men, even if they weigh the same and have the same drinking history. Apparently because men have a higher percentage of water in their bodies than women, alcohol becomes more diluted when ingested by men.

TEENAGE DRINKING

Corey started drinking after games. He felt like an insider, even as a sophomore, when the senior guys he played football with invited him along. At first it was just a beer or two, but pretty soon it was a six-pack every Saturday night. Only when he totaled his dad's car—but was lucky enough to walk away unscathed—did he have to explain to his parents *and* to himself how easy it had been to get into the habit.

Many teenagers drink experimentally. Kids may find older friends who will buy them beer, wine coolers, or liquor or—a classic American teenage trick—they'll pour a small amount from all the bottles in their parents' liquor cabinet into a jar and share the concoction with friends.

Many teenagers regard drinking as a desirably adult thing to do; getting drunk for the first time is often seen as a rite of passage into what they regard as a more mature, sophisticated state of being. But there's a good chance that many teens who drink frequently will drink excessively as they grow older. Estimates are that fully half of today's adult problem drinkers got their start as teens.

Alcohol is riskier for kids than they recognize. A teenager can become addicted relatively quickly, depending on a mass of variables. Among the factors are the teen's degree of social isolation, personal self-esteem, and ability to communicate with parents. Today, as ever, peer pressure *rules*, and today, as ever, peer pressure often says, "Let's go out and get a six-pack."

An obvious danger connected with teenage drinking that may have little or nothing to do with addiction is nonetheless an issue of critical importance: Every year in America, more than ten thousand young adults between the ages of sixteen and twenty-four die in alcohol-related automobile accidents.

CHILDREN OF ALCOHOLIC PARENTS

Statistically, children of alcoholics are more likely to become alcoholics than children of parents who drink in moderation or not at all. Predisposing genetic factors have been identified to explain this finding; in addition, drinking by children of alcoholics may also be a function of their environment.

We generally tend to behave much the way we saw our parents behaving, including all too often those behaviors we hated and swore we'd never emulate. Growing up with alcoholic parents is especially stressful and perplexing. The alcoholic parent may be quixotic— sometimes loving, sometimes distant, sometimes dependent, sometimes abusive—and his or her children rarely know what's expected of them or where they stand. They might regard their parent as weird or mean without even knowing exactly what the problem is since alcoholic parents are no more likely than any other alcoholics to admit their dependence, and a frank exchange of views is highly unlikely in their household.

An organization called Adult Children of Alcoholics (ACOA) has active chapters in many American cities. At regular meetings, members (some recovering alcoholics themselves) share their stories and find a degree of reconciliation in fellowship.

Fetal Alcohol Syndrome. As many as 300,000 children a year in the United States are born permanently brain damaged by fetal alcohol syndrome (FAS), a condition that would have been prevented completely if their mother had refrained from drinking alcohol during pregnancy. Tragically, it's almost impossible to help children disabled by prenatal exposure to alcohol. Many will never understand right from wrong, function independently, hold jobs, or plan a future. By their teen years, many enter a continuum of arrests for petty theft and other minor and occasionally major crimes. They act impulsively and are unable to comprehend the implications of their acts or feel any remorse for the pain they inflict on others. Ironically, some mothers of such children are themselves suffering from fetal alcohol syndrome and so are incapable of knowing that their drinking condemns their children to the same condition.

Although FAS is associated with large amounts of alcohol regularly ingested during pregnancy, all pregnant mothers today are urged to abstain from alcohol until they deliver because of concerns about adverse effects even from lower doses of alcohol (for more on FAS and other drug-induced fetal abnormalities, see *Hobbled by Habits*, page 145).

QUITTING DRINKING

It's hard for habitual drinkers, including those not technically alcoholics, to stop drinking. Many people spend their adult life trying to stay on the safe side of alcoholism by carefully monitoring their consumption; others who fear they're stepping over the edge will use the same watchful method to taper off. But controlled drinking usually doesn't work for alcoholics in the long term; the best intentions to drink moderately are usually overcome by the implacable need to drink more. A complete break with alcohol seems to be the only escape for most.

It's *possible* for alcoholics to quit drinking on their own; a fierce desire for sobriety occasionally enables some individuals to accomplish the task. Most often, though, alcoholics who want to stop join Alcoholics Anonymous. Newcomers who find their way to "the rooms," as AA meeting places are known, receive a warm welcome and complete empathy. All members have been in exactly the same trouble, all know how it feels, and all are ready to help as much as they can, often willing to go to any lengths to help a fellow alcoholic.

Newcomers to AA are introduced to the ingeniously modest and successful concept that it's best to abandon at once any idea of lifetime reform; instead, they're urged not to drink just "one day at a time." They're also introduced to the now-famous Twelve-Step program that has enabled so many generations of alcoholics to recover. The first of these twelve steps is tremendously difficult for many newcomers to accept, much less admit to a group, as they are invited to do: "We admitted we were powerless over alcohol, that our lives had become unmanageable." It's a difficult admission for most people, but acknowledging the truth of it—and it's factual enough for an alcoholic—is the beginning of the end of denial and the beginning of the return to reality. No one is forced to take this first step, or any other. But people are strongly encouraged to attend meetings, to keep coming back.

At AA meetings, which are held regularly in most cities and towns in the country, members "share" the experiences of their drinking years, study and "work" the steps, and pray hard. (AA is quietly insistent on the role of a "higher power" in recovery, but meetings for those who are nonbelievers do exist in major cities.) Alcoholics find a friendship and fellowship there that most say they've never known before. In the AA context, hundreds of thousands of despairing people have been able to achieve and maintain sobriety and have re-created their lives.

Alcoholics who apply to detoxification and rehabilitation clinics ("rehabs") operated by hospitals and other medical facilities or who are forced into them by family pressure or court mandate also encounter AA. The first part of their experience will be with detoxification or "detox," during which withdrawal from alcohol is conducted under close medical observation, typically with the help of tranquilizers, over a thirty-six-hour period. The remainder of a rehabilitation stay is filled with a mélange of psychotherapy, lectures, workshops, and encounter sessions based on the AA program. AA meetings are customarily held on the premises once or more daily. It's a kind of inculcation with AA thinking (all aspects of the rehab program are mandatory), and usually the patient will be encouraged to take the first step before departing. When people leave rehab, they are strongly encouraged to attend AA meetings on the outside.

Most rehabs accept drug addicts as well as alcoholics, and the treatment is the same in both cases. Rehabs are such a fixture in our society today that insurance coverage for them is sometimes included in medical health plans. Unfortunately, the long-term success rate is very mixed, variously reported at from less than 30 to 50 percent.

Some people will repeat the experience at least once, while others simply walk away after thirty days and resume their addiction. But many, many participants do decide to quit, accept AA principles, and achieve abstinence "one day at a time."

A newer option to AA is a controversial treatment program, Moderation Management (MM). The underlying belief of MM is that some (though by no means all) problem drinkers can learn to moderate their drinking. Some experts describe the approach as risky and dangerous, but some therapists report that the programs have been useful with certain of their patients. MM establishes limits—for women, no more than nine drinks a week, and no more than three on any one day. If the drinker cannot follow the regimen, however, then total abstinence from drinking is the only alternative.

HOW MUCH IS TOO MUCH?

So just how much alcohol is enough? Current recommendations are a maximum of one drink a day for premenopausal women who are not pregnant or lactating. Since this amount of alcohol can have beneficial effects on the heart by boosting high-density lipoprotein (HDL), the good cholesterol, and it inhibits potentially dangerous blood clots, thereby lessening the risk of heart attacks, a drink a day—as long as you can limit yourself to one—can be good for you. But once you reach your mid-sixties the body can't handle as much alcohol as it once could, increasing the risk of accidents and insomnia. If there is any family history of alcoholism or depression, or if you have liver disease, ulcer, gout, pancreatitis, sleep apnea, or chronic insomnia, avoid alcohol completely.

Be aware that regularly consuming three or more alcoholic drinks a day in combination with taking acetaminophen (Tylenol, for example) carries the risk of liver damage, and gastrointestinal bleeding may occur when taking aspirin or ibuprofen (Advil) along with three or more drinks daily. Of course, even small amounts of alcohol can be dangerous when used with sleeping pills and tranquilizers. Further, alcohol can reduce the effectiveness of anticonvulsants and beta-blockers.

DRUG ABUSE

Illegal drug abuse in the United States is believed to be half what it was in 1979, in part because of the widely publicized horrors of addiction to crack cocaine. But America is still the leading drug-consuming nation in the world: Some 60 percent of all illicit drugs are sold in the continental United States. And 41 percent of users in the United States are women—more than ever before.

Marijuana. According to the National Institute on Drug Abuse (NIDA), marijuana is the most commonly used illegal substance. NIDA estimates that three of five Americans between eighteen and twenty-five have used it at least once. "Grass" is usually smoked, but it sometimes shows up in baked goods, such as brownies.

Depending on one's mood and the type and quality of the marijuana, this drug is used for social interaction or private rumination or sexual enhancement. It's even used to mute the boredom of a long drive—but given the fact that marijuana slows reaction time and impairs both coordination and visual perception, popping a tape into the deck and singing along would be much less dangerous.

Marijuana's acceptability is entrenched among the current younger generation, who regard it as safe, natural, and organic—exactly as past generations of youth have thought of it. "Dealing," or selling, marijuana typically bears no stigma among young people.

Wise students, though, are cautious about smoking too much marijuana: Repeated use saps energy and motivation—which achieving students can't afford to be without—and marijuana interferes with the ability to think, make judgments, and solve problems.

Psychedelic Drugs. Lysergic acid diethylamide (LSD), or "acid," was the chemically invented drug that informed the mood, music, and art of the 1960s drug culture in America. A tiny dot of LSD dabbed on paper, when ingested, delivers a six- to eight-hour "trip." In the sixties and seventies, people "dropped a tab of windowpane" at rock concerts or on party weekends or with one or more friends in a shared ritual experience. LSD was regarded as spiritually illuminating and mind-expanding.

The posters, fashions, and general look of the hippie era reflected the visual experience of tripping: phantasmagoric images of wavy lines and amorphous, melting shapes and colors. In the 1980s, when hippie spirituality was out and *anything* reminiscent of the era was generally regarded as uncool, LSD more or less faded away. But LSD is making a comeback these days, showing up frequently on the current concert scene, though without its previous spiritual aura. Today it's just another recreational drug for seekers of sensation.

Psilocybin mushrooms ("magic mushrooms") are also popular again after a decade's virtual absence from the scene. They deliver a shorter psychedelic experience than LSD, but because they're an organic substance, they're preferred by the environmentally conscious.

Phencyclidine (PCP), another psychedelic agent, is actually a horse tranquilizer that, when ingested by humans, promotes extreme and sometimes violent behavior. Users, especially adventurous young males, are drawn to it because it fosters attempts at superhuman feats of strength or macho derring-do.

Cocaine. More than eight million Americans, half of them women, use cocaine. Coke has been called the most ladylike of drugs because it's slimming, it's sensual, and it inspires self-confidence and a sense of empowerment. In its customary powder form it's easy to carry, conceal, and use—"doing a line" means sniffing up a small amount that has been tapped out on a mirror—and it delivers a strong illusion of exhilaration, extra energy, intense concentration, and the impression of brilliant intellectual lucidity.

Once believed nonaddictive, cocaine, as a result of its widespread abuse from the 1960s onward, has disproved that dangerous assumption. Today recreational drug users know that a cocaine craving can override desires for food, water, sex, and sleep. A recent survey showed that 53 percent of young adults are well aware of the hazards of even casual use.

Crack cocaine began to appear in the inner cities in the 1980s and is probably the most horrifying addictive drug ever to come upon the scene. Once inhaled, it almost instantly hooks the user. Crack addiction is so severe and so instantaneous, it can clear out a bank account within days after the first trial hit. Crack addicts are willing to do virtually anything to get their fix: They've been known literally to sell all they possess to maintain their habit, and, when the possessions are gone, they either sell their body or commit robbery and even assault. Crack has ruined so many lives so quickly that its notoriety seems to have reduced overall drug abuse in the nation, while pushing up the crime rate almost exponentially. Crack is one drug that fully lives up to its negative publicity.

Heroin. A chemical derivative of opium, heroin has been a social scourge in America for half a century or more. Those addicted (and a demanding, driving addiction comes readily) find it nearly impossible to break the habit, to "kick." As a powder, heroin can be inhaled ("snorted"). When dissolved over heat, it's either injected under the skin ("skin popping") or into a vein directly into the bloodstream ("mainlining"). The word *fix* is used for a dose of heroin because addicts literally need fixing; too much time without a fix makes them physically ill. A fix makes them feel repaired, inducing a relaxed, drowsy, peaceful state for the hours during which the drug remains in effect.

Methamphetamine. Methamphetamine, known as "crystals" or "crystal meth," produces some of the compulsive behavior caused by heroin derivatives—addicts are constantly worried about supply and availability—yet it enjoys considerable currency in the middle class because many users maintain their habit for extended periods in complete secrecy while holding down good jobs and conducting relationships with their unsuspecting partners. Crystal meth reportedly lifts the spirits: It delivers a sense of intellectual superiority, of being on top of any problem or question that may arise. Users wonder how they ever got along without it. But when they *try* to do so, they find escape extremely difficult.

PRESCRIPTION DRUG ABUSE

Approximately half the drug emergencies dealt with in U.S. hospital emergency rooms are a result of abusing legal *drugs, either prescribed or over-the-counter.*

Probably the most commonly abused drugs are painkillers and tranquilizers. It isn't uncommon for postoperative patients or accident victims to seek more relief from pain by taking more—sometimes far more—of a painkiller than is prescribed. But some painkillers contain codeine, for example, and people may also use these drugs for recreation, to get high. Stimulants and antidepressants are mood-altering drugs, so these, too, are attractive to some people for reasons other than what they're intended for. And many tranquilizers are popularly used for sexual enhancement.

The related problem of overmedication may also arise from confusion. Many patients, especially the elderly, have difficulty remembering what pills they took when, making it easy to overdose or wrongly combine certain drugs meant to be taken at different times. Inexpensive pill dispensers with individual compartments for days of the week can be the solution when several medications must be taken every day or even several times a day and one's memory isn't quite what it used to be. These are available at most pharmacies and discount stores.

On another front altogether, anabolic steroids, which are prescribed legitimately for only a few ailments, are illegally used by both male and female athletes and body builders to enlarge muscles to prodigious proportions. Such use of steroids can have unintended and dangerous side effects like enlargement of the heart and an increased risk of other cardiovascular problems.

In women taking anabolic steroids male characteristics, including body hair, masculine voices, and higher blood level of male hormones than in normal men, may develop. These drugs also cause dangerous increases in artery-clogging cholesterol.

THE NAME GAME:
DRUGS ON THE STREET

Heroin. *Chemical name: diacetylmorphine, a.k.a. junk, smack, dope, horse, H, big H, express, boy, brown sugar, crap, skag. Users talk about "buying medicine," "getting well," or "getting straight" because an addict deprived of heroin becomes increasingly sick (chills, cold sweats, nausea, lack of appetite) until the next fix is "scored." Traditional use is through inhalation ("snorting") or hypodermic injection ("shooting up"), either into the skin ("skin popping") or into a vein ("mainlining"). But the risk of HIV infection and telltale needle marks, or "tracks," left in the skin has many users now burning heroin on aluminum foil and sucking in the vapor through tubes.*

Laughing Gas. *Chemical name: nitrous oxide, a.k.a. gas. Small, compressed cartridges of nitrous oxide purchased over the counter, marketed legally as a propellant for whipped-cream dispensers, are called "whippets." The most common form of use is piercing the cartridge with a small metal or plastic device known as a "whippetizer" and inflating a balloon, then inhaling the gas from the balloon.*

Cocaine. *Chemical name: 2 beta-carbomethoxy-3 deltabenoxytropane, a.k.a. coke, C, CO, blow, snow, lady, flake, gold dust, lines, rock, Bolivian marching powder. Said to be one of the original ingredients in Coca-Cola, cocaine was once used as a stimulant by Sigmund Freud. In powder form it's extremely addictive over time but not instantaneously so, unlike its hybrid form, crack. Cocaine is snorted by most users. However, aficionados developed a means of vaporizing the coke to provide a powerful initial rush. This method, known as "freebasing" with the product called "freebase," was eclipsed by the advent of crack, a form of ready-made solid freebase that can be smoked in a water pipe or in a small glass tube known as a "stem." Crack is called "base" when smoked from water pipes; it's also known on the street as "bubba."*

Marijuana. *Proper name: cannabis, a.k.a. pot, grass, reefer, bud, the green, smoke, herb, ganja, rasta, dope, weed, doob-age, hemp. The last person heard calling it "Mary Jane" was George Carlin in the early 1970s, though Louis Armstrong called it "Mary Warner." Street dealers call it "sens," mispronouncing* sinse, *short for sinsemilla, a seedless strain of the plant. Rolled marijuana cigarettes are called joints, J's, bones, reefers, spliffs, doobs, doobies, and sticks. The latest rage among the young is to smoke marijuana rolled in the outer leaves of cheap Phillies Blunt cigars, which is then known as "Blunts" or "Phillies." More commonly it's smoked in small pipes or water pipes called "bongs." Getting high is known as getting stoned, low, loaded, baked, fried, crispy-fried, wasted, burnt, lifted, buzzed, or zooted.*

Hashish. *Also known as boo, mezz, hash, and tar. It is a concentrated chunk of cannabis resin (see* Marijuana*).*

LSD. *Proper name: lysergic acid diethylamide, a.k.a. acid, windowpane, blotter trips, hits, doses, tabs, fry, double barrel. A powerful synthetic hallucinogen, LSD is taken in very small doses, or microdots. "Electric kool-aid" is Kool-Aid mixed with LSD. A "trip" can last up to eighteen hours.*

Mushrooms. *Proper name: psilocybin, a.k.a. magic mushrooms, 'shrooms, 'shroom-age, trips, caps, fungus. More "organic" than LSD, this hallucinogen is also shorter acting (about six hours).*

Ecstasy. *Proper name: 3, 4-methylene dioxymethamphetamine (MDMA), a.k.a. ex, Y, power, the party drug. Popular in the gay community and in large clubs, discos, and "raves." It enhances all tactile sensations, making them abnormally pleasant. Some Ecstasy is now being laced with heroin by dealers.*

Speed, Uppers, Crank. Proper name: amphetamines, all in various chemical combinations. Benzedrine is called Bennie, and methamphetamine, a.k.a. methadrine, is called crystal meth, ice, or glass. Most cases of amphetamine abuse in recent years are the result of legal prescriptions.

PCP. Proper name: phencyclidine, a.k.a. angel dust, dust, peace pill, hog. Sold in pills and powder, PCP is a horse tranquilizer. Sometimes smoked in marijuana or tobacco cigarettes, it reduces sensitivity to pain and has been said to facilitate great feats of strength.

Downers. Includes barbiturates, a.k.a. barbs, blues. A wide-ranging class of widely prescribed sedatives. Nonbarbiturate prescription downers include Quaaludes, Valium, Xanax, and Halcion.

Poppers. Proper name: amyl nitrite, a.k.a. amys, snappers, pearls. A chemical compound similar to medications used to relieve the chest pain of angina by briefly enlarging the blood vessels, amyl nitrite comes in small capsules. When crushed in the hand, they release a vapor whose inhalation provides a brief high and is also said to intensify sexual sensations. Butyl nitrite and isobutyl nitrite, less pure, are marketed as liquids in small bottles.

HARMFUL HERBALS

Nowadays a number of people are looking for natural ways to jump-start the body to run at optimal levels or to gain pleasure and stimulation, and they're turning to herbs, specifically, herbal extracts.

Touted as natural, safe ways to boost your spirits, your energy levels, your alertness, your sexual response, and your metabolism, and as a means of getting high or losing weight, these perfectly legal nutritional supplements are found for the most part in health food stores. Thus, of course, they appear to be not just a really terrific idea but actually good for you.

In fact, they can be downright dangerous.

They have names like Ultimate Xphoria, Trim-Maxx Burners, Cloud 9—and for a time, the popular Ecstasy. The ingredient that these herbal preparations have in common is the Chinese ephedra plant. More specifically, it's the crystalline alkaloid that's extracted from this plant, ephedrine (also known as ma huang*), which is a stimulant used in many decongestants for the relief of upper-respiratory maladies such as hay fever, asthma, and nasal congestion.*

In these herbal extract products, ephedrine is combined with caffeine to make a very potent upper. Soon after they are taken, the ephedrine-based pills prompt accelerated heart rate and elevated blood pressure that in some users cause heart attacks, strokes, and seizures, sometimes resulting in death when the pleasure seekers use them chronically or take a lot more than the manufacturer's recommended dosages. There have also been reports of liver failure associated with these herbal stimulants.

Some eighty companies produce these products; none of them is regulated by the FDA since vitamins, minerals, and herbs were reclassified by law in 1994 as food supplements, not drugs. That means that there are no controls on their manufacture or use. In response to the rising number of deaths, some states are now clamping down on some herbal stimulants. And although some companies put cautionary warnings on their ephedrine products, many don't. If you insist on taking them, never exceed the recommended dose.

TOBACCO USE

Up until the last several decades, American attitudes toward smoking were generally enthusiastic. Before World War I, tobacco in every form was extremely popular with men, who readily smoked cigarettes and cigars everywhere. Many chewed tobacco as well, and spittoons were a common amenity in the lobbies of the country's better hotels right into the late 1930s. On the other hand, before women got the vote in 1920, few of *them* smoked. It was considered "cheap," unladylike. Smoking was a thing men did.

With women's suffrage and political equality of the sexes came a social revolution. Skirts quickly rose from ankle to kneecap, and many young women took up smoking cigarettes. Shocked conservative elements condemned these widespread departures from propriety, but there was no returning. Many women saw smoking as a right, a means of expressing their daring new independence: Lighting up in public made them "modern," "smart," maybe even a little "fast." Then Lucky Strike weighed in with an ad campaign that urged women, "Reach for a Lucky instead of a sweet," and tens of thousands of women wanting to be svelte did exactly that.

By the late 1930s, cigarettes in the movies had become a metaphor for sex. Nearly all Hollywood love scenes showed the stars smoking in the initial stages of intimacy. As matters heated up between them—and because censorship prevented films from depicting anything specifically sexual—the camera discreetly cut away to the image of the two cigarettes, abandoned in an ashtray and smoldering together. Many movie stars (Bette Davis, notably) knew that their glamour was inextricably connected to their smoking. In fact, Davis later acknowledged that she couldn't have "existed" without a cigarette in her hand.

During World War II, cigarettes were rationed to civilians ("Lucky Strike Has Gone to War"), who stood in long lines to get their smokes. But free packs were distributed to the troops as fast and as often as they could be shipped to the front.

Through the 1950s and into the 1960s, America continued to be a nation of smokers. But, invisibly, the tide was starting to turn. Foes of smoking began to organize resistance and influence the powerful. Then in 1964 the U.S. Surgeon General issued a blockbuster report linking tobacco to cancer, heart disease, and other serious ailments, and Congress passed a law requiring cigarette manufacturers to print a warning to that effect on their products. In 1971 cigarette advertising was banned from TV and radio, and in 1988 smoking was banned on all domestic air carriers. This was the beginning of the end of smokers' dominance in American social life, setting off a pendulum swing away from the habit that had been so enthusiastically embraced by American culture.

Tobacco has been linked to oral cancers (mouth, lips, salivary glands, tongue, and throat), as well as esophageal, stomach, and lung cancers. While about 80 percent of smokers do not get cancer per se, many die of pulmonary diseases such as emphysema and heart and other circulatory diseases. In fact, smoking causes about one thousand deaths a day in this country.

Passive smoking—inhaling other people's cigarette smoke—was an unrecognized hazard until fairly recently. But research indicates that secondhand smokers, and children in particular, suffer from increased heart rate, elevated blood pressure level, and constriction of the airways in the lungs.

These hazards became the premise on which smoking in airplanes was disallowed. In 1993 the Environmental Protection Agency pronounced secondhand smoke a health hazard, and it's regarded as anyone's right to object to cigarette smoke in common spaces, even those in the designated smoking areas of sidewalk cafés.

The public response to the revelations about the health risks of tobacco to smokers and anyone near them has, over time, made smokers an embattled lot. Many city and state laws against smoking have driven smokers out of the workplace, out of hotel lobbies and waiting rooms of airports and train stations, and out of halls and restaurants. Smokers often feel like pariahs in their own community and express shame at their inability or unwillingness to quit. But many continue to smoke despite their guilt and fear. American smokers still number about fifty million strong, consuming some eighty million packs of cigarettes daily. To keep them loyal, tobacco companies spend more than $2 billion a year on advertising and promotion.

But they are definitely going against the tide. The longtime influence of legislators from tobacco-growing states has waned, and the tobacco industry has lost the federal clout it once enjoyed. Efforts are currently afoot to have nicotine declared addictive, thereby reclassifying tobacco and making it liable to control as a drug.

TEENAGE SMOKING

More than anything else, American teenagers want to be independent, to defy authority, and at the same time *to be just like their peers*. That agenda is, in part, a biological imperative, but, unfortunately, it is also one that makes cigarette smoking one of the most attractive things they can do, especially when authority figures are particularly down on the practice.

Young people know perfectly well that tobacco isn't an illegal substance, so it doesn't carry the dire consequences associated with illicit or street drugs. They also know it's bad for their health, and that makes it all the more attractive. Besides, at their age they think they're immortal, and they're also sure they couldn't possibly get hooked.

Past studies sought to prove that teenagers were more likely to smoke in households where one or both parents smoked. But many parents *don't* smoke anymore, so peer pressure seems to be the greater culprit now (and perhaps always was).

While smoking has been in steady decline since the 1960s, it's on the rise among teenage girls. Some studies show that it's tied to weight maintenance and loss, and that association often makes it harder for girls to quit than boys. Smoking is also, of course, a way for girls to seem sophisticated, just as it was for their flapper great-grandmothers.

More than half of today's smokers started before the age of eighteen, and about a million young people a year start smoking even earlier. These new smokers are deaf to warnings that lung damage and atherosclerosis can start early. Like generations of teenagers before them, they're sure it can never happen to them. But it can.

How can you help? Preventing smoking is easier than stopping smoking. You yourself can begin by being a good role model—when you smoke, that's almost like giving your teens license to do the same. So quit smoking if you are a smoker.

Teach your teens about smoking. Make sure they know what it means, in both the long and the short term, to their health. Help your youngsters recognize the power of peer pressure—teach them that strong people follow their own instincts. And make sure the limits are clear. If they start smoking, there should be a consequence. Maybe it's picking up every cigarette butt off the ground at the nearest teenage hangout. But your youngster should truly understand the consequences of his or her actions.

QUITTING SMOKING

It's said that quitting smoking is harder than quitting heroin, but in an increasingly smoker-unfriendly era, millions and millions of former smokers have managed it.

Significant aids have been developed to assist the smoker who wants to quit, notably nicotine gum and the nicotine skin patch. When chewed, the gum delivers a dose of nicotine just as smoking does. The patch does essentially the same job; applied every day, often to the upper arm, it delivers nicotine through the skin surface in controlled amounts while the smoker gets used to living without the behaviors and rituals that are part of smoking habituation: opening the cigarette pack, putting the cigarette into the mouth and lighting it, lighting up before making a phone call, after sex, and so on. Over time, the patch or gum become unnecessary.

A recent study has concluded that watching the clock may be the most effective stop-smoking program yet. The regimen begins with the smoker's counting the total cigarettes habitually smoked daily and evenly scheduling them throughout the day. The second week that number is cut by one third; the week after that they're cut by another third, and so on, until they're cut back to none. This strategy has produced a 44 percent success rate after one year, significantly higher than quitting cold turkey or using either nicotine gum or a nicotine patch.

A BITTER BEAN

You've finally made the decision to quit smoking, but the nagging need for oral satiety is a constant companion. You've tried gums, you've tried hard candies, you've tried everything short of sticking your thumb in your mouth, but nothing removes that cigarette craving. Maybe it's because you've been substituting the wrong taste.

The solution may be as close as your nearest supermarket, health food store, or Starbucks.

Dale was a heavy smoker—a very *heavy smoker: over three packs a day. She lit up virtually the moment her eyes opened in the morning, and the last thing she did at night was stub out a butt. So when she made the decision to quit, she knew she'd have to do so cold turkey; one puff and she'd be caught up in the whole mechanism of smoking again. Her resolve was fast; sticking to that resolve, though, was about the hardest thing she had ever done.*

A three-pack-a-day habit of more than twenty years' duration wasn't an easy thing to kick—and nicotine was only part of it. The rituals that go along with smoking are many and pervasive. And Dale hadn't realized how firmly attached to them she was until they weren't there any longer. She realized how automatic some of the rituals had become—such as lighting up whenever she made a phone call and, of course, those all-important after-dinner and postcoital cigarettes.

Recognizing and gradually eliminating the ritualistic aspects of smoking helped break some of its hold on her, but what she missed most was having something in her mouth that wasn't sugary. She had tried the whole panoply of usual solutions, but she was craving bitter, not sweet—that wonderfully awful taste from a cigarette is nothing *like what you get from a Chiclet. Then an idea hit her: whole coffee beans. To avoid ending up with an accelerated case of the jitters over and above that already provided by nicotine cessation, she used decaf coffee beans.*

Sucking (or chewing, for a really bitter hit) on a coffee bean or three was a great substitute for that foul, acrid taste she had grown so used to from tobacco and that can't be satisfied by a lemon drop. And it worked. Her last cigarette was over thirteen years ago—and she hasn't craved one in almost that long.

So give decaf coffee beans a try. They might nicely fill that empty place in your mouth. Moreover, they're inexpensive, handy, and (a nice bonus) completely noncaloric, so they're a good way to avoid the weight gain that often accompanies quitting smoking.

Cosmetic Surgery

CONTENTS

No one is immune to the changes wrought by time. But with the will—and the financial means—just about anyone who's unhappy with the wrinkling and sagging of old age can, with the assistance of modern medical technology, turn back the clock at least a little. For still-youthful men and women, there are ways to improve on Mother Nature's gifts, particularly where she has been too generous or too stingy.

In their quest for a more youthful face or beautiful body, more and more Americans of all ages and socioeconomic groups are visiting plastic surgeons; since 1981, the number of cosmetic surgeries performed in the United States has increased by more than two thirds.

Virtually any feature on your face can be altered by a skillful surgeon. If you simply can't live with those drooping eyelids, you can have the excess skin removed. A nose that's less than perfect can be remodeled. Skin scarred by teenage acne can be smoothed to a more pleasing appearance. And you need not confine your efforts to changes above the neck; that "jelly belly" that seems to have a life of its own can be nipped and tucked back into shape.

Of course, none of these procedures is inexpensive. Most cosmetic surgery is elective—not medically necessary—so unless a procedure *is* medically indicated (as with a nose that has been broken or interferes with breathing), insurance companies typically will not pay for it. But that does not seem to deter those bent on improving their appearance. Today an estimated 70 percent of households in which a member has had cosmetic surgery have incomes of less than $50,000 a year.

Once you have decided to investigate the possibility of plastic surgery, how do you go about finding the right surgeon? Plastic surgery is one of the fastest growing medical specialties in the country, and surgeons often advertise in local newspapers and the Yellow Pages of the telephone book. Unfortunately, these are probably the least reliable sources of information. A better idea would be to ask your health-care practitioner to recommend two or three, or to call a major hospital in your area for the names of plastic surgeons on staff who perform the procedure you are interested in. If a friend has had a good experience with a plastic surgeon and you like the results, you should probably consider that doctor.

Try to interview the physicians on your list, by phone or in person, before choosing one. Ask whether they are certified by the American Board of Facial, Plastic, and Reconstructive Surgery. While board certification in itself does not guarantee that a surgeon is proficient, he or she does have to pass an examination and meet certain standards to be certified. Also ask how often the surgeon has performed the operation you want (statistics suggest that a more practiced surgical hand is more skillful). Get a ballpark estimate of cost, too.

If you're seriously considering cosmetic surgery, bear in mind that no surgeon can guarantee results; living tissue does not behave in entirely predictable ways. Make certain your expectations are realistic. If you are plain or average-looking, a face-lift or eyelid reduction will not transform you into a beauty queen. Breast augmentation will not solve your marital problems. A session of liposuction won't turn you into the life of the party if your natural inclination is to blend into the walls. What cosmetic surgery *can* do, however, is make you look fresher, firmer, and younger, all of which can boost your morale and self-confidence.

To Lift or Not to Lift?

As a young woman Eileen was a knockout—big brown eyes, high cheekbones, beautiful skin. After she had a baby, at the age of forty-one, she felt her life was going downhill.

She lost her job, spent thousands of dollars on an ugly custody battle, and made the abrupt decision to move with her young son to another city. As the months dragged by and she couldn't find a job she wanted, depression set in, and her looks began to suffer as her spirits sank. As if that wasn't enough, she ran into an old college friend who looked fifteen years younger. Nothing mysterious or miraculous about it, the friend assured her; she'd had a face-lift six months earlier. Eileen dutifully took down the name of the plastic surgeon, but she was skeptical. She'd heard the horror stories of cosmetic surgery gone wrong and had long ago decided it was not for her.

But one day, staring glumly at herself in the mirror, she suddenly thought, "Why not?" and called the surgeon. They discussed at length her reasons for wanting a face-lift—a must in any consultation—before agreeing on the exact procedure itself. A month later she went into the hospital and, in addition to a classic face-lift, had both upper and lower eyelids reduced and her chin liposuctioned.

Although she had expected some pain when she woke up, Eileen was surprised by how incredibly tight her face felt. And, of course, when the bandages came off a week later, she was brutalized by the swelling and bruising she saw in the mirror. She thought she'd been prepared for it, both by her doctor and by what she'd read, but she wasn't. Her eight-year-old son, appraising her later, tried to console her with the reminder that Halloween was just a week away—and wasn't it great that she wouldn't need a costume?

She survived the Boris Karloff phase and decided that, overall, she did look better. Now, three years later, Eileen tells her friends that a face-lift may indeed help their looks and their spirits. "But it is major *surgery," she emphasizes. "If you really just need to get your eyes done, that operation's a snap. The eyes heal well, the scars are virtually invisible, the whole thing's fairly painless. A face-lift is a much bigger deal." She also tells women who ask that if they think a face-lift is going to make them look different, they should think again. It won't. "You've got to be clear on this. You'll still be the same you—looking less tired, more refreshed, maybe younger—but still* you." *(And that's if you've chosen a good surgeon; a less adept one can pull too tight and leave you looking like a Barbie doll.)*

Eileen would do it again, though, because although the face-lift didn't solve all her problems, it did give her enough of a boost to be able to see her options more clearly. Her looks have always been important to her, and now that she doesn't have to worry about them, at least for a while, she can focus on the bigger issues in her life. And that, to her, is worth a lot.

FACE-LIFT

One of the most frequently performed cosmetic surgeries is the face-lift, or rhytidectomy, which contours by removing excess, sagging skin from the jowls and upper neck, making the face appear firmer and younger.

Like all cosmetic surgery, a face-lift is not a panacea. It will not endow a perfect complexion on a woman who has finely wrinkled skin; chemical peel, laser resurfacing, or dermabrasion is a more appropriate remedy for such a problem (see page 173). Nor will a face-lift correct sagging eyelids or bags under the eyes; for that area *blepharoplasty,* a procedure often done in conjunction with the face-lift, is called for (see page 169). Those deep creases extending from the base of the nose to the corner of the mouth that affect most people as they age may be softened by a face-lift, but it will not eliminate them.

The ideal candidate for a face-lift has reasonably firm, smooth skin and stable weight. The latter is important because fluctuating weight can undermine the benefits of a face-lift, as skin stretches with weight gain and sags with weight loss.

At what age does a face-lift achieve the best results? As surprising as it may sound, many cosmetic surgeons say that anyone considering having only one face-lift should have it in her (or his) forties or fifties (depending on the type of skin that the individual has). At that time, the skin is healthier and more resilient.

If you decide to have a face-lift, your surgeon may hospitalize you or do the procedure in an outpatient setting. The operation can usually be performed with local anesthesia with intravenous sedation or with general anesthesia. Your blood pressure, heart rate, and respiration are monitored during the surgery.

With a marking pen the surgeon maps out the incision lines on the skin. The typical incision line runs downward along the natural creases in front of the ears, curves behind the cartilage in front of the ear (the tragus) and around the base of the ear lobe, and then follows the crease behind the ears. About two thirds of the way up the rear of the ear, the incision line will veer toward the hair-bearing scalp for about two inches. A traditional face-lift—also called a skin-supported face-lift—involves lifting a sheet of skin and subcutaneous fat, separating it from its underlying tissue. The superficial layer of muscles is tightened, the excess skin excised, and the incision closed. The unnatural pulled-back appearance that some people experience (sometimes producing a perpetually surprised expression) depends upon how tightly the surgeon performing the procedure stretches the skin.

While many plastic surgeons continue to use this method, others now employ a technique called a deep-plane or composite face-lift. This procedure moves not only the facial skin but the deeper structures such as deep muscles. The results can be dramatic, but this method *is* expensive—it's about twice as expensive as the skin-supported lift—and requires longer recuperation, four to six weeks instead of two.

At the end of the operation, the surgeon applies a sterile dressing to the face. You may be able to go home within a few hours or you may stay in the hospital overnight. Your face will be numb in some areas and may be painful in others; your surgeon may prescribe an analgesic to relieve the discomfort. You should regain feeling in your face within six to twelve weeks.

All sutures are generally removed by the tenth postsurgical day. Expect swelling and discoloration, some of which can be concealed by makeup. Most women who have had skin-supported lifts can return to work two weeks after surgery. During recovery, however, be sure to stay out of the sun for a few weeks to minimize swelling. Most people who undergo a face-lift do not suffer serious complications. Hematoma, a collection of blood under the skin, occurs in about 5 percent of face-lifts. In rare cases, the skin is injured or a facial nerve damaged.

Many people have repeat face-lifts as they age. How long does a face-lift last? While there are several variables—age at the time of surgery, heredity, condition of the skin, and weight stability—most face-lifts can be expected to last between five and ten years.

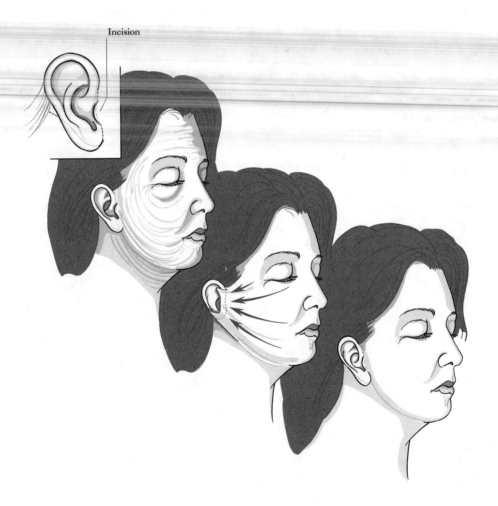

Working from an incision around the ear, the cosmetic surgeon will gently pull the skin across the face to tighten the tissues. Excess skin will then be removed before the incision is closed.

NOSE RECONSTRUCTION

Many people are unhappy with the size and/or shape of their nose, and it is true that, as the most prominent feature in the face, the nose plays a major role in the way one looks. Perhaps that is why *rhinoplasty*—surgery to improve the appearance of the nose—is one of the most common cosmetic surgical procedures.

Unlike most other facial cosmetic surgeries, rhinoplasty is generally performed during early adulthood, although an increasing number of middle-aged people have their nose fixed. Even older people are turning to rhinoplasty to reverse the drooping that typically occurs as the nose ages.

The shape of the nose is determined by a labyrinth of bone and cartilage. Trauma to the nose during childhood can result in a deformity that isn't apparent until adulthood. Any injury may heal in an abnormal position. Congenital problems may also result in an unsightly nose. And, of course, there is the heredity factor.

Most people who consult a surgeon about rhinoplasty do so because they don't like the way their nose looks, but in some cases medical reasons may dictate the need for correction. For example, a deviated septum—the partition that separates the nose's two cavities—can interfere with breathing. Psychological factors may also justify nose surgery, particularly in teenagers, for whom physical appearance and social acceptance are synonymous.

As a rule, it is much easier to make large noses smaller than to build up small noses. Noses with bumps generally benefit from rhinoplasty, but noses that look crooked from the front are more difficult to correct, as are extremely thick-skinned noses. In addition, many people who think their nose is too large actually have a chin that is too small, and this imbalance can be corrected by a chin implant, alone or in combination with rhinoplasty (see *Chin Surgery*, page 170).

Should you decide on rhinoplasty, your surgeon will take pictures of you beforehand and discuss the changes that he or she would recommend to improve the appearance of your nose, taking into consideration your age, facial anatomical features, and the quality of your skin. The surgeon will also discuss your expectations with you to make sure your goals are realistic. It is important to keep in mind that the goal of rhinoplasty is not to give you an ideal nose but a nose that you feel will better complement your face than does the one with which you were born.

Most rhinoplasty today is done in an outpatient setting under a local anesthetic, although your doctor will give you sedatives to relax you. During surgery, the skin of the nose is separated from the underlying bone and cartilage, usually from the inside of the nose (which makes it a difficult surgical procedure, because the surgeon has to proceed as much by feel as by sight). If it is necessary to make an incision on the outside of the nose, it is made in an inconspicuous spot to avoid a visible external scar. Then the surgeon reshapes the bone by cutting, trimming, fracturing, and augmenting. The skin is redraped, the nose is packed with gauze to prevent bleeding, and a metal or plaster splint is fashioned over the new nose.

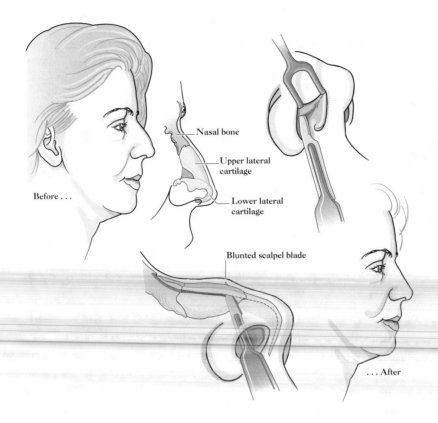

Nasal bone

Upper lateral
cartilage

Lower lateral
cartilage

Blunted scalpel blade

Before . . .

. . . After

Working from inside the nostril, the surgeon will first separate the skin from the structures within, the cartilage and bone. Excess nasal bone and cartilage are then removed to refine the external shape of the nose.

When you feel well enough to go home, you will be instructed to stay in bed with your head elevated for twenty-four hours to minimize swelling and discoloration. Cold compresses will also be recommended. While you may experience some discomfort, particularly in the first twenty-four hours, pain is usually not severe. Five to seven days after surgery, the splint is removed. Expect your nose to be somewhat swollen at this time; most of the swelling is gone by the end of the second postoperative week. Six weeks or so after the splint is removed, the bones in the nose should be completely healed. However, the final result, especially at the tip of the nose, will not be apparent for up to a year afterward because of the thickness of the skin tissue.

As for complications, the most common is the development of a fullness in the tip of the nose, the result of an accumulation of scar tissue. In most cases this can be treated with cortisone injections. Bleeding sometimes occurs but usually can be controlled by pinching the tip of the nose with the fingers for a few minutes. Infection, while rare, can be dangerous. In 5 to 10 percent of patients, a second, fairly minor operation may be necessary to revise or adjust the results of the first.

EYELID SURGERY

As people age, their eyelids begin to droop and the area below the eyes sags. This is a natural part of the aging process that happens to everyone eventually. But some people, because of a hereditary tendency, may experience these changes relatively early in middle age or especially severely. Aside from making one look perpetually tired and older than one's years, sometimes drooping upper eyelids can even interfere with vision.

The procedure most commonly performed on the eyes to correct the bags and sags of middle and advanced age is called *blepharoplasty*, and it is one of the oldest procedures in the history of cosmetic surgery. It involves the removal of excess fat and skin above and below the eyes and is often performed in conjunction with a face-lift. It is also frequently done alone, especially in younger people who do not yet need the more extensive procedure.

If you are considering blepharoplasty, you should understand that while it can significantly reduce baggy eyelids, it will not make fifty-year-old eyes look twenty-five again. Nor will it eliminate crow's feet at the corners of the eyes, though you may notice a slight improvement. Neither will it completely eliminate large bags under the lower lids.

Cosmetic surgery of the eyelids is usually done under local anesthesia in the plastic surgeon's office, in an outpatient center, or in the ambulatory surgery department in a hospital. After you are sedated and the area around your eyes has been anesthetized, the surgeon

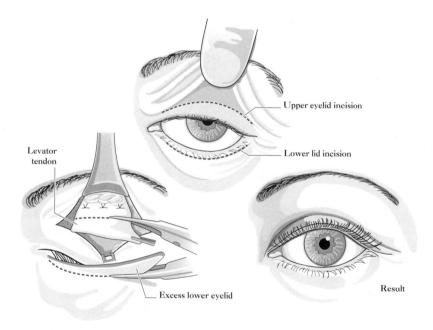

In performing a blepharoplasty, the cosmetic surgeon will make incisions in the lids above and below the eye. The doctor will tighten the tendon above the eye, remove excess fat from below, then tighten the skin before closing.

makes incisions in the fold of the eyelid and just below the lower lash line. Excess fat and skin are removed and the incisions closed with tiny stitches. After a few hours of observation, you are allowed to go home.

Expect to have some swelling, tenderness, and redness. Your surgeon may advise ice packs for a couple of hours to minimize swelling and bruising. Keep in mind that one eye may heal more quickly than the other. Since no one's face is perfectly symmetrical, don't expect the surgery to have made one side of your face a mirror image of the other.

While blepharoplasty has fewer complications than most cosmetic surgery procedures, problems do sometimes occur. During the surgery, minute blood vessels are disturbed, and the disturbance may create small hematomas (blood under the skin). In most cases, the hematomas last only a few days and then disappear. In the first few hours after surgery, you may also experience double vision, which is caused by the eye's reacting to its musculature's being disturbed. The problem should clear up within a few hours. Some people are also bothered by excessive tearing, but that should resolve itself in the first few days. Another phenomenon that plagues some patients is the inability to close the eyes completely when they sleep, but this, too, is almost always temporary.

A serious, albeit rare problem associated with blepharoplasty is ectropion, which occurs when too much skin is removed from the lower eyelid, which then turns outward. Tears fall directly from the lid instead of passing over the conjunctiva (the membrane that lines the eyelid and covers the front of the eyeball) and lubricating the eyeball. When ectropion is severe, it can be surgically corrected. Visual impairment or even blindness has occurred in a handful of patients who have had blepharoplasty.

After surgery, do not hesitate to call your plastic surgeon should you have problems. Signs of a potential problem include excessive swelling that does not subside gradually, redness that worsens over time, increased pain or tenderness around the eyes, and vision problems.

CHIN SURGERY

Aside from the nose, no facial feature is as important to the profile as the chin. Whether a chin is "weak" or unusually prominent, it can undermine what might otherwise be an attractive face. Of course, too much or too little chin is less of a handicap for men than for women; men have the option of disguising a weak chin with a beard, and a large chin is often considered a sign of strength or character. Women with a big chin, on the other hand, have no such compensations.

Like any other part of our body, the chin comes in various shapes and sizes, most of which fall into the acceptable range and do not seriously detract from one's appearance. The ideal chin position can be estimated by a line dropped perpendicular to the border of the lower lip. If, in profile, the chin aligns with this line, that is considered its ideal position. A chin that falls short of this imaginary line is considered receding or underdeveloped; one that juts beyond it is overdeveloped or prominent.

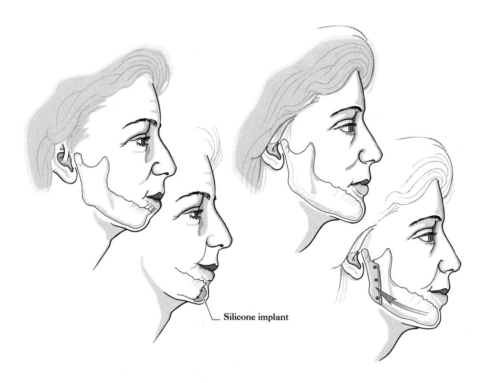

Silicone implant

To enlarge a chin, implants can be located under the skin either beneath the chin or below the lower lip (left); to reduce the size of the chin, a segment of the chin bone can be removed and the chin brought back and fastened in place (right).

In many cases people with chin abnormalities have other facial problems. A large nose is often associated with a weak chin and a sloping forehead; an estimated 15 percent of rhinoplasty (corrective nose surgery) patients could also benefit from chin augmentation. Protruding chins frequently occur in conjunction with lips that overlap. Problems with the teeth and jaws sometimes accompany overly large chins.

Years ago, weak chins were built up with living bone or cartilage. These days, surgeons have the added option of silicone rubber implants. This technique is generally considered superior to bone and cartilage grafts, which often decrease in size over the years as they are gradually absorbed into the body, although some surgeons believe the chance of success with grafts is higher because they use the patient's own bone. Chin implants are inserted through incisions made in the skin just under the chin or inside the lower lip. The primary advantage of the latter is that it leaves no visible scar. When the degree of chin recession is severe, many surgeons cut the bone and move it forward; this avoids the use of an extremely large implant, which is more likely to cause complications than a smaller one. Likewise, if a chin is very short, the bone is sliced horizontally and packed with wedges of bone graft.

If the problem is a chin that is too large, more extensive surgery is necessary. When the teeth are not involved, the surgeon may reduce the size of the chin by removing a segment of bone with an electrical saw, sliding the lower segment into position, and wiring it in place until it heals. The incision—three to four inches long—can be made either inside the mouth or under the chin. In cases in which a large chin is associated with a bite problem, more extensive jaw surgery, and sometimes orthodontia as well, is necessary.

Complications vary, depending on the exact procedure. Infection sometimes occurs with chin implants and may be serious enough to warrant removal of the foreign object. After the infection has cleared up, the implant can be replaced several months later, although often sufficient scar tissue forms to enlarge the chin naturally. Implants can sometimes erode the bone, making the recession more acute. Surgery to diminish chin size or realign bone or teeth also can be complicated by infection, but a more common side effect is numbness in the chin and front teeth, which usually subsides within six months.

CHEEK AUGMENTATION

One sign of classic beauty in many societies is high cheekbones, which with the eyebrows frame and accentuate the eyes. Not only are high cheekbones considered attractive, but women who are blessed with them tend to look younger longer than their flatter-cheeked friends.

It used to be that either you had high cheekbones or you didn't. Women who didn't learned to become adept with blushers and creams designed to fool the eye. Recently, however, increasing numbers of women have opted for surgery to reshape facial contours permanently.

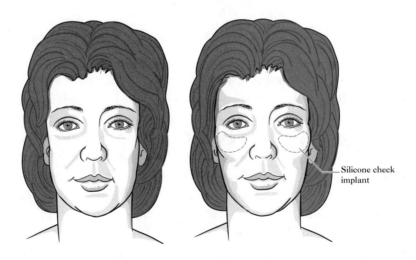

Silicone check implant

Silicone rubber implants can be inserted beneath the skin of the cheek to augment the appearance of the cheekbones.

Like a chin that falls short of one's ideal, cheeks that don't measure up can be enhanced with silicone rubber implants. Sometimes the cheeks are augmented in conjunction with a face-lift. Otherwise the implants are inserted through incisions made inside the upper lip or in the lower eyelid.

Cheek augmentation is generally performed in the doctor's office under local anesthesia. Afterward the face is bruised, swollen, and more numb than painful, but these discomforts usually subside within ten days or so. The implants themselves may be sensitive to the touch for several weeks.

Higher cheekbones may radically alter the shape of your face. If your face is long, it will appear more oval; if it is round, it should look less flat and more balanced. It is unrealistic to expect perfect symmetry—most people do not have perfectly symmetrical cheeks to begin with—but any differences should be minor and will probably not be noticed by anyone but you. If anything, that bit of subtle asymmetry often makes a face more interesting.

SKIN TREATMENTS

A woman can have virtually every feature on her face lifted or reshaped yet, if her skin is wrinkled or scarred, still not look young. To achieve that dewier, healthier-looking skin, many women are turning to a variety of cosmetic procedures.

Since ancient times people have sought ways to refine the skin by removing surface blemishes and wrinkles. The Egyptians tried such abrasive materials as salt, alabaster, and limestone. Sulfur paste and pumice have been used well into the twentieth century. The first power-driven abrasive tool, a wire brush, is still used, but diamond sanders are more common now.

Modern skin rejuvenation techniques work on the same principle—removing the outer layers of skin and sometimes part of the deeper dermal layer—with the result that imperfections such as acne scars, wrinkles, and age spots are diminished. The "new" skin that emerges is smoother, finer, and younger-looking. *Dermabrasion* removes skin mechanically, in a technique much like sanding. In a *chemical peel*, exfoliation is produced by application of a caustic solution. Cosmetic *laser surgery*, the newest technique, vaporizes the top skin layers with a very precise, controlled laser beam.

Facial pitting from acne responds well to all three techniques, although they are generally more effective for small and shallow scars than for larger, deeper pits. The fine lines and wrinkles of aging or sun damage are treated with deeper chemical peels and abrasion. Carbon dioxide lasers, which have been used for many years in other kinds of surgery, allow the surgeon a greater degree of control than the other techniques and are used widely in the treatment of birthmarks, warts, dilated capillaries, and benign tumors as well as the more common problems described.

Surgical skin treatments are generally performed on an outpatient basis in the doctor's office. Before dermabrasion, many doctors freeze the area to anesthetize it and keep it firm, making it easier to remove tissue uniformly. Otherwise, for all procedures, a local anesthetic

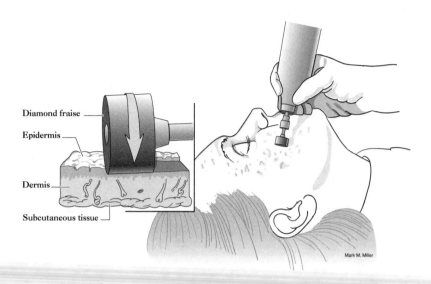

Diamond fraise

Epidermis

Dermis

Subcutaneous tissue

Mark M. Miller

Dermabrasion is a procedure that mechanically abrades or "sands" off the outer layer (epidermis) of the skin, causing a new and younger-looking layer to grow in its place.

is injected under the skin. At the end of the procedure, the area is either left exposed, treated with ointment, or covered with a light dressing. During the healing period the skin is puffy and red, as though sunburned. It is critical that the patient stay out of the sun for several weeks.

Superficial skin treatments are increasingly popular for minor skin problems, partly because they entail fewer risks than do deeper versions. Possible side effects of deeper chemical peels and dermabrasion are changes in skin pigment, scarring, and bleeding. Although laser surgery is preferred by some surgeons (who claim patients heal more quickly), the risks and benefits are still being evaluated. One caveat should be stressed: Laser surgery *must* be performed by a surgeon trained and certified to use carbon dioxide lasers.

A more important caveat, of course, is that none of these techniques can guarantee perfect skin. But the new skin under the old *will* be smoother and healthier looking, and for most patients that is more than sufficient.

EAR RECONSTRUCTION

While many cosmetic facial imperfections are not apparent early in life, big ears are unmistakable. Large, protruding ears, thought to be simply a hereditary trait, are hardly hazardous to one's health, but children born with this abnormality may soon know the ridicule of playmates. The impact on some children's developing egos can be significant and may lead to extreme self-consciousness and social withdrawal.

The medical solution is *otoplasty*, the repair or correction of unsightly ears, which can be performed on any patient above the age of four.

Like any body part, ears vary considerably in shape and size. But one characteristic that normal ears have in common is location. The average ear extends from eyebrow level to the base of the nose and projects from the head at a fifteen- to thirty-degree angle. Ears that project at a greater angle can be said to protrude, and thus become a distinguishing rather than unremarkable feature.

Three basic anatomical abnormalities cause prominent ears: lack of a fold in the outer ear, which makes the edge stick out; an excessively deep outer ear opening (the conchal bowl); or a protruding earlobe.

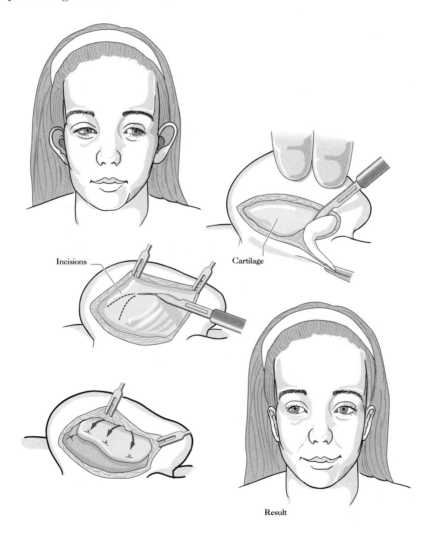

In an otoplasty, *or ear reconstruction, an ellipse of skin is removed from the back of the ears* (top). *Incisions are then made in the cartilaginous framework of the ear* (center), *allowing the cartilage to overlap upon itself, drawing the ear toward the head* (bottom).

Otoplasty is ideally performed when a child is five or six, when ear cartilage is sufficiently mature to withstand surgery but before the child enters school and is subjected to teasing by classmates. Most surgeons agree, however, that children should have some say in whether or not their ears should be "fixed"; parents should be alert to problems or complaints and encourage a child who's being teased to consider the operation, but they should not force it on a child who otherwise seems confident and well adjusted.

Most otoplasty on children is performed in the hospital. General anesthesia is typically used for young children and a combination of sedatives and local anesthetic for older children and adults. Reshaping techniques vary, but most involve modifying or removing cartilage and skin through an incision in the back of the ear and then using sutures to remold the remaining cartilage. After the new ears are in place, a sterile dressing is applied.

The first day or so after surgery is usually very uncomfortable. The surgeon will prescribe a pain medication and recommend bed rest with the head elevated. Usually the dressings are removed a day or so after the operation—so that the doctor can check for hematoma, blood accumulating beneath the skin surface—and then reapplied. Most swelling and discoloration subside within four to seven days, when the dressings and stitches are removed. Some swelling and tenderness may persist for a few weeks. To protect the ears from trauma, the patient must wear a tennis or ski headband for three or four weeks.

Most people who have had otoplasty do not experience serious complications. The most common problem is hematoma. Infection, while rare, can be very dangerous. Heavy scarring around the incision also sometimes occurs, particularly in dark-skinned individuals. Another risk is that the protrusion will recur. If this happens—though it rarely does—it is almost always within a few weeks of the procedure and is corrected with another operation. When otoplasty is successful, the results are permanent.

BREAST RECONSTRUCTION, REDUCTION, AND AUGMENTATION

Over the last few decades, cosmetic surgery designed to enlarge or diminish breasts—or even re-create a breast that has been removed—has become relatively common.

More recently, however, silicone implants used for both breast reconstruction and augmentation have been reported to rupture or leak into surrounding tissue, triggering concerns (as yet unconfirmed) about such adverse health effects as autoimmune disease. Other possible risks include hardening of the breasts (caused by calcium deposits or contracture of scar tissue), "gel bleed" (small, gradual leakage of silicone), and changes in nipple and breast sensitivity.

In 1992, the Food and Drug Administration declared a moratorium on the distribution and use of silicone-gel implants. While a panel appointed by the FDA ruled that allegations of safety risks were inconclusive and recommended that the products remain on the market, the panel also imposed severe new restrictions on their use.

Currently, the only women who may receive silicone-gel implants are those who were born with congenital deformities of the breast or those who desire breast reconstruction after cancer surgery and agree to be part of a clinical study to determine the implants' safety. This policy therefore excludes most cosmetic surgery for enlarging or reshaping the breasts using silicon gel (although saline implants are still available for cosmetic surgery of the breast). By 1992, an estimated two million women had breast implants; less than one in four was a breast cancer patient.

So what other options are available should you lose a breast to cancer? If you have had a mastectomy and are averse to reconstruction with a silicone implant, saline implants and

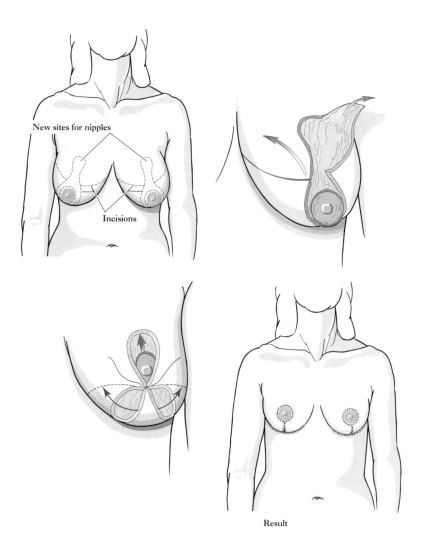

To perform a breast lift, the surgeon will make an incision around the aureolas (top left) *to allow for relocation of the nipples* (top right). *Excess skin is then removed and the central flap rolled up to high position, raising the breasts* (bottom right).

flap reconstruction are other alternatives. Reconstruction involves the removal of tissue from one part of the body, which is moved to the chest to re-create the missing breast. In one form of the surgery, a flap of skin from the abdomen—along with the accompanying muscle, fat, and blood and nerve supply—is "tunneled" under the skin and upward to the chest wall. Tissue for flap reconstruction may also be taken from the back or buttocks.

The advantage of flap surgery, which can be done either immediately after a mastectomy or years later, is that the body does not reject the tissue by forming a hard scar around it, as sometimes occurs with an implant. The breast is also softer and looks more normal than an implant and ages in the same way a natural breast would.

The disadvantage of flap surgery is that it is a major surgical procedure, both lengthy and expensive. Moreover, there is a scar both at the site of the tissue removal and around the breast. Since the surgery requires excess tissue (e.g., from a fleshy abdomen), it is generally not appropriate for very thin women who have little to spare; since part of the abdominal muscles is used in the surgery, abdominal weakness or hernia can be a problem. Women with health problems such as heart disease or diabetes, women who smoke, and women who are excessively overweight may not be good candidates for this surgery.

For women who desire breast augmentation, some doctors use silicone shells filled with a saline (salt water) solution instead of the silicone gel. There is no evidence that saline solution is harmful if it leaks out of the implant, though the implant will need to be replaced if it does leak. These devices are now under FDA scrutiny. As with silicone-filled implants, scar tissue can form around the implant, making it feel and look hard and unnatural. For

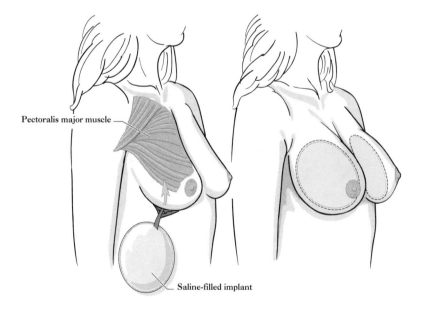

Pectoralis major muscle

Saline-filled implant

Breast implants are inserted over or under the breast through small incisions.

some thin women or those who have undergone a mastectomy, saline implants can be placed not only under the skin but also beneath the muscles for more lift.

A breast lift (or mastopexy), a procedure in which the surgeon removes excess skin to reduce sagging, is another option for women who want to change the shape or size of their breasts. The procedure involves the removal of skin above and next to the nipple, which is then moved higher up on the breast. The "lift" that results is often temporary, unfortunately, and there is scarring to contend with. If an implant is used in conjunction with the breast lift, the effect is more long lasting.

Another technique is breast augmentation mammoplasty by injection. This procedure involves the removal of excess fat from buttocks or thighs, which is then injected into the breasts. However, most surgeons are skeptical of this procedure, arguing that most of the fat will either break down, be absorbed into the bloodstream, or harden into a calcified mass, which will interfere with mammograms, and the injections would have to be repeated.

In general, augmentation procedures do not interfere with the capacity to breast-feed, although breast reduction may.

Many women have the opposite problem—breasts that are too large. Extremely heavy breasts not only are uncomfortable but also often cause back strain and can contribute to breathing difficulties and other health problems. Bra straps may cut uncomfortably into the skin of the shoulders. Participation in sports and other vigorous physical activities is hampered. Emotional problems may result as well, particularly during adolescence, when girls are painfully self-conscious about their bodies.

Oversized breasts are corrected with reduction mammoplasty, which is major surgery and requires hospitalization. Working on one breast at a time, the surgeon removes sections of breast tissue, fat, and skin; recontours the breasts; then centers them on the chest and repositions the nipples. After surgery, the patient has an inverted T-shaped or keyhole-shaped scar under each breast and scars around both nipples. Should she later have a child, she will likely not be able to breast-feed.

As with any surgery, patients can expect pain during the recovery period, as well as swelling, bruising, and sometimes a loss of sensation in the nipples and breast skin (usually temporary). They may not be able to lift their arms or sleep on their side for several weeks, although light exercise may be recommended as early as two weeks after the procedure.

For most women, the discomfort and scarring of breast reduction are a small price to pay for the rewards—physical relief, greater ease of movement, better fit of their clothes, and, for younger women especially, freedom from emotional and social distress.

BREAST IMPLANTS

Since their introduction thirty years ago, breast implants have been both popular and problematic. In that time, more than two million women have received implants, three fourths for cosmetic reasons, the rest for breast reconstruction after mastectomy or injury.

Kate, for example, just never liked her breasts. She always longed for big round breasts. Blanca, on the other hand, hated the thought of wearing a bra after her mastectomy and wanted a balanced, full look under her clothes.

While many women are delighted with their decision to have breast implants, both Kate and Blanca regret their decision. Kate eventually returned to her surgeons and had the implants removed—they had begun to harden. Blanca hasn't actually had problems with hers, but she's tired of feeling anxious about her breasts, and the furor surrounding implants seems to add insult to the injury of her breast cancer.

Few products in recent memory have been as controversial as breast implants. For years virtually everyone thought they were harmless. Then several years ago, along came the first of what soon would be many reports of women who believed they had suffered serious illnesses as a result of ruptured implants.

Early denials by implant manufacturers and many plastic surgeons that implants posed a health risk met with rebuttals from women with implants who felt seriously ill and from the doctors who treated them. In 1992, the Food and Drug Administration declared a moratorium on silicone implants, urging manufacturers to stop marketing the devices and advising surgeons to stop inserting them. A few months later a governmental panel of experts found evidence of safety risks inconclusive and recommended that implants remain on the market. The panel, however, urged doctors to restrict their use of silicone implants to women who need breast reconstruction after surgery. Subsequently two major manufacturers of breast implants agreed to establish a multibillion-dollar fund to help care for women with breast implant problems. After the collapse of the settlement, the lawyers went back into chamber, with a third manufacturer joining the negotiation. A final resolution may not be reached for all the women involved for a very long time.

The question of risk is based on the possibility that the silicone in the implant leaks from its envelope. There is speculation that the body's immune system, in an attempt to fight this silicone invader, produces inflammation and chest pain, and that the silicone can travel to the lungs, liver, and lymph nodes. Once there, silicone may trigger some autoimmune disorders as the body fights the foreign material. A virulent form of joint disease, rheumatoid arthritis; scleroderma (a rare connective tissue disorder that thickens and stiffens the skin and causes fibrous tissue to build up in the lungs and other organs); and lupus erythematosus (another disease of the connective tissues, which causes joint pain, rashes, and fatigue) are some of the ailments that may be linked to silicone implants. A study published in 1994, however, showed no increase in connective tissue disorders in women with silicone breast implants.

Breast implants make clear and accurate mammography difficult, and women with implants must use a special technique to allow mammography to detect small tumors. Whereas a woman with a breast implant—whether or not she has had breast cancer—is not at increased risk for development of cancer, any cancer that may develop may not be diagnosed as early as it would be otherwise.

Before the recent questions arose concerning its safety, silicone implant was the device of choice for 90 percent of women who sought breast reconstruction or breast augmentation. Today, an implant filled with salt water is considered a safe alternative for some. Should a saline implant leak, the solution poses no threat to the system. The drawback, though, is that the saline implant may shift or settle toward the bottom of the breast, causing the skin to stretch and tighten. Moreover, saline implants are not recommended for women who have small breasts or who have undergone a mastectomy because there is not adequate tissue to support the implant. An implant filled with peanut oil, which does not appear to interfere with mammograms, is currently being tested but is not yet available.

Some mastectomy patients may opt to have a new breast constructed with fatty tissue from their stomach or buttocks. This process, however, is time-consuming and expensive, and it isn't a suitable alternative for the thin woman who has very little tissue to spare. Because any health hazards that silicone implants may impose have not been confirmed, many reconstructive surgeons continue to offer them for women who have had mastectomies (see also Breast Reconstruction, Reduction, and Augmentation, *page 176).*

OTHER COSMETIC PROCEDURES

A range of other surgeries are commonly performed for cosmetic reasons. Among them are the following:

Sclerotherapy. Many women have spider-burst leg veins, a condition in which a pattern of bluish veins that resemble the shape of a spider is seen through the skin. Unlike varicose veins, twisted and enlarged veins that afflict one in ten women, spider veins are not painful, although they can be unsightly.

Since they cause no pain, spider veins are easy to ignore. But if they're making you self-conscious, there is a way to get rid of them. Called *sclerotherapy,* the procedure involves the injection of a solution into the visible veins that collapses them and prevents blood from entering them, so the discoloration eventually fades. The treatment does not impair circulation.

Liposuction. The liposuction technique uses a high-powered vacuum pump to remove fat from various parts of the face and body though a small incision. Developed in the mid-1970s by French surgeons, it has been used in the United States since 1982. The advantage of liposuction is that the surgeon gains access to fat deposits without subjecting the patient to a large incision. Areas of the body to which liposuction is commonly applied include the thighs, buttocks, and abdomen. On the face, it may be performed along with a face-lift to alleviate a double chin, heavy jowls, and deep folds between the nose and mouth. Liposuction will *not* cure obesity, eliminate cellulite (scientists have yet to come up with anything that will), or replace a weight loss regimen.

When surgeons in this country began using liposuction to remove extensive pockets of fat, several deaths from shock resulted. Since then, surgeons have made a practice of infusing patients with electrolytes, which are lost when large amounts of fat and fluid are removed. When performed by a doctor trained in the procedure, liposuction is generally considered safe.

Abdominoplasty. Colloquially referred to as a *tummy tuck*, abdominoplasty is often done in conjunction with liposuction but is far more complicated. It involves the removal of excess fat and skin in the abdominal area and tightening with sutures of the muscle wall underneath. The operation is generally performed in a hospital, leaves a linear scar (hipbone to hipbone, occasionally shorter), and entails a prolonged recovery period. Women whose tummy is slack after childbearing are the typical patients, but anyone in good health whose weight is reasonably stable is a good candidate, too. A "minituck" is a partial abdominoplasty performed below the navel, often on an outpatient basis. Recovery takes less time than with the full procedure.

Risks associated with abdominoplasty, which is major surgery, include blood clots (in about 1 percent of patients), bleeding, and infection. For women (and men) with a big, flabby paunch that just won't budge, the results may be well worth the pain and the risks.

CHAPTER 10

Mental Health

CONTENTS

The passages in a woman's life are marked by changes both in her body and in her societal and familial roles. Whether passing from childhood to adolescence, from adolescence to adulthood, or from premenopausal to postmenopausal maturity, each transition offers distinct challenges. Each life change also brings opportunities for profound emotional growth.

A woman's developmental journey begins early in life. It follows a unique and intricate map that, from the moment of conception, interweaves genetic, biological, environmental, social, and situational paths. Birth sets into motion a complicated process by which a child connects with caretaking adults, usually parents, and internalizes aspects of parental love and care. At the same time, the child is compelled to separate herself gradually from those adults in order to discover, create, and assert her own autonomy and mastery in the world. Simply put, birth begins a lifelong process of development along physical, cognitive, social, and emotional lines. As she develops, the average child comes to know and assert within her world an organized sense of self, all the while maintaining both a separateness from and connectedness to others.

The dramatic physical, cognitive, emotional, and social growth a child experiences during the first years of life is evident. By the time that same child reaches school age, the changes may not be so apparent. On the surface, development appears to slow. However, during what is commonly referred to as the latency period, a child's ability to think, learn, and socialize takes on greater sophistication and complexity. As a girl continues to accumulate such skills as reading, riding a bike, making friends, interacting with teachers, and doing arithmetic, for example, she gains a sense of mastery that forms the core of her evolving self-esteem.

During adolescence, the progress in a girl's physical, emotional, and intellectual development moves once again, as in the toddler years, at a conspicuous rate. As a girl goes through puberty and experiences the physical and emotional impact of hormonal changes—the onset of menstruation (menarche), the growth of body hair, the development of breasts and hips, and the surfacing of sexual feelings—she may appear very much a young woman. Yet, her emotional state may still be quite childlike.

Her social skills and preoccupations also shift as her relationships with peers and mentors take on greater importance, whereas her connection to her parents seems to recede in importance. Sometimes, family relationships take on contrary, combative qualities. In an attempt to try out, develop, and assert a personal identity, a teenager may steer abruptly away from her parents and toward her peer group. With all the changes agitating within and without, many teenage girls feel anxious and unsure of themselves. Nevertheless, a young girl negotiates a sense of self that will move her into womanhood. The quality of her relationships within her family and, more specifically, her family's ability to accommodate her developmental needs by gradually shifting the onus of personal responsibility to her help determine the ultimate success of this passage, as well as the degree of turmoil along the way.

Between her early twenties and her late forties, a woman ordinarily faces a variety of decisions that function to define and express further who she is. These decisions touch such areas as love, sexuality, coupling and uncoupling, motherhood, creativity, and work. Seldom, however, do these decisions chart out an uncomplicated, sequential path, and each requires adjustments in a woman's roles, responsibilities, and identity.

Midlife typically offers an opportunity for a woman to move deeper into life; to take stock of her successes and failures, her blessings and losses; and to develop a fuller sense of meaning for her own life. Simultaneously, as the time remaining shortens, sharper focus is brought to her limitations, inevitable disappointments, and mortality. Menopause, with its physical and emotional changes, inevitably brings some of the realities of growing older to mind. Many times, midlife also compels a woman to turn outward toward the community, as she seeks new venues in which to channel her talents, make a difference, and leave a legacy.

As old age approaches, self-esteem depends in large measure on a woman's capacity to accept both her life as it has been and her impending death with some measure of equanimity. The accumulation of losses, including parents, partners, siblings, friends, children, health and physical control, independence and youthful mastery, can be painful and disheartening. Nevertheless, as a woman comes to terms with life's triumphs and losses, with the gifts and the pain of her journey, she may see that, on balance, all the changes and struggles have made her life, and her, rich, meaningful, and alive.

A woman's development, even the most normal development, is propelled and frustrated, forged and determined, by a complex combination of physical, cognitive, emotional, and social forces. Obstacles can arise both from a woman's genetic blueprint and from the social, environmental context in which she finds herself or creates for herself. Good mental health isn't simply a matter of caring nurture or good genes—in many cases, a successful life and the ability to maintain a vital and competent sense of self over the years in the face of life's triumphs and tragedies require a hearty allotment of good luck.

For years, researchers and mental health clinicians noticed that some children emerge from horrific childhood experiences impressively intact, well equipped to meet adulthood's challenges. In contrast, others who came from privileged backgrounds and reasonably competent families find adult relationships and other adult developmental tasks impossible to negotiate.

We cannot explain mental illness, which has a strong genetic component, solely by looking at a woman's family or psychological dynamics. In the pages that follow, we will consider a number of common psychiatric disorders—depression, eating disorders, anxiety disorders, and others, too—that you or friends or relatives may experience. For whatever reason, a woman's personal, family, or psychological history may make her particularly vulnerable to stress, and psychiatric conditions may play a crucial role in her ability to handle stress, whether it originates outside, with, for example, a death or divorce, job loss, or relational disappointment, or within, with an illness or hormonal shift.

When all is said and done, however, a psychiatric disorder—depression, bipolar disorder, panic attacks, or psychosis, among others—is a disorder like diabetes or asthma or high blood pressure, which, in most cases, can be successfully treated.

THE BUSINESS OF MENTAL HEALTH

According to a 1993 study conducted by the National Institute of Mental Health, approximately fifty-two million adults in the United States—more than one in four—suffer from a mental disorder at some point during a year. Of these, only 28 percent seek help. Even though so many mental illnesses go untreated, close to $20 billion was generated in revenues by mental health organizations in 1986, the last year for which the U.S. Department of Health and Human Services has released figures.

As striking as this figure is, it does not paint a complete picture. It does not include expenditures for medication, prescribed and over-the-counter, used to treat mental illness. Nor does it reflect the number of people seeking help for emotional problems outside the mental health establishment. According to the 1993 study, 43 percent of those who sought help for a psychiatric disorder consulted doctors others than psychiatrists. Many others turned to Twelve-Step programs, self-help groups, encounter weekends, clergy, welfare workers, and ethnic healers for help. In addition, the 1993 study was concerned only with eight of the most common mental disorders: schizophrenia, drug and alcohol abuse, depression, anxiety problems, antisocial personality, severe cognitive impairment, and chronic complaints of multiple physical symptoms with no medical cause. Such problems as marital difficulties and bereavement, which send so many people to psychotherapists, were not considered in the study.

The mental health picture in this country has become considerably more convoluted and confusing as managed care organizations have become increasingly involved in shaping the kinds and duration of treatment offered. As a result, the mental health system is not always easy to negotiate, and that is especially unfortunate in that a woman who is seeking help may feel particularly vulnerable and stressed. This chapter offers a brief overview of the major mental illnesses as well as the most current thinking in the field concerning psychiatric problems and treatment options.

WHO ARE THE MENTAL HEALTH PRACTITIONERS?

A woman seeking help is faced with a wide array of choices: Does she need a psychiatrist, psychologist, psychiatric social worker, or therapist?

A psychiatrist *is a physician, a medical doctor whose training and education include at least four additional years of study, research, and clinical training in psychiatry beyond medical school. Psychiatrists have a thorough understanding of mental* and *medical issues and are licensed to issue prescriptions.*

Psychologists *have a master's degree or Ph.D. in clinical, educational, or experimental psychology. Typically, a psychologist has gathered knowledge about research techniques and psychological testing procedures.*

A social worker *has a master's degree in the discipline. The focus of the social worker is social environments, so they generally help people deal with social systems such as families, communities, and local and governmental social service agencies.*

Few states regulate the practice of psychotherapy, so almost anyone can call herself or himself a psychotherapist. *The name, as a result, doesn't imply a particular degree or training but indicates only that one is engaged in the professional practice of psychotherapy. Yet many who practice psychotherapy have professional degrees and/or have completed postgraduate training in one or more methods of therapy.*

Having one degree or another credential does not ensure that someone is a skilled and effective clinician, but the odds are that those practitioners who hold a state license or certificate will have more skills and training than those who have not met such standards. If you need assistance, talk to your health-care provider; ask him or her to refer you to an appropriate mental health professional.

WHAT ARE THE THERAPEUTIC OPTIONS?

For the woman seeking help with a mental disorder, there are a range of treatment options as well as mental health professionals available (see Who Are the Mental Health Practitioners?, *page 186). Among the possible approaches are the following:*

Individual psychotherapy *treats emotional problems and problems of everyday living by virtue of the special relationship between a patient and a psychotherapist, who may be a psychiatrist, psychologist, psychiatric social worker, or other therapist. Using a knowledge of psychological processes, the clinician attempts to relieve the patient's discomfort and suffering and help the patient to develop new ways of coping with problems and stress.*

Cognitive–behavioral therapy *attempts to guide a person toward more realistic and positive thinking. Especially effective in treating anxiety and mood disorders, these therapies work on the assumption that the way a person interprets events shapes her feelings and actions. The therapy focuses on how the distorted thinking leads to emotional and behavioral problems, and the patient is taught to identify, test, and correct specific distortions in her thinking.*

Group therapy *harnesses the power of group dynamics and the interaction of peers to create new understandings in individual members. Group therapy can be an invaluable treatment approach for a wide range of emotional, behavioral, and life problems, instilling hope and coping skills.*

Your mental health clinician can guide you to the therapy best suited to help you gain control over your life.

STRESS AND ITS MANAGEMENT

Stress, and especially its impact on women today, has become a hotly debated subject in the popular press. In many ways, *stress* has become the buzzword of the last decade. With every study reported in the papers, conclusions are reversed or contradicted. Stress is by turns denounced as increasing vulnerability to heart attacks or cancer or is lauded as an important factor in professional success and personal happiness.

Life by its very nature is stressful. Most women experience stress from time to time, and most handle it without giving much thought to it. Stress has been described as "the very salt and spice of life." Circumstances that are highly and negatively stressful for some may offer just the right kind of stimulation and excitement for others. For some, a quiet, contemplative life would prove intolerably stressful, while for others, balancing the often conflicting demands of a high-powered career with family obligations is unthinkable. Nevertheless, there are times when life's pressures become too much even for the most high-energy woman.

Stress can result from a variety—and usually a combination—of situations and experiences: an impending promotion at work plus a sudden trauma, such as an accident or death; the birth of a child plus the loss of significant income; a move to a new community plus the youngest child's leaving for college; prolonged marital difficulties plus a serious physical illness. As pressure builds, many women feel a deep need just to escape, to run away, as though avoidance is the only solution.

In most cases, however, burnout results not from the reality of the situations, but from the degree of control a woman feels in those situations. For this reason, effective coping with stress often arises from the process itself. The first step is to assess the situation objectively and consider ways of managing it. Coping may include setting more realistic goals and priorities, being more assertive about your needs, and seeking professional help.

When feelings of overload and burnout become intense, it's important to break problems down into manageable pieces; using pen and paper usually helps to sort things out: making a list of your stressors, then working on them one at a time.

Look around for a variety of solutions. Try to slow down the pace. Some women find meditation, relaxation techniques, and exercise particularly helpful in providing the time and distraction that help them to move away from the problem and back to themselves. Avoid alcohol and drugs, which tend only to blur and mute one's problem-solving capacities. Make time for people, activities, and interests that you value. Very often, time and a little bit of distance will dissipate enough of the pressure to render even the largest problem manageable.

As a rule, crisis presents an opportunity for growth. If you can meet it with humor, flexibility, imagination, and a sense of perspective, the next crisis may be easier to handle. Finally, when women discern and exercise the many smaller ways in which they do have power and control, having control over everything becomes less of an issue.

ANXIETY DISORDERS

Clinical anxiety is characterized by intense, recurring, and uncontrollable worry and fear. Persistent feelings of restlessness, of being on edge or all keyed up, coupled with fatigue, difficulty concentrating, muscle tension, and sleep disturbances indicate the presence of a psychiatric illness. The two most common manifestations of an anxiety disorder are panic attacks, *which are sudden, unexpected rushes of anxiety, and* phobias, *which are unaccountable fears around specific situations, activities, or objects.*

Anxiety is a natural emotion that everyone experiences at one time or another, usually in anticipation of a new, challenging, or stressful situation. A child, for example, feels anxious on the first day of kindergarten. A woman feels anxious when her company shows signs of downsizing. And everyone, of course, feels stirrings of anxiety when faced with a serious illness, divorce, or move to a new community.

Anxiety is rooted in the body's natural fight-or-flight response. This emotion functions as a signal to alert us to danger and elicit the appropriate reaction, in most cases, to confront or avoid. Sometimes, however, the feeling of anxiety is so intense or protracted that it interferes with our day-to-day functioning. When that happens, anxiety becomes a serious problem.

Understanding the Problem. Anxiety disorders take many forms. They may manifest themselves in inexplicable feelings of impending doom; unfounded or excessive worry about such things as one's health, a child's safety, the success of one's business, the fate of one's marriage; irrational fear of a situation, such as attending parties; an activity, such as driving; or an object, such as animals. Heart palpitations, profuse sweating, tightness in the chest, frequent urination, gas pains or diarrhea, nausea, muscle spasm, headaches, and neck pain are among the range of possible symptoms. Anxiety affects thinking, perception, memory, and learning; the sufferer can experience confusion and distortion of time, space, people's intentions, and the meaning of events.

Panic attacks constitute a common chronic illness that manifests as recurrent, sudden rushes of fearfulness accompanied by such symptoms as labored breathing, hyperventilation, rapid heartbeat, palpitations, and dizziness. A person who is subject to panic attacks often experiences feelings of unreality and fear of dying. These intense, unexpected surges of anxiety typically last less than an hour. After the panic attack passes, the person is often preoccupied with concern about recurrence, as well as the consequences and health implications of future attacks.

Unlike free-floating or generalized anxiety, panic attacks are experienced as discrete periods that reach full intensity within seconds or minutes and subside soon thereafter. Unlike phobic anxiety, they are not always predictable. Nevertheless, panic attacks may be associated with certain situations in which fleeing quickly may be impeded, such as riding on public transportation, driving across a bridge, standing in a crowd, or waiting in line. When this kind of anxiety results in avoidance and begins to circumscribe a person's functioning and activities, it flows into the condition known as *agoraphobia*.

Agoraphobia, one of the phobic disorders, is the fear of being in places or situations from which escape might be difficult or embarrassing or in which help might not be available should a panic attack occur. There are other kinds of phobias, such as the inexplicable fear of heights, dogs, or air travel. Phobias are the most commonly reported mental disorder; over twenty million Americans have at least one phobia severe enough to interfere with their daily functioning.

In general, anxiety disorders appear in late adolescence or early adulthood, sometimes with a second peak between the ages of thirty-five and forty. The tendency toward panic attacks and phobias is usually chronic and fluctuating, often resurfacing around life events such as loss through death or divorce. Women are two to three times more likely than men to be affected by anxiety disorders. Eight percent of American women experience agoraphobia in their lifetime. Although several effective treatments are now available, it is estimated that as many as half of all anxiety disorders are undiagnosed, misdiagnosed, or untreated.

Treatment Options. As part of the diagnosis, it must be determined that anxiety symptoms are not due to drug abuse, medication, or such general medical conditions as thyroid disorders and hypoglycemia (see pages 468 and 467, respectively).

Anxiety disorders can be treated in a variety of ways, although combined use of medication and cognitive–behavioral therapy has been found to be widely successful. Based on the assumption that how a person interprets events shapes her feelings and actions, cognitive–behavioral therapy guides a person toward more realistic and positive thinking. The focus is on how the distorted thinking leads to emotional and behavioral problems and the patient is taught to identify, test, and correct specific distortions in her thinking.

Antipanic and antidepressant medications are typically given to modify some of the more debilitating symptoms in dosages lower than for depression (see page 191).

Other common approaches used in working with anxiety disorders include teaching relaxation exercises and respiratory control techniques. Exposure techniques involve introducing the feared stimulation in a controlled and measured way so that it can be confronted. Systematic desensitization—visualizing anxiety-producing stimuli with the help of tranquilizers, hypnosis, and muscle relaxation techniques, then attempting to confront and cope with them—has been known to relieve symptoms. Flooding, or exposing the person to the feared object or situation for as long as she can tolerate until the fear is gone, is another approach.

MOOD DISORDERS

Mood disorders are a large group of psychiatric conditions in which a specific state, usually depression or mania, colors all of one's perceptions, thinking, functioning, and physical experiences.

The predominant feature of mood disorders is a sustained disturbance of an emotional state. When a woman suffers from a mood disorder, depression or elation persists regardless of life circumstances and colors her entire life.

Clinical depression *is characterized by depressed mood, lack of interest and pleasure in most activities, sleep disturbance, feelings of sluggishness or agitation, fatigue and loss of energy, feelings of worthlessness, excessive or inappropriate guilt, and a diminished ability to think, concentrate, and make decisions.* Elation, *or* mania, *is characterized by sustained elevated mood, a rush of ideas, hyperactivity, thoughts of grandiosity, irritability, anger, insomnia, and agitation.*

Eighteen million people in the United States suffer from depression or bipolar disorder each year. More than a persistent experience of sadness, depression is a cluster of signs and symptoms that represent a striking departure from a woman's habitual functioning, often recurring periodically or cyclically. Depressive illness features sustained feelings of deprivation or loss, low self-esteem and confidence, self-reproach, and disproportionate guilt, helplessness, and hopelessness.

Understanding the Problem. Women who are depressed may have trouble sleeping or, conversely, sleep much of the time. They may gain or lose weight. They often experience recurrent thoughts of death and suicide, decreased sexual interest, and a diminished capacity for pleasure of any kind. They may describe feelings of emptiness, self-loathing, and self-recrimination. At the same time, there may be a tendency toward angry and frustrated outbursts.

Psychiatric practitioners describe two basic types of depression. A *major depression* is the most commonly diagnosed mood disorder. It may appear as a single depressive episode or as recurring episodes. The course of a major depression may be protracted, lasting beyond several weeks to months if not treated. Milder depressive conditions are called *dysthymic disorders*: low-grade, intermittent, or chronic depressive states.

Mania, on the other hand, may look very different from depression in its symptomatic expression. Mania manifests itself in distinct periods of abnormally and persistently elevated, expansive, or irritable mood. Women who are in the grip of a manic episode have a decreased need for sleep, are more talkative than usual or feel pressure to keep talking, and experience a flight of ideas and racing thoughts. They are easily distracted, their attention easily drawn to the unimportant or irrelevant.

In manic behavior, there is a tendency toward goal-oriented activities in all aspects of life: social, sexual, work, and/or school. There tends to be excessive involvement in pleasurable activities that also often result in painful consequences. So, for example, a woman in a manic phase may engage in unrestrained buying sprees, sexual indiscretions, or unwise business investments. While it is true that milder forms of manic disorders can contribute to success in business, leadership roles, and the arts, recurrence of even the mildest mania can be disruptive. An elated mood, for example, can lead to impulsiveness and overoptimism concerning one's abilities, which can have unfortunate consequences.

Regardless of the different symptomatic picture, mania is closely linked to depression. Some of the symptoms—irritability, anger, insomnia, agitation, and a tendency toward outbursts—occur in both. Often women swing back and forth from one state to the other.

While occasionally women with mood disorders experience only manic episodes, most who experience mania also experience depression. Therefore, women who suffer from mania are usually diagnosed with bipolar disease, also called *manic-depressive illness*.

Bipolar disease differs from major depressive illness in that the diagnosis depends on at least one manic episode. More often than not, a woman with manic-depressive illness has numerous recurrences of alternating or cyclical phases. In about a third mixed states of simultaneous depressive and manic symptoms also develop.

The milder, chronic form of manic-depressive illness is called *cyclothymic disorder*. In this illness, there are numerous brief periods of mania alternating with numerous brief periods of depression.

Descriptions of melancholia and mania have been passed on to us from ancient times. Greeks and Romans hypothesized a temperamental origin for melancholia and mania. Today, mood disorders are thought to be determined by familial/genetic, psychosocial, and sociocultural factors.

Conceptualizations of mood disorders include the psychological model, which posits at the center the loss of a loved parental object or unsuccessful attachment to a nurturing object early in development. The cognitive model addresses the habitual pattern of thinking along negative lines. And the biogenic/neurogenic model points to chemical imbalances in the brains of people with mood disorders. Most researchers and practitioners, however, assume a multiplicity of factors that contribute to depressive or manic-depressive temperaments, including predisposing heredity (genetic factors), developmental predisposition (babies of depressed mothers naturally have more difficulty navigating complex developmental tasks), and life events.

While manic episodes are equally prevalent in men and women, there is a significantly higher prevalence of major depressive disorders in women. This gender difference remains consistent throughout life, though it becomes more pronounced in young adulthood and middle age. In general, women are at significantly higher risks for milder depressive states. This increased risk is often attributed to social and interpersonal variables. As a result, psychosocial explanations, such as the fact that women experience greater stress as they perform in multiple roles as homemaker, worker, wife, and mother puts them at greater risk, find prominence in today's popular notion of mood disorders. Nevertheless, it appears that biological factors are equally relevant, such as the influence of shifting hormonal levels especially around pregnancy and childbirth, around the time of menstruation, and around menopause. Many women are also subject to the depressive effects of steroidal contraceptives.

There is a clear but not completely understood connection between mood disorders and substance abuse. The fact that depression or bipolar disorder illness and substance abuse coexist so frequently likely reflects the attempt by the affected person to self-medicate. Also, there is some correlation between mood disorders and physical illness; physical illness, both minor and serious, occurs with greater frequency in people who suffer from depressive symptoms.

Treatment Options. Treatment for mood disorders typically includes cognitive therapy or medication or a combination of both. Many cases of mood disorders respond well to therapy.

Based on the assumption that how a person interprets events shapes her feelings and actions, cognitive–behavioral therapy guides a person toward more realistic and positive thinking. The focus is on how the distorted thinking leads to emotional and behavioral problems and the patient is taught to identify, test, and correct specific distortions in her thinking.

Antidepressants, and, in the presence of manic symptoms, mood stabilizers such as lithium are prescribed to treat depression and bipolar illness. If, during a major episode, there are strong psychotic features (see page 200) or suicidal behavior (see page 203), then additional approaches such as hospitalization, antipsychotic medication, and/or electroconvulsive therapy (ECT, below) may be necessary. After the acute phase has subsided, medications may be continued to decrease the likelihood of future recurrence. In cases of mood disorders, psychotherapy may also be recommended to complement treatment with medications.

ELECTROCONVULSIVE THERAPY

Also known as ECT, electroconvulsive therapy ("shock treatment" was its pejorative nickname) is used much less frequently today than it was in the early to mid-1900s. Yet ECT, as a safe and effective treatment for major depression, may be prescribed when medication or psychotherapy is ineffective and the depression is particularly severe.

Before treatment the patient is anesthetized and given a strong muscle relaxant. Then a short, low-intensity electrical current is passed through the brain, inducing a seizure. Current opinion is mixed, but the seizure is thought to increase the brain's production of norepinephrine, a neurotransmitter typically lower than normal in depressed people.

While the idea of "shock" treatment may be distasteful, ECT is actually quite safe. Side effects may include headaches, muscle aches, and temporary memory loss, but, compared to the symptoms of major depression, these are relatively minor. ECT offers, for many patients, relief from otherwise unrelieved depression.

CHRISTINA'S STORY

Christina thought maybe she was getting lazy. She knew she should be excited about her promotion to full professor in the English Department, but instead she felt fatigued and bored. If she could, she'd sleep all the time. Although it had always been something of a drag to get going in the morning, now it was a real struggle to get out of bed to make her eleven o'clock class. She felt irritable and seemed to be getting into little squabbles with the head of her department as well with a few of her colleagues. She was late getting her article written for the literary magazine and late getting her students' papers marked.

Christina mentioned her fatigue to her doctor, but a full general medical workup came back with negative findings. She admitted that she had lost interest in everything, including her dog. She had no drive, including no sexual drive. She went home every day after work and hardly went out on the weekends. Instead, she rented and watched old movies. She had gained fifteen pounds and began to wonder whether the reason she couldn't concentrate was that a brain tumor was developing. In fact, she was beginning to wonder whether life was really worth living. But suicide was out of the question since it was contrary to her religious beliefs. Still, the only writers she was interested in these days were the ones who successfully did away with themselves.

Her physician recommended a psychiatric consultation. After she had taken antidepressants over three weeks, her complaints began to reverse themselves. "It was like someone removed the film off my glasses. I began to see, to think more clearly, to view my future more hopefully." For Christina, the use of antidepressant medication was literally a lifesaver.

SEASONAL AFFECTIVE DISORDER

Seasonal affective disorder, or SAD, is characterized by fatigue, irritability, overeating, lack of concentration, and depressed sexual drive.

The daily cycle of light and dark that results from the twenty-four-hour rotation of the earth forms the basis for the circadian rhythm, the system of keeping time built into virtually all life. Bodily functions such as temperature, blood pressure, heart rate, and hormone production are tied to this internal clock.

The succession of the seasons and the corresponding shifts in the length of day and night introduce yet another, wider circular rhythm. While most of us welcome the coming of spring and summer, and many dread the shorter, colder days of winter, seasonal changes have a severe, deeply felt effect on some women. Many suffer from a seasonal accentuation or precipitation of depression called *seasonal affective disorder* (SAD).

Understanding the Problem. More prevalent in northern latitudes, where the climatic extremes are greater, SAD is specifically characterized by fatigue, sugar craving, overeating, and oversleeping. Insofar as oversleeping further disrupts circadian rhythms, depressive symptoms can be exacerbated.

While the exact cause of the disorder is not certain, some researchers think that the function of the light-responsive pineal gland causes SAD.

Treatment Options. Currently, light therapy, which extends exposure to bright light for measurable periods of time, is used in many cases to relieve symptoms. People with milder cases of SAD may respond positively to spending at least an hour a day outdoors, even in winter. Increase the amount of natural light in your house, and, if possible, take trips in winter to places that are warmer and sunnier. Antidepressants and psychotherapy may also be recommended.

MEDICATIONS FOR MOOD DISORDERS:
A PARTIAL LIST

The following list describes medications commonly prescribed to treat mood disorders. While most medications are effective, finding the drug and dosage that produce the desired results with fewest side effects often takes time and close cooperation between patient and psychiatric practitioner.

Tricyclics *are antidepressant drugs that affect the movement of certain stimulant brain chemicals (specifically norepinephrine and serotonin) to and from the nerve endings. These drugs alleviate symptoms in chronically depressed patients. Possible side effects include dry mouth, constipation, and weight gain. Generic (and brand) names are desipramine (Norpramin), amitriptyline (Elavil), doxepin (Adapin, Sinequan), nortriptyline (Pamelor), and clomipramine (Anafranil).*

Monoamine oxidase inhibitors (MAOIs) *work to block certain enzyme reactions within the body. These drugs have been found especially effective in treating more severe depression, anxiety, and phobias. Possible side effects include hypertension, weight gain, and sexual dysfunction. While on these medications women must adhere to a strict diet that precludes fermented, smoked, or pickled foods, as well as cheese, yogurt, processed meats, caffeine, chocolate, beer, and wine. Phenelzine (Nardil) and tranylcypromine (Parnate) are commonly used MAOIs.*

Benzodiazepines, *which up until the past few years were used to manage seizures, have a calming effect. Not surprisingly, the major side effects are drowsiness and sedation. Two major drugs in this class are alprazolam (Xanax) and clonazepam (Klonopin).*

Selective serotonin reuptake inhibitors (SSRIs) *and* selective norepinephrine reuptake inhibitors (SNRIs) *have become the mainstay of treatment for depression. They produce an antidepressant effect by preventing movement of the brain messengers serotonin and norepinephrine into nerve endings. Possible side effects include anxiety, mania, headaches, sexual dysfunction, and insomnia. Agents in this class include fluoxetine (Prozac), sertraline (Zoloft), paroxetine (Paxil), and venlafaxine (Effexor).*

Lithium *is a mood stabilizer used to manage manic symptoms and to prevent subsequent episodes. Possible side effects include hand tremors, mild and transient nausea, and general achiness. Other mood stabilizers include valproic acid and carbamazepine. All these mood stabilizers have been associated with a small increase in birth defects when taken during pregnancy.*

EATING DISORDERS

An eating disorder is a pathological preoccupation with food, weight, and shape and a desire for a thinner body. The most common types of eating disorders are anorexia nervosa, bulimia nervosa, *and* binge eating.

In a land of overwhelming plenty for most people, it is hardly surprising that psychiatric illnesses have emerged that center around food and its consumption. Food and dieting are frequent topics of conversation for many Americans, but anorexia nervosa, bulimia nervosa, and binge eating represent an all-consuming obsession with both.

Understanding the Problem. Eating disorders are firmly rooted in our society's prejudice against obesity and idealization of thinness. Moreover, they may actually reflect in a distorted manner the unrelenting pressure many women experience to perform at all times in diverse and often conflicting roles. A woman with an eating disorder may be thus expressing concerns about personal control that manifest themselves in weight regulation.

Eating disorders as a whole display varying progressions, ranging from a single, mild illness in adolescence to a lifelong disorder that either persists or tends to come and go.

Anorexia nervosa is a deliberate, self-imposed starvation in relentless pursuit of thinness and in fear of obesity, which leads to varying degrees of emaciation and even death. This disease appears ten to twenty times more frequently in women than in men. It is also found more commonly among the affluent and in those in occupations in which thinness is valued (dancing, for example, or modeling). Anorexia usually appears in adolescence, when girls' bodies change and breasts and hips develop.

Anorectics feel fat even though they are emaciated, diet all the time, and often abuse diuretics and laxatives in their determination to lose weight. Although the term *anorexia* means loss of appetite, anorectics, in fact, are obsessed with food. It is not unusual for someone suffering from anorexia to collect recipes and cook lavishly for others but refuse to eat. An anorectic may behave strangely around food, hiding it around the house, carrying candy in her purse, constantly rearranging the food on her plate. If she is unable to control completely her food intake, she may binge, often during the evening or night. Thirty to fifty percent of anorectics also suffer from bulimia nervosa (see page 71). Often rigid and perfectionistic, an anorectic may be obsessed with exercise and have little interest in sex. Moreover, anorexia leads to chronic malnourishment, which takes its toll throughout the body, particularly in the thyroid, heart, and digestive and reproductive systems.

Bulimia nervosa is an episodic pattern of binge eating that leads to a sense of loss of control, followed by efforts to control body weight through self-induced vomiting or use of laxatives. Like anorexia, bulimia is significantly more common in women than men. Some estimates put the incidence in college women as high as 40 percent; women in that age group are forty-five times more likely to suffer from bulimia than men.

Women with bulimia tend to be high achievers. Unlike anorectics, who may wish to deny or reverse their sexual development, many bulimics obsess about their sexual attractiveness. Although most are able to maintain control over their weight through purging, many women who suffer from bulimia manifest an obsession with food. They fast, diet too strictly, or exercise obsessively. The foods on which they binge tend to be treats or "comfort food"—sweet foods, high in calories, or smooth, soft foods like ice cream, cake, and pastry.

Binge eating disorder (BED), which is alarmingly pervasive, involves binge eating without subsequent purging. A woman who suffers from BED may binge on as much as ten thousand calories over a few hours and experience feelings of being out of control, as well as feeling self-reproach, guilt, and shame, like the bulimic. Because she does not purge, though, she may consider herself—and others may also view her—simply as an overeater. Many women who are binge eaters adopt purging years later after their weight has become a serious issue. It is not uncommon for binge eating eventually to evolve into bulimia.

Eating disorders spring from a variety of predispositions. Besides the links to social factors, there seem to be family connections. Where there is a family history of depression, alcoholism, obesity, or eating disorders, women are at higher risk. Psychosocial factors may also play a role. Women who manifest a sense of personal helplessness, a fear of losing control, self-esteem highly dependent on opinions of others, and all-or-nothing thinking seem to be particularly vulnerable to this kind of disorder. Finally, there may be a relationship between eating patterns, specifically dieting and starvation, and the neurological and hormonal systems.

Treatment Options. Unless a woman is being seen by a health professional for diagnosis and treatment of another illness, anorexia may not be identified until her weight is significantly lower than minimal normal weight for her age and height—around 85 percent of normal weight—or when a number of consecutive menstrual periods have been missed as the result of the anorexia.

Anorexia nervosa can be fatal. In extreme cases, the immediate goal of treatment will be to get the person to eat and gain weight. Because in general the anorectic, unlike the bulimic, does not consider her behavior abnormal, convincing her to eat may not be easily accomplished. As a result, many women with acute anorexia are hospitalized. In the hospital, the patient is weighed daily and monitored.

Once the immediate medical crisis subsides, and in more moderate cases of the illness, individual and often family therapy are recommended to address the underlying psychosocial contributors to the disorder. Medications, particularly antidepressants, may also be of help.

Because many binge eaters appear only to have a weight problem, it is not unusual for them to frequent diet centers rather than mental health settings. Often their eating problems will be addressed as general health issues by their clinicians. However, many are aided by such self-help organizations as Overeaters Anonymous.

More often impulsive and involved in other addictive behaviors than anorectics, many bulimics experience depression or "postbinge anguish" and subsequent remorse. They may sense that what they're doing is abnormal. And while they may try to keep their behavior a secret, once found out, many experience great relief. The ability to admit feelings in relation to their acting out may make them more willing to seek and respond to help.

There seems to be greater value in using antidepressants in the treatment of bulimia than in the treatment of anorexia. As with anorexia, individual and/or family therapy can be helpful in addressing the complicated emotional issues underlying the behavior.

In general, a woman with an eating disorder may be distrustful of health-care practitioners, suspecting them of being interested only in feeding her, breaking her will, and making her fat. Early on, education is valuable. Talking factually about body weight regulation, normal eating habits, and nutrition, and about the negative effects of starvation, vomiting, and laxatives, is usually a good place to start.

My Body Is Mine

Francine's eating disorder began as a reasonable attempt to lose weight. She was unhappy with the additional twenty pounds she had put on over the summer. But soon, she had shed more pounds than she had intended. At five feet, six inches, she now weighed one hundred and five pounds. Nevertheless, she still felt fat and continued to be preoccupied with losing weight.

Francine had begun to go out again, and she loved the bony look she was developing around her throat and through her pelvis. But when she looked in the mirror, she'd see a circus fat lady. It didn't matter what other people told her. Eventually, she took down all the mirrors in her bedroom.

In time, her dentist noticed signs of damage to her teeth and began to ask questions. The thought of losing her teeth and having an ugly smile drove Francine to take her dentist's advice and consult a therapist. As she began to understand her need for control, and the self-destructive nature of her behavior, she began to think, not merely act, whenever she approached food.

She also joined a group of other women struggling with similar issues. In addition to teaching her ways of sorting out feelings and coping with anxiety and stress, the group lessened her feelings of loneliness. The result of therapy, both individual and group, was the slow development of a positive sense of self based more on what was inside than outside.

Francine understands that she may well struggle with food issues for a long time, but she is beginning to see that she need not let food run her life and dictate her sense of self.

Sleep Disorders

The term sleep disorders *encompasses a variety of conditions that somehow disrupt a healthy sleep pattern. Specific symptoms range from the inability to get enough sleep at night to periodic cessation of breathing during sleep, from long periods of wakefulness at night to excessive daytime sleepiness, from loud snoring to difficulty in falling asleep, from morning headaches to dreamlike hallucinations, from nightmares and night terrors to sleepwalking.*

Sleep repairs and restores us physically and psychologically. It is as fundamental to good health as eating well. But for many, the benefits of a good night's sleep are elusive. Sleep disorders, whether *insomnia, hypersomnia, daytime sleeping problems,* or *parasomnia,* affect one third of all Americans. The cost to society, in terms of accidents and loss of productivity, exceeds that of AIDS and cigarette smoking combined.

Understanding the Problem. Sleep disorders include the dyssomnias (insomnia, or difficulty falling asleep; hypersomnia, or sleeping too much; and sleep–wake schedule disorder) and the parasomnias (sleepwalking, night terrors, or nightmares).

Insomnia, the inability to sleep enough or to fall asleep at night, is the most common sleep disorder. Each year, up to 30 percent of the population seeks help for insomnia, mostly in the form of sleeping medications. In fact, most people experience insomnia from time to time. Short-term insomnia may reflect anxiety, either before or after a worrisome or traumatic event such as a death or other loss, a significant life change, a job interview, or a final exam.

Long-term insomnia can develop into a significant problem, especially since worrying about sleep can further interfere with sleep. Insomnia is not in itself a disease, but it can be a symptom of a minor or serious illness. Insomnia that occurs over an extended period, for example, may stem from such medical problems as a painful or degenerative condition, a psychiatric disorder such as depression, or substance abuse. On the other hand, the exact cause may remain impossible to identify.

Hypersomnia is characterized by oversleeping, excessive daytime sleepiness (somnolence), and/or the tendency to fall asleep suddenly. Hypersomnia is a primary sign of depression. Menstruation, certain medical conditions, alcohol or drug abuse, and stimulant withdrawal can also trigger hypersomnia.

Daytime sleepiness problems are usually the result of inadequate nighttime sleep, but they are also associated with narcolepsy, sleep apnea (also called hypoventilation syndrome), and sleep–wake schedule disorder.

Narcolepsy is a chronic disorder that manifests in uncontrollable and recurrent spells of drowsiness and sleep that in turn can cause constant fatigue and lack of energy regardless of how well a person sleeps at night. Narcolepsy can also cause memory loss and hallucinations. Often, narcoleptics fall asleep abruptly, sometimes in the middle of a conversation, while watching TV, or, most alarmingly, behind the wheel of a car.

Sleep apnea is a neuromuscular problem in which the airway is partially blocked during sleep, causing breathing difficulties. Most people with this condition snore heavily and stop breathing for intervals that can exceed ten seconds, only to snort and gasp as they resume breathing. The cessation of breathing may occur dozens of times during the night, disrupting sleep. Although ordinarily harmless, for women with an impaired cardiovascular system, sleep apnea presents a risk of serious heart complications.

Sleep–wake schedule disorder typically afflicts people who frequently fly east to west across several time zones, or who often change work schedules or shifts. As a result, their internal clock is disrupted, and their sleep pattern becomes erratic.

Parasomnias, while most common among children, occur in all age groups. *Nightmares* may occur with particular frequency or intensity during periods of stress, uncertainty, or depression. *Night terrors*, which typically happen in the first third of the night, feature greater anxiety: Women who experience night terrors often sit up screaming and breathing heavily in bed, then forget the incident by morning. *Sleepwalking*, of course, is potentially the most dangerous of the three because of the sleepwalker's impaired ability to navigate stairs and obstacles.

Treatment Options Long-term insomnia may be particularly difficult to treat. If it stems from medical or psychiatric problems, treatment by a physician or therapist will target the precipitating condition. Otherwise, insomnia can be managed by addressing certain life-style issues.

Establish a regular bedtime, and get up at the same time every morning, even if you sleep badly all night. Relax before bedtime, maybe with a hot bath or warm milk, by listening to soothing music instead of watching fast-paced TV programs or working at the computer. If possible, don't take your problems into the bedroom with you. Work on unraveling them at some other time, in another part of the house. Use your bed for sleeping and sex and nothing else. If you do not fall asleep after twenty minutes, get up. Do something else until you feel sleepy. Relaxation tapes, meditation, deep breathing, or biofeedback may induce sleep.

Regular exercise, which is so beneficial to body and psyche, can be a great sleeping aid as well. Take long walks or do yoga or stretching in the late afternoon or early evening. More strenuous exercise, which is more stimulating, should be done before midday.

In addition to promoting overall health, such practices as eliminating large meals at the end of the day, stopping smoking, and reducing consumption of sweets, caffeine, and alcohol can help with sleep problems.

Although as yet there is no cure for narcolepsy, it can be managed to some degree with stimulants, such as amphetaminelike drugs, or antidepressants. It is important that women with narcolepsy establish sound sleeping habits. Allow plenty of time for sleep at night. Short naps and light meals during the day may reduce abrupt sleepiness.

Sleep apnea appears easier to correct. In many cases, changing sleeping position to one's side is all that is needed. Women who are overweight may find that losing weight brings with it significant relief. Devices to keep airways open during sleep are available, and in more severe cases, surgery may be required to remove the blockage.

For women bothered by nightmares and night terrors, psychotherapy may help.

While there is no specific treatment for sleepwalking, it is advisable to make the house safe for the sleepwalker. Also, reducing alcohol consumption may cause sleepwalking to abate.

PSYCHOSIS

The major symptom of a psychotic illness is an impaired perception of reality, often manifested in hallucinations, disordered thinking, delusions, deteriorating social and vocational functioning, disorganized speech, and grossly disorganized behavior.

Psychosis is a mental illness characterized by prominent and persistent disturbances in the way a person thinks, sees, and hears. Such cognitive and perceptual disturbances are often coupled with disturbances in mood. Psychosis can be either progressive or episodic. While this is a serious illness, the prognosis varies according to severity and type.

Schizophrenia is a psychotic disorder characterized by severe problems in a person's thoughts, perceptions, emotions, behavior, and language. Psychotic symptoms combine in various ways, creating considerable diversity among patients, but often include delusions and hallucinations. The cumulative effect of the illness, however, is always severe and usually long lasting.

Affecting just under 1 percent of the world's population, schizophrenia exacts an enormous personal and economic cost. Major symptoms that lead to diagnosis usually appear during late adolescence and early adulthood with the incidence in men peaking between the ages of fifteen and twenty-five and in women between the ages of twenty-five and thirty-five.

Understanding the Condition. While the exact causes of schizophrenia remain unclear, there are strong indications that genetic factors are involved. There is a tendency to presume that a person with schizophrenia will inevitably deteriorate in terms of functioning and symptoms, but, in fact, the long-term course of the illness varies among patients. Modern treatments produce significant relief from this severe disorder.

Treatment Options. During acute psychotic episodes, hospitalization is often needed to stabilize the patient. Antipsychotic medications are used to reduce the direct manifestations of the illness. Over time, drugs work to manage disordered thinking and behavior, maintain the achieved clinical effect, and prevent relapse. However, some antipsychotic drugs can produce severe side effects, including drowsiness, constipation, dry mouth, blurred vision, hypertension, and an involuntary series of muscle spasms called *tardive dyskinesia* or tremors.

Women suffering from schizophrenia often need continuing supervision or hospitalization to ensure that they continue on their medication. Because the illness is considered chronic, treatment usually involves training in social skills, vocational training, and supervised living to provide the support for the most normal day-to-day existence possible.

Schizoaffective disorder is a psychiatric illness that includes significant and enduring mood shifts, such as depression, euphoria (mania), or acute irritability, that overlap with prominent and persistent psychotic symptoms, such as hallucinations or delusions. This illness tends to be episodic rather than chronic or progressive. Schizoaffective disorder may be triggered by a combination of genetic, psychological, environmental, and interpersonal factors.

Understanding the Condition. If a woman experiences severe depression or mania (with its exaggerated elation, grandiosity, agitation, and accelerated thinking or speaking) or delusional thinking and hallucinations that have lasted for more than two weeks, her health-care professional will first want to rule out any drug abuse, medication, or general medical condition that could produce similar symptoms. Because the illness isn't usually progressive, the course and treatment outcome for schizoaffective disorder tend to be more favorable than for schizophrenia.

Treatment Options. Hospitalization is usually required during the acute phase of this disease. When mood symptoms include swings from depression to euphoria, drug treatment typically includes antipsychotics coupled with mood stabilizers such as lithium. In schizoaffective depression, the initial treatment of choice is usually antipsychotics alone, though in some cases, an antidepressant may also be recommended.

Antiparkinson medications to address tremor and drugs to reduce anxiety and insomnia can be helpful as well. Since the side effects of the antipsychotics can be disconcerting, clinical judgment is required to balance medicating effects against side effects. Electroconvulsive therapy (ECT) is sometimes used to treat mania, especially when other interventions have not proved successful.

Psychosocial therapy is usually advised to address family, social, and vocational needs; to identify and anticipate factors that could possibly trigger psychotic episodes; and to help manage stress.

Brief psychotic disorders are characterized by episodes in which psychotic symptoms are active for periods ranging from one day to one month. Typically, the psychotic period is followed by a full return to normal functioning.

Understanding the Problem. More than likely, the tendency to react to extreme stress by producing psychotic symptoms is rooted in combined psychological and genetic vulnerabilities. Unlike other psychotic disorders, here the stressor or stressors are usually identifiable, such as domestic strife, problems at work, an accident, illness, or death of a loved one.

Treatment Options. Treatment for brief psychotic episodes combines immediate and long-term interventions. In the short term, because the patient may pose a danger to herself or to others, she may be hospitalized where close observation and a full physical examination can rule out the existence of any medical condition that could produce similar symptoms. It is not unusual that once the patient is in the hospital, the structure and reduced stimulation help to relieve some of the active symptoms. Low dosages of antipsychotic medication are usually prescribed to address agitation and possible violent behavior. Once the acute episode subsides, medication may be continued and counseling recommended to clarify the patient's vulnerabilities to stress and to enhance coping skills.

SUICIDE

Caught in feelings of desperation and hopelessness, Rowena thinks taking her own life may well be the only solution to her intractable problems. Things seem so bad at times, and she feels so incapable of coping, that death somehow seems a reasonable way to get a rest. She feels empty, inert, pressured, and helpless, with nowhere to turn. She's not even sure she has enough energy to kill herself.

Each year, approximately thirty thousand people commit suicide in the United States. The number of attempted suicides is estimated at eight to ten times higher.

Suicide is the eighth leading cause of death in this country. Men commit suicide more than three times as often as women, although women are four times more likely to make the attempt. One reason men are more likely to complete the act, according to researchers, is that they tend to choose lethal methods: They hang themselves, shoot themselves, or jump from high places. Women seem to prefer to ingest an overdose of drugs or poison. Most men who commit suicide do so after age forty-five. Among women, the greatest number of suicides occur after age fifty-five.

Suicide is more common among women with a family history of suicide or attempted suicide, and among those who live alone with few social connections. People of higher social status are at greater risk, with professionals the most vulnerable. Overall, however, the risk is higher for the unemployed; during recessions, depressions, and periods of high unemployment, the suicide rate goes up. Other high-risk groups include alcoholics, other substance abusers, and people with depression and a history of schizophrenia and other mental illnesses.

A large majority of women who commit or attempt suicide have seen a mental health practitioner and have a diagnosed mental illness, most commonly depression. In fact, it is not uncommon for clinically depressed women to attempt suicide just as they begin to recover. As they get better, they regain enough direction and energy to act. For this reason, it is of critical importance that therapy continue and that the therapist monitor the patient as she recovers.

Women suffering from serious physical illness, including cancer, diseases of the central nervous system, and some endocrine conditions, are at high risk as well. In the chronically ill, loss of mobility, disfigurement, and unremitting pain often prompt suicidal thoughts. Suicide and attempted suicide are classified as crimes in some states. Providing assistance in a suicide, even to the terminally ill, is an ethical and legal question frequently in the news these days.

There are typically signs that someone is seriously contemplating suicide. If, for example, a woman who has recently experienced a significant loss is depressed, seems to lack a vision or plans for the future, gives away cherished possessions, makes a will, and talks with great specificity of killing herself, she is indeed at risk of committing suicide. A woman's psychiatric history and family history should also be taken into account.

Talking frankly with a woman about her suicidal thoughts and intentions will not necessarily encourage her. If she threatens to kill herself, such threats should be taken seriously. In addition to offering a warning, these kinds of threats are almost always a cry for help. Suicide prevention centers and telephone hot lines are available in most communities to help a suicidal woman move beyond an immediate crisis. However, medication and psychotherapy are necessary to address the underlying depression and life circumstances that lead women to contemplate such drastic solutions.

CHAPTER 11

Violence Against Women

CONTENTS

It's a tragic truth that violence at the hands of intimates has been a major threat to women's well-being for thousands of years. Fourteenth-century French law, for example, said a man was legally entitled to beat his wife if she failed to obey "reasonable" commands—though killing or permanently maiming her was considered wrong. One sage in fifteenth-century Italy advised husbands to show "restraint" with their wives, suggesting that women should be treated at least as well as fowl and livestock. And the expression "rule of thumb" is actually a vestige of an English common law that permitted a husband to beat his wife with a stick so long as it was no wider than his thumb.

The rules may have changed, but women still find themselves victimized by the men with whom they share their lives. Studies consistently show that a woman is more likely to be a victim of violence at home than on the street. Battering is the major cause of injury to women, resulting in more injuries than auto accidents, muggings, and rapes combined—an incident of physical abuse occurs every nine seconds in the United States. Nearly twenty-one million are verbally or emotionally abused by their spouse or partner. An estimated 4 percent of women and children are abused in their own family, whereas only about 0.04 percent of people falls victim to violent crime outside the home: In short, women are one hundred times more likely to be abused at home than outside it. Every day, four children in our country die of abuse or neglect. Every day nearly eight thousand children will witness an act of domestic violence, and since most severe child abuse occurs alongside domestic violence, the odds are that many of these children will themselves be beaten.

Why have so many societies legally sanctioned assault when it occurs in the confines of marriage and family? Why is violence against women still so frequent? One explanation is that violence enforces the status quo, with women and children legally considered little more than the male householder's property. Domestic violence has long been an inextricable part of the imbalance of power between husbands and wives. Historically, husbands have resorted to beating as a practical method of enforcing their legal rights. Until recently wives were taught that it was their religious and ethical duty not to resist or leave, but to obey their husbands. Even today, many marriage vows still instruct men to "love, honor, and cherish," while women are told to "love, honor, and obey"—sending a very definite message about who has the power and control. Contemporary child-rearing practices, many researchers point out, often reinforce this pattern, with boys encouraged to be strong and aggressive and girls told to be unselfish and nice.

Pointing to studies that indicate a decline in abuse in recent decades, some researchers suggest that the trend will continue as Americans gain increasing access to social services and family life education. But others fear that the isolation of today's nuclear household, with little of the daily contact with extended family members, boarders, or servants that characterized American home life a century ago, makes opportunities for violence behind closed doors more likely than ever before. In the privacy of their own homes, women and children are often hidden victims of unreported crimes. In fact, it is estimated that only one in seven wife assaults is reported to the police. Even so, we know that more than a million women in the United States each year seek medical help for injuries caused by battering, and more than four thousand a year die at the hands of their current or former partner. Twenty-eight percent of all adult women are likely to be abused at least once in an intimate relationship, and in as many as one of six couples, physical assaults are routine. Domestic violence is repetitive in nature. Once abuse begins, it often sinks deep roots in relationships, and left alone, it tends to get worse.

What defines domestic abuse? It includes physical attacks, verbal abuse, threats, humiliation and intimidation, withholding support and care, destroying personal property, and psychological and emotional abuse. It involves the systematic persecution of one partner by another. It is the abuse of power and control. It ranges from chronic verbal abuse to forced sex and threats of bodily harm to kidnapping, assault, and murder. Child abuse refers to neglect or inadequate physical care and supervision of children (including lack of food, clothing, or supervision, and inadequate medical care) and physical, emotional, and sexual abuse. Although in many parts of the world spanking children is illegal, Americans disagree on whether it's a form of abuse.

Physical abuse may include throwing things at a woman; pushing, grabbing, or shoving her; pulling her hair; slapping, kicking, biting, or punching; threatening her with a knife or a gun; or actually using a weapon against her. Emotional or psychological abuse occurs when a man uses words to hold power and control over his partner, humiliating, ignoring, criticizing, playing mind games, being threatening, isolating her from friends or relatives, and otherwise restricting her. Harder to define than acts of violence, this kind of abuse has drastic consequences. Many experts consider this one of the most hidden, least researched, and most damaging forms of intimate abuse. Sadly, emotional abuse is all too common among parents and children, as well. In fact, many parents consider criticism and threats perfectly normal and acceptable child-rearing "techniques."

Violence and abuse, in all forms, leave deep scars on their victims. Not surprisingly, children who have been abused by caregivers suffer from feelings of abandonment and loss of trust. As adults, they may feel alienated from intimate relationships, from community, and from their religious or spiritual roots. They are likely to feel disconnected from themselves and their own feelings. Survivors of childhood abuse are far more likely to become victims as adults—or do harm to themselves—than they are to harm other people. Yet the good news is that the great majority of survivors don't abuse their own children; in fact, worried that they'll become abusers, they may make a particular effort to prevent their children from suffering as they did or even avoid having children altogether.

Society has long had a tendency to blame the victim in violent crimes and abuse of women—less than one man in one hundred is convicted of spousal assault—and unfortunately the mental health field has been no exception. Much research has focused on the personality traits that make a woman ripe for an abusive relationship or vulnerable to attack, and there has been much bitter debate among mental health professionals on this topic. But the American Psychiatric Association has eliminated the diagnosis "masochistic" personality, in which an underlying personality disorder that led to abuse was identified. Clinicians now point to a characteristic pattern of symptoms *resulting* from chronic trauma, reassigning responsibility from the victim to the abuser. If you are seeking treatment to deal with abuse or trauma, be sure to choose a therapist who understands your rights and needs, someone who will reassure you that what happened to you is wrong and help you feel safe in the therapeutic setting. You shouldn't be blamed or humiliated or diagnosed as "sick."

Whether or not you have been personally victimized by violence, violence against women is a critical public policy issue. It's every citizen's responsibility to learn how and to whom to report instances of abuse and neglect that require legal or criminal intervention. In many states people whose job brings them into contact with children—teachers, clergy, therapists, and others—are legally mandated to report suspected abuse cases to child protective services. And every community needs a shelter or safe home for victims of domestic violence and their children, as well as access to rape crisis services.

RAPE AND SEXUAL ASSAULT

Rape is not a sexual act. It is a crime of aggression, humiliation, and power. A women who is raped was not "asking for it" because she was dressed seductively or was walking on a dark street any more than a person is asking to be mugged because he is wearing a gold watch.

What should you do if you are approached by someone intent upon sexual assault? There are a number of ways to respond. First of all, keep in mind that staying alive is the most important thing, even more important than resisting rape. Although women do succeed in resisting or escaping in some situations, trust your gut sense of the danger in the moment.

Try to stay calm and consider your options. If you scream, will someone hear? Is there a place to escape to? How likely is it that your attacker will hurt you if you try to escape? Running away is the most effective defense, and if you can get to a public place, that may discourage your attacker from following you. Make as much noise as possible to attract attention and get help.

Does your attacker have a weapon? Can you resist? If so, don't hesitate to get angry and fight back. Though you may worry that this will only lead to worse injury or murder, studies show that fighting back seems to be effective in many cases. Keep in mind that the goal is to incapacitate your attacker. Fight dirty: Kick him in the genitals, bite him, jab your fingers in his eyes, ram his nose with your fist.

If the worst happens and you are raped, afterward you may have symptoms of shock, including feeling numb and unable to cry, or shortness of breath and uncontrollable shaking. You may be in physical pain from the assault. You may have trouble believing the rape really happened or even deny that it did. You may worry what people think or feel ashamed to tell your family or partner.

In order to increase the chances that the rapist can be successfully prosecuted, go directly to a local emergency room. Do not shower or bathe first—that could wash away important evidence. The health-care providers there can treat and protect you, as well as help build a case against the assailant.

You may feel dirty or worry that you did something to make this happen to you. You may feel depressed, tired, hopeless, humiliated, guilty, overwhelmed, even suicidal. You may fear that you're pregnant or that you may have contracted a sexually transmitted disease, even AIDS. Over time, you may harbor a fear that you'll be raped again, that you may never want to be intimate again, that you're going crazy. Some rape victims report that for weeks, months, and even years they have flashbacks to the rape or reexperience the trauma through nightmares and intrusive thoughts. For a time, you may find it difficult to feel sexual or to express affection for a male. You may feel totally vulnerable and no longer in control of your life.

Sadly, many women attempt to gain control of their feelings after a rape by blaming themselves. The most important thing you can do for yourself afterward is to remind yourself that under no circumstances is a rape your fault. Keep in mind that although techniques for resisting rape often work, they're not always effective or practical. If you can't prevent a rape, remember that by getting help afterward, you take your first step toward recovery and gaining control over your life. A rape crisis center (see *Getting Help*, page 217) can help you find support and explore your legal options.

MARITAL RAPE

Marital rape is forced sexual activity with a husband or wife. Marital rape includes not only sexual activity by physical force but also verbal coercion like threats of beatings, threats that your children or other family members will be harmed if you resist, or threats that financial support will be cut off unless you submit.

Statistics vary, but one study reported that 14 percent of married women are forced to engage in intercourse and other sexual acts against their will. (Since marital rape is rarely reported to criminal justice authorities, it's likely that this figure is far too low.) Fortunately, our legal system no longer supports the notion that husbands have the "right" to sex. Marital rape is not a private matter strictly between husband and wife to be dealt with in the couple's bedroom, nor is it your wifely duty to submit to unwanted sex. In more than half the states, a husband can be prosecuted for rape even while he's living with his wife, and many more states allow for prosecution if the spouses are living apart.

Unfortunately, as frequently happens when the rapist is the husband, the victim is reluctant to go to the police, fearing either physical reprisals or withdrawal of financial support from her partner, or she is emotionally bound to this man and so her concern for him skews her sense of judgment.

But rape is a crime, whether the rapist is a complete stranger or the man who promised to love, honor, and cherish you.

DATE RAPE

Rape or sexual assault by someone the victim knows happens far more often than rape by a stranger. Some 84 percent of all sexual assaults are committed by an acquaintance of the victim, according to one study. It is defined as rape, rather than as aggressive sex or passionate seduction, because the sex is not consensual. If you as a woman dress attractively and agree to go on a date with someone, go for a ride with him, allow him into your home or dorm room, kiss him, or indulge in heavy petting, that doesn't automatically mean you're willing or obligated to have sex. If at any moment you decide you don't want to have sex and say no but the man proceeds anyway, the act is defined as rape.

As with any crime, there are precautions you can take to avoid becoming a victim of date rape. First of all, stay away from men who like to be in control, men who don't view you as an equal, who put you down or make insulting or disparaging remarks about women, or who are jealous or intimidating. If you go out with a man you don't know well, take your own car and stay sober. Consider double-dating. If you find yourself feeling uneasy or uncomfortable with a man, trust your instincts and steer clear of him.

What can you do if an acquaintance attempts to rape you? As with any potential rape, fight back. Some experts suggest that you may be able to stop a date rape by disrupting his fantasy of a seduction scene. You might tell your attacker you have your period, for example, or have a sexually transmitted disease. Or pretend you're about to throw up, and gag as disgustingly as you can.

A victim of date rape has many of the same feelings as the victim of any sexual assault as well as some specifically related to date rape. She may worry that no one will believe what happened. She may doubt her own judgment, find it hard to trust others, and feel strong guilt, fear, and disbelief. As with any rape, seeking help at a rape crisis center can be the first step toward getting the emotional and legal support and advice you need.

Sexual assault is one of the most underreported of all violent crimes (estimates are that only 16 percent of all rapes are reported to the police), often because the victim has feelings of shame and because many women fear they will be made to feel, even by the authorities, that they brought the attack on themselves.

If you are raped by an acquaintance, you must try to remember that you have done nothing wrong and you have nothing to be ashamed of. You are a victim, no matter what may have preceded the assault.

JUST SAY "NO!"

Many women, especially younger women who are less sure of themselves, are pressured into having sex by their date or boyfriend. A man might tell you that he finds you beautiful and that he wants to feel closer to you. Or he might tell you that you make him really hot—and what are you going to do about it?

Or he might tell you that if you really love him, you'll prove it by having sex. Or he might tell you that you led him on—perhaps you have dressed in an alluring fashion

and maybe you were kissing him back enthusiastically—so, he says, you're obligated to
go through with it. Don't. Not unless you, *too, really, truly want to.*

It's your body and yours alone. Don't let anybody coerce you or shame you or
blame you. To borrow that dictum about drugs, Just say "No!" Loudly and clearly. A
decent guy will respect your decision and, in the long run, respect you.

DOMESTIC VIOLENCE

The sad news is that the American family can be a dangerous place. You're far more likely
to be assaulted, injured, raped, or killed by someone you know than you are by a stranger.
Statistics on violence vary tremendously, and family violence is believed to be substantially
underreported throughout the country. Even so, we know that an act of adult domestic violence occurs more frequently than any other crime in the United States.

Battered women account for roughly 35 percent of women seeking care in hospital emergency rooms. At least two studies concluded that there is regular and repeated violence
between spouses in some 20 percent of all marriages, and violence will occur at least once in
two thirds of all marriages. Some four million women are beaten each year by their present or
former partner. Four thousand women a year die as a result of domestic violence. (Between
1959 and 1975, fifty-eight thousand American soldiers were killed in Vietnam; during that
same period fifty-one thousand women were murdered by their male partner.) When a
woman is murdered, it is most likely at the hands of a member of her own family. When
women kill, the victim is often her abuser. The abuse generally escalates, and the women
adjust to higher and higher levels of violence until the abuse goes beyond what the woman is
willing to put up with. Frequently, when the abuser threatens her child, she kills him.

Battering cuts across socioeconomic and racial lines. Time and again the media report
patterns of domestic violence among celebrities, sports figures, and other highly successful
people, making it clear that battering is not just found among the uneducated or the poor.
Several studies have suggested that pregnant women are at greater risk than nonpregnant
women of being abused. Others point out that women thirty and younger are about twice
as likely to be battered as their older counterparts.

To the popular way of thinking, alcohol abuse is often associated with domestic violence. We tend to think of the man who comes home after a night out in bars and beats his
wife. But domestic violence is *not* caused by alcohol or drug abuse or, for that matter, by
unemployment, poverty, money worries, or mental illness. In fact, some researchers
believe that alcohol consumption may be used as an excuse because some men believe
that society will blame them less for beating their wife if they say they were intoxicated at
the time. Others seem to get drunk in order to become violent; for them, drinking serves
as a trigger for arguments that, in the mind of the abuser, justify violence. However, alcohol, high stress levels, and money problems may create special risks and worsen an already
abusive situation.

But abuse is basically about power and control. We know our partner's vulnerabilities and frailties better than anyone. We know exactly how to hurt and how to make a conflict escalate. Even the smallest everyday issues can become the focus of power struggles: Who gets to use the bathroom first in the morning? What video are we going to watch? What are we having for dinner? How clean does our home need to be?

Then there are the larger questions, like how to raise the children, or whether to relocate for a husband's or wife's job. Men's explanations for beating their wife vary from complaints about meals of leftovers to sloppy housekeeping to sexual rejection. A 1986 study found that relationships in which one spouse was dominant and needed to win daily power struggles had the highest likelihood of violence. Relationships defined as equal, on the other hand, with a willingness and capacity for give and take, could tolerate the most conflict before they erupted into violent outbreaks.

Why do women stay with men who batter? They stay for a variety of reasons, primarily fear, guilt, anger, emotional dependence, economic dependence, isolation, and acceptance. Fear dominates the lives of most battered women, who live each day worried about their safety and the safety of their children. Such grinding fear and insecurity paralyze many battered women. They also make it even easier for abusers to manipulate and dominate their victim, since fear erodes the ability to choose and then act on choices.

Many battered women hold fast to traditional sex roles and believe that ending a marriage or being without a man means failing as a woman. They may believe that staying in a marriage is a moral or religious imperative, no matter how unpleasant or damaging, and would feel tremendous guilt and self-blame for shirking responsibility as a nurturing, loving wife. At some level all abuse victims are angry about their treatment, but they are unable to express it, as doing so would incur horrible consequences. So they turn their anger inward, into self-destructive behavior.

Some women stay because they are unable to nurture themselves and need their partner for approval; this dependence in turn is encouraged and fostered by the abuser, who can then manipulate his power over her. Some women stay in the belief that their children are better off living with their father, and the abuser uses this knowledge and makes her feel guilty for even thinking about leaving.

Women also stay for financial reasons. Often in abusive relationships the abuser controls the finances and all the assets are in his name alone (while all the debts may be in *her* name alone). Many battered women think they're incapable of living independently, especially when children are involved. Women fear the effects of poverty on their children, and an abuser often convinces his wife that child custody is given to the parent with the higher income. With affordable child care hard to come by in most of the country, and with women still earning on average substantially less than men, battered women often don't think they have any choice but to stay. Most battered women gradually become increasingly isolated from family, friends, community support, even independent income, with the abuser exercising control over a woman's comings and goings. At the same time, having ceded her power in the relationship, a woman may isolate herself because of shame over being abused.

Women who stay in abusive relationships may be living out a pattern of relationship, low self-esteem, and helplessness learned in childhood. Women who saw their mother victimized by their father or who were physically and sexually abused as children may see victimization as a normal part of family life. Some people, even friends and neighbors, look away when such violence occurs, especially when it's a result of "justifiable" reasons like job stress or financial trouble.

Finally, women who stay in abusive situations have good reason to fear leaving their abusers. Though comprising only 10 percent of American women, separated or divorced women report 75 percent of violence by a spouse or ex-spouse, a rate *fourteen* times that of married women. About 75 percent of the visits to emergency rooms by battered women occur after separation. About 75 percent of calls to police for intervention in domestic violence occur after separation from batterers. Women are at high risk for homicide after they leave their abuser or make it clear that they're leaving for good. One study in Philadelphia showed that 25 percent of women murdered by their partner were killed while trying to separate.

The Children of Family Violence. The children of homes troubled by violence are at high risk to suffer from physical, emotional, and sexual abuse. Child abuse, like wife beating, has a long history as an accepted part of family life and cuts across all socioeconomic, educational, and ethnic lines. Hitting, whipping, and switching have been used as methods of discipline for thousands of years. Yet this only fosters compliance in a child, not moral decision making or the self-esteem that will enable a child to stand up for what is right in difficult situations. An abused child learns to connect love with pain, learns that hitting those you love means you care and violence is a permissible way to handle conflict.

If you suspect a child is being physically abused, look for signs of injury or neglect. A neglected child may beg or steal food, hoard food for siblings, seem listless or overly compliant. The child may not attend school regularly, or there'll be signs of inadequate medical or dental care. Look for bruises, welts, bite marks, lacerations or abrasions, cigar or cigarette burns, fractures or head injuries. If parents' explanations of the injuries don't ring true, trust your instincts. A child who has trouble relating to others, or is very aggressive toward other children or animals, or is very withdrawn, or inflicts injury on himself or herself may be a victim of physical abuse.

Emotional battering is, of course, a lot harder to spot, and often the effects aren't readily obvious, perhaps not until years later, when the now-grown child repeatedly ends up in demeaning relationships, both personally and professionally. It's difficult to counteract the harm done by a parent who regularly calls his child stupid or worthless or who has little regard for the child's needs. Many psychologists and psychiatrists feel that scars left by verbal and emotional abuse take much longer to heal than broken bones. How can you tell whether such abuse is going on? Usually emotionally/verbally abused children have low self-esteem and few friends, exhibit depression and hopelessness, and do poorly in school.

Even if they aren't victims themselves, children who witness violence in their homes are tremendously affected. Family violence causes fear, anxiety, guilt, and stress, which may translate to learning or language problems, developmental delays, and physical ailments such as headaches and stomachaches. Boys who witness family violence are far more likely to batter their own partner as adults; conversely, girls who witness their mother's abuse are far more likely to be battered themselves as adults. And children of violence have a higher risk of alcohol and other drug abuse and juvenile delinquency.

Taking Steps to Change. If you are experiencing violence in your marriage or relationship, how can you end it? First you need determination. Women who have successfully stopped the abuse in their own relationships advise that you must be determined that the violence has to stop. Know that you do not deserve to be abused. Know that even if you are not employed now, you don't need to be dependent on your partner. Know that you can leave the situation if there is a threat of violence. You don't have to put up with being attacked. Once you have made up your mind that you'll no longer take abuse, you can get help from social service agencies. If you choose to go into counseling, do so on your own. Couples counseling is *not* advised as a treatment method. If you don't have the resources for a private therapist, most departments of social service offer individual counseling on a sliding-scale basis. They'll also encourage your partner to enroll in group therapy (often the most effective approach). If you decide to leave without benefit of counseling, enlist the help of friends, relatives, and social service agencies.

Approaches to family violence can be divided into two types, which have been described as focusing on *control* or *compassion*. Approaches to control of the abuser's behavior include arrest, court action, and imprisonment. Arrest, according to some research, doesn't necessarily reduce or eliminate beatings. Some critics are concerned that arresting abusers simply hands over the fate of victims to the judicial system rather than empowering them to change their situation themselves. Compassionate approaches treat the entire family as a system in need of help, support, or education and may include helping in stress management, job counseling to improve household finances, and psychotherapy.

For many years in cases of child abuse, the priority among social service agencies was to protect the child but keep the family together. This is now being reassessed. All too often headlines prove that there are dangerous cracks in the system that can end tragically for the child. Family therapy can place women and children at greater risk of violence because discussing a batterer's behavior in front of the abuser may risk retaliation after the therapy session. Others point out that compassionate intervention may draw an inappropriate distinction between family violence and street violence: If offenders who attack strangers receive a clear message that their behavior is wrong, why should those who do violence within the family escape prosecution?

For all these reasons, many experts recommend a mixture of compassion and control, combining restraining orders and shelters, for example, with psychotherapy and education.

PORTRAIT OF A BATTERER

Men who batter and abuse are of all ages, races, religions, and socioeconomic backgrounds. Some have white-collar jobs, others blue-collar jobs, and still others are unemployed. Some batterers abuse alcohol and drugs, but many don't. In short, there's no typical profile.

There are, however, common behaviors, and if you want to avoid being involved with someone who'll be physically or emotionally abusive, there are definite warning signs to be on the lookout for. If a person exhibits three or more of the following behaviors, there's a strong potential that emotional abuse will escalate to physical violence; the last four are already battering behaviors. Though some of them may resemble signs of love and concern and be flattering, as time goes on, the behaviors usually become more severe and serve only to dominate and control.

- Jealousy. *Jealousy isn't a sign of love; it's a sign of possessiveness and lack of trust. Your partner may start showing up at your job, calling you frequently during the day, or dropping by unexpectedly, checking up on you and even embarrassing you in public.*

- Control. *Watch out for controlling behaviors such as making decisions for you ("for your own good") or demanding to know where you've been or why you're late. An abuser may insist on taking control of your finances, using an excuse that it will "free up your time."*

- Breaking promises and abusing trust. *An abuser won't follow through on commitments or take a fair share of responsibility. And he'll lie, withhold information, and cheat on you.*

- Emotional withholding and disrespect. *An abuser won't express his feelings or give support, attention, or compliments. He'll interrupt or change the topic when you're speaking or not listen or respond to you. He won't respect your feelings, rights, or opinions.*

- Quick involvement. *Abusers come on like whirlwinds, claiming, "You're the only person I could ever talk to." Many battered women knew their abuser for less than six months before marriage or moving in together. The abuser may pressure you to commit yourself or instill guilt if you try to slow things down.*

- Unrealistic expectations. *An abuser may expect his partner to meet all his needs. Beware of lines like "You're all I need; if you love me, I'm all you need."*

- Isolation. *An abuser will often try to cut off his partner from all resources, including friends, family, job. He may monitor your phone calls and your freedom. He may want you to live way out in the country, sometimes without a phone or a car.*

- Blame of others for his problems and feelings. *Someone is always doing the abuser wrong or is out to get him. Usually the abuser's partner is at fault for anything that goes wrong: If he makes a mistake, it's because you upset him and prevented him from concentrating on his work. If he's angry, it's because you made him mad.*

- Hypersensitivity. *An abuser is easily insulted and takes the smallest setbacks as personal attacks, be it having to work overtime or getting a parking ticket.*

- Cruelty to children or animals. *Abusers may expect children to be capable of doing things beyond their ability. He may spank or even beat a baby for wetting its diaper, for example, or he may tease and taunt children until they cry. Abusers are brutal to animals and are insensitive to their pain and suffering.*

- "Playful" use of force in sex. *Abusers may want to act out sexual fantasies that are degrading or in which his partner is helpless, like rape. He may use force or coercion to obtain sex or get you to perform sexual acts. An abuser won't care if you don't want to have sex—even if you're ill or tired—and he may start to have sex with you while you're sleeping.*

- Rigid sex roles. *An abuser will expect you to serve him, saying that women must stay at home and obey men in all things. He'll consider you inferior to him, stupid, and not a whole person without a relationship.*

- Verbal and psychological abuse, destructive criticism, and disrespect. *An abuser will systematically destroy his partner's self-esteem by using cruel and hurtful words and degrading her (whether alone or in front of others), belittling her accomplishments and abilities. He'll manipulate and play head games on you, often using your children to make you feel guilty.*

- Economic control. *An abuser will try to prevent his partner from getting or keeping a job. He'll take her money or make her ask for money, giving her an allowance to maintain control.*

- Dr. Jekyll and Mr. Hyde. *Abusers may exhibit contrary personalities, loving one minute and exploding the next. Moodiness and explosiveness are characteristic of abusers.*

- Past battering. *An abuser may tell you he has hit women in the past—because they made him do it, he'll say. But situations don't make a person an abusive personality. A batterer will beat any woman if she's with him long enough for the violence to begin.*

- Threats of violence. *These can include any threats of physical force to control you, even saying something like "If you talk that way to me again, I'll break your neck." But a batterer will make light of the threats by saying that everyone talks like that.*

- Physical intimidation. *An abuser will instill fear by using looks, actions, gestures, shouting, sometimes smashing something that his mate especially loves to punish her. But usually throwing or breaking something or pounding on a table is a terrorist tactic meant to frighten you into submission.*

- Any force during an argument. *An abuser may hold you down, physically restraining you from leaving the room, or push or shove you against a wall, demanding, "You're going to listen to me!"*

Other forms of abuse involve manipulations such as threatening to harm themselves or others (you, your children, your friends, your relatives) or threatening legal

action, usually an attempt to gain child custody. A batterer may promise to get counsel-
ing or may make promises in general, saying he'll never hit you again or he'll never
drink again or he'll get rid of his guns.

The desperate batterer may try to flush out his wife from her place of safekeeping
by faking a report that he's been in an accident or by filing a missing person report
with the police, enlisting them as unwitting accomplices to track down his partner. He
may have a friend call, saying he's the woman's lawyer or doctor and needs to meet
with her right away. In short, he'll do anything to maintain the status quo.

Why do men batter and abuse? Above all else, an abuser is determined to main-
tain power and control over his partner. Most are not out of control when they abuse,
and they're not angry men suffering from low self-esteem. A batterer believes he's enti-
tled to control his partner, who is obligated to obey him. He believes he's a moral per-
son, even if he uses violence against his partner. He believes he'll get what he wants by
using violence. And he believes he won't suffer any significant adverse legal, economic,
or personal consequences as a result of his battering.

Battering isn't a mental illness; it's a learned behavioral choice. And what has
been learned can be unlearned. If an abuser sincerely wants to change his behavior,
counseling programs try to teach batterers how to end their violent, controlling, abu-
sive behavior; hold batterers accountable for their behavior; and provide treatment
and education.

GETTING HELP

If you're a victim of rape or battering, getting help is the first step to recovery and control of your life.

If You've Been Raped. The first thing to do if you've been sexually assaulted is to go to a safe place. Then get medical attention. You can get immediate response from authorities by dialing 911 in most areas, or calling the operator, or going to the nearest hospital emergency room. Medical attention will determine whether you have sustained physical injuries, contracted a sexually transmitted disease, or become pregnant; collect medical evidence for possible prosecution; and be the first step toward concentrating on yourself and your health.

Avoid destroying evidence that may be important should you decide to press charges against your attacker: *Do not shower, bathe, wash your hands, brush your teeth, douche, or use the toilet. Do not change your clothing. Do not clean up the scene of the assault.*

Contact a trusted friend or family member or call your local rape crisis hot line for information and support. A trained volunteer from a rape crisis center may accompany you to the hospital and stay with you through the physical examination, which can be frightening and uncomfortable in the aftermath of a rape.

If you don't contact the police after a sexual assault, most hospitals automatically do so once you visit the emergency room. This doesn't mean you have to make a crime report, which may be emotionally difficult and require repeating the story many times to police and in court. But keep in mind that by doing so you may protect others from being raped by the same attacker, you may help substantiate another victim's report, and you may be eligible for state financial compensation.

A rape crisis center or shelter for battered women can be a lifesaver. Support groups for survivors are sponsored by rape crisis centers; women who've had the same experience will offer you support, give you practical help with getting your life in order, and listen to you and care about your ordeal and recovery. One word of caution, however: Some researchers advise that recent victims' needs may not be served by being in groups in which women describe their rapes in graphic terms. If you find the group upsetting or traumatic, trust your instincts; treatment should not be experienced as a reenactment of the rape. A trained counselor or psychotherapist working with you individually can also be helpful.

If You've Been Abused. If you're the victim of domestic violence in any form—be it physical attack or verbal abuse and intimidation—your safety and that of your children come first.

- If you're in physical danger or are being emotionally harmed, go to a safe place and only tell those you trust completely where you're going.
- If you've been physically attacked, get medical attention as quickly as you can. An injury may be worse than it seems, and you may not be aware of how badly you've been hurt or what complications or long-term effects may result from the beating. When you're examined, be truthful about what happened to you. Both the police and the courts are there to help you.
- If you're in an abusive relationship, talk to someone you trust or call a domestic violence hot line for confidential counseling and information. Find out what your options are, what resources are available, and what are the likely consequences of your decisions.
- Make a safety plan. Memorize emergency phone numbers if 911 isn't yet available in your area, and plan an escape route if you need to get out of your house or apartment in a hurry. Make sure your children know how to use the phone to contact police.

Select a code word you can use with your children, family, or friends that will alert them to call for help. Keep some money, changes of clothes for you and your kids, and copies of important documents and keys hidden somewhere that your partner doesn't know about but that you can get to quickly, maybe at a friend's house or neighbor's or even in the trunk of your car. Keep your purse and car keys in a place where you can grab them fast and easily.

- If you decide to leave, even for a short while, take your children with you if doing so won't expose them to harm. If you can, plan ahead by packing birth certificates and other important documents such as marriage or divorce papers, passports or green cards, social security cards, school and vaccination records, bank account numbers (including cash machine numbers) and credit card numbers, house deed or rental agreement, driver's license and car registration/title, medical information and prescription numbers, plus any money you've managed to set aside.

Pack several changes of clothes and some of your children's favorite toys or security blankets as well as your own pictures, jewelry, and irreplaceable items of sentimental value. Any evidence you might have that substantiates the abuse done to you—such as threatening letters or phone message tapes—will aid police in making a case against your abuser. But remember that personal safety comes first; leave without these things if you can't get them without risking harm.

• Call 911. The police can arrest your abuser, help you get medical attention, and get you and your children to safety. Be sure to write down the name of the responding officer; it may be helpful to you later.

• Get an Order of Protection. While an Order of Protection can't guarantee your safety, it will legally require that your abuser leave you and your children alone—at home, school, and your workplace—and if the order is violated, he will be arrested and jailed. If you have left your home, an Order of Protection makes it easier for you to get the police to go with you to get your personal belongings. Also, a protective order may require your abuser to undergo drug testing, get counseling, and pay for any medical and legal costs that his violence has created. You don't need a lawyer to get a protective order. You can get one on your own, or a domestic violence victim advocate will help you.

Get help. Get safe. Stay safe.

SEXUAL ABUSE OF CHILDREN

Child sexual abuse is the involvement of children and adolescents in sexual activities that they don't fully understand, that violate social taboos, and to which the children cannot give informed consent. This may include touching, masturbating, oral sex, exposure, undressing, photographing or videotaping, and other forms of sexual activity, with or without penetration.

Sexual abuse is damaging not only to a child's body but to her or his sexual attitudes. Repeated trauma becomes part of the child's total developing personality. The abuse itself, as well as the child's efforts to cope with it and adapt, affect his or her ability to participate in relationships, cope with anxiety, trust her or his instincts, and even distinguish reality from fantasy.

Whether by a parent or a sibling, relative, baby-sitter, teacher, member of the clergy, or anyone else in a position of authority over the child, sexual abuse is an abuse of power and attachment. That these acts are inflicted by people to whom the child looks for love and protection makes the child feel shame and betrayal. If she or he tells others of the abuse and isn't believed or even is punished for "lying" when the abuser refuses to admit to the abuse or threatens the child for telling, then the child learns to doubt her or his own perceptions.

Children who are abused often get through the ordeal by escaping mentally, pretending their mind and spirit go to a safer or happier place, leaving only the body behind to endure the abuse. They may pretend they're asleep or do simple arithmetic in their head or study wallpaper patterns. This survival technique is called *dissociation* and persists later in life. Survivors may have difficulty experiencing their own sexuality, instead engaging passively and sometimes promiscuously in sexual activity. They may have trouble "feeling their feelings." They may experience flashbacks or a whole range of symptoms termed *complex posttraumatic stress disorder,* a combination of flashbacks and anxiety.

It's hard to know whether the actual incidence of sexual abuse of children has increased dramatically in this country or whether it's just the reporting of that incidence that has increased. Whichever the case, it is clearly, tragically, not a problem that's going away.

Incest. Incest—sexual abuse by family members—that occurs in childhood is never forgotten. An incest survivor may have terrifying nightmares that seem almost real. She may be highly anxious, with psychosomatic complaints that may be hard to understand. She may have flashbacks or notice that hearing certain words or phrases or thinking of particular places or ages of her childhood or being in particular situations as an adult makes her sad or uneasy. She may reenact the trauma in disguised ways, such as risk taking or sexually promiscuous behavior. She may be unaware of a lack of feeling, numbness, or a tendency to *dissociate*—not feel present in her body—especially during sex.

Sexual boundaries are important to children's well-being, not only for moral reasons but also because when a child's boundaries are respected, she learns to contain and control her feelings. When her boundaries are violated, she experiences very strong feelings that are likely to be overwhelming. As a result, adults who experienced incest in childhood may have difficulty controlling their emotions, including anger and sexual feelings, and expressing them appropriately. In their intimate relationships they frequently follow an on-again, off-again pattern, either searching for a rescuer who will meet all their needs or running away in anger and hopeless despair when the relationship fails to live up to these expectations.

If you are an incest survivor, seek help. Find a therapist with the experience, understanding, and commitment to provide effective treatment. Exploring past experiences is never easy and often painful, but your therapy or group work should help you feel empowered, not reenact your childhood abuse by controlling or overwhelming you.

Effective therapy helps you to explore your past in meaningful ways and to know and trust your own feelings, instincts, and experiences in the here and now. You will need to feel the therapeutic situation is a safe place in order to remember the abuse, mourn the loss, and restore your connections to the community.

ABUSE OF THE ELDERLY

Old age, even for people who have lived an active and productive life, is usually a time of greater dependence and vulnerability. The ancient, traditional idea that elders deserve honor and respect, and that a long life brings not only a decline of vigor but also a richness of wisdom and experience to be shared, has served to protect older people in many cultures. In the United States today this view has been replaced by the idea that the "golden years" are a time to enjoy golf, gardening, and grandchildren—a prospect that has its appeal but is, unfortunately, only possible for seniors blessed with relative affluence and good health. Among older people who are frail and in need of protection and care, abuse is, sadly, all too common.

More often than not, "elder abuse" (elders are usually defined as people older than sixty) occurs at the hands of their caretakers: a spouse, a sibling, a child, or someone employed in a nursing home. The term refers to various kinds of mistreatment of an older person by someone with whom the victim has a special relationship.

Elder abuse includes not only physical attack but also any crime perpetrated by a caregiver against an older person because of his or her frailty. Sometimes the abuse is sexual, as, for example, in the case of marital rape. It may be psychological, taking the form of intimidation or verbal threats to the older person. Elder abuse can also be financial, in cases, for example, in which an older person's social security checks are misappropriated or his or her property or funds are used without permission.

Sometimes elder abuse takes the form of neglect or failure to fulfill a caretaking obligation to which the abuser has voluntarily agreed. Neglect includes both active abuse and a willful failure to provide care. Such passive abuse may result from the lack of knowledge or illness of the caretaker.

Elder abuse often is unnoticed and unreported because the elderly are often isolated, and their injuries may not be easily recognized in public, unlike a child's, whose injuries are likely to be spotted by a teacher or school nurse. Elder abuse is, surprisingly and sadly, all too common—and getting more so. Between 1986 and 1988 elder abuse reports increased by almost 20 percent nationally. Research studies indicate that only one in four elder abuse incidents are reported, suggesting that *two million* incidents occurred in 1988.

Some studies show that the older person's dependency is a major factor contributing to abuse. Older people in poor health may be three to four times more likely to be abused than those in good health. The abusive caretaker may be part of the "sandwich generation," under high stress from obligations to parents *and* children; the caretaker feels burdened by responsibilities and ill equipped to devote the time, money, and energy to caring for the older person.

As people live longer, it's rapidly becoming true that older people may be dependent on their grown children longer than their children were dependent on them. In families without close ties of love and friendship or with unresolved childhood resentments and conflicts still smoldering in the parent-child relationship, the dependence of an aged parent may lead to frustration and anger that can result in abuse by the now-grown child. Some studies suggest that caretakers who were abused as children are more likely to inflict violence on elderly parents later in life, but this point is in debate.

Whether older men or older women are more likely to be abused is also disputed; some studies suggest that men are at greater risk because older women are more likely to live alone and therefore be less vulnerable to abuse. Abuse is almost three times more common among those living with someone than those living alone. Others say the most likely victim is a female eighty years or older, especially one suffering from physical or mental impairments. Abusers are often the victim's middle-aged daughters, but more elders are abused by spouses than by their children.

The physical consequences of abuse include pain, bruises, fractures, burns, wounds, and malnutrition. But there are also emotional consequences of elder abuse, especially fear and a sense of helplessness.

If you are a victim of elder abuse, or if you suspect that someone you know is being abused, contact the police or, if you prefer to keep matters out of the courts, call your local Department of Social Services.

SEXUAL HARASSMENT

Just what *is* sexual harassment, anyway? It's a hotly debated topic with much disagreement as to exactly what it is.

Sometimes it's easy to recognize. If a superior makes promises of employment benefits in exchange for sexual favors—say a promotion, a raise, or a job offer in return for sexual acts—that's a pretty obvious example of sexual harassment. But sometimes more insidious forms of harassment create a hostile work environment.

If you work in a place where sexually explicit drawings or photographs are hung up, for example, or where suggestive remarks, teasing, or jokes are all part of a day's work, you may have legal grounds to consider this harassment. What makes harassment different from an attraction or an office romance is the difference in power between the harasser and the victim plus the fact that sexual advances and remarks are an unwelcome part of business as usual. Because most working women have male supervisors, it isn't surprising that women feel intimidated when the relationship is sexualized.

Despite the stereotype of the executive chasing his secretary around the desk, sexual harassment is an issue for women in every profession and salary level. The hearings on the behavior of Supreme Court Justice Clarence Thomas, accused of harassment by the attorney Anita Hill, won't be soon forgotten. And a female brain surgeon at Stanford University School of Medicine resigned as a tenured professor because, she alleged, she had been sexually harassed for years, with colleagues calling her "honey" in the operating room and stroking her legs under the operating table. It can happen at any level of business or academia.

If you are being sexually harassed, immediately make your feelings and wishes clear. But saying no is only a first step. Clearly confront your harasser. State in no uncertain terms that you do not like the way he is speaking and you do not want to be talked to in such a manner. Don't hesitate to make your statements in the presence of coworkers; should you decide to bring charges, having witnesses may be important.

Make it clear that you mean business. Don't worry about being "nice." Don't smile. If the problem continues, report it to your supervisor or the personnel manager. Learn your company's grievance procedures. If there is none, propose that a process be put in place. Keep in mind that you have leverage: Not only are allegations of sexual harassment bad publicity for your company, but the company may also be financially liable.

CHAPTER 12

Occupational and Environmental Issues

CONTENTS

If you're like many Americans, you've become an active participant in your own good health. You've cut the fat and increased the fiber in your diet; no week is complete without several good workouts; and, as a woman concerned about the risk of breast cancer, you practice self-examination and have periodic mammograms as recommended by your doctor. In short, you are making a real effort to prevent disease and prolong your life.

All of this makes it even more disconcerting to know that external forces over which you have little or no control can have a negative, even dire, impact on your health.

In this chapter we'll discuss the ways in which the environment as well as your occupation may be a threat to your health and what you can do to minimize that threat.

CLEAN AIR

If you live in or around a city, you need only look up to see that something isn't quite right. In many cities, even on a sunny day you're likely to see not blue sky but yellow haze.

That sickly looking sky is caused by pollution, a major by-product of an industrialized society. On its worst days, this pollution can be hazardous to your health, especially if you have heart or lung problems or other chronic diseases. Carbon monoxide lowers the oxygen-carrying capacity of the blood; nitrogen and sulfur dioxide, when combined with water, form acids that damage lung tissue; ozone damages body tissue directly; and particulates (airborne particles) decrease lung capacity and function by accumulating in the lungs.

The following are the main sources of pollution:

- *Motor vehicle exhaust.* Carbon monoxide, oxides of nitrogen, and lead are the main pollutants released by cars and trucks into the atmosphere. Oxides of nitrogen from car exhaust are one of the main causes of acid rain.
- *Industrial and power plants.* Sulfur-containing fuels like oil and coal that are burned by factories and power plants are the primary source of industrial pollution. Oxides of sulfur are another major cause of acid rain.
- *Chlorofluorocarbons.* We've all heard that the ozone layer of the atmosphere, which protects our planet from the sun's ultraviolet rays, is gradually being depleted. Chlorofluorocarbons, used in air conditioners, refrigerators, and dry cleaning solutions, are believed to be the culprits. An increasing incidence of skin cancer is thought to be one result of this depletion.

In recent decades, much concern has focused on air pollution. The Clean Air Act of 1970 (which established maximum levels for sulfur and nitrogen dioxide, particulates, hydrocarbons, ozone, and carbon monoxide, the primary urban pollutants), the establishment of a toxic waste "superfund," and private and government efforts have helped improve air quality, but clean air is still a long way off. Even with increasingly stringent controls on auto emissions and industry, air quality in urban areas sometimes doesn't meet minimum standards.

You can do your part by making sure your car's pollution control devices are functioning well. Many states mandate a yearly inspection. If yours does not, take it upon yourself to have your car checked.

THE WATER YOU DRINK

The water that comes out of your faucet may taste fine. But is it safe?

At the turn of the century, public health programs practically eliminated the widespread threat of infectious diseases caused by drinking contaminated water. Thus, diseases such as cholera and typhoid almost disappeared in the United States, and our water was thought to be perfectly safe.

Today, the greatest threat is still bacteria but pollutants such as heavy metals, polychlorinated biphenyls (PCBs), and pesticides are added risks. These pollutants come from many sources and contaminate streams, lakes, and ground water in both rural and urban areas.

How do these pollutants find their way into water supplies? One source is agricultural tracts, whose fertilizer- and pesticide-containing runoff fouls streams, lakes, reservoirs, and ground water (underground water sources). Landfills sometimes contain hazardous materials that leech into the soil and contaminate ground water. Faulty filling station gas tanks and septic tanks are two other routes for contaminants to enter our water system.

The water pollutants that pose the most serious risk to your health are the following:

- *Trihalomethanes.* Public water supplies are cleaned of potentially harmful bacteria with chlorine and fluoride, the levels of which are regularly monitored. But chlorine reacts with certain pollutants to undergo chemical changes that result in trihalomethanes (THMs). Animal testing has shown these chemical compounds to be potential carcinogens.
- *Nitrates.* High levels of nitrates from fertilizers may be found in well water in irrigated agricultural areas. Nitrates are suspected carcinogens.
- *Asbestos and heavy metals.* Lead from old plumbing pipes and paint in older homes and apartments, as well as from ground contamination from vehicle exhaust, and asbestos from older construction (both asbestos–cement water pipes and insulation) all can pollute water. Asbestos exposure by inhalation can result in lung cancer, and high lead levels in the blood can cause nervous system impairment and anemia.
- *Mercury and PCBs.* Discharged into water in industrial effluent, mercury becomes concentrated in the food chain (as does any waterborne pollutant that doesn't rapidly degrade) and may be hazardous if you eat large quantities of contaminated fish. Shellfish glean nutrients from water and can concentrate PCBs and pesticides. Metals like lead and mercury remain toxic indefinitely.

How Can You Avoid Drinking Polluted Water? Some people have turned to bottled water to reduce their risk of pollutants, but this pricey water source may be no better than what your own tap offers. If bacteria are a concern where you live, you can always boil your water, but this won't eliminate pollutants.

Public water supplies are, of course, monitored by the Environmental Protection Agency (EPA) and local and state organizations, and their pollutant levels must fall within an acceptable range. But if your water comes from a well, have it tested yearly to ensure your safety. Filtration systems may be useful for certain contaminants, but sometimes exaggerated claims are made about their efficacy. If you plan to purchase a water filter, check with an independent consumer testing agency for their findings before you buy.

SUN EXPOSURE

No matter how good it feels on your skin, the sun is one of your skin's worst enemies. That's not to say you must spend your life indoors, but your days of basking in the sun in search of the perfect tan should be over.

It wasn't very long ago that sunbathing was considered healthy, a good way to soak up vitamin D. Maybe you spent your summers outdoors with nothing between you and the sun's powerful rays but a tank top and pair of shorts. That was before we knew the extent of the sun's adverse effects on skin.

Our understanding of the sun's role not only in aging but also in skin cancer has come a long way in recent years. Chronic overexposure to the ultraviolet radiation in sunlight is, in fact, the leading cause of skin cancer. Moreover, more than 800,000 Americans will have some form of the disease this year alone. We now know that people who received severe sunburns when young are more likely to have malignant melanoma, a potentially fatal form of skin cancer. The deep tan that made you look so healthy when you were twenty gives you premature wrinkles when you're forty.

Of course, there's no practical way to avoid being in the sun—not that you would want to, anyway. But you can protect your skin from overexposure to harmful ultraviolet rays.

Always Use a Sun Screen. Use one with a sun protection factor (SPF) 15 rating. This rating means you can stay in the sun fifteen times longer than you could without sun screen. Thus, if your unprotected skin could take twenty minutes of sun exposure before starting to burn, an SPF 15 sun screen theoretically allows you to stay outside for five hours. If you're particularly sensitive, use a sun block on the delicate skin around the eyes, nose, and lips in particular.

The sun lotions of yesteryear (coconut oil, baby oil, and cocoa butter) might keep your skin feeling smooth, but they provide no protection against sunburn and the harmful effects of ultraviolet radiation. Choose a sun screen containing either para-aminobenzoic acid (PABA, to which some people are sensitive), cinnamate, or benzophenone. Remember, though, that sun screen comes off when you are swimming or when you perspire, so you need to reapply it frequently if you're outside for any length of time.

Remember, too, that water and sand reflect light, intensifying the effects of the sun. And sun screen isn't just for summer. Winter radiation hazard is highest on cloudy days just after a snowfall, and the higher the altitude, the higher the radiation—so skiers should always use a sun screen or sun block.

For optimal results, apply your sun screen at least thirty minutes before going outside. Alcohol-based products may provide the best protection since they seem to penetrate the skin more deeply.

Stay out of the Sun When the Rays Are at Their Strongest. That's between 10:00 A.M. and 3:00 P.M. So mow your lawn and enjoy other outdoor activities either early in the morning or in the later afternoon.

During Prolonged Sunlight Exposure, Protect Your Face. Wear a broad-brimmed hat (in addition to sun screen). Cover your body, too, with loose-fitting pants and long-sleeved shirts made of a tightly woven fabric. Loosely woven material may look and feel cool, but it allows too much penetration by ultraviolet rays.

Besides damaging your skin, excessive exposure to sunlight, especially when there's little breeze and high heat and humidity, can result in heat stroke or heat exhaustion. Both are medical emergencies that require immediate attention.

To prevent heat exhaustion (characterized by weakness, dizziness, nausea, headache, and even collapse) or heat stroke (an acute and dangerous reaction to heat exposure, characterized by high temperature, rapid pulse, confusion, and even coma), don't drink alcohol when you must be outside on a hot day. Make sure you have access to adequate water. And wear a hat and loose-fitting, light-colored clothing to reflect the sun off your body.

PHOTOSENSITIVITY

It's a beautiful summer day and you'll be spending most of it outdoors. Being an intelligent person, you've put SPF 15 sun screen on your exposed face, arms, and legs. So no need to worry, right?

Not quite. Without realizing it, we occasionally put ourselves at risk of sunburn or even blistering and rashes as a result of combining certain medications, food, even skin preparations, with ultraviolet light—natural and artificial. This heightened reaction is called photosensitivity, *and its symptoms are similar to those incurred from prolonged exposure to the sun, including redness, rash, and blistering.*

Among drugs known to cause photosensitivity are certain antihistamines, tranquilizers, tetracycline, sulfonamides, antidiabetics, antihypertensives, antidepressants, and anticancer drugs. Some antibacterial deodorant soaps, shampoos or soaps containing coal tar, skin-bleaching creams, after-shave lotions, topical antiseptic creams, even perfumes with sandalwood, lavender, or citron oils are known sensitizers. If you're having an outdoor picnic and may be photosensitive, you might think twice before eating carrots, celery, parsley, or limes or putting mustard on your hot dog. All of these foods commonly promote sunlight reactions.

There are two types of photosensitive reactions. A photo allergy *is a result of changes in your immune system and will occur whenever you're exposed to sunlight. Symptoms of a photoallergic reaction are red skin (though not sunburn) with a rash similar to poison ivy and sometimes discolored patches, blisters, and swelling.*

A phototoxic *reaction has the same appearance and feel as a severe sunburn, showing redness, blisters, and sunburn pain. You might have this reaction whenever a sensitizing drug or food that you've taken (or a substance worn on your skin) is exposed to sufficient sunlight.*

To prevent photosensitive reactions, find out from your health-care provider or pharmacist whether any of your medications may cause photosensitization, and, if so, either avoid prolonged sun exposure or wear light-colored protective clothing, including a broad-brimmed hat.

EXPOSURE TO TOXIC MATERIALS

It would indeed be difficult to live in today's world without some exposure to a potentially dangerous substance. You break your arm and need an X ray. Your old house was painted with lead paint and has lead solder in the pipes. The soil under your lush, green lawn is contaminated with permanent residue from lead gasoline additives of twenty years ago. You work in a factory and are exposed to industrial solvents that are known carcinogens. Your carpets release carbon-based organic compounds and your comfortable foam-stuffed couch contains formaldehyde, which can be irritating to the lungs.

We've all been exposed to materials that have the potential, under the right circumstances, to make us sick. Most of the time the exposure is limited, with no noticeable adverse effects. But in cases of prolonged or intense exposure, problems may result.

The following are some common toxic materials:

Radiation. Most of us have been exposed to radiation as a result of having an X ray, which is a valuable diagnostic tool. The amount of radiation in a diagnostic X ray is very low, the risk minimal, and no radiation remains in your body after the X ray is taken. In fact, we're exposed to more radiation from the rocks and soil and the air around us than through our average yearly exposure as a result of X rays.

X rays, of course, should be done only when medically necessary, whether you're pregnant or not. The risk to the unborn child from diagnostic X rays is minimal, and pregnancy is not a reason to avoid X rays that are otherwise indicated.

Far greater radiation exposure—especially in some parts of the country—results from radioactive radon gas formed by decaying uranium. Uranium is found in soil and rocks that contain granite, shale, and phosphate. Aside from the soil and rocks themselves, bricks and concrete are formed from these materials, making your home a potential radon repository. When released by the soil and/or brick, it can accumulate inside your house, seeping in via cracks in the foundation and mortar, open sump pumps, or pores in concrete block.

Radon poses potential health risks. The radon decays to radioactive atoms that can attach themselves to dust particles. When radon is inhaled over an extended period, the radioactivity may damage your lungs and eventually may cause lung cancer. This risk is primarily seen in people who smoke.

The Environmental Protection Agency recommends that you test for radon (using a readily available radon detector available in hardware stores) since one survey found one in three basements contained potentially dangerous radon levels. It's also recommended that you make the necessary changes to prevent radon from entering your home. Usually the changes are fairly minor—sealing dirt floors in your basement or crawl space, covering and venting sump pumps, or caulking cracks in the basement floor and walls. Avoiding cigarettes is an important means of decreasing radon risk.

Hazardous Substances. It would be impossible to list within this section all the chemicals and substances that can do you harm. Most often a person comes into contact with one or more hazardous substances in the workplace, especially when that workplace is a factory. Organic chemical compounds, many acutely toxic, total 60 percent of the hazardous waste generated by industry. Toxic fumes, gases, particles, and smoke are a fact of life in many of our factories. Typically, a worker is exposed to low levels of a toxicant at levels regulated by the Occupational Safety and Health Administration. Unless accidents that expose a worker to a high level occur or a worker ignores prescribed safety measures, serious health problems caused by these exposures are rare.

If you work in an occupation that exposes you to dangerous materials, use recommended safety precautions to minimize your risk. Wear proper clothing and eye protection. Use an air-filtration mask when appropriate and make sure the area you work in is well ventilated. If you think you're being placed at unnecessary risk, call the Occupational Safety and Health Administration (OSHA), which oversees workplace safety.

Remember, your home also contains hazardous substances such as those found in cleaning supplies. If you have children, be careful to keep these products out of reach.

Pesticides. The fruits and vegetables you buy at the supermarket may look beautiful and taste equally good. But are they safe to eat?

Pesticides have been a boon to agriculture, but the growing concern is that the chemicals sprayed to prevent insects from devouring our produce may make these products dangerous to humans, too. The Food and Drug Administration monitors the amount of pesticide found on food and has determined that low levels of these chemicals aren't hazardous to health.

Many people question whether these levels should be lower—though there's no agreement on just how low. The objections to pesticides are often based on superstitions; some people believe that chemicals by definition must be harmful. It is important, however, to balance the use of pesticides against the risks of food-borne disease from spoilage that would occur in untreated food. In addition, some of the most harmful chemicals in the environment are perfectly natural, made by plants themselves or by the organisms that live on them.

As a precaution, always wash your fruits and vegetables thoroughly before eating them. While this may not get rid of any pesticide that has permeated the fruit, it'll certainly remove surface contaminants. Eating organically grown produce is another, though more expensive, option.

THE DELICATE BALANCE: ALL WORK AND NO PLAY

You're on the fast track at work, logging seventy-hour weeks as you slowly climb the ladder to the senior executives' floor.

Non-business-related meals are wolfed down between phone calls, the only exercise you get is running to and from meetings, and your spouse—if you've had time to find one—has been relegated to a snoring lump in the bed, asleep when you get home and still oblivious when you leave in the morning.

If part or all of this description hits home, you're not alone. More and more women today are speeding down life's fast lane as they race to be the first and best: the company's first female CEO, the top salesperson, the copywriter demanded by all the major accounts. And it usually isn't enough to succeed at work. We all know someone who's the model employee, the mother who volunteers for school committees even when she's about to keel over in exhaustion. She never seems to order pizza but cooks nutritious meals nightly for her family. She's superwoman, a woman who can do everything and—as it appears from the outside looking in—the woman who has everything.

But at what cost?

When you're just starting out, it's easy to be single-minded in your determination to succeed in your chosen path. You have the seemingly endless energy of youth on your side, your body is relatively healthy and fit, and not many things are competing for your attention. But for many women the situation changes as they grow older. They develop a loving relationship that requires effort if it is to flourish. Children, with a constant need for time and attention, may enter the picture. Other interests begin to compete with work.

Somewhere along the way, most of us realize there's more to life than work, however satisfying a career may be. Childhood passes with lightning speed, and a parent too busy to notice and appreciate every nuance is likely to be filled with regret. Muscles long neglected eventually sag in protest. Backyard roses left unattended succumb to infestation and disease. In short, a satisfying life is constructed of many parts. One that's all work is just as incomplete as one that's nothing but play.

From a health standpoint, the inability to attain a good balance in your life may be doing you harm. Stress is a normal part of everyone's life, but if you're driven, you have more than your share of stress. Stress itself can cause a plethora of side effects such as headache, insomnia, upset stomach, and digestive problems. Or you may feel constant fatigue or lose interest in sex.

Many people learn relaxation techniques to cope better with stress. One of the best ways not only to reduce stress but also to strengthen your cardiovascular system and improve the way your body looks is exercise. We now know that exercise has a calming effect that lasts long after your workout. Schedule at least twenty minutes of vigorous aerobic exercise at least three times a week (see Exercise, *page 72) and see whether you feel calmer.*

Though setting aside time for exercise will make you feel better, it won't bring balance into your life. A life that's all work and no play may be a busy one, but it isn't a rich one. It's up to you to recognize the importance of a well-rounded life and to institute the changes that will make that possible.

HOUSEHOLD POLLUTION

You'd think that if there were any place you could go to be safe it would be inside your home.

Unfortunately, that may not be always true. Many houses—particularly newly constructed ones that are tightly sealed to prevent the loss of heated or cooled air—are filled with substances that can make you sick. As a result of prolonged exposure to these indoor pollutants, increasing numbers of people are experiencing allergic symptoms such as rash, eye irritation, cough, and sore throat. A far more serious risk of exposure to some household pollutants is cancer.

Many things can pollute your home. The most common are the following:

• *Cigarette smoke.* If you or someone else in your household smokes, your home is hazardous for everyone living there. We've long known that smokers are at high risk for development of cancer and serious lung diseases. But we've recently learned just how damaging the effects of secondhand smoke are.

Secondhand cigarette smoke in an enclosed environment poses nearly the same threat of lung cancer and emphysema to people chronically exposed to it as to the smokers themselves. If you even visit a house where cigarettes are smoked, you're exposed to high levels of tar, nicotine, carbon monoxide, and cancer-causing compounds including 3,4-benzpyrene. Your heart rate will increase and your blood pressure will rise. If you have respiratory problems, you may find it harder to breathe.

Studies have shown that the children of smokers have a higher incidence of pneumonia, bronchitis, and tonsillitis than those of nonsmokers. Moreover, babies during their first year of life are more likely to be admitted to the hospital for respiratory illness when they live with one or more smokers (for further information on the dangers of smoking to babies and fetuses, see *Tobacco Use*, page 158).

• *Carbon monoxide.* This deadly odorless gas is produced by the incomplete combustion of carbon-based fuel. Many stoves (both cooking and wood-burning), lamps, space heaters, engines, and furnaces produce it. Carbon monoxide is most likely to build up if you have a defective pilot light or control valve on a stove or heating unit. Your risk of carbon monoxide poisoning is greatest during cold weather when your home is sealed tightly against the elements.

When the carbon monoxide level in your home is too high, it replaces oxygen in your red blood cells. The initial symptoms of carbon monoxide poisoning are vague. You may have a headache and feel nauseated. Vomiting, fatigue, and dizziness also may occur. When the concentration of carbon monoxide is very high, you'll become unconscious.

To prevent carbon monoxide poisoning, make sure your wood stoves, space heaters, and flame-burning appliances have been properly installed and adjusted. *Do not* use ovens or gas ranges to heat your home.

Carbon monoxide detectors are available at hardware and housewares stores. They sound a warning if the level becomes high.

• *Formaldehyde.* Construction materials such as particle board and urea-formaldehyde foam insulation and some synthetic carpets and curtains contain formaldehyde. In most cases, when the materials are installed properly, formaldehyde levels are very low and thought to be harmless. But high concentrations of this irritating gas—which is found more often in mobile homes because of their greater use of formaldehyde-containing materials—can result in chest pain and irritation of the respiratory tract.

SICK BUILDING SYNDROME

Until a few years ago, no one had ever heard of "sick building syndrome." This condition causes large numbers of people in one building to suffer respiratory illness, headaches, and impaired concentration. Today, experts estimate that as many as 30 percent of our country's four million commercial buildings are in poor health. And a sick building ultimately causes sick people.

The Environmental Protection Agency, in fact, ranks indoor air pollution—both in the home and in the office—as one of the five most urgent environmental issues facing us today. The EPA estimates that between thirty and seventy-five million workers are at risk of illness because of the buildings in which they work.

The most commonly reported symptoms caused by a sick building include headaches, dizziness, nausea, burning eyes and throats, and skin rashes. Some people experience asthma or other serious respiratory complaints. In more extreme instances, outbreaks of such potentially deadly illnesses as legionnaire's disease have been traced to working in a sick building.

Unfortunately, a sick building, unlike a sick person, can be hard to spot. Many of the culprits are newer office buildings, constructed to be energy-efficient—so efficient that they're virtual fortresses against the environment, the result of which is that little fresh air circulates; that means breathing in recirculated air.

Another common problem, especially in the first six months of a building's life, are the fumes and by-products of construction materials. Harmful compounds in paints, adhesives, cabinets, and carpeting can cause a wide range of respiratory and other ailments.

In many buildings, old and new, an improperly maintained ventilation system is to blame. In an attempt to save money, for example, a building manager may shut down outside dampers, impeding the flow of fresh air. Or building management may allow dust and microbial matter to accumulate in the ventilation system. Investigations of sick buildings commonly turn up dead mice, insects, mold, mildew, pesticides, and bits of building materials lurking inside ventilation systems. These substances, of course, then end up in the air everyone breathes. Another potential problem source is a ventilation system that draws in air from a polluted environment like a loading dock: Instead of pulling in a fresh air supply, it's drawing in quantities of carbon monoxide.

Determining whether your building is sick isn't easy. The majority of symptoms associated with sick building syndrome are common flulike complaints that typically affect everyone once in a while. Probably the best way to determine whether it's your building or simply nature that's making you sick is that your symptoms improve after you've left your office. Victims of sick building syndrome typically find that their symptoms decrease at night and on weekends. But by Monday afternoon, they feel terrible again. Another tip-off is a large percentage of your coworkers experiencing similar problems. When more than 20 percent of a building's workforce isn't feeling well, something is wrong.

If you suspect sick building syndrome, keep a log of your own and your coworkers' symptoms. Take a look around your work area. Check the ceiling, walls, and floor to see whether each room has an independent air source. Look at the air vents. When you hold a piece of tissue paper in front of a vent, does it move with a flow of air, showing evidence of circulation? Make sure furniture isn't blocking an air vent. Inquire about the ventilation system and how often it's cleaned. If you find what you think are problems, take your suspicions to your employer. If that doesn't yield results, call the National Institute for Occupational Safety and Health's Hazard Evaluation and

Technical Assistance Branch, which investigates only the most serious cases of sick building syndrome but can refer you to state and local agencies.

Once your building's problem is diagnosed, the cure won't be overnight. Generally it takes anywhere from three to six months for the air to clear—and in very poorly ventilated buildings as long as a year.

VIDEO DISPLAY TERMINALS: WHAT ARE THE RISKS?

More than fifteen million Americans spend a good part of their day staring at video display terminals, or VDTs.

If you're among them, you may be wondering just how safe it is to be exposed to an electrical field for so many hours.

VDTs themselves are not dangerous to your health. The exposure levels to radiation from the screens are negligible. With the exception of hand and eye strain, no major health problems have been confirmed. There is little evidence that pregnant women who constantly work at VDTs face any increased risks.

If you spend your workweek in front of a video monitor, you can minimize your risk of eye and muscle strain:

1. Sit so that the screen is at eye level, about twenty-two to twenty-six inches away from you.

2. Keep your neck relaxed and your head facing forward.

3. Bend your elbows at a ninety-degree angle to the keyboard, so that you don't have to bend your wrists to type.

4. Make sure your chair offers adequate back support.

5. Take a fifteen-minute break every two hours, more often if your workload is heavy.

REPETITIVE MOTION SYNDROME

Repetitive motion syndrome—also called repetitive stress injury—was first reported three centuries ago. But it's an occupational hazard that's steadily increasing today. Workers who pluck chickens, cut meat, work on assembly lines, or do any repetitive, fast work have always had a high incidence of neck, elbow, shoulder, back, and hand injuries. Any body part subject to constant, selective hard use may develop problems, but one of the most common is damage to nerves in the hand, wrist, and forearm due to repetitive rapid hand movements.

Statistics show that repetitive motion syndrome accounted for 56 percent of the 331,600 gradual-onset, work-related illnesses reported by the Occupational Safety and Health Administration in 1992, an *eightfold* increase since the previous decade. In terms of missed work and medical costs, this illness is taking a toll: In 1990 this problem cost some $20 billion.

While there are many forms of repetitive motion syndrome, the most widespread work-related hand injury today is carpal tunnel syndrome, a nerve problem that affects the wrist. Carpal tunnel syndrome has become a major problem in the workplace during this age of computers, with countless numbers of people sitting all day in front of keyboards, punching tens of thousands of strokes.

Carpal tunnel syndrome results when the median nerve that passes through a narrow tunnel of wrist bones (carpals) is compressed by tissue or excess fluid. It most often occurs with activities requiring prolonged bending of the wrist or constant repeated hand motions—such as typing, assembly-line work, knitting and sewing, golf, tennis, and canoeing. Hormonal changes due to pregnancy may cause fluid accumulation in the carpal tunnel, and diseases such as rheumatoid arthritis, diabetes mellitus, and Raynaud's syndrome may promote carpal tunnel syndrome.

Early symptoms of carpal tunnel syndrome are numbness, tingling, and eventually pain in the fingers and hands; pain, often worse at night (sometimes to the extent that it wakes you up), in the hand, forearm, or shoulder; and weakness in the hands and fingers, often so severe that it's hard to hold on to or pick up objects. The disorder most often affects women between thirty and sixty. For discussion of the treatment options for carpal tunnel syndrome, see page 595.

Part III

❧

PREGNANCY AND CHILDBIRTH

The four chapters that follow are devoted to the complex and remarkable process of having a baby. The focus here is on the normal, healthy events that every woman might expect to experience in the process of having a child, but also on the concerns and special challenges that pregnancy can present to the mother-to-be and the child within her.

Much of the advice and guidance offered here addresses specific concerns: from proper prenatal care to breast-feeding; how to distinguish Braxton Hicks contractions from the real thing; from concerns like preeclampsia to placenta previa; from pain-control issues to the midwifery option. Childbearing can be an emotional and physical roller-coaster ride, but it is an experience that can be made easier when you have a sound understanding of what to expect.

CHAPTER 13

❧

Planning for Pregnancy

CONTENTS

No amount of thinking, planning, talking, or reading can prepare a woman and her partner completely for the changes that having a child will bring. For a woman, the experience of conceiving, producing, and nurturing a child is a complex one. At times, it may seem that she has tossed all aspects of her identity—her body, her marriage, her career, her relationships, and all assumptions about who she is—into the air like so many colored pick-up sticks, and the way the pieces rearrange themselves as they fall down may well surprise everyone, including the woman herself.

That's why it's a good idea to think and plan and talk and read about pregnancy and childbirth. The clearer a woman is about the path she charts, the more she can anticipate steps and detours along the way, the better she can weather the changes and meet the challenges.

Until the 1960s, when oral contraceptives and intrauterine devices were introduced and became widely available, women who were sexually active had little control over the decision to start a family. More often than not, family planning was a matter of luck, abstinence, or resignation. Even with some form of birth control, contraceptive failure was fairly common. Countless children were conceived (and still are) regardless of a couple's readiness for and commitment to a family. Not coincidentally, a woman's role until a few years ago was generally circumscribed by family responsibilities. The expectation was that a girl would, naturally, grow up to marry, have children, and devote her life, like it or not, to the duties of a mother and housewife.

Today there are a variety of safe, easy-to-use, and effective contraceptives (see *Birth Control*, page 101). In addition, societal attitudes tolerate more open and honest discussion about sexuality as well as a greater range of professional and emotional options for women. A woman is able to determine whether and when to accept motherhood as part of her life and identity. She can embrace both motherhood and career. She can postpone having a baby well into her late thirties or even her early forties. She can stay home and care for children. She can remain unmarried and have children. She can choose not to have children whether she's married or not. In short, the choices a woman makes these days can be based on who she is. And she will find that pregnancy and childbirth are, for each individual woman and her family, complex, personal, and unique experiences.

Despite the availability of options and information, many children are conceived without much thought or preparation. As with other life decisions, the changes involved in creating a family are more likely to be for the better when careful thought has been invested. Even in the most thoroughly considered pregnancies, though, there is only one certainty: Ambivalent feelings will surface and the unanticipated will happen.

To Be or Not to Be

Like so many other couples, Helen and her husband have talked about having a child—over and over and over again. All their friends are having babies, their parents want grandchildren, and they are secure in their marriage and comfortable with their finances. Emotionally and financially they feel ready to take on the rigors of parenthood, good and bad, come what may. Or so they think.

Both are in their late twenties, and now's the time. Or so the societal pressures they feel seem to be saying. They really shouldn't wait much longer. Yet, before Helen starts consulting the calendar to determine peak fertility days, there are a number of practical matters concerning health and life-style that she and her husband should consider.

General Health. It's a good idea for any woman planning to get pregnant to schedule an appointment with her health-care provider. A comprehensive physical examination can identify and address health issues that could interfere with a successful pregnancy and delivery. If you are currently taking medication, whether prescription or over-the-counter, now is the time to discuss the possible effects on pregnancy and fetal development.

Some women have chronic health problems, such as asthma, depression, and diabetes, which should be brought under control before pregnancy. Other problems that would not necessarily manifest themselves until pregnancy, such as high blood pressure, anemia, or pelvic tumors, may be detected during a prepregnancy exam. Since such problems can complicate pregnancy, a health-care professional may recommend a special diet or medication or may adjust current medications to anticipate the developing fetus. In some cases, health problems can be corrected before conception. In other instances, a physician who specializes in these kinds of pregnancies may be consulted.

Rubella. Also called *German measles*, the normally benign childhood disease rubella can have serious consequences on a developing fetus. If a woman contracts rubella during pregnancy, an infant can be born with severe birth defects such as cataracts, deafness, heart defects, and central nervous system problems.

A woman who had rubella during childhood need not worry since she has likely established an immunity to the disease. For women who never had German measles and for those who are unsure of their childhood medical history, a blood test can determine immunity. If there is no immunity, immunization given before pregnancy will guard against dangerous exposure.

Genetic Concerns. A physical examination will include questions about family history and genetic vulnerabilities. If there is a history of such defects as Down's syndrome, Tay-Sachs disease, sickle-cell anemia, or thalassemia, genetic counseling may be advised for both partners. A genetic counselor will look at genetic probability, that is, the likelihood that a given genetic abnormality will be passed on to children. In addition, he or she will provide information on further diagnostic testing (see *Identifiable Abnormalities*, page 292).

DINA'S STORY

Whenever they discussed starting a family, both Dina and Homer worried that their children would have sickle-cell disease, an inherited blood disorder commonly found among African Americans. They discussed their fears with Dina's health-care provider before she became pregnant. Her clinician recommended a test to determine whether one or both carried the gene responsible for this chronic disease.

Together, Dina and her husband visited a genetic counselor, who explained that although having the gene does not necessarily mean a person will have the condition, they were wise to be concerned. From the tests, Dina and Homer learned that because they both have the recessive gene, any child they produced would have a 25 percent chance of having sickle-cell anemia. They decided to go ahead with plans to conceive with the understanding that once Dina was pregnant, she would have a fetal test to determine whether in fact the baby would have the disease. Genetic testing and counseling provided them with the information and time to make informed choices about whether to terminate the pregnancy or, should they elect to give birth to a child who needs special medical care, to make adequate preparations.

LIFE-STYLE ISSUES

Examine your life-style for areas that could influence the developing baby *before* you get pregnant. Healthy habits increase the likelihood that your baby will be born healthy.

Katherine, for example, is overweight. She wisely understands that losing the extra pounds before she becomes pregnant is the healthy way to go. Her health-care provider advised her to lose weight by decreasing calorie and fat intake and increasing her activity level, rather than relying on a crash diet, which might upset her nutritional balance and therefore could adversely affect her fetus once she does become pregnant. Because Katherine has watched many of her friends go through pregnancy and childbirth, she knows that extra pounds don't melt away magically on the way back from the delivery room, so it's preferable to be in good physical condition even before becoming pregnant.

Diet. While the chances of having an uncomplicated pregnancy and healthy baby are quite good for most women, those chances improve dramatically when a woman is conscientious about eating an appropriate, healthy diet during pregnancy. A varied and ample diet of cereal, grains, fruits, and vegetables, containing adequate amounts of protein, vitamins, calcium, and iron, increases the likelihood that your child will be born in good health. Recent studies have shown that having a sufficient amount of folic acid, which is found in leafy vegetables, in the diet decreases the incidence of spina bifida, an open or malformed spine that causes paralysis in the baby. A healthy diet may guard against gestational diabetes, hypertension, and preeclampsia during pregnancy. Often, a multivitamin will be prescribed to assure that a woman receives adequate levels of vitamins.

Starting at a Sensible Weight. Not long ago, an obstetrician would admonish his or her patient if she gained more than fifteen pounds during pregnancy. Today, it is widely recognized that a gain of only fifteen pounds is insufficient. Babies whose mother gains less than twenty pounds are more likely to suffer growth retardation in utero.

On the other hand, it is not a good idea to eat without regard to weight gain. Too much weight gain can cause greater fatigue, backaches, leg pains, and varicose veins. It increases the risk of diabetes and high blood pressure and may complicate delivery.

For many women—even those who are thin to begin with—it is difficult to avoid gaining more than the twenty-five to thirty-five pounds that most health-care providers recommend.

Smoking. Despite the fact that cigarette smoking is an acknowledged health hazard, millions of Americans continue to smoke. The fastest growing segment of the smoking population is young women of reproductive age. In addition to having a higher risk of cancer, heart disease, stroke, and lung ailments, women who smoke decrease their fertility and jeopardize their unborn children in a number of ways.

Smoking has been linked to a range of prenatal complications, including miscarriage, stillbirth, premature separation of the placenta, premature rupture of the membrane leading to premature delivery, and bleeding in the first trimester. In addition, there is considerable evidence that smoking causes serious damage to the developing fetus. Smoking a pack or more of cigarettes each day affects the baby's birth weight; a woman who smokes is more likely to deliver a baby whose weight is lower.

Some evidence indicates that the effects of maternal smoking are long-term. One study done as early as 1958 in the United Kingdom compared the seven-year-old children of women who smoked more than ten cigarettes daily during pregnancy to children of nonsmokers or light smokers. It found that by the age of fourteen the children of the heavy smokers tended to be 0.4 inch shorter and lagged four months behind the control group in reading ability. Other studies have shown that children of smokers were more vulnerable to respiratory problems.

Passive smoking poses a similar threat to fetal development and health. Babies born to families in which only the father smoked showed blood quantities of thiocyanate, a derivative of cyanide commonly found in increased levels in the blood of smokers. Studies show that parental smoking, no matter who smokes, causes respiratory problems and impaired lung function in children, which can follow them into adulthood.

Fortunately, there is no clear evidence that a history of smoking before pregnancy poses significant danger to the fetus. Because smoking during pregnancy causes low birth weight and increases the risk of miscarriage and prematurity, as well as other serious complications, quitting *prior* to conceiving is the safest approach. Nevertheless, some studies show that women who quit in early pregnancy—before the fourth month—reduce the risk of prenatal damage almost to the level of a nonsmoker. No one will argue that cigarette smoking is an easy habit to break, though some women luckily have a natural aversion to tobacco during pregnancy. If quitting won't be easy for you, ask your health-care provider to recommend methods of quitting that have proved effective.

Alcohol. Fetal alcohol syndrome (FAS), caused by maternal alcohol consumption during pregnancy, affects an estimated two infants in every one thousand born. In addition to being responsible for a high neonatal mortality rate, FAS can produce a range of developmental problems, including stunted growth (both before and after birth), facial abnormalities, heart defects, joint and limb problems, learning disabilities, and mental retardation. Invariably, FAS is a serious and irreversible condition.

Fortunately, not every woman who drinks during pregnancy produces a child with fetal alcohol syndrome. There is no evidence that moderate consumption—a drink or two on a couple of occasions—will harm your baby. However, the more a woman drinks during pregnancy, the greater the effect on the developing fetus. As many as 33 percent of infants born to heavy drinkers have some congenital defects as compared to less than 5 percent whose mother did not drink.

The best time to give up alcohol—and to make modifications in your life-style for those activities and times when a drink or two seems natural—is before you are pregnant, and before fetal development begins. It may mean finding new ways of relaxing at the end of a day or attending Alcoholics Anonymous meetings. In all cases, the sooner a pregnant woman stops drinking, the better it is for her baby.

Drugs. The use of recreational and illegal drugs during pregnancy has become alarmingly widespread in recent years, with devastating effects. Heroin, cocaine, amphetamines, and barbiturates do serious harm to the fetus and threaten the pregnancy itself. Infants born to drug-using mothers are two to six times more likely to be premature and/or have growth retardation. As many as one half of the infants born to heroin addicts are drug-addicted themselves and must go through a painful withdrawal process after birth.

Studies show that women who use marijuana during pregnancy run an increased risk for fetal distress; *hyperemesis,* a severe and chronic vomiting which can cause prenatal malnutrition; insufficient weight gain; and anemia. In addition, labor tends to be more difficult and problematic as a consequence of marijuana use.

While most pregnancies are successful and, on the whole, trouble-free, there is no doubt that the process is a partnership between you, the mother, and the developing child. It is important to recognize and consider your responsibilities in the partnership at all times. In so doing you can help the process along and increase your chances of having a normal pregnancy *and* a healthy baby.

GETTING PREGNANT

Nina used to joke that all she had to do to get pregnant was pass her husband in the hall. With each of their three children, conception seemed practically effortless.

For Maria, on the other hand, getting pregnant was such an arduous process, involving calendars and temperature charts, that it took all the romance out of making love. When she found she was pregnant after years of trying, she and her husband felt blessed. But not wanting to go through the anxiety and heartbreak again, they stopped with one child.

Lauren will be satisfied with one child. She and her husband have tried to conceive on their own for years. But after a number of miscarriages and with Lauren moving closer to her fortieth birthday, they decided to seek the help of aggressive medical intervention. With in vitro fertilization, Lauren is now pregnant.

Franny, however, was not so lucky. Even with the latest technological methods of conception, she wasn't able to conceive, much to her disappointment. Now, she and her partner are looking into adoption.

It's seldom apparent why it's relatively easy for some women to get pregnant and so difficult for others. Of all the times when it is possible to conceive, a child is produced only 20 percent of the time. Generally, it's a simple matter of sperm meeting egg; other times, it's clearly not so simple.

A man is capable of fathering children well into old age. For him, reproductive health means having plenty of healthy, potent, and mobile sperm to connect with the female's egg and the ability to achieve penile erection followed by orgasm in order to ejaculate that sperm into the vagina. When a man ejaculates within a woman's vagina, sperm is delivered within a sticky, milklike liquid called *semen*. The average amount of semen ejaculated during an act of intercourse measures one teaspoon or less. Yet this small amount contains more than 100 million microscopic long-tailed spermatozoa, which are produced by the testes.

For her part, a woman releases each month during ovulation one of the approximately 200,000 eggs contained within her two ovaries. During a woman's life, many of these eggs atrophy or are absorbed elsewhere in the body. Others survive within the ovaries, surrounded by cells that form a capsule or follicle. Under normal circumstances, women ovulate every month between the years of puberty and menopause. Ovulation begins when the pituitary gland secretes a substance called follicle-stimulating hormone (FSH), causing the follicles to develop. Some follicles fatten and bulge; others wither. Then one—sometimes two—of these fat follicles grows so large that another pituitary hormone, luteinizing hormone (LH), stimulates the follicle to burst through the surface of the ovary and release its egg down the thin, five-inch fallopian tube, usually on the same side as the ovary from which the egg has exited (see *The Menstrual Cycle*, page 404).

Conception is most likely when intercourse occurs on the day of ovulation or within five days before. A sperm cell remains able to fertilize an egg for at least seventy-two hours after it is ejaculated. An egg's susceptibility to conception, however, appears to end on the day of ovulation.

Fertility can be estimated, therefore, by determining the time a woman ovulates. The normal menstrual cycle is twenty-eight days, with ovulation typically on the thirteenth or fourteenth day, counting the first day of menstrual flow as day one. Most women are con-

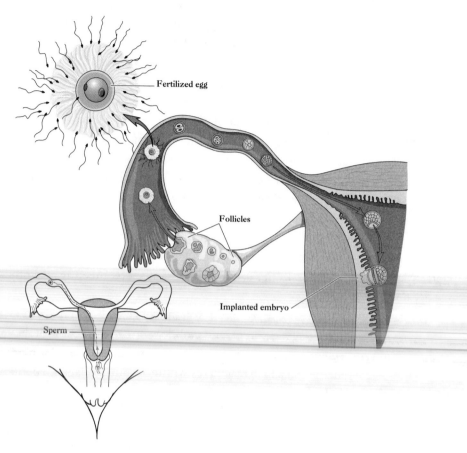

For fertilization to occur, two events are required. An ovarian follicle in the female ovary must release an egg, or ovum, that travels down the fallopian tube. There it must meet a male sperm, which has moved upward through the cervix and uterus into the tube. If fertilization is accomplished, the resulting embryo implants into the wall of uterus.

sidered most fertile between days ten and fifteen of their menstrual cycle.

For a few days during midcycle, a woman may notice an abundance of watery, colorless vaginal discharge. This fluid creates a slippery environment that facilitates the sperm's progress. At other times the fluid becomes less abundant and more sticky, actually impairing sperm advance and the chance of fertilization.

After sperm are ejaculated, they enter the cervix. Some never find their way into the cervical canal, dying in the acidic environment of the vagina. Most, however, reach the alkaline confines of the cervix, which is more conducive to sperm survival. Here, the sperm swim in every direction, bumping into each other, finding their way into crevices from which later they can be released into the upper genital tracts. Many travel up the wrong tube. Of millions of sperm that enter the vagina initially, only a few hundred reach the middle part of the tube containing the egg. The sperm must then penetrate a capsule (zona pellucida) around the egg. Once through the zona, the sperm fuses with the egg. Several sperm may begin to enter the outer egg capsule, but only one is able to penetrate the egg and pair its twenty-three chromosomes with those of the egg.

When you consider all the genetic possibilities launched in the single act that made you and will make your own children, you see that chance is a leading player in the creation of every living thing. Look at yourself in the mirror. Perhaps you have black hair, a cleft in your chin, high cheekbones, and freckles on your nose; all those attributes and, perhaps, your passion for music or talent for putting together machinery are the result of your genetic heritage. Yet prior to the moment you were conceived, any one of many other genetic scenarios could have come to pass. Had a different sperm cell reached the egg, you might have had red hair instead of black, dark skin instead of light, been tall instead of short, a man instead of a woman, or had a lawyer's love of logic instead of an artist's eye for color. In short, you would be a very different person.

SELECTING A HEALTH-CARE PROVIDER

Thirty years ago, when Marguerite was pregnant, she, like most women at that time, gave very little consideration to who was going to deliver her baby. Pregnancy seemed a rather straightforward process. Doctors were doctors, weren't they?

There were few procedures and tests to consider, and she assumed that she would be unconscious during labor and delivery. Her husband wasn't really involved in the process—occasionally he went out to get her a food she craved in the middle of the night, and he worried about driving her to the hospital when the time came. Marguerite herself didn't feel much more like a participant. Like most women of her generation, she obediently accepted her doctor's advice and never really questioned the choices he made on her behalf. It didn't matter that they had no affinity for each other. When she thinks about it in the light of today's greater awareness and information, Marguerite feels that luck more than anything accounted for the fact that her pregnancy and delivery were uneventful. She shudders to think that there could have been problems of which she was never aware.

Today, there are so many choices and tests that Marguerite never had to think about. She's relieved that her own daughter, Penny, is so much more actively involved in her pregnancy, as is Penny's husband. It appears to Marguerite that Penny, her husband, and their practitioner have formed a responsible working partnership.

Given the opportunity—almost the imperative—to choose a health-care provider, many women today are a bit overwhelmed at the thought of beginning. Indeed, how do women go about choosing the right health professional for this very important partnership?

Nine out of ten women choose to work with obstetricians, *specialists trained to handle complications in pregnancy and childbirth should they arise. Most women who use obstetricians, however, have normal pregnancies and deliveries. There are also obstetricians who specialize in specific types of pregnancies with a higher risk of complications. They are called* perinatologists.

About 10 percent of women choose family practitioners. *These are physicians who are trained in several areas of primary care and provide medical services for the entire family.*

About 1 to 2 percent use certified nurse–midwives, *who are trained to care for women with low-risk pregnancies and to attend uncomplicated births.*

There are also different kinds of practices to consider. A solo practitioner *has his or her own practice and relies on other providers to cover when he or she is unavailable. Some women like the fact that with a practitioner in solo practice, they come to know the health professional and feel that he or she knows them. They feel relatively confident that their practitioner will be the one to deliver the baby. However, it may happen that her clinician is not available when a woman goes into labor, in which case her baby may be delivered by someone she does not know.*

A group practice *is typically made up of two or more medical professionals who care jointly for patients. A group practice may include one or more nurse–midwives as well as obstetricians or family practitioners. Frequently, you will see a different practitioner from one visit to the next. As a result, you get to know everyone in the practice so that when labor comes, you will know the clinician who delivers your baby. You may not like all the practitioners equally, however, and you may be disappointed with the clinician who shows up when you go into labor. Because you will see different clinicians, you may also receive differing points of view concerning your pregnancy and your options. This may be helpful in rounding out your understanding, or it may be confusing.*

Frequently nurse–midwives group together and work with a physician on-call to form a maternity center. *These centers usually operate out of a distinct facility or in a hospital. Many women appreciate the more natural and sensitive childbirth experiences these centers promote. However, because not all kinds of pregnancies are handled in these centers, if a complication develops, the pregnancy will be referred to the doctor on-call. Up to a fifth of all deliveries that start out in maternity centers are shifted in midlabor to a hospital because of an unforeseen complication.*

Given all these choices, how does a woman make a choice?

• *First, consider your own personality and the kind of patient you are. It may be that you prefer to be able to put your trust completely in the professional expertise of another. Perhaps you would feel better having your doctor make all the decisions with only minimal consultation with you.*

• *Or you may be uncomfortable with the idea of working with a medical professional who seems resolute about certain obstetrical practices and philosophies. You may have clear ideas and opinions about pregnancy and childbirth and may feel better working with someone who will provide medical information and support, let you make the decisions, and step forward only when it becomes medically necessary.*

• *Or perhaps you fit somewhere in between. You may look for a practitioner who creates a balance of his or her own medical experience and knowledge, your ideas and wishes, and your specific pregnancy needs.*

- *Put together a list of names. Ask your internist, gynecologist, and/or family practitioner for referrals. Perhaps your current practitioner does deliveries. Ask friends. Consult the* Directory of the American Medical Association *or the* Directory of Medical Specialties *in your local library. Write to the International Childbirth Education Association. Call La Leche League or other childbirth organizations.*

- *Schedule consultations with one or more of these clinicians. Have a list of questions ready. Figure out which aspects of pregnancy and childbirth interest you. What is his or her thinking about childbirth? About pain medications and anesthesia during childbirth? How about breast-feeding, episiotomy, and induced labor? Or the use of fetal monitoring, enemas, forceps, cesarean sections, home delivery?*

What are his or her recommendations for diet and medication? Does he or she encourage childbirth classes? Ask whether he or she is available for over-the-phone questions, and if not, whether there is someone in the office, such as a nurse practitioner, who is? Ask about hospital affiliation. Does the hospital use birthing rooms? Does it encourage rooming-in and the inclusion of fathers in labor and delivery? In the case of cesarean sections? Does it have a neonatology intensive care unit? Do they encourage breast-feeding immediately after delivery?

Once you've chosen the right practitioner for you, the relationship will develop steadily for about nine months. If along the way it seems that it is not a productive partnership, you can always consider changing clinicians. However, having the best prenatal care will surely be less likely if you jump from doctor to doctor.

PREGNANCY TESTS

Linsey thinks she might be pregnant. Her period is a few days late and she feels, well, different. The surest way for her to end the guesswork is to have a pregnancy test.

Pregnancy tests—which analyze either blood or, more commonly, urine specimens—measure the hormone human chorionic gonadotropin (hCG) in the body. A fertilized egg begins to secrete this hormone from its earliest days. hCG is found first in the blood if you are pregnant and in your urine and body tissues shortly thereafter.

The most accurate pregnancy test and the one most adept at detecting pregnancy soon after the embryo implants is a blood test. However, because it costs more and takes longer to produce results, it is not used as often as a urine test. In cases in which, on the basis of symptoms and the physical exam findings, a health professional suspects a complication such as an ectopic or tubal pregnancy, a serious condition in which the embryo has implanted outside the uterine cavity, a blood test may be recommended.

A urine pregnancy test can be done at your health professional's office or at home with a pregnancy test available at the pharmacy. Most home pregnancy kits require that you mix a solution with your urine in a test tube. Some companies are now marketing devices that you hold directly under your urine stream, which do away with mixing. After an interval—usually within minutes—a change in color or the formation of a dark ring indicates pregnancy.

The accuracy of a home pregnancy test depends on gestational age. Blood tests are highly accurate and sensitive within about a week of conception. Urine tests require a few additional days. Nearly all urine tests are accurate after a period is ten days late. If you decide to use a home pregnancy test, you must follow the instructions closely. It is best to use the first urine of the day.

Even when your home pregnancy test registers a positive result, an appointment with your health provider is necessary to confirm the results and begin your prenatal care. If the pregnancy is unwanted, this is the best time to discuss options with your clinician.

No test is foolproof. Although a positive pregnancy reading is almost always reliable, a negative reading is less so. If you have symptoms of pregnancy but the test result is negative, it may be too early in the pregnancy for hCG to appear in your urine. Wait a few days and then repeat the test. If a new test result comes up negative and you still haven't started your period, see your health-care provider.

PREGNANCIES WITH COMPLICATIONS

For a new parent, the birth of a child can be a momentous event. Luckily, from a medical standpoint, most births are uneventful. The large majority of pregnancies proceed in a normal fashion without the kinds of complications that could put the mother or child at risk.

The most common concerns during pregnancy are nausea and/or vomiting during the early weeks, frequent urination, heartburn, backache, fatigue, insomnia, and varicose veins. A small number of women, though, have chronic conditions that, in general, make their pregnancies problematic. In others serious problems develop during the course of the pregnancy.

Women who have a thorough physical examination before pregnancy have the opportunity to identify problems that could add complications to the normal strains placed on the body by a full-term pregnancy. Few problems will prohibit a woman from bearing a child. However, problems and conditions that can complicate a pregnancy—including those discussed in the next section—require more careful monitoring and, in some cases, special treatment.

In many cases the doctor or midwife will be able to manage the condition sufficiently. Sometimes, though, a specialist may be called in. A woman, for example, with a preexisting heart condition may be referred to a cardiologist. There are also perinatologists/obstetricians, who have secondary training in specific pregnancy-related complications.

Diabetes. Before the discovery of insulin in 1922, most diabetic women were too sick to conceive. Those who did often miscarried. Many died during the pregnancy. Today, diabetic women are able to control their condition and, as a result, are capable of both conceiving and delivering healthy babies. But both the woman and the infant require special care if they are to come through the process in good health.

Diabetes is a chronic condition that arises when the body is unable to generate adequate levels of insulin to regulate the rate of production and absorption of blood sugar. Pregnancy impedes insulin's effect and thereby ensures that enough sugar remains in circulation for transport to the fetus. Women who are diabetic or have diabetic tendencies are particularly vulnerable to problems as a result.

For diabetic women, there is nothing more important—pregnant or not—than controlling their blood sugar level. In most circumstances, blood sugar level is controlled through a combination of diet and insulin injections. If a pregnant woman's blood sugar level becomes high, excess sugar crosses the placenta and causes an increase in the fetus's blood sugar level. The fetal pancreas then produces insulin, which acts as a growth hormone. The babies of diabetics whose blood sugar level is not controlled can be excessively large at birth. This can complicate both labor and delivery. If, on the other hand, diabetes-related vascular disease affects the uterus or placenta, the baby may be born small and undernourished. Infants born to diabetic mothers have a greater chance of development of diabetes themselves. Congenital malformations, stillbirth, and metabolic problems are seen more often in diabetic pregnancies.

Not only is the infant of a diabetic mother at risk from the condition, so is the mother. A diabetic mother has a higher risk of infection, postpartum hemorrhage, and heart and lung problems. Moreover, she is four times more likely to have preeclampsia, a dangerous condition characterized by hypertension, protein in the urine, and swelling (see page 303).

About 2 percent of women who have not been diabetic before pregnancy experience *gestational diabetes*, and the risk for this condition becomes greater with age. This form of diabetes usually abates after the baby is born, although it may recur later in a woman's life. Women with gestational diabetes (in which the characteristic elevated blood sugar level of diabetes mellitus occurs), like those with chronic diabetes, must be scrupulous about their diet. However, they may not need to take insulin shots. Gestational diabetics do not have the same increased risk of stillbirth or birth defects in their babies.

Hypertension. About 2 percent of all pregnant women have gestational hypertension; that is, their blood pressure becomes elevated during pregnancy. If treated, this condition seems to pose little danger to the health of the pregnancy and usually disappears after delivery. Women whose blood pressure is chronically high and untreated are at significant risk during pregnancy, as are their babies. Hypertension can be an especially insidious problem because it often exists without symptoms. Fortunately, high blood pressure is easily detected with a blood pressure check that is part of every routine prenatal examination.

Women whose blood pressure rises throughout the pregnancy above what is considered normal are more likely to have *preeclampsia*. Occurring after the twentieth week of pregnancy, preeclampsia is found in about 1 percent of all pregnancies in the general population. There are usually a sudden weight gain and severe swelling in hands, face, and ankles. Other symptoms may include headaches, blurred vision, and abdominal pain. One in fifteen hundred women goes on to develop a blood infection called *toxemia*. To guard against this condition, which can be dangerous to both the mother and her baby, partial or complete bed rest, hospitalization, medication, and delivery may be advised.

Babies born to mothers with untreated hypertension tend to be small and have a small placenta. The incidence of fetal death is slightly higher than in the general population. But in most cases, women with high blood pressure can have a normal delivery and normal baby.

Heart Disorders. Even under the best of circumstances, pregnancy puts extra strain on the heart. For most women, this extra strain poses no problem. But for women who have a history of heart disease, the extra cardiac load imposed by pregnancy can increase the chance of heart failure.

In most cases, heart disease will not prevent a woman from becoming pregnant or from having a healthy baby. However, one of the safest approaches includes the joint care of an obstetrician and a cardiologist during the pregnancy.

Some women aren't aware that they have a heart disorder until the extra demands of pregnancy bring the problem to light. A pregnant woman with a heart disorder must be monitored carefully. It is important to watch weight gain in order to limit the stress on the heart. Your provider will also watch closely for any signs of excessive water retention or anemia. While health professionals advise any pregnant woman to give up cigarettes, women who have a heart condition put themselves at much greater risk if they continue to smoke during pregnancy.

Depending upon your particular condition and its severity, bed rest may be recommended for some or all of the pregnancy. If there is a history of rheumatic fever, antibiotics may be prescribed to circumvent another attack.

Labor and delivery naturally stress the heart, especially during the pushing stage. Your health-care provider will want to make the final stage as expeditious and efficient as possible.

Asthma. Asthma affects about 5 percent of adults. As long as asthma is brought under control by medication and the medication is closely supervised, sometimes by an allergist or a pulmonary (lung) specialist, as well as by an obstetrics professional, the chances of having a normal pregnancy and healthy baby are almost as high as for women who do not suffer from asthma.

The effect of pregnancy on asthmatic women, however, is not always the same. In about a third of all cases, there is no change in the severity of the illness. In another third, the illness will worsen, and for the last third, it will improve.

Asthmatics are more prone to respiratory infections in general, and pregnancy may increase the incidence of infection.

It is important that asthma be brought under control before conception or as early into the pregnancy as possible. If you are currently taking allergy shots, they can be continued safely throughout the pregnancy. It is not likely, however, that your health-care professional will begin allergy shots during pregnancy. Treat asthma attacks immediately with prescribed medication in order to prevent oxygen loss to the fetus. Studies show that current asthma medications will not harm the developing infant. However, continue to discuss medication and its use with your practitioner.

Epilepsy. Seizure disorders such as epilepsy generally do not interfere with a healthy pregnancy. However, children of epileptic women have a slightly increased risk of birth defects. Some women have severe nausea and vomiting, especially in early pregnancy, that make it difficult to keep medication down. This, of course, increases the risk of having a seizure.

Medications used to control seizures have been associated with an increased incidence of birth defects. If you have epilepsy and are thinking about having a child, discuss your medication with a neurologist and with an obstetrics clinician. Be sure to review a *complete* list of medications with the medical professionals you consult.

Age. Women at both ends of the reproductive spectrum—teenagers and women over the age of thirty-five— are at increased risk for complications during pregnancy, labor, and delivery.

A pregnant teenager has a higher risk of miscarriage, premature birth, and stillbirth (a condition in which the infant is born dead) than women in their twenties. This age group also is more prone to development of preeclampsia and eclampsia (toxemia), which are potentially life-threatening.

One would think that a young woman, simply by virtue of her body's youth and resiliency, would have a trouble-free pregnancy. Many researchers suspect that the problems in teen pregnancies are related to poor diet and inadequate prenatal care. When teenagers receive good medical care and cultivate good health habits, their pregnancies are usually normal and their babies healthy.

This is also the case for older mothers. As a group, women who delay pregnancy until their thirties and increasingly until their forties tend to be both highly motivated and well educated. Older mothers, aware of the age-related risks, often adhere to a schedule of prenatal visits, eat right, avoid alcohol and cigarettes, get appropriate exercise, and participate in childbirth classes.

The majority of these women have healthy pregnancies and babies. Some, however, despite their diligence, have problems related to age. Pregnant women over the age of thirty-five, for example, are more likely to have diabetes and hypertension. The rates of miscarriage and stillbirth are somewhat higher.

If you are in your late thirties or early forties and are considering motherhood, don't let age deter you. But make sure you have a prepregnancy examination so that you and your health-care provider are aware of any health problems you may have *before* you get pregnant. Moreover, because the chance of chromosome abnormalities increases with age, you may also want to consult a genetic counselor or your health-care provider about your child's risk of birth defects. There are a number of diagnostic options for determining fetal abnormalities once the pregnancy has commenced (see page 289).

SHANNON'S STORY

Throughout her life, Shannon had periodic bouts with asthma. In childhood, her asthma was quite severe, and several times, she ended up in the hospital after acute attacks. By the time she reached adolescence, however, her asthma seemed to abate and when it reappeared in a milder form as she neared thirty, she paid little attention to it.

Shannon remembered with apprehension the awful feelings—palpitations, giddiness, and dry mouth—induced by the asthma medications of her youth. Now, there was talk about asthma's being psychosomatic, so she felt guilty and embarrassed even to admit she was asthmatic. Instead, even with her health-care provider, she acted as though it were a minor problem and played down the symptoms. Each time she had an attack, especially after a cold, she'd use the bronchodilator her internist had prescribed—probably more than she should have. In time, she'd feel okay.

When she got pregnant, however, her asthma got worse. Twice in the first trimester, she went to the hospital emergency room. Luckily, her oxygen level remained high enough to ensure the baby's safety, but she felt really frightened by being unable to breathe. Once she could breathe again, though, she ignored her doctor's advice that she take her medication regularly. She worried about taking aspirin during her pregnancy, let alone anything more potent.

In her eighth month, Shannon had a bad cold, which led to a sinus infection, which in turn went to her chest. Her doctor prescribed antibiotics and a regular regimen of her asthma medicine. All seemed to clear up a couple of weeks before her due date, and she discontinued her asthma medicine. The delivery went well and her daughter was healthy and active. Relieved that her illness had not affected her baby, still Shannon did not feel particularly healthy. She felt a chronic tightness in her chest and a general fatigue that failed to diminish even after she stopped nursing her baby at ten months.

Finally, Shannon went to a pulmonary specialist, who was concerned at the compromised level of Shannon's breathing. It seemed that she had never fully recovered from her earlier asthma attacks and her lungs were constantly inflamed and therefore easily irritated. It's not surprising, the doctor explained, that the slightest irritant triggered asthmatic reactions.

The doctor readjusted Shannon's medication and urged her to treat her asthma as a chronic nuisance, something to be managed on a daily basis, not just when it pre-

sented an acute crisis. Once Shannon assumed responsibility of her condition and took her medication as the doctor had advised, she was surprised how much better she felt. And she felt great regret that she hadn't taken her asthma seriously and gotten it under control before it became a crisis and detracted from the pleasure of her pregnancy and her child.

INFERTILITY

Few things are as frustrating as the inability to conceive a child once you and your partner have decided to become parents. Unfortunately, infertility today is a relatively common problem, affecting an estimated 10 to 15 percent of couples.

The normal monthly conception rate in a group of fertile couples is 20 percent; that is, one fifth of women will conceive after one month of unprotected intercourse. Eighty-five percent of fertile couples will become pregnant within one year of trying. Couples who have tried for a year and still failed to achieve pregnancy are considered to be infertile.

Infertility is not synonymous with sterility. In some cases, infertility may mean that it simply takes longer to conceive; in essence, it could be described as underfertility. Many couples try for years, never seek treatment; then suddenly, for no apparent reason, conception takes place. Other infertile couples are unable to conceive until a problem with one or, sometimes both, partners is successfully corrected. And there are those who, despite all the advances medical science has to offer, still are unable to have children.

Although there have always been couples who, for a variety of reasons, have been unable to have children, infertility is more widespread today than in the past. In 1988 an estimated 4.9 million married American couples were infertile. Of this group, 2.2 million had no children and thus were said to have primary infertility, while 2.7 million had at least one child but were having difficulty conceiving another (secondary infertility). Not all of these couples sought medical treatment. But experts estimate that one half of all couples with primary infertility and one fifth of those with secondary infertility consult a doctor. As a result, in recent years visits for infertility services swelled from 600,000 in 1968 to 1.6 million in 1984.

One reason for the increase in infertility is the higher incidence of such sexually transmitted diseases as gonorrhea (see page 445) and chlamydia (see page 444). In women these are often insidious infections. Because they don't necessarily have uncomfortable or active symptoms, these infections can exist for long periods without treatment. Without treatment the infection may travel up the female reproductive tract, typically settling in the fallopian tubes, causing scarring, blockage, and often infertility.

Another factor in the marked increase in infertility is delayed childbearing. As a woman's body ages, conception becomes more difficult. For a woman between the ages of twenty-five and thirty, the chance of getting pregnant is 6 percent less than between the ages of twenty and twenty-four. The decrease is 14 percent for women between thirty and thirty-four; fertility is reduced by 31 percent between thirty-five and thirty-nine. After the age of forty, one in four couples is infertile.

Most health professionals recommend that a couple try to conceive for a year before seeking help. There are some situations, however, in which it might be advisable to get help earlier. If, for example, a woman is in her forties, time is a more pressing factor. After the age of forty-five, the likelihood of monthly ovulation decreases significantly, and that makes conception even more difficult. Thus, if you have been trying for a few months without luck, it might be to your advantage to discuss your options with a health professional sooner rather than later, particularly if you have irregular periods, which make it more likely that you are not ovulating or are ovulating irregularly.

Causes of Infertility. There are many reasons that couples have difficulty conceiving. In about 40 percent of cases, the man is the infertile partner; in another 40 percent, the problem stems from the woman. Sometimes both partners have problems that, combined, result in an inability to reproduce.

Most male infertility arises from a problem with the sperm. Disorders of the testes, inadequate hormone levels, and infections all can adversely affect a man's sperm, rendering them less able or completely incapable of fertilizing an egg. Some men, upon examination, are found to have *azoospermia*, an absence of sperm, which is usually due to a problem with the testes or a blockage in the passage that leads from the testes. A man with *oligospermia* has some sperm in his semen, but the count is so low that fertilization is less likely to take place.

In a woman, the causes of infertility are often more varied and complex. About 10 to 15 percent of female infertility is the result of a woman's inability to ovulate (anovulation). This happens in women who have never menstruated, have stopped menstruating, or have infrequent periods. In these cases, there may be a developmental problem with the ovaries or uterus. In other cases, anovulation is the result of hormonal dysfunction, such as *hyperprolactinemia*, in which the blood contains too much of the hormone prolactin, which inhibits ovulation. Or a woman may have an undiagnosed condition such as thyroid disease that interferes with the ovaries' ability to release an egg. Some woman ovulate but the egg fails to develop normally, frequently because of hormonal abnormalities.

For many women a problem arises when something blocks contact between the egg and sperm. This will happen if the fallopian tubes have been damaged by pelvic inflammatory disease (see page 449). Endometriosis—a condition in which uterine tissue plants itself within other reproductive organs—can cause infertility (see page 545).

Uterine and cervical defects also contribute to infertility. A small proportion of women produce cervical mucus that is hostile to sperm, making the chance of any sperm's reaching the egg less likely. Sometimes a woman is actually allergic to sperm and her body will produce antibodies which destroy them long before penetration of the egg.

EVALUATING INFERTILITY

Martha and Norman have been trying to get pregnant for more than a year. They have a nagging worry that there might be problem, so they have decided to ask Martha's health-care provider to do an infertility evaluation. But they had no idea when they began the process of the commitment of time and money involved in infertility testing.

They had to be candid with strangers about their sex life. Weeks went by when they felt that if they had to make love one more time they'd scream—and not out of pleasure. Sex became a regimented chore in the service of baby making. The vast array of tests and diagnostic procedures were intrusive, uncomfortable, embarrassing; some were even painful.

Early in the diagnostic process, Martha and Norman were referred to an infertility specialist. Norman had always assumed it was Martha's problem, so he was surprised that he had to be tested as well. He was asked to ejaculate into a container. The semen was then analyzed at a laboratory for quality and quantity of sperm as well as for the presence of inflammatory cells.

Martha's process began with a thorough medical history and physical examination. To determine whether she was ovulating, she was asked to take her temperature each morning before she got out of bed and to record the results on a chart. This allowed the clinicians to measure the normal rise in Martha's body temperature that follows ovulation. She was then subjected to a series of blood tests to assess hormone levels.

There are a number of other tests that health professionals advise in cases like Martha's and Norman's, including a postcoital cervical mucus test, *which typically is performed within twelve hours of intercourse around the time of expected ovulation. In a painless procedure, a small sample of cervical mucus is removed. The specimen is then examined to see whether the mucus is hospitable to sperm.*

An endometrial biopsy *samples uterine tissue. Tissue is removed just prior to the beginning of menstruation to determine whether ovulation occurs and hormonal preparation of the uterine lining is adequate to allow it to receive a fertilized egg.*

If a woman is not ovulating or if sperm are not able to survive the cervical environment, treatment may begin without further diagnostic tests. Often, however, other, more complicated tests may be recommended.

There are several procedures for investigating problems with the uterus and fallopian tubes. A hysterosalpingogram, *for example, generally takes about ten minutes in a radiology unit. A liquid contrast medium is injected through a small tube into the uterus and fallopian tubes. X rays then reveal whether there are obstructions, tumors, or adhesions (scar tissues) that could impair fertility.*

A laparoscopy *uses a small lighted telescope inserted through a small abdominal incision to inspect reproductive organs for abnormalities (see also* Laparoscopy, *page 554).*

Few women evaluated for infertility have every test, of course. Sometimes the cause of the problem is discovered early in the course of evaluation; at other times the cause is never determined, even after every diagnostic test available is used. The tests used in your evaluation and their sequence will depend upon your clinician's recommendation and on how far you want to proceed.

Given the extraordinary costs and the cycle of hope, loss, and despair that can be involved in fertility treatment, couples should begin with a clear idea of how far they are willing to go. It is also helpful to have an idea of what life will be like if the treatment is not successful. Is adoption an alternative? How would the future be if there were no children? Many couples find that with couples' therapy, they are better able to handle the stresses, disappointments, and uncertainties during protracted treatment.

In the case of Martha and Norman, after many months of tests and raised hopes, the clinicians still don't know what is interfering with their ability to have children. But in 90 percent of all couples who are evaluated for infertility, the problem is uncovered. In most cases, these couples are able to go on to bear healthy babies. Despite all the difficulties and the lack of guarantees, Martha and Norman are committed to going to great lengths as long as there is the slightest chance that they could have their own biological child.

TREATING INFERTILITY

Treatment depends upon the source of the infertility. Many infertility problems that once were untreatable can be treated successfully today. Even those problems that are beyond repair do not necessarily render pregnancy impossible. The advent of assisted reproductive technology procedures has enabled many couples to become parents. In this section, we will look at ways of treating infertility problems.

Most health-care providers begin by counseling a couple on ways of maximizing the chances of pregnancy by having intercourse on certain days in the woman's cycle when she is likely to be ovulating.

Treating the Male. Some conditions affecting the testes can be surgically corrected. If a man is infertile because an infection has impaired sperm function, antibiotics will be prescribed. In cases in which there is a pituitary gland disorder, hormones may be used to help return sperm production to normal levels.

Treating the Female. In women, the treatment options are several.

MEDICATION. If tests determine a lack of ovulation, your clinician may prescribe "fertility drugs." Of all female fertility problems, the failure to ovulate is the one most responsive to treatment. In one study, 96 percent of women treated with medication for anovulation (failure to ovulate) and amenorrhea (failure to menstruate) became pregnant within two years.

Clomiphene citrate is the drug most frequently prescribed to induce ovulation. It works by stimulating the release of follicle-stimulating hormone (FSH). Other drugs include human menopausal gonadotropin (hMG) and gonadotropin-releasing hormone. Typically, a drug such as clomiphene citrate is taken for five days, beginning three to five days after the onset of a woman's natural period or, if she is not menstruating, after hormones have induced bleeding. Studies have shown that most women who have no infertility problem other than anovulation typically conceive within four to six cycles of clomiphene treatment once they start ovulating, if they are going to conceive at all on this medication.

Some fertility drugs are expensive. And, as with most drugs, there can be side effects. Transient ovarian cysts form in about 5 percent of women treated with clomiphene citrate. Other side effects, found in fewer than 10 percent of all women who take the drug, include hot flashes, blurred vision, abdominal pain and bloating, and temporary hair loss.

The chance of having twins is increased to 8 percent if you take clomiphene. However, the incidence of miscarriage, ectopic pregnancy, fetal death, and malformations is not significantly increased. Injectable ovulation-inducing drugs, such as hMG, carry a higher risk of birth of twins and higher-order multiples (triplets, quadruplets, etc.), but no increased risk of birth defects.

Even if anovulation is not the problem, drugs may be part of the treatment. If, for example, an infection or underlying illness has been identified as contributing to the inability to conceive, your clinician will prescribe the appropriate medication. Endometriosis, a common cause of infertility, is often treated with oral contraceptives, other hormonal medications, or surgery (see page 545).

Surgery. Many women with blocked fallopian tubes, endometriosis (see page 545), or uterine tumors can become pregnant after surgery. Often the procedure is performed with a laparoscope, a lighted instrument inserted into the pelvic cavity through a small incision in your abdomen (see *Laparoscopy*, page 554). A laser or electrocautery device is then inserted to destroy the abnormal tissue.

An estimated 85 percent of women treated for mild and 50 to 60 percent of women treated for moderate endometriosis conceive; the fertility rate for women treated for severe endometriosis is about 30 to 40 percent. About half the women who conceive after surgery do so within six months; the rest, within fifteen months. Because endometriosis is a progressive disease that tends to recur after treatment, it is best to try to become pregnant as soon as you have recuperated from surgery.

Health professionals are now able to reconstruct damaged or blocked fallopian tubes with microsurgical techniques. Whether such surgery can enable a woman to become pregnant depends upon the degree of tubal damage and the site of that damage. The overall conception rate after surgery to reconstruct the fallopian tubes is about 30 percent, although when the tube is partially blocked, the pregnancy rate jumps to 65 percent. Women who do get pregnant after tubal repair have a higher rate of ectopic (tubal) pregnancy than the general population, however.

Assisted Fertilization. As more and more couples know, there is more than one way to have a baby. Increasingly couples are turning to techniques that even a generation ago would have appeared only in the pages of science fiction. When other approaches to conception prove unsuccessful, there are a number of options available.

ARTIFICIAL INSEMINATION. In the relatively common and simple technique of artificial insemination sperm from a woman's partner or an anonymous donor is injected into the cervix a day or two before ovulation. Sometimes the sperm are injected directly into the uterus to facilitate their journey to the fallopian tubes.

Artificial insemination is used when the male cannot ejaculate into the woman's vagina or when his sperm count is low. Artificial insemination allows the sperm to travel a shorter route, thus maximizing the chance of reaching the egg. When there is a problem with sperm count, however, pregnancy rates with artificial insemination are generally low.

In cases in which a man's infertility cannot be treated, he carries a serious genetic abnormality, or the partners have Rh incompatibility (see page 301), using donor sperm is an option. Though this means that any child conceived will not be the biological child of the woman's partner, it is possible to find a close match in terms of such physical characteristics as race, coloring, and build. However, while most sperm donors are carefully screened, there is a risk that genetic abnormalities, the AIDS virus (see page 451), gonorrhea, and other sexually transmitted diseases (see page 440) can be passed on. If you decide to use donor sperm for insemination, your health-care provider or a fertility clinic can help you locate sperm from a sperm bank that strictly screens donors for these and other health factors.

IN VITRO FERTILIZATION (IVF). Normally, fertilization takes pace in the fallopian tubes. But if the tubes are obstructed or damaged and surgery cannot correct the problem, fertilization cannot occur. In this case, the egg can be removed from your ovaries and fertilized in a laboratory with your partner's sperm.

Developed in 1978, in vitro fertilization has been used by many couples—whether their infertility stems from endometriosis, low sperm count, or an unknown source. The media popularly refer to babies conceived through IVF as "test tube" babies. Yet the truth is that these infants, like any other, develop in their mother's uterus. The only things that occur outside are fertilization and the first few cell divisions.

In vitro fertilization is costly and success rates vary. First, a woman is given hormones to stimulate the number of mature follicles within the ovaries. When the eggs are ripe, several eggs are removed; ultrasound guides the clinician as he or she inserts a needle through the vagina into the ovary to retrieve the eggs.

The eggs are then incubated in a laboratory. After six to twelve hours, the eggs are

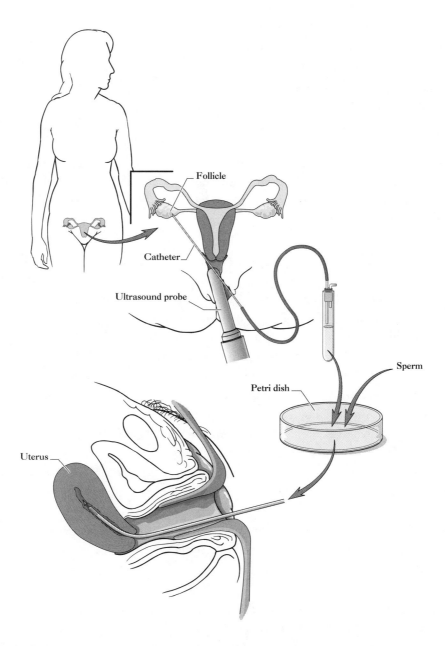

Follicle

Catheter

Ultrasound probe

Sperm

Petri dish

Uterus

To accomplish in vitro fertilization, the mother-to-be will take fertility drugs to stimulate follicle development. When she is ready to release ovum (eggs), they are retrieved using a needle. Ultrasound guides the procedure. The eggs are then mixed with semen in a petri dish and, once fertilization is observed through a microscope, one or more embryos will be transferred to the uterus.

mixed with sperm (either your partner's or, if he is infertile, donor sperm). After fertilization, embryos begin to develop, and the eggs are implanted within the uterus by means of a small catheter placed through the cervical canal. Because most embryos fail to attach, they perish. Therefore, to increase the chances of attachment, anywhere from one to four embryos are transplanted.

Chances of success decrease with the age of the mother. For women forty years old or younger whose infertility is tied to tubal blockage, the rate of successful pregnancies after one in vitro attempt is around 25 percent. Only 10 to 20 percent of women with endometriosis, a subfertile male partner, or unexplained infertility have a child after one try. Many couples have in vitro fertilization several times before a pregnancy occurs; some never become pregnant despite repeated attempts. Because several embryos are placed into the uterus, in vitro fertilized mothers have a greater chance of delivering more than one infant (see also *Twins and Multiple Births*, page 295).

Gamete Intrafallopian Transfer (GIFT). Similar to IVF, GIFT is used when at least one of a woman's tubes is healthy, and it usually addresses such problems as low sperm count or sperm motility difficulties. In many instances, when artificial insemination has not worked or when the cause of infertility is not clear, GIFT will be used.

In this procedure, ripe eggs are removed from the ovary, mixed with sperm, and immediately injected back into the fallopian tube. Bringing the egg and sperm into direct contact encourages fertilization within the woman's body. A few weeks after the procedure, an ultrasound is usually conducted to make sure that an ectopic pregnancy, in which the egg implants within the fallopian tube, has not occurred.

Approximately 23 percent of women who have GIFT deliver infants, compared to an overall rate of 14 percent for in vitro fertilization.

Zygote intrafallopian transfer (ZIFT) combines elements of IVF and GIFT. Fertilization takes place in a laboratory and the fertilized eggs are then transplanted back into the fallopian tubes. This method is used when there is some doubt as to the sperm's ability to penetrate the egg. In the lab, it is possible to expose a number of eggs to sperm and to transplant only those that have been fertilized. Although not widely offered, ZIFT has produced a delivery rate of 22 percent after one cycle.

Sperm/Egg Donor. Fertilization or artificial insemination with sperm from a donor other than a woman's husband is an accepted practice. Donor sperm are used in such procedures as in vitro fertilization, GIFT, and ZIFT when the man has a problem with sperm count or motility or carries a troublesome genetic abnormality.

In cases in which a woman's ovaries are inactive because of menopause, inaccessible because of such diseases as endometriosis, or absent because of surgery, if her fallopian tubes and uterus are intact, egg donation, used in such procedures as IVF, GIFT, or ZIFT, allows a woman to become pregnant with her partner's sperm. The possibility that grave genetic defects will be passed on from the mother also presents a reason for using egg donation.

Some eggs are donated by friends and relatives or through egg banks. While only around 40 percent of clinics use egg donation, this method has produced a 29 percent delivery rate.

SURROGATE PARENTING

Like adoption, surrogacy is one solution to infertility. A relatively recent phenomenon, surrogate parenting refers to the arrangement made for a fertile woman to carry and deliver a baby for another couple. This option typically is considered when a hysterectomy or anatomical defects render pregnancy impossible. The surrogate is, in some instances, a relative, but more often a paid donor.

The surrogate is artificially inseminated with the prospective father's sperm. After birth, the surrogate relinquishes her rights as the child's biological mother. The man is the biological father, and the woman, the adoptive mother.

Although many couples have found surrogacy to be a fortunate solution to infertility, there are many legal and ethical issues that remain unresolved. In some cases, surrogate mothers have become attached to the baby during pregnancy and find it hard to give up him or her after birth. Some of these cases have ended in court settlements. In addition, there is the question of responsibility if a child is born with a serious defect.

If you decide to use a surrogate, proceed cautiously. There are agencies that specialize in surrogacy, and, of course, some are better than others. Typically, the agency screens surrogate candidates and matches them with couples. The couple then pays a substantial fee to the agency and the surrogate, as well as money to cover the surrogate's medical expenses.

Should you want to investigate surrogate parenthood, consult a lawyer about the legal implications and ask your health-care provider to recommend a clinic.

ADOPTION

Until World War II, orphanages brimmed with infants needing loving families. But now legal abortion and the loosening of taboos against single mothers have rendered adoption a more complicated process. The available children are fewer in number, and their special needs are greater.

For many of the one million American couples who currently await adoption through standard channels, the process is often time-consuming and frustrating. Only one in thirty of those couples will become parents this year. And for these people, the expense of adopting a child can be stunning, on average about twenty thousand dollars.

In 1970 there were 89,000 adoptions, less than two thirds of which involved infants. By 1986 (the latest year for which figures are available), the number had dropped to 51,000.

While there are a dearth of available infants, the same cannot be said for adoption agencies. There are thousands of agencies whose business it is to place unwanted children. Some are listed in the Yellow Pages; some advertise in newspapers and magazines. Some are responsible and ethical; some are not. In recent years, as the supply of healthy babies has diminished, a quasi-legal market has sprung up offering babies from the United States and from abroad. The practices and methods of those involved in this trade are more than questionable.

Adoption is a process that all must enter into cautiously and knowledgeably. Adoption laws vary from state to state. Marketing practices used by some agencies in some states would be considered illegal in others. And some adoption counselors, even if they operate within the letter of the law, can be unscrupulous. It will prevent a lot of later heartache if you contact an independent lawyer before you start in order to review your rights and anticipate legal difficulties.

Most people who want to adopt initially contact a not-for-profit agency. However, the number of babies available through agencies has decreased significantly in the last few decades. The wait to adopt a healthy white baby may be up to seven years. Many of the children who are placed with these agencies are older and have severe health, learning, or emotional problems. Nevertheless, there are plenty of couples who happily adopt children with special needs or older children. Many adopt children of color or children from other countries. But in recent years the number of foreign adoptions has declined as governments have set limits on the number of children who can leave the country. Moreover, as the debate around the effect of differences in ethnicity and culture on children has heated up, interracial adoption has become more difficult.

In the last decade or so, couples have tried to sidestep the bureaucracy and long waiting lists associated with agencies by arranging adoptions independently. They place advertisements in newspapers, specifically in states that allow private adoptions. In many cases, a pregnant woman searching for a suitable home for her baby, and perhaps for payment of her maternity expenses, will respond.

There are community and support groups that offer help and advice in arranging independent adoptions. Some physicians and lawyers specialize in private placement, but be aware that, because they profit from these adoptions, they may not always act in your best interest. Frequently, this process can be complicated, exploitative, and disappointing, involving strong and often ambivalent feelings, vulnerabilities, hopes, and anxieties. Some couples have been quite lucky in adopting through private channels; many have not been so lucky.

In recent years, some for-profit adoption agencies have begun marketing their services to pregnant women. They provide housing, medical care, and other resources a woman might need to get her through her pregnancy. In some states, however, any payment to a birth mother is construed as "buying" a baby. As such, it is against the law. A couple wishing to adopt from a for-profit agency pays an initial fee. At some agen-

cies, the birth mother is given profiles of several couples from which to choose. Meetings between the birth mother and the prospective adoptive couple often take place before she makes her decision.

In most cases, significant pain and confusion are involved in giving a child up for adoption. For many prospective parents, there is the heartbreak of an adoption gone awry. Adoption experts say that only between 10 and 30 percent of pregnant women who consider adoption actually go through with it.

Before you consider adoption, acquaint yourself with the laws of your state concerning the birth mother's rights. In some states, the mother has seventy-two hours after the baby's birth to decide to cancel the adoption agreement. Some other states allow mothers ninety days in which to make up their mind.

REPEATED MISCARRIAGES

More than half of all fertilized eggs die before a woman knows she is pregnant. The egg may undergo a few cell divisions in the fallopian tube, then cease developing. Or for some reason the embryo may fail to implant itself in the uterus. The natural termination of a pregnancy prior to the twentieth week of gestation is called a *spontaneous abortion* or miscarriage.

Between 10 and 20 percent of pregnancies miscarry after a woman learns she is pregnant. Most of these happen during the first twelve weeks of pregnancy, usually between the sixth and eleventh weeks. A few miscarriages, however, happen between the twelfth and twentieth weeks of pregnancy (see *Late Miscarriage*, page 295).

The great majority of miscarriages are due to arrested or abnormal embryonic development. About half are the result of a genetic abnormality in the embryo, usually an abnormal number of chromosomes. In these cases, miscarriage is simply the body's reaction to a nonviable pregnancy.

Once a woman knows she is pregnant and begins to plan for the birth of a child, miscarriage is a difficult emotional as well as physical event. Many women feel guilty. They wonder whether the loss could have been prevented had they taken better care of themselves. The reality of miscarriage, however, is that in virtually all instances, miscarriage is beyond a pregnant woman's control.

The majority of women who suffer miscarriages subsequently go on to carry a pregnancy to term and produce a healthy child. Although many women who have miscarried once are understandably nervous, having one miscarriage does not preclude successful pregnancy. The anxiety usually recedes once a woman moves beyond the point in the current pregnancy when the last miscarriage occurred.

When there have been three or more consecutive miscarriages or one miscarriage beyond the first trimester, however, there is more cause for concern.

Certain conditions seem to increase the incidence of miscarriage. Women over the age of thirty-five miscarry more often than younger women. The more miscarriages a woman has, the more likely she is to have another. Women whose mother took the drug diethylstilbestrol (DES—a powerful synthetic estrogen thought to prevent miscarriage and prescribed heavily between 1941 and 1971) are more likely to miscarry than those who were not exposed to the hormone (see *DES-Related Disorders*, page 526).

Once aborted, many of the embryos are shown to have genetic abnormalities. However, in between 80 and 90 percent of women who have three or more miscarriages fetuses with no apparent chromosomal abnormality are expelled. This raises the question of maternal disease or structural defect. Spontaneous abortion can result from infection during pregnancy, abnormalities in uterine development, benign uterine tumors, or incompetent cervix (in which the cervix opens during the second trimester of pregnancy, expelling the fetus before it is capable of living outside the womb). Environmental factors that may be responsible for recurrent miscarriages include smoking and excessive alcohol consumption during pregnancy, both of which introduce into the womb toxic agents that can destroy a normal fetus.

Many health-care providers recommend a number of tests to determine the cause of recurrent miscarriages. These may include a complete blood workup and a hysterogram, which can detect problems in the shape or size of the uterine cavity. If these tests do not reveal a cause for repeated miscarriages, your health-care provider might analyze both your and your partner's chromosomes for evidence of an abnormality.

In some cases of recurrent miscarriage, a cause can be diagnosed and treated successfully. Studies have shown, however, that most often, no cause is identified. Fortunately, the majority of women who miscarry eventually have a normal pregnancy.

NUTRITION AND EXERCISE

Eating well is one of the nicest—and perhaps most important—things you can do for yourself when you're pregnant. If you eat well, you will be healthier. Your risk of such complications as infection, anemia, and toxemia will be lower. Good nutrition helps to ensure that the baby will grow to its full potential and weight.

In order to secure the nutrients you need, eat a wide variety of food. If eating makes you uncomfortable, you may want to eat five or six smaller meals instead of three large ones. In addition, an empty stomach may make you feel worse, so eat healthy snacks between meals if you have morning sickness or indigestion.

In general, pregnancy increases your need for calories and protein. Many health-care providers prescribe a daily vitamin supplement that contains folic acid and iron (see *Folic Acid and Neural Tube Defects*, page 289). However, take vitamins only in consultation with your clinician; large doses of certain vitamins can cause harm to the fetus.

The Basics. The following outlines the basic elements of a well-balanced diet.

Protein is necessary for the repair of your tissues and the growth of your developing baby. Meat, poultry, fish, eggs, milk, and dried beans all are good sources of protein. A pregnant woman should have two or three servings of protein each day (from 75 to 100 grams).

Carbohydrates are good sources of energy. This food group includes breads, noodles, pasta, rice, whole grains, and potatoes. Cereals and grains are rich in vitamins and trace minerals. Starchy food seems to curb the discomfort of morning sickness.

Minerals are contained in many foods. Usually it is necessary to supplement a pregnant woman's dietary intake of iron since iron stored within the body is often insufficient to meet the increased demands of pregnancy. Iron is vital to the baby's developing blood supply. As with any vitamin or mineral, too much iron can be as dangerous as too little. So make sure you follow precisely your health professional's advice, which is likely to include a multivitamin supplement taken daily in capsule form.

Calcium is found in milk, cheese, ice cream, yogurt, and many vegetables. It contributes to the formation of strong bones and teeth. It also serves a vital role in the development of the heart, nervous system, and muscles. A pregnant woman does not need to drink milk to satisfy her calcium requirements, which may be met with other dairy products, vegetables, or supplements.

Vitamins, organic compounds in the foods we eat, are essential to the growth and maintenance of your body. Balanced diets, especially diets that depend heavily on fruits and vegetables, contain sufficient vitamins. Your health-care provider, though, may prescribe a supplement during your pregnancy.

Salt is needed to maintain sufficient body fluids and blood volume. It also maintains osmotic pressure and regulates muscle and nerve irritability. There is sufficient salt in foods; thus, no salt needs to be added in cooking or at the table. Avoid highly salted foods, such as cured, processed, and prepared meat; salty snack foods; and seasoning salts.

A pregnant woman can eat almost anything unless it disagrees with her or a special diet has been prescribed for a medical condition. Some foods, however, should be eaten in moderation. Many obstetricians recommend limiting caffeine consumption to three cups of coffee a day or the equivalent of tea, cola, and chocolate drinks. Desserts tend to be high in calories and low in nutrition, and it's a good idea to avoid empty calories as much as possible.

Weight Gain. The issue of weight and weight gain during pregnancy can be highly charged for a woman. In a society that consistently places pressure on women to be thin, and at the same time, pushes food at them, a woman can feel guilty and anxious about eating. Many women worry, not about eating well, but about gaining too much weight during pregnancy. If a health-care professional puts too much emphasis on weight without much regard to nutrition, a woman may anticipate her prenatal visits with considerable dread.

In recent years, the thinking behind weight gain in pregnancy has changed. Today the minimum recommended gain is twenty-five pounds. In most cases, weight gain between twenty-five and thirty-five pounds will mean that most women will not have gained excessive fat and will be able to lose the weight after the baby is born.

Exercise. As part of a normal pregnancy and the development of a healthy baby, it's important that you not only eat right but exercise as well. Although studies show that a lack of exercise doesn't adversely affect your developing child, in general mothers who are physically fit have more stamina. Unfortunately, contrary to popular belief, fitness is *not* reflected in a shorter and easier labor.

Don't go overboard. If prior to your pregnancy, you have been relatively sedentary, now is not the time to begin a heavy training program. Anyone—pregnant or otherwise—should ease into an exercise program gradually.

During pregnancy, a woman's body undergoes hormonal changes that can make it more vulnerable to injury. Connective tissues now stretch more easily to accommodate the growing fetus, making joints more unstable and subject to injury. Then, too, as a woman becomes larger, her balance becomes a bit more precarious as a result of a shift in her center of gravity. This makes her more prone to falls.

Because of these changes, exercises that are hard on the joints, such as high-impact aerobics, should be avoided. Certain racquet sports are not an ideal form of exercise for a pregnant woman since it is easy to become unbalanced and to invite joint damage or falls. Scuba diving below thirty feet, skiing, and parachute jumping should be avoided until after childbirth.

There are many ways a pregnant woman can safely exercise. Walking increases cardiovascular strength with little risk of injury. Many communities offer low-impact and water aerobic classes specifically for pregnant women. If you jogged or rode a bicycle prior to getting pregnant, there is no reason not to continue, although you may find that you fatigue more easily now and need to cut back on the amount of time you work out.

During your workout, remember never to overdo it. Drink fluids when you exercise to prevent dehydration. If the weather is hot and humid, postpone a workout outdoors until conditions are more comfortable.

Before embarking on any exercise program, check with your health-care provider. He or she probably will encourage your plan unless there is a medical problem that could make the extra exertion dangerous.

TEENAGE PREGNANCY

Damian was sixteen when she discovered that she was pregnant. Neither she nor her boyfriend was ready to marry, and Damian didn't want to have an abortion. Her mother and grandmother were willing to help. She could remain at home after the baby was born and they'd baby-sit when Damian went back to finish high school.

Damian paid little attention to her pregnancy. Her habits were typically adolescent. She ate as she always had—lots of fries and diet Coke. She continued to smoke, although now that she was pregnant, she hid her smoking from her mother. She drank beer when she hung out with friends, and she smoked marijuana on occasion. Damian was well into her third trimester when she began to worry enough about the pain of delivery that she visited the local clinic.

Damian's story, unfortunately, is fairly typical. Every year in the United States more than one million teenage girls become pregnant. Most are not married. Although some choose abortion, the majority go through childbirth and either give up the baby for adoption or, more commonly, raise the children themselves or with the help of their families. One third of these girls get pregnant again while still in their teens.

Developmentally, adolescents naturally have one foot in childhood and one in adulthood. They look as though they should know better, but often they do not. They are old enough to engage in adult behavior, but usually they are not ready to assume adult responsibility. More often than not, teenagers act with little thought to or understanding of the consequences. So a teenage boy will urge his girlfriend to have sexual intercourse without using contraceptives—without thinking about what pregnancy and fatherhood would mean in his life. And a teenage girl will become pregnant without thinking what pregnancy will do to her body and what motherhood will mean.

In general, once they find themselves pregnant, teenage girls don't take very good care of themselves. Poor nutrition, smoking, alcohol, drugs, and venereal disease are all factors that can compromise a young women's pregnancy as well as her baby's health. Moreover, many teens delay seeking prenatal care, if they seek it at all.

Teenage girls, as a group, are more likely to have specific pregnancy-related problems. Anemia, probably as the result of a poor diet, affects an alarming number of pregnant girls. One study revealed that 95 percent of pregnant teens had a diet deficient in iron, protein, calcium, and vitamin A.

A large number of teens suffer from preeclampsia and eclampsia during pregnancy. This pregnancy-related toxemia is always serious and sometimes fatal when not brought under control (see page 303).

The incidence of premature births and infant mortality is higher in babies born to young mothers. This appears to be a function of poverty and poor prenatal care rather than age. Congenital malformations of the neural tube occur more often in the children of teens than in the general population, among them spina bifida, anencephaly, and meningomyelocele. Most health-care professionals attribute this to the fact that while folic acid supplements during early pregnancy have been associated with a lower incidence of these neural tube defects, teens are less likely than older women to take vitamins (see page 289).

In the best of all circumstances, if a teenage girl and boy are not prepared for the responsibility of parenthood, they should approach sex knowledgeably and cautiously. Two thirds of sexually active teens in this country do not regularly use birth control Using a condom will protect against pregnancy as well as such sexually transmitted diseases as AIDS, gonorrhea, syphilis, or chlamydia (see *What Is Safe Sex?*, page 442).

If you are a parent of a teenager, it is important that, however embarrassing and uncomfortable it may be, you take the time to talk to your child about sexual feelings, behavior, and responsibility. If it were up to most parents, their children wouldn't become sexually active until they were adults. In addition, there is always the concern that if you talk openly about sex, it will seem to your child that you are condoning the action. But the truth is, talking to your kids about sex won't make them sexual, but it will help make them responsible (see *Talking About Sex with Your Teenage Daughter*, page 21).

Many parents have the idea that they need to explain the facts of life only once. However, talking about sex is not a one-time event; rather, it should be an ongoing dialogue, the content of which will naturally change as the child's developmental curiosity and needs change. By opening the subject up to candid discussion early in the child's life—conversation about where babies come from can take place before the child begins kindergarten—discussions about sex will be natural when it is an active issue in his or her life. In addition, if an atmosphere of candor and safety is created around the subject, there's a good chance your child will be able to approach you with any questions and confused feelings he or she may have. If your daughter discovers that she is pregnant, she may feel comfortable coming to you despite her feelings of guilt, fear, and conflict.

Should a teenage girl suspect that she is pregnant, the first step is to make an appointment with a doctor, midwife, or community health-care provider. The earlier the pregnancy is confirmed, the more time there is to consider options.

What are those options? Abortion—the termination of pregnancy—is a safe and legal procedure. Abortions are most easily and safely performed in the first trimester of pregnancy.

For many women, having an abortion is not as painful and difficult as having an unwanted child; for others, it simply isn't an acceptable ethical or emotional choice. When a girl does choose to carry the pregnancy to term, she can either put the infant up for adoption or decide to raise it herself. No matter which of these two options she chooses, good prenatal care will keep her and her baby healthy.

PREGNANCY AFTER THIRTY-FIVE

When Michaela and her husband moved from the city to a house in the country, they were warmly greeted by their neighbors Dana and Matthew. Both couples were in their late thirties, and on the surface, they seemed to have much in common. However, within a few weeks, it became apparent that Michaela and Dana were on conflicting schedules, and their idea of leisure time was quite different. Michaela was the mother of a two-year-old son and was in the early stages of her second pregnancy. She was preoccupied with naps and diapers and making sure that her toddler didn't choke on the things he picked up. Dana's daughter was applying to law school, and her son was graduating high school. Dana had a lot of extra time and frequently invited Michaela on long walks and days at the mall. Michaela had neither time nor energy to go along. Despite the fact that they were close in age, Dana and Michaela soon discovered they didn't have much in common because they were at different stages in their family life.

A generation ago most women in their middle thirties were anticipating the day when the last child would be packed off to college or join the workforce. Today, an increasing number of women that age are comparing the safety of infant car seats and weighing the benefits of breast-feeding over bottle feeding instead. College, to these new mothers, is practically as remote as retirement.

There are a number of factors that have contributed to the trend these days to delay starting a family: effective methods of birth control, later and second marriages, involvement in work and career, and in some cases, infertility, among others.

Today, with a woman's average life expectancy at eighty-two, a thirty-five-year-old woman is a long way from old age. Compare that to a woman born in 1841, who was likely to live only forty-two years. But even though a woman at thirty-five feels as strong and healthy as ever, from an obstetrical standpoint she's approaching the end of her reproductive years. Nevertheless, with good prenatal care, pregnancy at that age is quite safe. There can be, however, specific age-related considerations.

Fertility decreases as a woman grows older. It becomes more difficult, therefore, for her to conceive once she decides to have a child. Those who do conceive have a higher risk of having a child born with Down's syndrome, a birth abnormality caused by an extra chromosome. The risk of this genetic abnormality is 1 in 1,205 in a twenty-five-year-old woman, 1 in 365 in a thirty-five-year-old, and 1 in 140 in a thirty-nine-year-old woman. Children born with Down's syndrome have some degree of mental retardation and often have heart and gastrointestinal defects as well. If you are thirty-five or older, your health-care provider may recommend chorionic villus sampling or amniocentesis, prenatal tests in which a sample of placental tissue or amniotic fluid is removed from the womb and studied for chromosomal defects. These tests can detect other chromosome abnormalities as well as Down's syndrome (see *Prenatal Testing, Monitoring, and Other Procedures*, page 289).

Older mothers are more likely to experience hypertension (high blood pressure) or gestational diabetes, either of which can complicate pregnancy and compromise the infant. First-time mothers over the age of forty, along with pregnant teenagers, are most prone to preeclampsia and eclampsia (see page 303). The rates of miscarriage and stillbirth also are slightly higher in this age group.

As a group, older mothers tend to be better educated and highly motivated when it comes to prenatal care. With good prenatal care, about 95 percent of women over thirty-five have uncomplicated pregnancies and deliver healthy babies.

PERIMENOPAUSAL PREGNANCY

Sandy, age forty-two, was in her obstetrician's office soon after her daughter's birth. They were talking about birth control. "Well, we could consider putting you on the pill, but only for a few years." He paused, then continued. "Menopause is just around the corner."

"Menopause!" Sandy thought. "I just had a baby." She found herself a little surprised at her doctor's insensitivity.

Even today, with many women delaying pregnancy much later than in previous generations, the majority have their last child years before they begin to think about menopause. But there are women—although relatively few—who become pregnant in their fifties.

Pregnancy after the age of forty-seven is uncommon. By the time a woman is forty-five ovulation is more erratic, making it increasingly difficult to conceive. The median age of menopause in the United States—that is, the age when the average woman ceases to menstruate—is fifty-one. But menopause is actually a process that begins with a decline in ovarian function and culminates in the cessation of menstruation. This process can take five years from start to finish and during that time some women become pregnant.

Women who begin to exhibit the symptoms of menopause often think that they are no longer capable of pregnancy. While pregnancy becomes more unlikely as a woman gets older, if she has regular periods, chances are she's ovulating. And there is, therefore, a risk of perimenopausal pregnancy (a pregnancy that occurs about the time of menopause). In one study of women between the ages of forty and fifty, doctors found that ovulation was related more to the regularity of a woman's periods than to her age. The women who menstruated regularly ovulated during almost every cycle. Yet even erratic periods and severe menopausal symptoms were no clear sign that ovulation had stopped. There are examples of women conceiving two years after they stopped menstruating. Thus, a woman approaching menopause should continue using contraception, unless, of course, she wants to get pregnant.

In the event you do become pregnant—either by design or by accident—you, like any older mother, will be more prone to problems such as hypertension, diabetes, and preeclampsia and eclampsia. Miscarriage, stillbirth, and low birth weight also are more common in pregnancies among older women. However, responsible prenatal care usually means that a perimenopausal woman can have a successful pregnancy and healthy baby.

CHAPTER 14

Being Pregnant

CONTENTS

When Carnie announced to her family that she was pregnant, her mother sat her down. Martina hugged her daughter, then shook her head. "Don't think this is just about bearing, delivering, and nurturing a baby," she warned. "That's only the most basic level of the experience. Pregnancy is not just a physical process. Pregnancy begins a stage in your life that will extend throughout and touch all parts of your life. Some things," Martina added, "will be changed—possibly forever."

Carnie received this advice in silent horror. Wait a minute, she thought to herself; can't I have a little time to get used to the idea of being pregnant? To be relieved of the worry that maybe I couldn't get pregnant? And to take pleasure in the reality of my pregnancy? Do I have to start worrying already about what it will mean to be a mother? I can hardly face all the choices and details of pregnancy as it is, without thinking about the abstract questions.

Both women are right. Pregnancy and motherhood are experiences that involve all aspects of a woman and her existence. Pregnancy sets in motion—in the blink of an eye— a process that, in most cases, spans the balance of a woman's life.

THE FIRST TRIMESTER

Tamara and her husband had been trying to get pregnant for months. But even before she missed her period, Tamara had a feeling that finally they were going to have a baby. She had a queasy feeling and slight nausea during most of the day. Her breasts were tender and fuller—even more than was normal around her period. Her nipples hurt. In addition she had to urinate a lot. Tamara didn't feel especially well, but she felt really happy.

The first three months of a woman's pregnancy is in many ways the most important, especially in terms of embryo development. Many woman, though, do not become aware that they are pregnant until well into their first trimester. As a result, they are not as careful as they might be otherwise. Nevertheless, this is the time that judicious health habits really count—including good nutrition, reasonable exercise, avoidance of smoking and alcohol, and prudent drug use (which means no recreational drugs and use of medication only on the instruction of a health professional).

It is during the first trimester that the basic embryo form begins to develop: By the end of this period, your fetus will be around three inches long and weigh about an ounce. In many ways, the fetus will resemble the child he or she will become.

FERTILIZATION AND
EARLY FETAL DEVELOPMENT

Fertilization begins when a single male sperm penetrates the female egg. One out of the hundreds of millions of sperm ejaculated into the female reproductive system, the successful sperm attacks the firm capsule (zona pellucida) of the egg. Approximately 266 days later, a baby will be born.

The egg and the sperm each contribute twenty-three chromosomal pairs. These forty-six chromosomes, in turn, contain thousands of genes, which dictate the basic out-line for the new person being created. The genetic material establishes, for example, eye, hair, and skin color; body size and type; facial features; and, to some degree, tempera-ment, character, and intellectual style and capability.

The sperm and egg merge to form a one-cell embryo (zygote). After fertilization, the zygote begins an intricate process of division. Every twelve hours, the number of cells doubles, adding to the complexity of the organism. Slowly, the fertilized egg travels down the fallopian tube, and it reaches the uterus within four to five days. At this point, it has also transformed itself from a solid mass to a group of about five hun-dred cells centered around a fluid-filled cavity called a blastocyst. *One section of the blastocyst will become the embryo and the other section will become the placenta, which provides nourishment.*

Meanwhile, the ovaries have begun secreting progesterone, which causes the uterine lining to swell with secretions, thus preparing itself for the embryo's implantation. Firm implantation is completed around the twelfth day of gestation.

The average length of normal gestation is 266 days from conception to full term. However, a woman's due date is typically measured from the first day of her last period, which is about two weeks before actual fertilization. This means that the esti-mated length of a full gestation is 280 days, though it may be as short as 266 days and as long as 294. Gestation is, then, roughly forty weeks from the last menstrual period.

PRENATAL CARE

One of the most important things you can do for yourself and your baby is to seek prenatal care as soon as you suspect you are pregnant. During your first visit your health-care provider will take a detailed health and family history and ascertain whether there are any preexisting conditions or problems than may require special attention during the preg-nancy.

He or she will also be able to determine an approximate due date, based on the date of your last menstrual period. Blood will be taken to determine blood type, Rh type, and the existence of anemia, rubella antibodies, and syphilis. A urinalysis will be done to check for glucose, protein, and white blood cell levels, and for bacteria.

A thorough physical examination will include an assessment of your general health. A baseline blood pressure measurement will be taken, height and weight will be recorded, and the presence of edema (swelling) and varicose veins will be noted. During a pelvic examination, a Pap smear will be performed. Typically, your health-care provider will spend some time advising you on nutrition, weight gain, and exercise and will prescribe prenatal vitamin supplements. Follow-up care usually includes monthly visits for the first seven months, bimonthly visits during the eighth month, then weekly visits until delivery.

During subsequent visits, your weight and blood pressure will be monitored. Each visit usually includes urine tests to measure protein and sugar levels as well. Your clinician also will feel your abdomen to measure the rate of fetal growth and examine your hands and feet for edema.

At these visits, you will be asked whether you are having such problems as headache, nausea, vomiting, swelling, or vaginal bleeding. It is also the best time to pose any questions or worries you have. It's a good idea to keep a list of questions between visits.

Around the twelfth week of gestation, the fetus's heartbeat can be heard with the help of an amplifying device called a Doppler instrument. The moment at which a woman can actually hear the life that's stirring within her is often a joyous one. It is during the first trimester that the basic fetal form begins to develop: the body, arms, legs, and internal organs. By the end of this period, your baby will be around three inches long and weigh around an ounce. In many ways, the fetus will resemble the child he or she will become.

After the egg implants in the uterine wall, it doubles its size every day. The placenta has begun to form, as has the fetal spinal cord. In addition, eyes and heart have begun to develop. In the third week after fertilization, around the time a woman's period would normally begin, an embryo has formed—the head and intestinal tract begin to develop. At the end of the sixth week, the brain becomes noticeable and arm and leg buds appear. Genital cells—those that will later become ovaries or testes—also appear. By the seventh week, the abdomen and chest are fully formed and lungs begin to develop. Facial features, finger, and toes begin to form around the eighth week, and a boy's penis begins to appear around this time. By the end of the second month, your baby looks like a baby—though very tiny. By the tenth week, the face is developed and the heart, complete with four chambers, is beating between 120 and 160 beats per minute. At this point, your embryo becomes a fetus in medical terms.

COMMON CONCERNS DURING THE FIRST TRIMESTER (AND PERHAPS THEREAFTER)

There are a number of minor discomforts that often accompany pregnancy. Most of them are simply passing irritations; others may require a consultation with your health-care provider.

Anemia is a condition that arises from a deficiency of one or another nutrient in the blood. In pregnant women, the most common type of anemia is *iron-deficiency anemia.*

Early prenatal blood analysis looks for anemia, but most women are not anemic when they begin their pregnancy. By the end of pregnancy, however, 20 percent of all pregnant women suffer from anemia. The lack of iron affects the mother rather than the fetus; serious anemia can leave a woman feeling tired, weak, shaky, breathless, and light-headed. Women who have a number of pregnancies in quick succession, those who have trouble eating or keeping food down because of morning sickness, women who begin pregnancy poorly nourished, and those who are carrying multiple fetuses are at particular risk for development of anemia.

Anemia is easily prevented and corrected through good diet and a daily iron supplement, which is included in most prenatal vitamins.

Morning Sickness. One third of all pregnant women in America suffer from some form of morning sickness during their pregnancy. Usually ending by the twelfth week, the symptoms of morning sickness seem to be triggered by higher levels of pregnancy hormones. These higher levels influence stomach emptying. Also, as the uterus expands rapidly, a woman may experience extra sensitivity during digestion.

Typically there are good days and bad days. Early morning is usually the worse time—hence the name morning sickness. During the early hours, the stomach is empty, blood sugar level is lower, and stomach acids have accumulated. Unfortunately, morning sickness does not necessarily limit itself to the morning hours; some women experience nausea and digestive discomfort throughout the day. For a few, this discomfort lasts throughout the nine months of pregnancy with some ebb and flow in its severity.

Some women find that by guarding against an empty stomach they can curb the discomfort of morning sickness. Protein and starch or sugar—milk, cheese, fruit, or juice—eaten just before bed seem to diminish stomach irritation the next morning. Keep crackers or dry toast next to your bed so that you can nibble before you rise. Give yourself time to wake slowly and get out of bed gradually.

Avoid fatty foods at breakfast and greasy foods throughout the day. Some women find spicy foods a problem. Avoid coffee, sweets, and processed foods. Fruit and fruit juice, which are acidic, are best consumed at the conclusion of a meal. For some women, vitamin B_6 seems to prevent vomiting. Yogurt seems to help some women, as does a high-carbohydrate, high-protein diet.

In order to prevent your stomach from getting empty, have five or six smaller meals throughout the day instead of three large ones. Snack on nutritious foods between meals. Carry bananas (which seem to help some women) and crackers so that you are not caught unprepared by a wave of nausea.

Unquestionably, it's harder to eat once you are nauseated; if you find it impossible to hold food down over a short period, be sure to drink a lot. Very hot or very cold liquids can make you feel better. Ginger ale and colas are helpful because they are rich in carbohydrates and carbonation can settle the stomach. Some women find that herbal teas—peppermint, spearmint, chamomile, peach leaf, and red raspberry leaf teas—relieve nausea and vomiting.

If you cannot keep food down, your health-care provider may prescribe medications. These are typically prescribed when there is a very real risk that your baby is being deprived of the nutrients it needs. *Fatigue* is most pronounced in early pregnancy. Just as in adolescence, when your body needed more sleep to accommodate greater growth and development, in pregnancy, the body needs more energy. If you are naturally an energetic, active person, you may find this increased fatigue disconcerting. Yet, you might as well get used to the extra demands that the baby is making on you—and will continue to make throughout his or her life.

Respect your need for more sleep; make time for naps, even if that means closing your eyes for five or ten minutes at periods during the day. Go to bed earlier. Avoid criticizing yourself as being lazy. And be prepared to experience impatience, irritability, difficulty in concentration, and loss of sexual interest—all possible side effects of fatigue.

Frequent urination is another sign of pregnancy. In the early months, because of hormonal changes, a woman may find herself needing to urinate frequently and without warning. Later on in the pregnancy, as her uterus expands, a woman will have to urinate often because there is increasing pressure on the bladder.

Swelling (edema) affects close to 40 percent of all pregnant women. Just as the rise in hormone production prior to a woman's period naturally causes water to build up in her body, the same hormones that are now being produced by the placenta cause fluid retention. In pregnancy, there is a significant increase in blood volume and circulation, and fluid retention facilitates this increase.

About one fourth of the weight that a woman gains in pregnancy is fluid. Anything more than mild or occasional edema should be discussed with your health-care provider.

In the old days, clinicians prescribed diuretics. Such water pills are not helpful. In fact, diuretics may harm the mother and fetus. Diuretics can decrease the ability of the body to add needed fluid to the circulation. Avoiding excess salt and prolonged standing or sitting is the best remedy for swelling. Mild exercise such as walking and swimming can also reduce edema. If your fingers and feet get puffy, remove your rings and avoid standing or sitting in one position for extended periods. Lying down on your side will help your kidneys get rid of excess fluid.

Teeth and gums are often affected during pregnancy as increased levels of hormones cause swelling of periodontal tissue. Gums may bleed easily, and bacterial infections can occur and recur. Attention to brushing, flossing, and gum stimulation is helpful. It's also a good idea to see your dentist at least once during the pregnancy and to have your teeth cleaned professionally.

Backache often occurs in pregnancy as your posture changes to compensate for the shift in your center of gravity and for the increased weight. Moreover, your ligaments become more elastic, allowing the pelvis to expand in order to accommodate the fetus. This elasticity means that your joints are more prone to strain and injury.

A pregnant woman may experience backache—especially lower back pain—when she is tired or after she has been lifting, bending, or walking. Some women experience a pain that radiates down to their legs, called *sciatica*. Many may have pain in the area around the abdomen, caused by the stretching of those ligaments, especially in the second trimester.

Backache is most effectively relieved by eliminating as much strain as possible. Your clinician may recommend specific stretching and strengthening exercises to ease the discomfort.

Varicose veins occur when the valves in the veins break from the increase in back pressure caused by the enlarging uterus. As a result, the veins in the legs can become swollen and uncomfortable.

Varicose veins appear in approximately 20 percent of all pregnant women. They usually worsen in the later stages of pregnancy, although they appear earlier and are more pronounced with each subsequent pregnancy. Older women and women who stand for extended periods are more likely to have varicose veins in pregnancy. Heredity also seems to play a role.

If you have varicose veins, wear comfortable, nonbinding clothing. Support hose may lessen the swelling and discomfort. Whenever possible, stay off your feet and elevate your legs.

Constipation, difficulty in passing stool, occurs because increased pressure from a growing uterus makes it more difficult for the intestines to contract and the bowel to expel its contents. Women who are normally constipated may experience greater problems during pregnancy.

Fluids, exercise, and a diet rich in fruits, vegetables, and grains will more than likely alleviate the problem. Fiber laxatives can also be helpful.

Hemorrhoids are the result of increased pressure on the veins in the anus. Women who have hemorrhoids find that taking warm baths and applying cold compresses soaked in witch hazel are comforting. If you have hemorrhoids, avoid getting constipated and straining to have a bowel movement.

Heartburn arises when stomach acid flows upward into the lower esophagus, causing a burning sensation. This happens as increased levels of progesterone relax all the smooth muscles, including the cardiac sphincter of the stomach, the muscle that would otherwise block the acids as they push back up. In addition, the growing uterus pushes the stomach upward, increasing the pressure.

Half of all women experience heartburn during pregnancy. If you are one of them, avoid greasy, spicy food; large meals; alcohol; and coffee. Drink milk and buttermilk. An antacid may also help relieve the discomfort, but discuss the selection and dosage of antacid with your clinician.

Sleeping with your head elevated is another strategy that may reduce some of the symptoms of heartburn.

WHAT'S OKAY—WHAT'S NOT OKAY

The embryo is vulnerable in the first trimester to birth defects caused by drugs and alcohol, although the risk continues into later stages of development.

Alcohol consumed in large amounts may cause nerve and brain damage in the fetus. According to the National Institute on Alcohol Abuse and Alcoholism, more than two drinks a day (one ounce of hard liquor, two mixed drinks, two glasses of wine or beer, for example) can harm your unborn child. Six or more drinks a day—throughout the pregnancy or at critical stages—put your child at significant risk for fetal alcohol syndrome, an alcohol-related grouping of defects that includes facial and heart abnormalities, body deformities, and diminished intelligence. Even with fewer than six drinks, there is a significant risk of some of these defects. Binge drinking also can be harmful.

Drinking also interferes with the absorption and utilization of nutrients. It decreases a woman's appetite and substitutes empty calories for real nutrition.

Baths are safe at all times during pregnancy except when your membranes have broken, at which time the chance of infection increases. Hot tubs, however, can be dangerous during pregnancy if the mother's body temperature rises too high. Soaking in a tub longer than ten minutes at a temperature higher than 104 degrees Fahrenheit (104°F) can raise a mother's temperature to the point where there is an increased risk of miscarriage or birth defects.

Clothes should be comfortable. Even in the early stages, avoid clothes that are binding and tight. However, wear a bra throughout the pregnancy. Your breasts will gain substantial weight during the first trimester. Wearing a bra will support the extra weight and prevent sagging when you lose the weight after childbirth and nursing. Because your breasts will continue to grow throughout the pregnancy, buy only one or two bras at a time.

Caffeine crosses the placenta and can stimulate the fetal nervous system. It has been suggested that high doses of caffeine may be linked to miscarriage. Current recommendations are to decrease caffeine consumption to less than three cups of coffee per day; you need not eliminate caffeine altogether.

Diets that are varied and based on unprocessed foods, vegetables, and fruits provide the best sustenance for a normal pregnancy and healthy baby. A diet that is insufficient in both quantity and nutrition increases the risk of having a low-birth-weight baby. Most health-care professionals recommend that a woman gain between twenty-five and thirty-five pounds during pregnancy. Inadequate weight gain can have a negative impact on your pregnancy and on the baby—possibly causing growth retardation and long-term developmental problems. If, on the other hand, you overeat, you may gain too much weight, adding more stress on your body, increasing your discomfort, and making it harder to lose the extra weight after the baby is born (see page 357).

On average, a pregnant woman needs between 2,200 and 2,400 calories each day. A healthy daily diet will include two or three servings of protein (meat, poultry, fish, eggs, milk, dried beans), four or more servings of carbohydrates (breads, pasta, rice, and potatoes), and five servings of fruits and vegetables that are rich in vitamins and minerals. Many clinicians recommend a vitamin supplement that includes iron and folic acid, which has been found to prevent spina bifida, an open or malformed spine.

Drug exposure puts the fetus at risk of injury throughout pregnancy, although popular belief has it that the first trimester is the most dangerous time. Although few drugs are known to cause birth defects, any drug, even those considered necessary, should be discussed with your health-care professional. Ask whether it is advisable to eliminate the drug; it may actually be in your best interest and the best interest of the baby to continue treatment.

Exercise has become accepted as a regular part of a healthy life-style. If exercise is part of your life, there is no reason to stop once you become pregnant. It is important, though, to take your pregnancy into consideration when you engage in any physical activity.

Discuss necessary limitations or moderation in your routine with your health-care provider. As you become bigger, you will experience a shift in your center of gravity and your sense of balance may feel more precarious. Exercises that include deep bending or stretching around your joints therefore might not be a good idea. High-impact aerobics or such sports as tennis and racquetball which require abrupt changes in direction and could result in falling are also not recommended at this time unless you have been conditioned for them.

The most suitable exercises during this time include swimming—which offers good cardiovascular stimulation as well as the protection against injury afforded by water buoyancy—and walking, jogging, and cycling. In many communities, there are special low-impact aerobic classes for pregnant women.

If you were not particularly active before, pregnancy is not the time to embark on a vigorous exercise program. However, it may be a good idea to develop some kind of fitness regimen with the guidance of your health-care provider. There are advantages to regular exercise in terms of stamina and cardiovascular health.

At no time should you exercise to the point of exhaustion. Drink plenty of fluid to prevent dehydration. And always be aware of how your body is responding to your exercise; if it feels as if you are overdoing it, you probably are.

Food additives that are found in snack foods, cured meats, cake mixes, breakfast cereals, and canned foods have no apparent effect on the baby. These include sodium nitrates and nitrites that are used to cure meats and fish and are found in hot dogs, bacon, salami, and other processed meat. These foods are often high in sodium, however, and can increase swelling. Saccharin and aspartame (Nutrasweet) are artificial sweeteners; they have not been shown to harm the fetus. However, for general health reasons, foods containing many additives should be consumed in moderation.

Harmful and toxic environmental products have been identified as harmful to the embryo in some cases, and those that are harmful are also dangerous to adults. For example, carbon monoxide poisoning from faulty heaters or lead poisoning from stripping of old paint can produce developmental problems.

Smoking during pregnancy can result in having a smaller infant, increase the chances of miscarriage and stillbirth, and predispose the baby to serious health problems throughout his or her life (see page 243). Quit smoking before, during, and after pregnancy.

Stamina, strength, and balance change during pregnancy. As a result, don't lift or push heavy objects, climb ladders and step stools carefully, don't exhaust yourself, and accept help whenever it's offered. Ask for help when you need it.

Toxoplasmosis is produced by a parasitic organism transmitted through cat feces and raw meat. Though normally a disease so mild its symptoms—slight achiness, rash, and swollen glands—can go unnoticed, if contracted in pregnancy, it can inflict everlasting harm to the fetus. This infection can result in fetal brain damage, blindness, malformation of the head, or even death of the fetus. Retardation and other neurological problems can occur if the fetus is exposed in the last months of pregnancy.

Luckily, this infection is both uncommon and preventable. In most cases, a woman who contracts the disease does not pass it on to her baby. If she does, in most cases, the baby will show no ill effects. Health-care professionals can test their pregnant patients for systemic immunity to the infection. If you are not adequately immune, there are ways of avoiding infection.

Since heat kills the organism, avoid raw or rare meat. If you have a cat, feed it only cooked, canned, or dry food, never raw meat. Have another member of the household clean the litter box. Your cat can avoid being infected if you keep him or her indoors and unable to eat infected meat such as mice and birds. Wear gloves when gardening and wash your hands afterward.

Travel is an issue that comes up frequently during pregnancy, especially as women's jobs require that they travel, pregnant or not, and many women wish to visit family and friends or to get away as a couple before the baby arrives.

In the early months of pregnancy, when many women experience morning sickness, travel may exacerbate feelings of nausea and digestive discomfort, but there is no indication that travel prompts either labor or miscarriage. Still, the possibility remains that either can happen with little or no warning, and that possibility may make being away from home worrisome.

If you have a history of spontaneous abortions (miscarriages) or premature delivery, you may want to be somewhat conservative about unnecessary travel. If you have other high-risk factors such as high blood pressure or diabetes, your doctor may not think travel is a good idea. In the last six weeks of pregnancy, you may be urged to limit your trips to within fifty miles of home.

Although flying has no effect on labor, the chances of going into labor increases as your due date approaches. Some airlines recommend restricted travel for women after their seventh month. Sit over the wings or toward the front of the plane, where you will feel less of the plane's motion. Eat lightly when flying because pregnancy makes you more prone to motion sickness. Go to the bathroom before boarding, since there may be long periods of time on the plane when you cannot safely leave your seat. Fasten your seat belt below your belly, across the bony pelvis.

Car trips can be exhausting, so if you can, limit car travel. If you take a long trip, get out of the car and walk around at least every hundred miles or every two hours of travel to ensure good circulation. Fasten your seat belt across the bony pelvis and use the shoulder harness.

Vaginal products, such as douches and gels, should be avoided during pregnancy. Those that contain povidone iodine can cause thyroid defects in the fetus. Moreover, there is a risk of creating a life-threatening embolism through douching; bulb syringe douches can be especially dangerous in this regard.

Diagnostic X-ray procedures do not use enough radiation to harm the baby. Of course, all X rays should be avoided if they are unnecessary, but needed X rays should not be withheld on the basis of pregnancy. The fetus will not be harmed by dental X rays.

Working while you are pregnant is the same as working when you're not pregnant. Nevertheless, there are physical changes and discomforts that need to be respected and accommodated. There is no reason not to work when you are pregnant unless your job involves heavy physical labor or is in an industry with potentially harmful materials and fumes.

SEX DURING PREGNANCY

Sexual relations during pregnancy—as well as after you become parents—will no doubt change. You may find yourself apprehensive and unsure. Sex can become better than it's ever been—or nonexistent.

People differ in their reactions to conception and the idea of parenthood. These reactions often get played out in the bedroom. In addition, over the nine months of your pregnancy, there will be emotional and physical swings; a woman who experiences nausea, vomiting, fatigue, tender breasts, and/or backache may not feel strong sexual desire. On the other hand, as her hormones surge, so may her sexual drive. All this variability need not be problematic, especially if you and your partner talk to each other about it.

Some women understandably worry that sex will harm the fetus. The baby actually is protected by a bag of fluid (amniotic sac) on the other side of a closed cervix. Seminal fluid cannot infect the fetus. Nor can the baby be crushed.

Some people worry that the baby is watching. While a fetus does experience sound waves, its mother's movements, and rocking caused by uterine contractions during orgasm, it neither sees nor understands.

It is not uncommon for women to worry that sex and orgasm might lead to miscarriage. Yet this doesn't seem to be the case. Even in the first trimester when most miscarriages occur, a woman should take things slowly, at her own pace, and massage, caress, and move past the anxiety. But there is really no need to avoid intercourse.

Bleeding may accompany intercourse, especially in the first few months. Usually this occurs when a man thrusts his penis deeply up against the cervix (mouth of the uterus). Because the cervix is softer during pregnancy and there are extra blood vessels at the mouth of the uterus, pressure may cause a small amount of bleeding. These bruises heal quickly, and most of the time, they are no cause for worry. If, however, bleeding causes you anxiety, it may be a good idea to avoid deep penetration. Talking to your health-care professional may assuage the anxiety and rule out the possibility of miscarriage or other problems.

In the last months of pregnancy, the degree of physical discomfort and a woman's sense of herself as she becomes larger may interfere with satisfactory sex relationships. In a country where fat is a dirty word, a woman may feel that she is undesirable as she becomes larger. Chances are, though, that your mate will not find you unattractive. In fact, many men find their partners particularly sexy in the fullness of pregnancy.

Often there is concern that sex in the last trimester will bring on labor. Labor, however, will not be triggered merely by intercourse, although nipple stimulation may produce contractions.

If a couple is able to manage the variety of feelings—guilt, anxiety, anticipation—during this time, sexual enjoyment is often enhanced by the lack of contraceptive worries as well as by a woman's hormonal changes. It is important, therefore, to keep communications open and honest between you and your partner. Sincere and gentle reassurance during this time can strengthen your intimate and sexual relationship as you ease into your new roles as parents. If you overcome any reticence you may have about discussing or experimenting, pregnancy may usher in a new depth and fullness to your sex life, which will continue to grow well after the baby is born.

DRUGS TO AVOID AND DRUGS TO USE CAUTIOUSLY

Although nearly all drugs cross the placenta to reach the developing baby, very few have been shown to produce developmental damage. Most birth defects appear to be due to spontaneous errors of embryo development rather than to noxious influences. Some are due to genetic abnormalities, a minority to exposures. Of those caused by foreign agents introduced to the body, the most common substance is alcohol.

Still, there are some medications that are not used during pregnancy because they produce birth defects. Other potentially harmful drugs are used in spite of the possibility of fetal harm, because the consequences of leaving certain diseases untreated pose graver risks to the mother and baby than do the potential side effects of the drugs.

- Isotrenoin, *a medication used for severe cystic acne, causes miscarriage and defects of the head, face, heart, and other organs. It is recommended that this medication never be used during pregnancy.*

- Anticonvulsants *can produce cleft palate, heart defects, and neural tube defects. However, most exposed fetuses are unaffected. In addition, the consequences of untreated epilepsy for mother and baby are generally worse than the risk of the drug treatment.*

- Iodine-containing medications *can cause damage to the fetal thyroid gland and are to be avoided during pregnancy.*

- Aspirin *in high doses has been associated in some (though not all) studies with a small increased risk of birth defects. More important, use of aspirin prior to delivery by the mother increases the risk of abnormal bleeding in the newborn, particularly in premature babies.*

- Lithium, *a drug used in some psychiatric disorders, has been suspected of producing a small increase in congenital heart disease.*
- Methotrexate, *an antiproliferative drug used in some cancers and rheumatic disease, can increase the risk of birth defects, primarily those involving the head and face.*
- Angiotensin-converting enzyme inhibitors *are a special class of antihypertensive medications that can produce renal failure, skull defects, and death in the fetus after use in the second or third trimester.*
- Warfarin, *a blood thinner, produces abnormalities of the bones and of brain structures.*
- Tetracycline, *an antibiotic, can permanently discolor teeth and can cause underdevelopment of some bones.*
- Streptomycin, gentamicin, and kanamycin *represent a class of antibiotics that produce hearing loss in some exposed fetuses.*

In spite of the relatively small number of medications for which adverse effects have been shown, there are a number of exposures for which information is incomplete or studies contradictory. It is a good idea to have all medications assessed by a health professional trained in evaluating the pregnancy effects of exposures. Help is available through national organizations that provide this kind of information.

One such resource is
The Reproductive Toxicology Center
2440 M Street NW
Washington, D.C. 20037
Phone: (202) 293-5137

MISCARRIAGE

Also called spontaneous abortion, *an early miscarriage typically is signaled by abdominal cramps, vaginal bleeding, and, at times, passing of clots and bits of tissue.*

The developing fetus is most vulnerable to miscarriage during the first trimester. Three fourths of all miscarriages occur in the first trimester, usually between the ninth and eleventh weeks of gestation. More often than not, a miscarriage is the body's natural reaction to an embryo that is not—for a wide variety of reasons—viable. Approximately half of all fertilized eggs abort spontaneously—most of these before a woman knows that she is pregnant.

In the large majority of first-trimester miscarriages, the embryo or fetus has died before it is spontaneously aborted. In an estimated 60 percent of these, a chromosomal or developmental abnormality is apparent. Other miscarriages at this point may be due to chronic infections or uterine defects.

Understanding the Problem. Usually vaginal bleeding is the first warning that a miscarriage may be happening. Often, the bleeding is accompanied by cramping. It's important to note, however, that vaginal bleeding does not always mean miscarriage. Almost 20 percent of all pregnant women have some bloody discharge during the first trimester, and miscarriage happens in fewer than half these cases. If you do experience bleeding at any point in your pregnancy, call your health-care professional.

When an embryo or fetus dies, miscarriage is inevitable. Usually a woman will feel cramps in her lower abdomen or back. The pain may be dull and relentless or acute and intermittent. Bleeding will be heavy and the fetus and placenta may be expelled. If it is possible, collect this clotlike material so that your clinician can examine it for cause of death. If fetal material is only partially expelled, in what is called an *incomplete abortion*, pain and bleeding can continue for days. If the fetus has died but has not been expelled, this is called a *missed abortion*. Often when this happens, a woman experiences no pain or bleeding, but all the symptoms of pregnancy dissipate.

Treatment Options. Usually the pregnancy tissue will be expelled, but sometimes a health-care professional will recommend dilation and curettage (D & C) (see *Dilation and Curettage,* page 539) or vacuum suction to remove from the uterus any remnants of the pregnancy after a miscarriage. It is not necessary to wait before trying to conceive again, although some couples do not feel emotionally prepared to start over right away.

As most obstetrics practitioners will tell worried women, a pregnancy goes well until it stops going well. Very little can be done to avert a miscarriage. And it does no good at all for a woman to blame herself.

ECTOPIC PREGNANCY

Symptoms of ectopic pregnancy, which usually appear in the early weeks of pregnancy, include cramps and pain in the lower abdomen, typically beginning on one side and radiating out; brown vaginal spotting or scant bleeding; nausea and vomiting; dizziness; shoulder pain; rectal pressure; or general weakness.

Ectopic pregnancy, or tubal pregnancy, results in early pregnancy when the fertilized egg implants outside the uterus, sometimes in the ovary or abdominal cavity, but most of the time in the fallopian tubes. Many ectopic pregnancies are diagnosed before a woman knows she is pregnant and most are discovered by the eighth week of pregnancy.

There are a number of factors that predispose a woman toward tubal implantation, including incomplete or reversed tubal ligation (sterilization surgery), scarring from pelvic inflammatory disease or surgery, and previous ectopic pregnancies.

Understanding the Problem. Ectopic pregnancies occur in about one of every hundred pregnancies. If an ectopic pregnancy continues, the tube can burst. When this happens, usually between the eighth and twelfth weeks, symptoms can be quite severe. A woman who has any of the symptoms—which include vaginal bleeding, pain in the lower abdomen, weakness, and fainting—should call her doctor immediately.

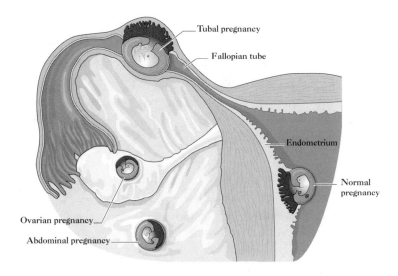

Normal pregnancies occur when the embryo is embedded in the lining of the uterus, the endometrium. *When the fertilized egg implants elsewhere, it's called an ectopic pregnancy.*

Before the tube ruptures, however, signs of an ectopic pregnancy are negligible. An ultrasound (see page 290) or laparoscopy (see page 554) can confirm the existence of an ectopic pregnancy.

Treatment Options. In the event of an ectopic pregnancy, quick medical attention is necessary to save a woman's fallopian tubes and fertility. Surgery or medication therapy will be offered. If the tube has not ruptured, the embryo and placenta can be removed from the tube. Sometimes the affected fallopian tube can be rebuilt; at other times, it has to be removed. When rupture leads to hemorrhaging, a blood transfusion may be necessary and blood vessels may need to be clamped off.

The chance of being able to conceive again after a tubal pregnancy is 50 percent. Subsequent pregnancies have a good chance of progressing normally, although there is a higher risk for another ectopic pregnancy in women who have had one than in those who have not.

HYDATIDIFORM MOLE

As this cyst develops around an embryo, the uterus expands rapidly, and a woman may experience vaginal bleeding, nausea and vomiting, and high blood pressure. She may pass bloody grapelike tissue.

In rare cases, a benign growth develops from the tissue surrounding the fertilized egg. When this hydatidiform mole forms instead of the placenta, the embryo rarely develops. A woman will then experience vaginal bleeding, severe nausea, and vomiting, and she may expel bloody grapelike tissue. It is important that a woman who experiences these symptoms contact her health-care provider. The tumor will have to be removed.

Hydatidiform moles develop in about one in two thousand gestations. This condition becomes a medical concern not only because it results in an aborted pregnancy, but also because the tumor can become large and potentially dangerous.

Eighty percent of the tumors are benign. If left untreated 15 percent will develop into invasive moles, which embed deeply into the uterine wall, causing hemorrhaging and other serious problems. In 2 to 3 percent of cases, hydatidiform moles precede a choriocarcinoma, a fast-growing, fast-spreading malignancy.

Understanding the Problem. If a woman's symptoms point to the existence of a hydatidiform mole, her clinician will order ultrasonography (see page 290). A urine or blood test will also be ordered to measure levels of human chorionic gonadotropin, a hormone produced by such moles.

Treatment Options. A hydatidiform mole usually is removed by suction in a procedure similar to a D & C (see page 539). Afterward, follow-up analysis of human chorionic gonadotropin levels yields indications of recovery. If hormonal levels do not return to normal, this may indicate an invasive mole or a choriocarcinoma. Chemotherapy is the treatment of choice for both these conditions. In rare cases, though, some health professionals may recommend a hysterectomy, a procedure in which the uterus is surgically removed. Nevertheless, the prognosis for a full recovery is excellent. For a choriocarcinoma, complete cure rate is 85 percent.

ABNORMAL BLEEDING

Many women experience bleeding or bloody discharge at some point in their pregnancies, and most women experience considerable anxiety at the appearance of blood. In most cases, though, a bit of bleeding is not an indication of trouble. In some cases, however, it is. So if you notice vaginal bleeding during your pregnancy, you should notify your health-care professional immediately.

During the first days of pregnancy as the egg is implanting into the uterine wall, there may be some spotting. However, in the first trimester, when most miscarriages happen, bleeding may indicate that a spontaneous abortion is about to occur.

After the twentieth week of pregnancy, bleeding may signal a number of problems, including placenta previa (see page 302), miscarriage (see page 285), or the onset of premature labor (see page 299). Any severe hemorrhaging poses a threat to mother and baby.

After the first months of pregnancy, if you begin to bleed, contact your clinician. He or she may recommend ultrasonography (see page 290) to determine the cause of the bleeding. You may also require hospitalization or bed rest.

FOLIC ACID AND NEURAL TUBE DEFECTS

Folic acid is a nutrient found in leafy vegetables. Essential in early pregnancy for synthesizing deoxyribonucleic acid (DNA), folic acid aids in fetal blood and cell formation. Recent studies show that sufficient amounts of the nutrient ingested through diet and vitamin supplements can reduce by 70 percent the incidence of spina bifida. This congenital defect in the walls of the neural tube usually manifests in an open spinal chord.

Women who have folic acid deficiencies tend to be anemic. Maternal vitamins include folic acid so that regardless of a woman's supply, she will receive the amount necessary to promote fetal health

Because the neural tube closes only twenty-eight days after fertilization, women may not have a chance to start vitamin supplements if they wait for a diagnosis of pregnancy. It is recommended that all women who are sexually active and who are not using contraception consume adequate folic acid, either in the diet or by supplements, even if they do not know they are pregnant.

PRENATAL TESTING, MONITORING, AND OTHER PROCEDURES

Just a generation ago, women had to wait out the entire nine months before they knew whether their baby was a boy or a girl, had fair or dark skin—or had ten fingers and ten toes. However exciting it was to anticipate what the child would be like, there also was usually an undercurrent of apprehension: Will my baby be okay? *Today, questions about the baby's health—as well as about his or her gender—can be answered early in the pregnancy thanks to a range of prenatal tests and procedures.*

For 95 percent of all women who undergo prenatal diagnostic procedures, there are no apparent fetal abnormalities. For the rest, early discovery of a problem, though certainly upsetting, offers time to make critical choices. As a result of prenatal testing, some women choose therapeutic abortions. Others choose to continue the pregnancy while making adjustments to their expectations and life-style to accommodate a child with special needs. In a few cases, with diagnostic information in hand, they may have the option of prenatal treatment, as in the case of fetal surgery to drain an obstructed bladder or fetal blood transfusion to treat Rh disease (see page 301).

Here are the most commonly used methods of prenatal diagnosis:

• Chorionic villus sampling (CVS), *usually performed between the sixth and eighth weeks of gestation, involves the removal of a small piece of the placenta for analysis. In addition to determining the gender of the fetus, this analysis can detect such genetic abnormalities as Down's syndrome.*

The test itself can be a bit uncomfortable but is rarely painful. Using ultrasound, the clinician inserts a catheter into a woman's cervix to suction out placental tissue. Though certainly safe in the majority of instances, CVS has been linked to a slightly higher risk for miscarriage than amniocentesis (below). Also, CVS may, in rare cases, trigger uterine infection.

 • Ultrasound *uses high-frequency sound waves to produce a computerized image on a video screen. Through this technology, it is possible to visualize an embryo as early as six or seven weeks after a period has been missed. This noninvasive, painless diagnostic tool has become all but commonplace in prenatal care. It is recommended when a woman has had earlier tubal (ectopic) pregnancies, a hydatidiform mole (see page 287), or a baby with genetic defects or disorders. It can be used to determine causes of spotting and bleeding, to verify due date, and to detect the existence of multiple fetuses. It allows close monitoring of fetal growth, development, and positioning. Fetal brain and organs can be examined for abnormalities and defects.*

While the mother lies on her back, her abdomen is covered with a gel that conducts sound. Then a transducer is moved over her belly, recording echoes as the sound waves bounce off the baby. Ultrasound therefore can provide one of the more exciting moments of early pregnancy—the moment when it is transformed from a cluster of vague symptoms to the realization that there's a baby in there. A mother can actually see on the screen her baby—its tiny head, hands, heart, and sometimes its genitals. She may even walk away with a computerized picture to show all her friends.

 • Amniocentesis *is a technique usually performed between the fifteenth and eighteenth weeks of pregnancy that provides a reliable measure of fetal chromosome abnormalities. In this procedure, a small amount of fluid that surrounds the fetus (amniotic fluid) is removed for examination. This test can diagnose such conditions as genetic defects and neurological, kidney, and metabolic problems. Gender can also be determined from this test.*

During this outpatient procedure, a woman's abdomen may be anesthetized with local anesthetic. Then, guided past the fetus by ultrasonography, the clinician inserts a long, hollow needle into the uterus and draws a sample of amniotic fluid which contains fetal cells. These cells are then cultured and analyzed in a lab. Most women experience only mild discomfort during the procedure. On rare occasions, a woman will have some vaginal bleeding or fluid leakage. Fewer than one in two hundred women experiences more serious complications—miscarriage or infection—after amniocentesis.

Amniocentesis is indicated by a number of factors. It is routinely recommended for women who have reason to suspect genetic defects such as Down's syndrome. Women who have already given birth to a child with genetic defects and women who carry the gene for such disorders as hemophilia are also advised to consider amniocentesis, as are couples who may carry the genes for such congenital disorders as Tay-Sachs disease or sickle-cell anemia. Amniocentesis is also used to assess the maturity of fetal lungs when early delivery is being considered. In these cases, as in many others, the benefits of reliable diagnosis usually outweigh the risk of complication.

• Maternal triple screen testing *uses blood analysis to detect an increased risk of neural tube defects and chromosomal abnormalities. Often recommended as a matter of course in all pregnancies, this noninvasive blood test carries no risk to mother or child and is usually performed around the sixteenth week of gestation.*

Specifically, this test measures levels of alpha-fetoprotein (AFP), human chorionic gonatropin (hCG), and estriol. AFP, hCG, and estriol levels can be used to calculate the risk of chromosomal defects such as Down's syndrome. If the risk appears high enough, amniocentesis can be used to make an accurate diagnosis. Elevated levels of AFP may leak into the mother's blood, indicating such fetal neurological defects as spina bifida (open spine) or anencephalus (absence of part of the brain). Because false-positive results are common, when analysis registers an elevated reading, the test will be repeated and other explanations will be sought. If, for example, the gestational stage is more advanced (the fetus is older) or there are multiple fetuses (twins, for example), AFP levels will be high. Roughly fifty women out of a thousand tested will have high (positive) readings. In most cases, the second screening comes back with a negative finding. When the second test result is positive, an ultrasound typically follows to view the fetus. Should the ultrasound fail to discover any defect, an amniocentesis will be recommended. Of the fifty women who originally receive a positive reading, only one or two turn out to have affected fetuses.

• Percutaneous umbilical cord sampling, *most often done in the third trimester, takes fetal blood from the umbilical cord for measurements or testing for genetic conditions. The clinician will insert a needle through the abdomen and uterus to the umbilical vein. Results often are available within hours or a few days.*

• Fetoscopy *uses a small telescopelike device that is inserted through a large needle into the amniotic cavity to view and photograph the fetus. It also gathers tissue and blood samples for analysis in diagnosing blood disease and certain skin disorders.*

Performed after the sixteenth week, fetoscopy carries higher risk to the pregnancy than many other procedures. There is a 3 to 5 percent chance of fetal loss with this technique.

In addition to these high-technology, high-profile tests, there are a number of routine analyses that are done, often without the woman's awareness, during regular prenatal visits. After perhaps the first visit, once pregnancy has been confirmed the clinician will order an early blood workup. Typically this early blood work will provide a reading on conditions that could affect the pregnancy including an Rh profile (see page 301) and indicating the presence of sexually transmitted diseases (see page 440) and anemia (see page 276).

IDENTIFIABLE ABNORMALITIES

Parents-to-be often wonder about the color of a child's eyes, the hue of their baby's skin, or the temperament of the child. They wonder whether the child is a girl or a boy and whether the baby will be born healthy or will meet life with a birth defect or chromosomal disorder.

The answers to these questions lie in the intricate, and in many ways mysterious, interplay of genetic material—the biological basis of heredity. At conception the mother's egg and the father's sperm each bring twenty-three chromosomes; the union produces a fertilized egg with forty-six chromosomes. The way in which these chromosomes interact, along with the genetic material they carry, determine the kind of person who emerges, not only in terms of appearance, and, in large part, temperament, but also in regard to basic health.

Occasionally, such environmental agents as radiation, viruses, and chemicals cause genetic defects. At other times, genetic disorders are passed on from one or both parents. For example, *Tay-Sachs* disease is an inherited disease that results from the deficiency of an enzyme (hexosaminidase A). The disorder affects the function of the nervous system. Infants born with Tay-Sachs disease appear normal, but as the disease progresses, development slows. Mental and physical retardation, blindness, spasticity, convulsions, and other disorders of the nervous system follow. Few children with this disease live past the age of four.

Tay-Sachs disease is transmitted when both parents pass on the gene. It is found most commonly in the children of Jewish couples whose families come from Eastern Europe and in French Canadians. Blood tests can determine whether a couple is at risk for producing an infant who has Tay-Sachs disease. Amniocentesis can also determine in utero whether the fetus is affected (see *Prenatal Testing, Monitoring, and Other Procedures*, page 289).

Sickle-cell anemia is also transmitted when both parents are carriers of the gene. It occurs in about one in five hundred African Americans. It is also prevalent in Mediterranean populations. Symptoms, which may be apparent in childhood or may develop later in early adulthood, include jaundice, poor physical development, abdominal pain, lowered resistance to infections, swelling and pain in joints and muscles. Pregnancy can exacerbate symptoms: A pregnant woman with sickle-cell anemia may find that circulatory problems and fatigue become worse. She is also at higher risk for miscarriage.

Thalassemia is a group of hereditary anemias occurring with greatest frequency in Asian and Mediterranean populations. The severity of the disease varies, but it can be fatal. It usually appears in childhood. Symptoms include facial features resembling those of the Down's syndrome child, severe fatigue, and heart enlargement.

Other conditions that are passed on genetically by both parents include *cystic fibrosis*, characterized by chronic respiratory infection and pancreatic insufficiency; *phenylketonuria*, caused by a failure to metabolize an amino acid, which, if untreated, can result in brain damage and retardation; and *color blindness*, characterized by an absence or defect in the perception of color.

Hemophilia, a blood disorder in which a failure to clot causes excessive and often dangerous bleeding, is passed on by a single gene from the mother to the son. *Huntington's chorea*, an inherited disease of the nervous system, is passed on from the affected parent.

Chromosomal abnormalities, such as *Down's syndrome*, arise from the lack, excess, or abnormal arrangement of one or more chromosomes. Birth defects caused by genetic disorders occur in about one in 250 newborns. Moreover, over half of early miscarriages are due to chromosomal abnormalities.

Other disorders or defects seem to stem from the interaction of a congenital predisposition with environmental factors. Environmental factors that act on genetic vulnerability include drugs or alcohol taken during pregnancy, smoking, and such chronic maternal diseases as diabetes. Other factors are not so easily identifiable. Conditions such as hypertension, coronary heart disease, schizophrenia, cleft palate, and spina bifida seem to be linked with the interplay of environmental and genetic factors.

When a couple consults a genetic counselor, the counselor will determine the odds of bearing a healthy child, which are based on a trained analysis of family history, blood test results, and the couple's current health. The best time to see a genetic counselor is *before* conceiving. Then, if tests reveal a high likelihood of passing on a genetic defect or disorder to future children, the genetic counselor can help the couple make informed choices. Even after the pregnancy is confirmed, a genetic counselor can guide the parents, should the tests uncover a serious defect, through the complicated and often painful options of terminating the pregnancy or having a special needs child.

THE SECOND TRIMESTER

For Claudia, the fourth, fifth, and sixth months of her pregnancy were the best. Feelings of nausea and fatigue had all but disappeared. She was no longer so worried about miscarriage and felt enough confidence to begin telling family and friends.

She could look into the mirror and see a little bulge around her middle. She began to buy maternity clothes. People all around her began to notice and pay attention to her pregnancy—sometimes offering excited congratulations, sometimes unwanted advice. But best of all the baby started to move about, making his presence known. The reality of Claudia's pregnancy was beginning to take shape for her.

Claudia's experience in the second trimester is not uncommon. For many women, this is the best part of their pregnancy. In most cases, the pregnancy is moving forward in a relatively uneventful, unintrusive way.

By the end of the fourth month, the fetus is about four inches long. Such reflexes as sucking and swallowing have developed. Tooth buds appear. By the end of the fifth month, the fetus is about ten inches long and strong enough to make its presence known. Hair begins to grow on its head, and eyebrows and eyelashes appear. At the end of the second trimester, the fetus is around thirteen inches long and weighs around two pounds. Eyelids begin to part and eyes are wide open. If born now, most fetuses can survive outside the womb with special neonatal care.

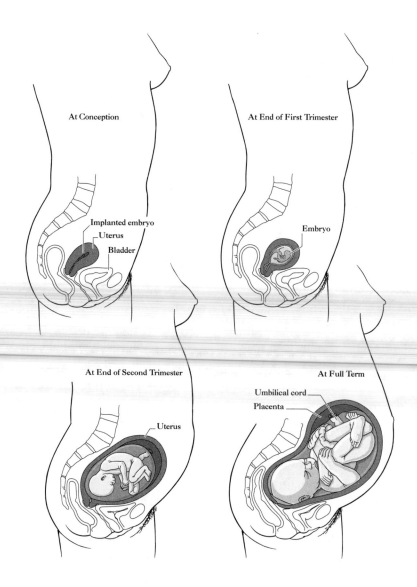

During pregnancy, the female body experiences changes in overall shape and organ position and size. As the fetus develops, it requires more and more space, distending the abdomen.

Unless there is a medical reason for more frequent visits, a woman continues to see her doctor once a month. The clinician will continue to monitor blood pressure and sugar level, protein level in the urine samples, fetal heartbeat, size and shape of the uterus, height of the top of the uterus (fundus), and signs of water retention (edema). He or she will also note the amount and rate of maternal weight gain. The average woman should gain approximately three to four pounds during the first trimester. In the second trimester, a healthy weight gain is around twelve to fourteen pounds. In the last trimester, the standard is eight to ten pounds: about one pound a week in the seventh and eighth months, and only one to two pounds total in the ninth month. But more important than the numbers is the rate at which a woman gains—a steady weight gain without sudden jumps or drops is best.

LATE MISCARRIAGE

Midtrimester miscarriages are often signaled by pink or brown vaginal bleeding over an extended period. There may also be vague labor-related symptoms including cramping and abdominal pressure.

Miscarriages are rare past the third month of pregnancy, but occasionally a fetus is lost between the twelfth and twenty-fourth weeks. Late miscarriages account for less than a fourth of all spontaneous abortions.

The popular notion is that miscarriages at this stage are caused by sudden physical trauma, but in fact, accidents account for very few miscarriages. Whereas miscarriages in the first trimester usually involve fetal health and viability, those in the second trimester most often involve aspects of maternal health. Problems such as serious infection, uterine tumors, a misshaped uterus, or an incompetent cervix that opens prematurely (see page 302) all seem to contribute to late miscarriage. In many of these situations, the threat to pregnancy can be addressed through prompt and appropriate medical care.

A midtrimester miscarriage may be signaled by scant brown discharge for a period of weeks or pink bloody spotting over a few days. It's important that once a pregnant woman notices vaginal bleeding or discharge she contact her medical practitioner. If the cervix has begun to dilate, the clinician may speculate that the cervix is weak (see *Incompetent Cervix*, page 302) and suture it closed until the pregancy is closer to a viable delivery date. This procedure, which works to prevent miscarriage, is called *cerclage*.

If incompetent cervix is ruled out, the clinician will likely advise, "Watch and rest." If, after a few days of bed rest, the bleeding stops, it was probably not related to miscarriage. If bleeding becomes heavier and is accompanied by cramping, a miscarriage may be inevitable. Often, hospitalization is recommended to control hemorrhaging. If cramping and bleeding do not stop once the fetus is expelled, in all likelihood, the miscarriage was incomplete. Then a D & C (see page 539) may be necessary to evacuate the uterus.

Ordinarily, medical practitioners try to determine the cause of late miscarriage in order to avert future miscarriages. If an incompetent cervix is suspected, cerclage early in subsequent pregnancies can prevent repeat miscarriages. Tumors and some abnormalities in uterine structure can be corrected surgically.

Delivery after the twenty-fourth week is considered premature birth rather than miscarriage because survival outside the womb is possible.

TWINS AND MULTIPLE BIRTHS

There is not a woman who, while contemplating her largeness in pregnancy, wonders what it would be like to carry twins—or, on those days when the baby seems particularly active, whether in fact there isn't a dialogue going on in there. For women who have a family history of fraternal twins, women who have already had a pair of twins, and women who have taken fertility drugs, the possibility of giving birth to and raising twins is not just a matter of whimsical thinking.

Twins occur either when more than one egg is fertilized, producing fraternal twins, or when one egg splits after fertilization, producing identical twins.

Twins are the most common form of multiple births. One in every ninety births in America involves twins. One in every eight thousand involves triplets, although the rate is higher with fertility treatments. In most cases, the multiple pregnancy is discovered before labor. It is usually signaled by unusual weight gain or size, or the sound of more than one heart. An ultrasound will confirm the suspicion.

Because carrying and delivering more than one fetus pose increased risks, prenatal care and special consideration of pregnancy-related habits—rest, nutrition, and exercise, for example—are especially important for women who expect twins. There is a higher incidence of toxemia (see page 303) in pregnancies involving more than one fetus. In addition, there is a greater likelihood of premature labor.

On the average, multiple pregnancies tend to be around twenty-one days shorter than single pregnancies. As with all premature deliveries, there is a greater chance of neonatal complications. The mortality risk for twins is four times greater than for single births—usually because twins are premature. Unless there is a medical indication for cesarean, twins are commonly delivered vaginally. In vaginal births, unusual presentations are not uncommon (one baby can be positioned head first, or cephalic, and the other rear first, or breech), although the head-first position for both babies is the most common presentation.

THE THIRD TRIMESTER

Karen can count the weeks until her due date on her fingers. Even her maternity clothes are getting tight. Walking resembles waddling. Her skin is stretched and itchy. The idea of bending over to tie her shoes exhausts her. Her ankles are swollen, and her insides feel squished.

She can't get comfortable in bed at night. When she does fall asleep, she wakes up a couple of hours later to urinate and then can't fall back to sleep. She feels fat and cranky. She can't believe a baby's coming—but the baby's coming, and soon.

Accordingly, Karen and her husband have started buying things for the nursery. They are going to childbirth classes, where they've met other couples who are expecting around the same time. Their social circle has begun to expand to include their new role as parents.

Karen has begun to imagine what labor will be like. Is it really as painful as she's heard? Should she ask for medication or will that hurt the baby and deprive her of the full experience? Will she be able to nurse?

And what about handling the demands of motherhood?

Karen is relieved to have gotten this far in her pregnancy. There's no need to worry about miscarriage now. Even if something should happen, her baby could be delivered and in all likelihood survive and be healthy. All she has to worry about, if she were so inclined, is labor, delivery—and motherhood.

For many women, all the experiences of pregnancy—both physical and emotional—reach a crescendo in the final months. Discomfort, anxiety, anticipation, excitement, and ambivalence intensify and become more focused. Prenatal visits become more frequent. After the thirtieth week, most women see their clinician every two weeks, and every week after the thirty-sixth week. Around the thirty-eighth week, the visit will include an internal examination to check for cervical effacement and dilatation.

By the end of the seventh month, the three-pound fetus can suck its thumb, hiccup, cry, taste sweet and sour, and respond to light, sound, and pain. A woman's uterus becomes very large and quite hard to the touch, and a woman can feel and see as the fetus flips over. There are other times when it's clear that the baby is asleep. As the fetus begins to descend toward the birth canal, activity seems to diminish.

By the end of the eighth month, the fetus weighs around five pounds and is about eighteen inches long. Birth can take place safely any time around the end of the ninth month. The average baby will be twenty inches and seven and a half pounds at term.

CHILDBIRTH CLASSES

There is much to be said for childbirth education classes, not least of which is that they provide an excellent opportunity for pregnant women to meet other pregnant women. In addition, most classes encourage involvement of a woman's partner, affording a chance for couples to develop greater intimacy and openness around the experience of childbirth as well as forging a productive relationship between laboring mother and coach.

By offering clear, accurate information, most childbirth classes work to reduce anxiety about delivery, improve a woman's ability to cope with pain, and encourage a woman's (and a partner's) involvement in the decisions made during the course of labor and delivery. Most teach specific techniques for relaxation, distraction, muscle control, and respiratory activity in order to increase participation and control during the process of childbirth. In addition, many offer nutritional counseling. Most provide an excellent arena for sharing experiences and airing concerns.

Unfortunately, the advent of childbirth education may have led to the idea that labor and delivery are events for which a couple must take lessons. Some women experience considerable anxiety that they will make mistakes along the way. The fact is that regardless of how well or ill prepared you are, things almost always go just fine.

The benefits of a childbirth class depend largely on the match between the woman's attitudes and values and those of the teacher. In general, some classes work better than others, and some women work better in groups than others. However, by including the partner in the process, and by teaching coping skills that decrease a woman's perception of and increase her tolerance for pain, and that manage stress before and during labor, these classes have moved childbirth away from the old-fashioned model—the mother anesthetized to unconsciousness and the father pacing the waiting room outside. Today, a mother is much more likely to be awake and participating with her partner throughout the childbirth experience.

Ask your medical practitioner to recommend classes or teachers on the basis of his or her knowledge of your feelings, values, and inclinations. In some communities, there may not be many choices. Larger communities may offer a wider range of options. Some classes are offered through hospitals. Others are offered privately by nurses, midwives, physicians, or childbirth educators. In general, smaller classes are better as teachers can give more individualized attention, and camaraderie can develop more naturally in a group of, for example, six or fewer couples.

Although in recent years childbirth preparation classes have begun to be offered all over the map, especially in larger communities, there are three major philosophies at the root of most.

- *Lamaze has become synonymous with childbirth preparation. This popular natural childbirth (psychoprophylactic) method was developed in the 1950s by the French obstetrician Fernand Lamaze. Relying heavily on the involvement of a labor coach (usually the father of the baby), this approach teaches disciplined ways of breathing, focusing, and relaxing during labor and birth. Lamaze works to prepare women so that they can anticipate the full experience of childbirth and use relaxation techniques to combat pain. It also works to condition women to work with labor contractions instead of against them to facilitate each contraction's efficiency.*

- *Grantly Dick-Read, a British obstetrician, pioneered in 1914 the concept of childbirth as a natural process rather than as a medical condition. His psychophysical approach combines relaxation techniques and prenatal education to break the fear–tension–pain cycle of labor and delivery. Women are taught to assume an attitude of passivity and acceptance toward childbirth; in that way, the Dick-Read method resembles yoga. Moreover, women are encouraged to maintain close communication with the obstetrics staff during labor.*

- *The Bradley approach evolved out of a concept of husband-coached natural childbirth. It emphasizes good diet and exercise to ease the discomfort of pregnancy and to prepare the muscles for birth and breast-feeding. It rejects the use of drugs during childbirth. Women learn to breathe deeply and slowly as if they were asleep and to concentrate on the work of their body as they are laboring. Many Bradley-based classes begin as soon as pregnancy is confirmed in order to take advantage of the full nine months to prepare a woman for childbirth. Because Bradley emphasizes nonmedicated participation during childbirth, this method has been embraced for home births and by many birth centers.*

Preterm Labor: Signs and Symptoms

There are a number of signs that announce the possibility of preterm labor. If you experience any of these, contact your practitioner immediately:

Rupture of the membranes*: The key symptom is a leak or even a gush of vaginal fluid.*

Bloody show*: A vaginal discharge that appears streaked with pink or brown blood.*

Contraction*: A rhythmic hardening of the uterus, sometimes with menstrual-like cramps.*

A baby is considered preterm if delivery takes place before the thirty-seventh week of gestation. Most preterm deliveries occur in high-risk pregnancies. Women living in poverty are at greater risk for preterm deliveries (thirteen out of one hundred); the explanation is likely such factors as poor diet and insufficient prenatal care.

Understanding the Problem. Factors responsible for preterm labor that can and should be eliminated early in the pregnancy include smoking, drug abuse, insufficient nutrition, and poor medical care. Other factors are not so easily eliminated, but their effects can be tempered: uterine malformations, urinary tract and vaginal infections, venereal disease (see page 440), placenta previa (the placenta is implanted over the cervix, see page 302), and a history of premature deliveries.

Every day that a baby remains in the uterus before term increases the chances that he or she will be born alive and healthy. Except in the event that the mother and/or child is endangered, such as when the placenta prematurely separates from the uterus (abruptio placentae), every effort will be made to delay preterm childbirth.

It is possible to have any or all of these symptoms and still not be in premature labor. However, only your health-care clinician can say for sure. If he or she suspects that labor is beginning, there are a number of steps to postpone or prevent the onset.

Treatment Options. Initially, you may be advised to limit your sexual activity and to stay in bed. In the face of some symptoms (for example, if the membranes have ruptured), your doctor will admit you to the hospital, where every step will be taken to delay active labor. Medications may be administered to relax the uterine muscles and halt contractions. These medications include betamimetics and magnesium sulfate. Other medications such as betamethasone may be given to prompt the development of fetal lungs for survival outside the uterus.

If, despite all efforts, labor proceeds and the baby is born prematurely, the chances that the baby will be healthy and normal depend on the degree of prematurity. Most hospitals now have fully equipped neonatology units capable of providing the most sophisticated care to even the smallest of newborns.

Braxton Hicks Contractions

Throughout pregnancy, many women notice uterine contractions that may cause them considerable anxiety and, toward the end of the term, discomfort. These are called *Braxton Hicks contractions.*

As childbirth approaches, a woman may feel her uterus hardening. In this way, the uterus begins to prepare for actual labor, when the muscles of the uterus contract to dilate the cervix. Unlike real labor, Braxton Hicks contractions do not occur at regular intervals, nor do they increase in frequency and intensity. Typically, there is a tightening that begins in the upper uterus and spreads down. Braxton Hicks contractions usually last between thirty seconds and two minutes.

Braxton Hicks contractions will subside if you change your position or walk around. In most cases, when the "real thing" comes along, a woman knows it—even though for months she may have been worried that she won't. Nevertheless, if you suspect you are in labor, call your health practitioner. He or she can determine whether the cervix is beginning to dilate.

PROLONGED PREGNANCIES
Will this pregnancy ever end?

That is a common lament among women in the last weeks of pregnancy. However, some pregnancies do stretch beyond forty-two weeks and become more than just an inconvenience.

When pregnancies go beyond forty-two weeks, the condition is called *postmaturity* or *postterm pregnancy* and is a cause for medical concern. Like prematurity, postmaturity can be dangerous to the child. In cases in which the baby continues to grow, it will have more difficulty in passing through the pelvic channel. In cases in which the placenta has aged to the point that it fails to provide sufficient nutrition, the fetus will stop thriving. The baby may lose weight and, in very rare cases, begin to starve.

Most clinicians make a thorough evaluation of the course of the pregnancy around the fortieth week. Some postmature pregnancies are actually normal-term pregnancies, the gestational age of which have been miscalculated. Therefore, the original due date will be checked against other dating techniques such as ultrasound. Then the practitioner likely will run tests to monitor placental function (see *Tests in Preparation for Childbirth*, below). If it appears that the fetus continues to thrive in the womb, the clinician will probably let the pregnancy progress a bit longer. Fetal health tests may be run again in a couple of weeks. If there is any indication, however, that the fetus is not thriving or that there is placental insufficiency, the health-care practitioner will induce labor. Sometimes clinicians offer induction in place of doing testing.

TESTS IN PREPARATION FOR CHILDBIRTH

There are a number of tests that are performed in the latter part of pregnancy and in postterm pregnancies to determine fetal position and to estimate fetal condition in anticipation of childbirth.

Ultrasonography is often recommended during the latter part of pregnancy to measure fetal growth and position, to locate the position of the placenta, and to determine the amount of amniotic fluid around the baby. This noninvasive procedure uses high-frequency sound waves to compose a computerized image of the fetus in utero. In the event of growth retardation and placenta previa (see page 302), ultrasonography can uncover the problem before severe damage is done.

Electronic fetal nonstress tests gauge fetal heart rate to assess placental transfer of oxygen. Lying on her side, the pregnant woman wears an electronic monitor around her abdomen, and fetal heart rate, movements, and uterine contractions are measured.

In the last few weeks of pregnancy, many practitioners conduct a *biophysical profile*, an assessment process which looks at five aspects of fetal physiological features: heart acceleration rate, fetal breathing, movement, tone, and amniotic fluid volume. These indicators are measured through ultrasonography and with a device to record fetal heart rate. These findings constitute another estimate of placental adequacy.

RH INCOMPATIBILITY

The question of blood compatibility between mother and fetus is posed early in pregnancy. Among other information, early blood tests determine a woman's Rh factor, that is, the existence of certain proteins on the surface of the blood cell. If tests reveal that a woman has the dominant Rh-factor, and is therefore Rh-positive, or if both she and her husband are Rh-negative, and therefore the fetus will also lack the factor, there is no concern. If on the other hand, the baby is Rh-positive and the mother is Rh-negative, there is a risk, especially in second and successive pregnancies, that in the mother antibodies will develop to combat the baby's blood. Accordingly, when a woman is Rh-negative and her husband Rh-positive, the pregnancy is potentially at risk.

Rh factor does not usually present a problem in first pregnancies. The Rh factor enters into the mother's circulatory system only during delivery, abortion, or miscarriage of a child who has inherited the positive factor from the father. In an immunological reaction to the foreign substance, antibodies then develop in the mother. In subsequent pregnancies, these antibodies can cross the placenta into the fetal system. If that child is Rh-positive, the antibodies will attack fetal red blood cells, causing anemia that can range from mild to severe.

Although there is not a high risk of Rh-related problems in first pregnancies, in rare cases, fetal blood leaks through the placenta into the mother's circulatory system during first pregnancies, stimulating production of antibodies.

At around the twenty-eighth week, an Rh-negative mother who shows no antibodies in her blood is given a shot of Rh-immune globulin. This should prevent sensitization to any leakage of fetal blood. Another dose is administered within seventy-two hours of delivery, abortion, or miscarriage. If the woman shows that she has Rh antibodies, an amniocentesis (see page 290) is ordered to assess fetal blood breakdown.

Severe anemia that results from Rh incompatibility is usually treated by replacing the fetus's Rh-positive with Rh-negative blood. Occasionally, fetal transfusion can take place in utero. If the fetus is not severely affected, the transfusion can wait until after delivery.

INCOMPETENT CERVIX

The term *incompetent cervix* describes a condition in which the aperture at the lower part of the uterus is weak and likely to open prematurely. Often, an incompetent cervix is responsible for second-trimester miscarriages.

Understanding the Problem. Women who have structural defects as a result of exposure to DES (the synthetic estrogen used in previous generations in an attempt to prevent miscarriage; see *DES-Related Disorders*, page 526) and women who have undergone a number of D & C procedures (see *Dilation and Curettage*, page 539) seem to have a higher incidence of weak cervix.

Treatment Options. If a woman has a medical history that points to this condition, a surgical procedure called cerclage can be done to keep the cervix closed during pregnancy. Successful approximately 90 percent of the time, cerclage is typically performed after the first trimester and under general or epidural (spinal) anesthetic. It involves stitching around the cervix with strong thread to prevent it from opening. In the ninth month, the thread is cut, allowing for normal delivery.

PLACENTA PREVIA

The key symptom of placenta previa is painless bleeding from the vagina. The bleeding may be slight, though it can be severe.

In normal pregnancies, the placenta, the organ that nourishes the embryo, implants high in the uterus. In cases of placenta previa, it implants in the lower uterine segment, often covering the cervix partially or completely.

Understanding the Problem. The risk of this condition arises in the seventh through ninth months of pregnancy as the uterus prepares for labor. As the cervix opens, the placenta can be torn loose. When this happens, a woman can experience painless bleeding from the vagina. The bleeding is sometimes mild, though it can be severe. Sometimes the bleeding will stop on its own.

Placenta previa occurs in approximately one of two hundred pregnancies that go beyond the seventh month. The chance of its happening increases with each subsequent pregnancy. Women who have delivered babies by cesarean section and older mothers are at higher risk of this complication.

An ultrasound will confirm placenta previa. When placenta previa exists, sexual activities may be restricted so as not to dislodge the placenta. In addition, complete bed rest may be advised to forestall premature labor.

Treatment Options. If the placenta covers the opening only partially and hasn't begun to separate from the uterine wall, vaginal delivery may be attempted with the help of fetal monitoring. When the placenta completely covers the cervical opening, cesarean delivery is necessary. If a woman's due date is near and detachment of the placenta has begun, a cesarean section may be recommended by her doctor in order to prevent bleeding. In rare cases, severe bleeding can cause fetal death. Occasionally, a woman must undergo a blood transfusion.

PREECLAMPSIA AND ECLAMPSIA

Preeclampsia is characterized by high blood pressure, swelling, and protein in the urine. As the disease progresses, a woman may experience abdominal pain, convulsions, and unconsciousness; the latter two qualify the problem as eclampsia. Preeclampsia and eclampsia when present together are sometimes called toxemia.

No one knows exactly why some women experience preeclampsia, a serious condition that if left untreated will develop into eclampsia, a disease that can pose a grave threat to mother and child. Eclampsia can cause convulsion, stroke, and even death.

Preeclampsia occurs in about 1 percent of pregnancies. There is also some speculation that preeclampsia is linked to poor nutrition and insufficient dietary calcium. Teenage mothers and older mothers, women in their first pregnancy, and women carrying twins are at higher risk for preeclampsia.

Understanding the Problem. Preeclampsia typically manifests near term. Its existence is indicated by a rise in blood pressure; edema (swelling due to water retention) of the hands, face, and ankles; and protein in the urine. Women receiving good prenatal care will likely be diagnosed as having preeclampsia. With prompt treatment, the disorder should present no further complications.

If, however, preeclampsia is allowed to progress, more serious symptoms will arise, including blurred vision, headaches, and severe abdominal pain. Finally, it can evolve into eclampsia, a condition characterized by seizures and coma. In rare instances, the disease can be fatal to the mother or fetus.

Treatment Options. Once diagnosed, preeclampsia is treated with complete or partial bed rest, hospitalization, and/or medication. High blood pressure will be brought under control with medication. Resting as much as possible lying on one's side takes some of the weight off the major blood vessels, improving blood flow to the kidneys.

In more severe cases, admission to a hospital is required. There, a woman will receive medication to lower her blood pressure and to remove excess fluid. Continuing the pregnancy may be risky if it seems that preeclampsia is becoming more severe. When the pregnancy is near term or there is a good chance that the fetus will survive outside the womb, labor may be induced or a cesarean section may be performed. After delivery, the disease resolves and the symptoms abate.

PREGNANCY AND PREEXISTING CONDITIONS

There are a number of medical conditions that both complicate pregnancy and are complicated by pregnancy. Usually, when a woman who has a serious medical problem becomes pregnant, she will need to work with a specialist in the area of concern as well as with an obstetrics practitioner.

A partial list of such conditions follows.

Breast Cancer During Pregnancy. The course of breast cancer is seldom influenced by pregnancy. In most cases, if cancer is discovered during pregnancy, it is not necessary to undergo a therapeutic abortion since an abortion will not improve prognosis. The chance of surviving breast cancer beyond five years is dependent primarily on the stage at which the disease is diagnosed. This is true in both pregnant and nonpregnant women.

Although survival is stage-dependent, pregnancy may pose serious delays in clinical assessment, diagnostic procedures, and treatment of a breast tumor. Hormones triggered in pregnancy cause changes in the breast which tend to obscure masses. As a result, breast cancer may be detected at a later stage in pregnant women.

The diagnostic approach in pregnant women with breast tumor is no different from that in nonpregnant women. Any suspicious breast mass found during pregnancy should prompt an aggressive plan to determine its cause, whether by needle or open biopsy. The risk of mammography to the fetus is negligible. The dense breast tissue engendered by pregnancy, though, makes mammography less reliable.

If a cancer is detected, surgical treatment to remove the lump is not usually delayed. Neither modified radical mastectomy nor total mastectomy seems to present a significant risk to the pregnancy or to fetal health. Radiation therapy, however, usually is not recommended during pregnancy. Whether chemotherapy is advisable depends on the aggressiveness of the cancer and on the stage of pregnancy (see also *Breast Cancer*, page 390).

Pregnancy Following Treatment for Cancer. Ten percent of women treated for breast cancer subsequently become pregnant. There is little evidence that pregnancy that follows cancer treatment adversely affects the mother's survival. However, it is important that the obstetrics practitioner be kept up to date with a woman's treatment and that the pregnancy also be followed by her oncologist.

Diabetes. In the past, diabetes prevented most women from conceiving, and those who did had little chance of having a successful pregnancy. Most pregnancies were problematic throughout, babies were usually not robust, and in many cases, neither mother nor baby survived. Today, with insulin injections and dietary modifications, a diabetic woman can enjoy a normal pregnancy and deliver a healthy baby.

Left on its own, a diabetic woman's body does not process sugar effectively. Consequently, there is always the risk that excess blood sugar will cross the placenta into the fetal blood supply. This can result in excessive fetal growth, which in turn complicates child-birth. Higher-than-average rates of birth defects and a predisposition to diabetes are associated with maternal diabetes. There is also a greater chance of stillbirth.

Diabetes that is not sufficiently controlled can predispose the mother to infection, post-partum bleeding, and preeclampsia (see page 303).

Gestational Diabetes. Some women experience gestational diabetes during pregnancy; it is found in about 3 percent of pregnant women and is more common in women who are overweight, are over thirty-five, or have a history of stillbirths or large babies. This form of diabetes also needs to be strictly controlled, with blood sugar levels carefully maintained, but usually does not require insulin injections. Normally, it subsides right after delivery, although some women go on to have chronic diabetes.

Gastrointestinal Disorders. Some gastrointestinal conditions, including Crohn's disease and ulcerative colitis, can produce symptoms that pose risks during pregnancy. It is vital that these conditions be managed before and followed during pregnancy. If Crohn's disease and ulcerative colitis are not controlled, for example, the diarrhea, cramping, abdominal pain, and dehydration associated with these can develop into serious problems in pregnancy and present a danger to the health of the fetus.

Heart and Lung Ailments. Disorders of the heart and lungs are considered significant pregnancy-related complications. They do not, in most cases, preclude having a normal pregnancy and a healthy baby. They do, however, necessitate careful monitoring and, at times, special treatment. Because the heart naturally works harder in pregnancy, the extra stress put on an already vulnerable organ may exacerbate heart disorders or lung disease. Be sure that you discuss your medical history with your practitioner. Also, medications used to manage the condition should be reviewed. Finally, weight gain, water retention, and anemia are factors that affect the way the heart works and should therefore be closely watched.

Hypertension. Hypertension (high blood pressure) is easily detected in routine prenatal visits. Some women enter pregnancy with high blood pressure; others experience it in the course of the pregnancy. Mild or intermittent hypertension is usually not a problem in pregnancy. Nevertheless, hypertension can lead to preeclampsia, which as it progresses poses an increasingly serious threat to the pregnancy, the mother, and the baby (see page 303). Hypertension is managed by monitoring blood pressure, adjusting dietary sodium consumption, and, at times, taking medication. Usually blood and urine tests will assess kidney function. In some cases, an ultrasound will be recommended to evaluate fetal growth.

Kidney Disease. Kidneys function as the body's filter. As blood volume grows to nourish the developing fetus, a woman's kidneys increase in size and work harder to process waste created by both the mother and fetus. Any compromise in renal function, therefore, can interfere with the mother's health and may increase the risk of preeclampsia.

Pregnancy predisposes a woman to urinary tract disorders and other renal problems. If a woman already suffers from kidney disease, kidney dysfunction may worsen during this time. When renal disease is not brought under control, women experience a higher rate of miscarriage, preterm delivery, fetal growth retardation, and fetal death. Moreover, most women with chronic renal insufficiency are also anemic, and anemia brings with it other complications (see page 276). Consequently, it is essential that pregnant women with any type of renal or urinary tract disease consult practitioners familiar with these disorders.

Lupus. Systemic lupus erythematosus is a chronic, progressive inflammatory disease of connective tissues that affects skin, joints, kidneys, nervous system, and mucous membranes. Although the exact cause of this autoimmune disorder is uncertain, pregnancy can trigger lupus. As with other autoimmune disorders, the body's immune system reacts to normal stimulation defensively, producing antibodies against parts of the body, inflicting injury to tissue.

Lupus is often difficult to diagnose in pregnant women because many of its symptoms mimic those of pregnancy. With lupus, a woman will feel unusual fatigue, which is often difficult to distinguish from pregnancy-related fatigue, and general inflammation, which may be confused with pregnancy-related edema. Other symptoms include a butterfly rash on the cheeks, mouth ulcers, anemia, and convulsions. The disease may begin suddenly with fever, joint pain, and malaise, or it may develop over a period of years with intermittent fever and malaise.

Women who enter pregnancy with lupus or who experience it in pregnancy face a higher-than-average risk for miscarriage. In addition, the disease can intensify after childbirth.

Women with lupus are usually considered to have high-risk pregnancies. It is a good idea, therefore, to consult a specialist in the area of autoimmune diseases as well as an obstetrics practitioner (see page 460).

PREGNANCY AND SEXUALLY TRANSMITTED DISEASES

There are a number of diseases that arise when bacteria or viruses are transmitted during sexual contact. While these sexually transmitted diseases (STDs) can cause considerable problems for adults, they pose serious risks in pregnancy and childbirth.

Genital herpes is, at present, an incurable venereal disease. In adults, this prevalent disease is painful but basically harmless, manifesting in lesions around the genitals and sometimes in the cervix and upper vagina. In newborns, though, it can be deadly if the baby comes into contact with the infection during delivery. It can damage the baby's nervous system and eyes. It can also result in fetal death.

Some women carry the virus without symptoms; others have sporadic attacks. If active lesions are present at the time of labor, the clinician likely will recommend cesarean section so that the fetus will avoid the journey down the birth canal and exposure to the virus. In the meantime, women with the virus should avoid sexual intercourse when the infection is active, wash their hands frequently, bathe daily, and keep lesions clean and dry. Some clinicians recommend the use of acyclovir in late pregnancy to decrease the risk of virus activation and cesarean section.

Hepatitis B is a liver infection transmitted though sexual intercourse. This virus can cross the placenta and infect the fetus, often causing liver failure in children. If tests show that a pregnant woman has antibodies to the virus, her infant will be injected with antibodies soon after birth. Many practitioners now recommend immunization of all infants against hepatitis B, whether or not the mother is infected.

Syphilis is a dangerous sexually transmitted disease that can lead to serious fetal problems including stillbirth, bone and tooth deformities, progressive nervous system damage, and delayed brain damage. Early prenatal blood tests screen for the infection. If a woman tests positive for syphilis or if the infant is born with the infection, penicillin will be prescribed.

Gonorrhea is another venereal disease that responds well to antibiotics. However, as an infant moves through the birth canal, contact with the infection can result in serious problems, such as eye damage and blindness. Accordingly, all newborns are treated with an antibiotic ointment immediately after birth. Penicillin will be administered if it appears that the baby has gonorrhea.

Chlamydia can cause eye infection or pneumonia in a baby born to a mother with the infection. This, too, can be successfully treated with antibiotics or prevented if the mother undergoes antibiotic therapy before childbirth.

Cytomegalovirus (CMV), a herpes-related virus, affects a high number of infants each year, causing death and such defects as blindness, seizures, anemia, and neurological disorders. It is also difficult to treat. Although some women contract CMV in pregnancy, it is fortunate that serious fetal damage is uncommon.

Genital warts are both painful and highly infectious. They tend to grow faster during pregnancy. Treatment is less effective during pregnancy, although most current treatments do not hurt the fetus. If the warts grow large enough, they can interfere with the baby's passage through the birth canal, usually prompting surgery to remove the obstruction.

AIDS is a deadly disease. Women can contract the disease through sexual intercourse with a man who is infected with the virus, through blood transfusion, or through intravenous drug use with an infected needle. The virus can also be transmitted through artificial insemination with contaminated semen. Women with AIDS pass it on to the fetus in utero less than half the time. To date, there is no cure for the disease, and babies who are born with it die within a few years. However, treatment of pregnant women and infants with azathioprine (AZT) has been known to reduce the incidence of prenatal transmission dramatically.

CHAPTER 15

❧

Labor and Delivery

CONTENTS

For almost nine months, Sandy has become increasingly absorbed by her pregnancy. She has developed a more sensitive awareness of her body, its changes and responses. She has made a conscious effort to eat well and to keep regular prenatal appointments with her obstetrician.

As her due date rapidly approaches, she is even more preoccupied with the direction of her career, on the one hand, and with baby clothes, nursery supplies, and equipment, on the other. She's ever more conscious of families with young children: On the street, Sandy's always encountering mothers behind strollers; she's forever spying baby-sitters in playgrounds and children in school yards.

She has passed through morning sickness to lower back pain, and from anxiety to relief, with each prenatal test and procedure she's undergone. Her speculations concerning what her baby will be like, how her relationship with her husband will change, what her life will look like once the baby is born have evolved, too. In a couple of weeks, her pregnancy—which at times seemed to stretch out endlessly but which now seems to have happened in little more than a blink of the eye—will end, and her baby will be born. Before that occurs, however, she adds to the many preoccupations of pregnancy an almost palpable worry about labor and delivery.

For the vast majority of women, the course between conception and childbirth is both predictable and personal, joyous and unsettling. Like Sandy, most women find that the many and varied concerns, changes, preoccupations, and speculations of pregnancy serve to prepare them for childbirth and parenting. While doubts and questions surface at each point along the way and touch each aspect of a woman's experience, there are times when these misgivings, however natural and understandable, seem a bit overwhelming.

The time immediately before childbirth can be particularly fraught with anxiety. Despite the considerable distress of labor, the odds are tremendously reassuring. For most, the conclusion of the nine-month process is both positive and fortuitous. As Sandy said after her baby was born, "My pregnancy was hard. I was sick much of the time, and, though I don't think people could really tell, I worried a lot, mostly about how my baby would be affected by just about everything. And then there was labor. It was long and painful. I never knew anything could be so intense. But then it was all over.

"The minute they placed my beautiful, healthy, sparkling daughter in my arms, all the pain and difficulties were forgotten."

THE CURRENT CHILDBIRTH ENVIRONMENT

The last quarter of a century has witnessed dramatic shifts in childbirth attitudes and practices in this country. It has been only since the late 1960s that resources such as childbirth education, natural childbirth techniques, full participation of fathers or coaches in the delivery process, birthing rooms, and nurse–midwives have become elements of the medical environment. Each has enriched the birthing experience for many women.

In numerous ways, these changes in the shape of childbirth practices represent a return to a more woman-centered, natural model. At the same time, this renewed emphasis on natural childbirth is complemented by myriad medical advances and refinements. For women with particular pregnancy complications, the development of prenatal testing, ultrasound imaging, and fetal monitoring has enhanced the likelihood of having a healthy baby. Introduction of local and regional anesthesia enables mothers to be fully conscious during delivery and, at the same time, experience minimal pain. Moreover, many medical settings have eliminated or modified such standard prep practices as pubic shaves and enemas, as well as the routine use of intravenous lines (IVs), fetal monitors, and episiotomies.

Today, most pregnancies utilize the best of both natural childbirth and medical technology. Even the most conservative doctors encourage women and their partners to explore natural childbirth classes and techniques. In almost all settings, pregnancy is regarded as a natural process that women can manage quite well, especially with sufficient information and support, and one that no longer requires a period of "confinement."

In this new era of enlightenment and cooperation, prospective mothers are encouraged to plan and prepare for their pregnancies, to educate themselves about their options, and to discuss their preferences with their health-care providers. All this contributes to richer, more satisfying birthing experiences for mothers and their partners.

DECIDING WHERE TO DELIVER

As the time comes for Sophie to consider where to have her first baby, she is inclined to be in a hospital room when her time comes. Besides, her local hospital offers birthing rooms and so many other accommodations that she has begun to feel confident that, guided by her obstetrician, childbirth can be both safe and natural.

Sophie's best friend, Toby, is due around the same time as Sophie. Her priority is that her pregnancy and childbirth be treated as a natural process rather than an illness. After talking things over with her health-care provider and her partner, she has chosen to deliver at the nearby birthing center with her nurse–midwife, who has a history with her and her family and will continue to be involved with them after birth. In addition, Toby likes the feeling that should something go wrong in the process or if things become at all complicated, the nurse–midwife will surely know how to handle it. That way, she believes that she has all bases covered.

Sophie's sister, Gretchen, is about to deliver her third child. Her first two babies were born in the hospital, and in both cases, her experiences were positive and predictable. Nevertheless, this time, because she is healthy and her husband is eager to be more involved, she has chosen to have this child at home. She will be assisted by a nurse–midwife and attended by her husband, her children, and her sister.

Even a casual awareness of the recent developments in prenatal and birthing practices can make the decision of where to deliver your baby seem difficult, if not altogether overwhelming. The truth is, though, that if a woman engages in early and regular prenatal care, the options become easier to sort out.

By the time they reach the final months of their pregnancies, most women have established a working partnership with their health-care providers. The majority of women choose to go through their pregnancy with the help of a gynecologist who also practices obstetrics. Some use family practitioners, who follow the pregnancy, deliver the baby, and then provide medical care after the birth. In pregnancies that present no risk factors and proceed without complication, women can choose to work with a nurse–midwife, a registered nurse who is also trained in gynecology and obstetrics (see *The Midwifery Option*, page 333).

Usually, when a woman chooses an obstetrics practitioner, she is choosing a place to deliver as well, as most providers associate themselves with hospitals or other facilities. Conversely, since services and procedures, approaches and technological supports, may vary from site to site, these days some women take into account *where* they want to deliver as they select their maternity-care provider.

Just as most women favor doctors, most prefer to deliver in hospitals. In general, hospitals provide a full range of technological supports that can address nearly all delivery-related complications. In addition, for many couples, especially first-time parents, the availability of a wide range of medical options—many of which may never be used—alleviates their natural apprehension and doubts. Furthermore, for those women who have a possibility of serious complications, such as diabetes, high blood pressure, and multiple births, a hospital setting is the safest choice, regardless of philosophical preference.

Whereas in the past, hospitals treated most pregnancies in the same methodical manner, in recent years, many settings have expanded their services and methods beyond a strict medical model. They may offer more individualized care. Many hospitals have added *birthing rooms* or *alternative birthing centers*, for example. Rather than placing a woman in one room for labor, then moving her to another room for delivery, these alternative maternity centers offer one place for a woman and her partner to experience all stages of labor and delivery. Typically decorated to replicate many of the comforts of home, these rooms may have full showers or baths, rocking chairs, and accommodations for rooming in, that is, keeping the baby nearby in the room rather than off in the nursery. When special equipment is required, it is generally wheeled into the birthing room; this eliminates the need to take a laboring woman to the equipment and install her in a starkly technological environment. At best, these birthing centers combine aspects of minimal-interventionist, natural childbirth with the security of having highly trained medical personnel at hand. Some hospital maternity floors, however, have only a few birthing rooms; therefore, it is possible that once a woman arrives at the hospital, she will find that the birthing rooms are in use.

In recent years, as interest in natural childbirth has grown, *freestanding birth centers* have become an increasingly viable alternative in some communities. Usually staffed by certified nurse–midwives who are trained to handle all aspects of uncomplicated births, these centers provide a homelike environment, a noninvasive approach to childbirth, and access to medical consultation and hospital acute care services when needed. Should problems arise during pregnancy or labor, referrals are generally made to staff obstetricians or family practitioners. In these freestanding maternity centers, obstetrical interventions, such as electronic fetal monitoring (see page 323), anesthesia (see page 318), or episiotomy (see page 326), are not used routinely. Family and friends can remain with a woman during labor.

Prenatal care and deliveries at such centers tend to be less costly than in hospitals. Although most freestanding birthing centers work in cooperation with local hospitals, there can in some cases be a lapse of time in transferring a woman to a medical setting when complications arise; in rare cases, this lapse can result in delivery-related problems for mother or child or both.

Home birth offers the woman the opportunity to go through labor and childbirth with the people she chooses in familiar surroundings. Generally monitored by nurse–midwives or lay midwives, home births represent the return to a woman-centered, woman-attended manner of childbirth in its purest form. In the unusual event that complications arise during labor and delivery, though, there can be delays in obtaining the medical assistance that might be necessary, in which case at-home births can put the mother and child at increased risk (see *The Midwifery Option*, page 303).

NATURAL CHILDBIRTH

In the early decades of this century, childbirth gravitated away from being a natural woman-centered process, garnering the impersonal qualities of a medical phenomenon. Only a generation ago, for example, a pregnant woman readily put her pregnancy, herself, and her baby entirely in the hands of her doctor.

Her husband, if not altogether excluded from the process, would be relegated to a very minor role. Once labor began, the mother-to-be would be driven, according to the 1950s stereotype, by her anxious, helpless husband, to the hospital, where she was put under general anesthesia. Lying on her back, her legs in stirrups, the woman remained immobile as her baby was extracted from her womb. Thus, the involvement of both mother and father was essentially passive. Today, the return to many natural birth practices has altered the picture and the process of labor and delivery. As a result, it has extended the cast of characters and enriched the experience for all involved.

In its purest form, natural childbirth embraces the normal course of spontaneous labor and birth. Medical intervention is used only when necessary—never routinely. Throughout labor and childbirth, a woman remains fully conscious and unanesthetized. Instead of medication, special relaxation techniques and breathing are used to relieve pain. Most commonly, these techniques are taught in childbirth class and through childbirth groups (see *Childbirth Classes*, page 297).

In addition to teaching methods of breathing and relaxation, most natural childbirth classes impart a comprehensive understanding of the stages of labor, thereby encouraging women to be as involved, aware, and active during childbirth as they choose. Most women who follow a natural approach choose, by the very nature of their involvement, to participate in the process and in all decisions that arise along the way. Moreover, in most cases, natural childbirth facilitates the active participation of the father or the mother's partner.

LABOR DEFINED

Throughout pregnancy, a woman's body has been preparing itself for labor. During labor, uterine muscles gradually stretch the cervix open to allow the baby to be pushed down into the vagina and out. In many cases, the cervix begins to efface (thin and draw up) and dilate (open up) before there are other, palpable signs of labor. Some women, in fact, walk around with the cervix slightly dilated for weeks before labor begins. For others, contractions start before dilation begins.

It is, however, the combination of contractions *plus* cervical changes that constitutes labor. Neither alone is the real thing.

Many times, as the due date approaches, contractions become stronger and resemble menstrual cramps. *False labor*, as it is sometimes called, plays an important role in moving dilatation and effacement along. Although these contractions can last for hours, they usually stop on their own after a while or if you walk around. They resemble Braxton Hicks contractions, which can occur much earlier in the pregnancy (see also *Braxton Hicks Contractions*, page 299).

SIGNS OF LABOR

As her due date approached, Hester worried that she wouldn't recognize the signs. She was afraid that she'd be involved in her work or that she'd be on her way somewhere—and the baby would come all of sudden. After all, so many babies on television are born in taxicabs.

Although some women have no clear signs, others experience symptoms that leave little doubt that labor has begun. Nevertheless, with or without undeniable signs, most women do know when true labor begins and are able to judge when to call their clinician.

There are three signs that labor may begin soon:

Bloody Show. Many women expel blood-tinged mucus just before or during labor. This small mucus plug, which has sealed the cervical opening, comes out as the cervix begins to stretch.

Water Breaking. At some point during labor, the membranes containing amniotic fluid break. As the membranes break, water trickles or rushes out. The fluid is usually odorless and appears clear or slightly milky. A woman cannot hold the water back, like urine, by squeezing her abdominal muscles. Although some women trickle for days or weeks, labor will likely begin within twenty-four hours of the membranes' rupture.

Most health-care providers recommend that once the membranes have ruptured, a woman go immediately to the hospital to be evaluated.

After the membranes break, a woman should not bathe, have sexual intercourse, or insert anything into her vagina, any of which could result in infection. Often, if it has not started on its own, labor will be induced within twenty-four hours of rupture. If a woman does not go into labor and her labor is not induced within that time, her health-care provider will keep an eye on her temperature and possibly monitor her white blood cell count to make sure there is no infection. He or she may also want to assess the baby's heartbeat periodically.

If the membrane ruptures suddenly, your health-care provider may check the position of the baby's head to determine the presenting position and the position of the umbilical cord. Also, any brown or green staining in the fluid could indicate that meconium, the fecal substance from the baby's bowels, has squeezed out. This sign is common when a woman has passed her due date and is not usually a sign of trouble.

Contractions. In most cases, uterine contractions become progressively stronger and more regular. At first they may feel like gas pains, menstrual cramps, a backache, or pressure and straining in the pubic area. During early labor, when contractions can be either regular and unremitting or sporadic and slight, most women can get on with their daily routines. Many enjoy taking a walk, finishing chores around the house, or napping. Unless the membranes have broken, most women can stay home until contractions are frequent and strong. Most women find the comfort and familiar distractions of home preferable to long hours waiting for something to happen at the hospital.

During active labor, contractions become strong and rhythmic. Building like waves, they pull and tighten throughout the uterus around to the back and groin. Then they ebb. By relaxing between contractions, you can prepare yourself for the next one and reduce the sensation of pain. There may be time after each contraction to rest, nap, walk around, and carry on conversations.

Some signs, such as the rupture of the amniotic membranes, are indisputable; in almost all cases, these announce the approach of labor. The exact significance of contractions is usually less obvious; however, the closer a woman comes to her due date, the closer she should attend to contractions. Contractions are especially meaningful if they occur at regular intervals, if the time between contractions shortens, and if the contractions themselves become longer and more intense. For each woman, however, the onset of labor is gradual.

When any of these indicators occurs, contact your health-care provider. An examination will determine the degree of cervical dilatation and effacement.

Just how long it will take for labor to progress—just when the baby will be born—is impossible to predict. In general, labor takes longer with first babies primarily because the uterus and birth canal are less flexible. While the time of labor varies, the average, from the time a first-time mother goes into active labor until the baby is born, is thirteen hours. For women who have given birth before, the average time is four to eight hours.

STAGES OF LABOR

From the first contractions to the delivery of the placenta, most obstetrics clinicians identify three stages in the progression of labor. While these stages are convenient for understanding the dynamics of labor, during the actual experience they tend to be less distinct.

First Stage. The first stage describes the period of time during which the cervix effaces (thins) and dilates (opens) to the full ten centimeters (about four inches). When labor begins, the cervix is about an inch long and almost completely closed. Contractions work to dilate the opening so that the baby can pass through the birth canal. As each contraction forces the baby against the cervix, the opening stretches. This happens until the cervix opens to a diameter of ten centimeters. At the same time, contractions cause the cervix to thin until it merges with the uterine wall.

The first stage of labor can be divided into two phases. The *latent phase* represents the time the cervix takes to efface completely. On the average, this takes from six to eight hours. Contractions tend to be short, from thirty to forty-five seconds, and irregular, from two to thirty minutes apart. Depending on a woman's individual history (second and subsequent babies typically come faster, and some women just naturally deliver quickly), and the degree to which the cervix is found to be dilated, a woman who goes to the hospital at this point may well be advised to go back home. In her own surroundings, she might use her time to go for a walk, soak in a warm tub (if her membranes have not ruptured), rent a movie, play with her other children, or take care of last-minute details before the baby comes.

After complete effacement, a woman is considered to be in *active labor*. This is the point at which most women set off for the hospital. Once a woman reaches the hospital, a healthcare professional will conduct a pelvic examination to determine progression of dilatation and effacement. Many hospitals use monitors to record the infant's heart rate and the rhythm of the mother's contractions (see *Fetal Monitoring: The Debate and Limitations*, page 323).

Active labor usually takes seven to eight hours, at which point the cervix has dilated from three to ten centimeters. Many women find that this is the time to use the breathing, relaxation, and distraction methods learned in childbirth classes (see *Childbirth Classes*, page 297). Others find that they need some kind of medication to take the edge off the pain (see *Anesthesia Options and Pain Relief*, page 318).

Some hospitals recommend that an intravenous drip be started at this point to ensure that a woman receives adequate fluids for the work that needs to be done. Moreover, if an emergency cesarean section becomes necessary, many clinicians find that an IV presents a convenient way of administering medications. Oxytocin, the hormone used to speed up contractions, can also be given through the IV if it becomes necessary to establish a normal labor pattern or to help the uterus contract after childbirth in order to stem any heavy bleeding that may ensue (see *Postpartum Hemorrhage*, page 322).

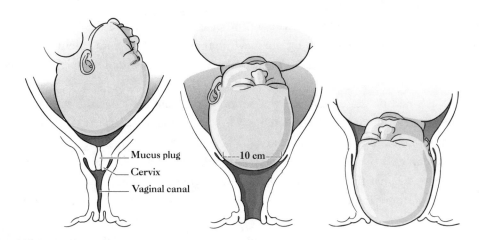

Mucus plug
Cervix
Vaginal canal

—10 cm—

As labor begins, the cervix begins to dilate. As labor progresses, the cervix dilates and, when it reaches ten centimeters, the baby can begin to travel down the birth canal.

Second Stage. Once the cervix opens to ten centimeters, the woman is fully dilated. This point marks the beginning of the second stage of labor. As a woman achieves full dilatation and effacement, she may feel herself opening up. Full dilatation and effacement mean that the cervix no longer offers resistance. Propelled by the mother's pushing efforts, the baby begins its five-centimeter journey down the birth canal. As the baby moves downward, the uterus involuntarily contracts to facilitate the movement out.

In some cases, labor slows, and contractions become further apart. More commonly, though, full dilatation is accompanied by intense, rapid contractions. Often a woman feels a tremendous, uncontrollable urge to push down, as though she were having a bowel movement. It is important, though, that she wait until her maternity attendant guides her to push in order to prevent bruising the cervix and tearing the tissue between the vagina and rectum.

As much as possible, a woman should relax between contractions. By remaining as composed as she can, a woman reserves her strength. She therefore may not tire as quickly. Moreover, the perineum, the area between the vagina and rectum, has more time to stretch around the baby's head, and that may prevent tearing. Some women are able to distract themselves between contractions; others become more focused and concentrated. It is not unusual for women to experience at this point nausea, shaking, trembling around the thighs and legs, chills, and irritability. However, most women also experience a heightened sense of excitement and relief at the growing awareness that they are nearing childbirth.

As the mother is directed to push, the baby continues to move out, and the vaginal opening bulges. Unless she is already in a birthing room, a woman will be moved at this stage from the labor room to the delivery room. If it appears that the vaginal opening will not provide adequate room for the baby to pass through, and that the tissues will likely tear, an episiotomy will be performed. This vaginal incision creates a larger opening for delivery (see *Episiotomy*, page 326).

With first babies, it takes an average of two hours or more to push the infant out; with second and subsequent babies, labor usually progresses more quickly. The perineum begins to bulge as the baby's head pushes against it. When the full circumference of the head is visible, a position which is called *crowning*, birth is imminent. Unless the baby is in breech position (see page 321), the baby's head will be born first. Then, the baby rotates a quarter turn before the shoulders emerge. Last, the body is born.

As the baby emerges, the health-care provider will check to see whether the umbilical cord is around the baby's neck, then suction mucus from its nose and mouth. The infant will appear bluish and still until regular and sustained breathing is established. Contrary to the popular notion that all babies wail upon delivery, many actually enter this world quietly. Some have oddly shaped heads at birth as a result of their passage through the vagina; this is temporary.

Many practitioners cut the umbilical cord once the baby breathes or cries. Some wait until the cord stops pulsating, usually five or ten minutes. There is no evidence that the timing of cord clamping makes any difference. Frequently placing the baby on the mother's abdomen, the health-care provider clamps the cord and cuts it a few inches from the navel. The remaining bit of cord generally turns black within a week or two and falls off.

Ordinarily a birth attendant cleans the baby, removing the wet, waxy substance, called *vernix*, that covers it at birth. Most hospitals treat the baby's eyes immediately upon birth with an antibiotic or silver nitrate to guard against gonococcal and chlamydial infection. If left untreated, these bacterial infections can lead to blindness (see page 307). In some settings, vitamin K is administered to help blood clotting factors develop in the newborn.

Immediately after birth, practitioners evaluate the baby's well-being. Most use the Apgar scale to assess general health. This test rates the baby's heart rate, color, breathing, crying, and muscle tone; a low score indicates the need for immediate medical intervention to help establish normal breathing and heart rate. The baby also will be weighed and footprints made.

Third Stage. The delivery of the placenta or afterbirth usually takes anywhere from five to thirty minutes, completing the birth process. After the baby is born, you may feel a contraction, have a rush of blood, and expel the placenta.

If the placenta is not expelled entirely, the blood vessels remain open, and women are vulnerable to infection and hemorrhage. Once the placenta is born, blood vessels close off, and the uterus clamps down and begins to shrink. If the placenta does not come out on its own, the birth attendant may give you a shot of oxytocin, pull gently on the cord, or extract it manually.

INDUCING AND AUGMENTING LABOR

For Patty, who is thirty-eight years old and two weeks past her due date, the fact that labor will be induced in two days if it has not begun on its own is a great disappointment. She counted on having natural childbirth, and induction, as she understands it, often necessitates the use of painkilling drugs, fetal monitoring, forceps, and episiotomy. In contrast, for Charlotte, whose baby seems to be at risk from an inadequately functioning placenta, induction promises real relief.

Although there are times when a woman and her health-care professional elect to induce labor for the sake of convenience, as a rule, labor is triggered artificially only when there is an identifiable risk if the pregnancy continues. Reasons to plan for inducing or augmenting labor include the following:

- The mother has severe preeclampsia or eclampsia (see page 303).
- Infection is likely as a result of premature rupture of the membranes.
- There are signs the baby is not getting enough oxygen.
- Labor has failed to begin spontaneously or the pregnancy is prolonged. If the baby is fourteen days past the due date, for example, there is a concern of placenta insufficiency, which means that it will no longer support the baby.
- The cervix fails to dilate because the contractions are not strong enough.

Induction is almost always planned. Sometimes a woman is admitted to the hospital on the night before induction is scheduled. A health-care professional will examine her cervix to determine whether it is soft and partially dilated. If her cervix is not ripe, and labor does not appear imminent, a medication may be given to soften the cervix.

Amniotomy. Sometimes labor can be brought on at term once a health-care professional ruptures the membranes. A crochet hook–like tool is inserted into the cervix, and the bag is punctured. Usually painless, amniotomy often hastens dilatation.

Oxytocin. A hormone naturally secreted by the pituitary gland, oxytocin stimulates labor. Often better known by the brand name Pitocin, it can bring on or enhance contractions.

Oxytocin, administered through an intravenous drip, is controlled by a pump. The dosage therefore can be adjusted to maintain normal contraction strength. Oxytocin can, however, increase contraction force to the point that placental blood flow is impaired. For that reason, monitoring of contractions and fetal heart rate is recommended as a precaution. If the contractions become too strong, the oxytocin rate can be decreased.

ANESTHESIA OPTIONS AND PAIN RELIEF

Helaine always imagined that she'd adhere to the principles of natural childbirth and really felt that she could go through delivery and childbirth without the benefit of artificial painkillers. When the time came, however, and her labor stretched out for hours only to become intense and unremitting, she pleaded for some kind of pain relief.

Stephanie, on the other hand, gave pain relief very little thought; she hated pain and made the decision to have an epidural anesthetic way before she felt the first pang of labor.

Rose thought she would just wait and see how things progressed. When labor began, she found that the methods of relaxation and breathing she had learned in her childbirth classes were sufficient to get her over the rough spots of childbirth. Furthermore, her partner's support and encouraging words helped the process along, and she delivered her baby without any kind of painkiller.

The threshold of pain varies from woman to woman. Thus, it isn't an easy or obvious decision whether to rely solely on breathing exercises and relaxation techniques or to take advantage of painkillers to counteract the pain and anxiety of childbirth.

It is probably best to talk over the options with your partner, friends who have gone through childbirth, and your health-care professional. In addition to calming anxiety and dulling the pain, painkillers can make a woman feel groggy and light-headed. Some actually induce sleep. As a result, they may interfere with a woman's experience of and participation in childbirth. Moreover, many drugs cross the placenta to the baby, although the method of administration has little effect on the newborn.

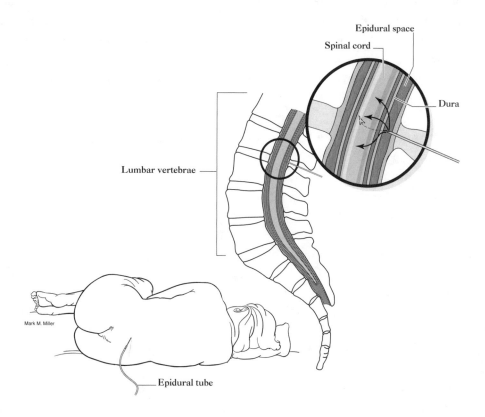

To relieve the pain of childbirth, an anesthetic may be delivered via an epidural tube. It delivers the pain reliever into the epidural space that surrounds the spinal cord.

It was only a generation or so ago that women in labor were routinely given general anesthetics. A couple of hours later, they awoke to behold, often in a haze, their baby boy or girl. Today most women prefer to be alert and involved during childbirth. However, it is impossible for a woman to enter labor with complete knowledge of her own ability to withstand pain as well as the full force of labor. It is not uncommon for women to begin labor with an open mind or a general idea of their preference only to make a clearly different choice as labor progresses. It is important that a woman seriously consider pain relief when it is offered.

More often than not, though, a woman who is committed to the idea of natural childbirth can get through the most arduous stages of labor with a few encouraging words from her partner or health-care professional.

For those who elect medication, there are a number of choices for pain relief during labor and delivery.

Narcotics, such drugs as nalbuphine, are usually given by injection. They help a woman in labor to relax and tolerate the pain by numbing the pain centers in the brain and spinal cord. While they do not eliminate pain totally, some women find that these medications take the edge off the pain and therefore enable them to focus more easily and to work more calmly with their contractions. Because they pass through the placenta and can slow a baby's breathing, these drugs are usually not considered appropriate for women nearing delivery.

An *epidural* is the most widely used obstetrics anesthesia. It dulls the conscious sensation of pain and brings about the closest thing there is to pain-free childbirth. Basically safe for both mother and baby, this method leaves the mother alert and able to participate in both labor and childbirth. It is used in cesarean deliveries as well.

An epidural increases the technological aspects of childbirth, bringing with it the need for an intravenous drip to maintain fluid levels in the event blood pressure drops and often necessitates use of a fetal monitor. Once a woman is in active labor and her cervix has begun to dilate, an epidural anesthetic can be injected via a thin tube into the spinal column outside the dura, the hard outer membrane that protects the spinal cord itself. The dosage can be modulated, allowing the anesthetic's effect to be gradually diminished as delivery approaches. This permits the woman to feel enough sensation that she can push the baby out.

Like an epidural, a *spinal anesthetic* is injected into the spinal canal and does not interfere with the mother's alertness. However, it is generally administered just before delivery and therefore does little to alleviate the pain of labor. Most often, it is used in cesarean sections.

General anesthesia was the method of choice a generation ago. It involves the use of drugs that bring on unconsciousness. Today general anesthesia is used almost exclusively in cesarean sections, in delivery of a baby in breech position, multiple fetuses, or a retained placenta.

ABNORMAL FETAL POSITIONS

As birth approaches, most babies assume the normal fetal position: head down, face to the mother's back. Some babies, however, present in a way that poses difficulties and increases risk during childbirth.

About one in twenty babies present at the time of birth in the *occiput anterior position* (head first, face down); the other 5 percent present in other ways. Most of these fetal positions require special measures during labor and delivery. Some pose slight risk to mother and baby.

Understanding the Problem. In the breech presentation, for example, the baby's feet or rear is seen first. Because many babies do not assume the head-down position until the last

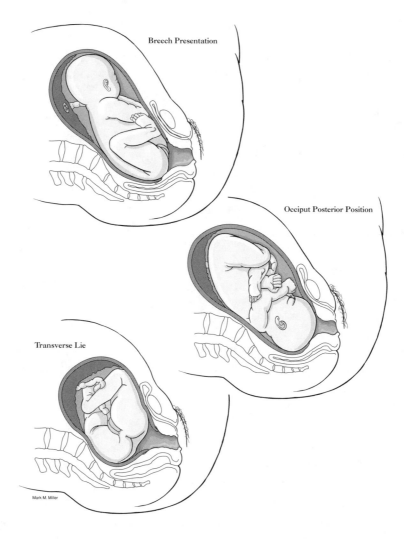

Most babies descend the birth canal head first, face down. Some babies present in other ways, including breech (bottom first), occiput posterior (head first, face up), and transverse.

few weeks of pregnancy, breech is particularly common in premature infants. Other factors that predispose women to breech birth include multiple fetuses, uterine abnormalities, tumors, hydramnios (in which an excess of amniotic fluid accumulates), and placenta previa (see page 302).

A baby who presents in the occiput posterior position is sometimes called a "sunny-side up" baby because its face is up toward the mother's front. This position often impedes movement down the birth canal.

Most common in cases of prematurity and placenta previa (see page 302), the infant may lie horizontally across the uterus (*transverse lie*). With an infant in this position, vaginal delivery is usually not possible and a cesarean section is required. Moreover, there is an increased risk that the umbilical cord will fall through the cervix and become obstructed, cutting off the infant's oxygen supply.

Treatment Options. If, during the last prenatal visits, your health-care provider determines that your baby is in the breech position, he or she may try to turn the baby manually. In the case of this presentation or other abnormal fetal positions, a range of strategies may be available. Discuss the various options—which may include cesarean section—with your practitioner.

PROTRACTED LABOR

There are times in normal labor when many women begin to feel that the process seems endless. In most cases, everything is normal, but labor can be exaggeratedly drawn out and inefficient, and when a woman's labor continues without much advance, she is said to be experiencing *protracted labor*.

Understanding the Problem. Lack of progress during labor can be caused by poorly coordinated or weak contractions. Occasionally, passage through the birth canal is impeded by the baby's presenting position or by the size of its head.

Treatment Options. If the problem lies in contractions, the uterus can be stimulated by an intravenous infusion of oxytocin (see *Inducing and Augmenting Labor*, page 317). In cases in which the position or size of the fetus interferes with childbirth, vaginal delivery may be helped along by the use of forceps if the cervix is completely dilated. Otherwise, a cesarean will be performed.

POSTPARTUM HEMORRHAGE

All women experience some bleeding after childbirth. In most cases, careful hygiene, sanitary pads, and time will address the problem. Sometimes, though, there can be excessive bleeding and blood loss. Hemorrhaging may involve massive flow or a steady seepage over time. Once in a while, rather than escaping through the vagina, blood collects inside the uterus, which in turn becomes distended.

Understanding the Problem. There are a number of reasons that can account for excessive postpartum bleeding. The uterus, exhausted and weakened after pregnancy, may be unable to contract firmly enough to control the bleeding once the placenta separates. Bleeding may result from vaginal trauma after episiotomy. The uterus may have ruptured during labor. Excessive bleeding may also be caused when the expulsion of the placenta is incomplete.

Postpartum hemorrhage is more common in women who have delivered an exceptionally large baby or more than one child. Delivery after several previous deliveries can predispose a woman to excessive bleeding. Hydramnios (in which an excess of amniotic fluid accumulates) and drug-induced labor can also result in postpartum bleeding.

Treatment Options. As a rule, postpartum hemorrhage can be controlled through drugs that work to help the uterus contract. If it appears that tissue has been torn, it will be repaired under local anesthetic.

OTHER DELIVERY-RELATED PROBLEMS

Although the large majority of deliveries proceed without significant problems, in a small number of cases, problems that require special attention do arise:

Placental Abruption. When, in rare instances, the placenta separates prematurely from the wall of the uterus, there is an immediate danger that the baby will be deprived of oxygen. This condition, signaled by heavy bleeding, will necessitate rapid vaginal delivery, if possible, or emergency cesarean section (see page 327).

Placenta Previa. When the placenta lies low in the uterus in front of the fetus, it can block, either partially or completely, the cervix. This condition is also marked by heavy bleeding and necessitates a cesarean section (see page 327).

Meconium. Meconium is the feces produced in the uterus by the baby. When it is present in the amniotic fluid, it changes the otherwise colorless appearance to brown or green. The appearance of meconium in amniotic fluid is common after the due date. It is in some instances a sign of inadequate oxygen supply to the baby.

FETAL MONITORING: THE DEBATE AND LIMITATIONS

Once a laboring woman checks into the hospital, the evaluation procedure often includes an assessment of the relationship between uterine contractions and the baby's heart rate. While the fetal heart rate can be monitored through the use of a hand-held Doppler ultrasound device or stethoscope, many hospitals and birthing centers use electronic fetal monitoring (EFM) equipment to record the unborn baby's heartbeat during labor. Through such monitoring, many obstetrics practitioners believe they can determine whether the baby is getting enough oxygen.

Monitors are often used when there is a specified cause for concern. If, for example, labor is to be induced or augmented (see Inducing and Augmenting Labor, *page 317) for any reason, a woman will be attached to a monitor. Pregnancies that involve diabetes or hypertension (see* Pregnancies with Complications, *page 250) will likely entail EFM, as will the use of an epidural (see* Anesthesia Options and Pain Relief, *page 318).*

As the uterus contracts during labor, the blood flow through the placenta slows. If the baby continues to get enough oxygen, the heartbeat will remain steady. With lack of oxygen, a specific pattern of heart rate decrease may occur. Most decelerating patterns, however, are not associated with any problem with the baby.

External monitors are the most widely used. Two belts are strapped around the mother's abdomen; one measures the frequency of contractions while the other utilizes ultrasound to measure the baby's heart rate. External monitors are less invasive than internal monitors. Moreover, they can be used before the amniotic membranes rupture. However, the information they provide is somewhat less detailed.

The use of monitors can be a mixed blessing. The presence of the instruments may lead to a tendency to intervene medically in response to even the smallest of changes that show up on the monitor rather than letting labor take its natural course. Statistics

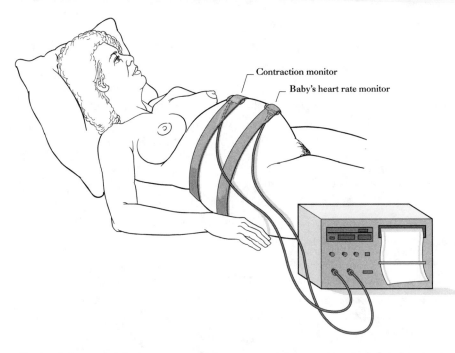

During labor and delivery, your practitioner may wish to monitor the baby's heart rate as well as the progress of your contractions. External monitors are belted to the mother's abdomen, while internal monitors are inserted through the cervix into the uterus.

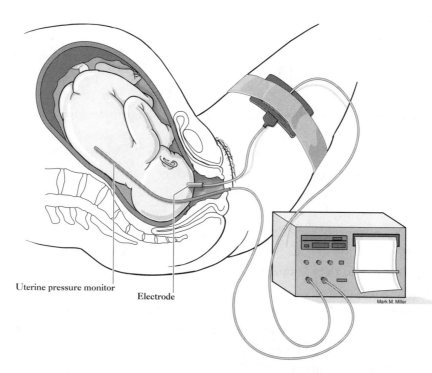

Uterine pressure monitor

Electrode

Mark M. Miller

With internal monitors, a thin catheter is inserted between the baby and the wall of the uterus to measure the pressure inside the uterus as it contracts. In addition, a tiny electrode is clipped to the baby's head through the mother's vagina and cervix. During labor, after the membranes have ruptured on their own or have been ruptured by a clinician, the rate and pressure of contractions as well as the baby's heartbeat are recorded on a paper printout.

show that babies who are monitored electronically are three times more likely to be delivered through cesarean section.

Recently, some hospitals have begun using monitoring equipment that employs telemetry. This kind of monitor relies on radio waves. Strapped to the mother's thigh, the telemetry monitor dispenses with wires or belts, therefore freeing the mother to walk around as she wishes during the early stages of labor.

Fetal Blood Sampling. *A method of estimating how much oxygen the baby is getting during labor, fetal blood sampling is a procedure by which blood is extracted from the fetus in utero. In order to extract the fluid, an endoscope is inserted through the mother's dilated cervix. Tiny incisions are made in the baby's skin, most commonly the scalp, and a small amount of blood is drawn into a tube. The sample is then measured for its pH content. The pH of the blood—whether it is alkaline or acidic—reflects the level of oxygen that the baby is getting.*

EPISIOTOMY

Whenever Carol thinks about delivering her baby, she is struck by the fact that it will emerge from her vagina. She wonders how an opening so tight and tiny—it's small enough that sometimes intercourse can be painful and her tampons always seem to fit so snugly—will be able to accommodate a creature so large. It is hard for her to believe that her vagina is so elastic, but Carol's doctor assures her that after childbirth, the vagina will return pretty much to its original size.

In fact, a woman's vagina is made up of accordion folds that stretch and open for childbirth, in most cases permitting a baby of seven or eight pounds to pass through without tearing. The area between the vagina and rectum, the perineum, though, is not so elastic. For many women, this area will stretch without tearing. For others, an episiotomy, a minor surgical procedure that widens the perineum, may be done to prevent tearing.

Using local anesthetic just before the baby's head emerges, an incision is made either directly back toward the rectum or slanting toward the side away from the rectum. After delivery, the incision is sutured closed. The stitches can cause some discomfort; hot baths, ice packs, pain medication, and anesthetic sprays can help to ease the pain as the area heals. This procedure was at one time routine. Today there is considerable evidence that argues against performing episiotomy with such regularity.

Conventional wisdom cites several reasons to recommend the procedure. Customarily, episiotomies were performed during premature labor to prevent the baby's head from bumping up against the perineum, when a forceps delivery was necessary, and during first pregnancies (episiotomies were performed in 80 to 90 percent of first births, and in about

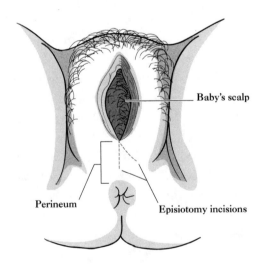

Baby's scalp

Perineum

Episiotomy incisions

A common surgical procedure done during delivery is episiotomy, *in which a small incision is made in the perineum, the area between the vaginal opening and the rectum, in order to ease the baby's exit.*

50 percent of subsequent births), although none of these indications has been shown to be absolute. In general, some practitioners make an incision whenever there is a chance of perineal tears because ragged tears tend to be more difficult to repair than straight incisions, and because they believe that a well-timed incision can reduce injury to the perineal and vaginal muscles. Also, this procedure can shorten the second stage of labor by some fifteen to forty-five minutes.

On the other side of the debate, there is the argument that episiotomies work against the natural process of childbirth. Some claim that the cuts tend to be more extensive than any tearing would be, that they result in excessive bleeding, that the postpartum discomfort following an episiotomy is great and unnecessary, and that they invite infection. Some assert that episiotomy distorts sensation later during intercourse. Instead, those who argue against the procedure offer as an alternative Kegel exercises and local massage to prepare and strengthen the perineum before labor. In addition, an upright birthing position, massage, warm oils, and wet compresses during delivery minimize and, in many cases, prevent tearing.

The fact is, though, that only when the baby's head crowns (that is, when the full circumference of the head becomes visible) can the need to assist perineal stretching be objectively assessed. Episiotomy is one of the many aspects of childbirth that should be discussed with your health-care provider. He or she can help you decide what approach suits your needs better.

CESAREAN SECTION

A surgical procedure that involves lifting the baby out through abdominal and uterine incisions, cesarean section accounts for more than 20 percent of all U.S. births.

Unquestionably, cesarean sections save lives and avert many dramatic birth-related complications. On the other hand, there has been a groundswell of criticism of the frequency of "C-sections"—are they necessary in one of five births?

There are a number of reasons for a baby to be delivered by cesarean section. Among them are instances in which a woman ready to give birth has active herpes lesions (see page 306); when the infant is too large or the mother's birth canal too narrow; when there are abnormalities of the uterus or vagina that obstruct the birth canal; when there are placental abnormalities such as placenta previa (see page 302); when the umbilical cord falls out before the baby; when there are more than two fetuses; when the baby presents in a transverse lie (see page 322).

The very fact that a baby will be delivered by cesarean changes the nature of the childbirth experience. Labor and delivery are shaped by medical procedure—drugs and anesthesia, antibiotics and blood transfusion equipment, catheters and pubic shaves, and, of course, the surgery itself.

Cesarean section has become, over the last few decades, an increasingly viable and prevalent birthing alternative. With improvements in anesthesia and antibiotics, the proce-

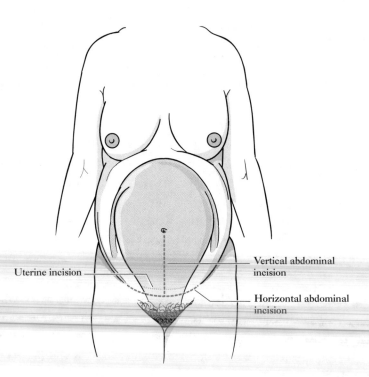

When performing a cesarean section, the physician may make a vertical or a "bikini-line" incision in order to reach the uterus, where another incision is made, and then remove the baby.

dure itself has become safer. The widespread use of fetal monitoring now provides health-care professionals with an estimate of the fetus's ability to withstand labor. If there are indications that there might be problems during vaginal delivery, cesarean section may well be the most prudent solution.

At the same time, there is a debate around the dramatic increase in cesareans over the past decade. As with any operation, there is an increased risk of death related to cesarean sections. In addition, some researchers have identified possible links between this procedure and transient respiratory distress in infants.

The Procedure. Unless factors indicate the necessity of general anesthesia, most surgeons prefer to use epidural or spinal anesthesia (see *Anesthesia Options and Pain Relief*, page 318), which allows a woman to stay alert and, at the same time, diminishes her sensation of pain. Most hospitals permit a woman's partner to stay in the operating room during a cesarean.

In a surgical procedure that usually takes a little less than an hour, an abdominal incision is made; it can be either a horizontal bikini cut near the pubic hairline or a vertical cut from the navel to the pubis. Once the incision reaches the uterus, another incision is made. In most cases, the surgeon uses a lower uterine transverse incision, which tends to heal better and is less likely to cause uterine rupture in a subsequent pregnancy. In the event greater access to the uterus is needed—when, for example, the infant is premature or is lying across the mother's body—a vertical incision will be used to open the uterus.

After the uterus is opened, the baby is taken out. The placenta is then extracted and the incision stitched closed.

Complications. Most women who undergo cesarean sections recover promptly and completely from the operation. As with any major surgical procedure, however, cesarean sections introduce the possibility of specific complications. Cesarean-related deaths occur two to four times more often than deaths related to vaginal deliveries. This risk, though, is strikingly lower than it was a generation ago and, in most cases, involves preexisting medical problems.

Recovery. As a rule, women are encouraged to move around soon after delivery and to eat a regular diet when intestinal function returns. As soon as a woman feels well enough, she can hold and breast-feed her baby. Hospital stays tend to be several days longer, as the woman recovers from what is major abdominal surgery.

Future Pregnancies. Years ago, the fact that a woman delivered a baby through cesarean section predetermined all subsequent deliveries; it was thought that to attempt vaginal birth after cesarean section risked rupture of the uterine scar. Today, there is no longer an absolute prohibition. Instead, health-care professionals encourage future vaginal births.

The course of the first cesarean influences decisions concerning subsequent deliveries. If a lower transverse incision was made, chances are higher that a vaginal delivery will be successful. Today, half to two thirds of women who have had cesarean sections can go on to deliver subsequent babies vaginally.

ALTERNATIVE OPERATIVE STRATEGIES

Although the trend these days is toward noninvasive natural childbirth, there are times when medical intervention is necessary to ensure successful delivery. Such strategies include the following:

Forceps Delivery. Forceps, a tool consisting of two blunt tonglike blades, are sometimes used to guide the baby out of the vagina when delivery is not progressing as it should or when there is concern about the fetus's heart rate. Forceps are also used to assist in vaginal breech deliveries. Sometimes they are used when a woman does not have the strength to push the baby out.

If a forceps delivery is necessary, an episiotomy may be done, but it is not always necessary (see page 326). Though complications from forceps deliveries are rare, use of the instrument may cause temporary bruises on the baby's face and, in extremely exceptional cases, facial nerve damage, which is usually temporary.

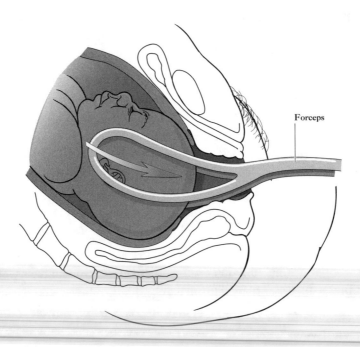

One method of delivering a baby quickly is through the use of forceps. Obstetric forceps both protect the child's head and allow force to be applied to remove the head from the pelvis. Forceps may be used in case of fetal distress or failure to progress down the birth canal.

Vacuum Extraction. Used to address many of the same problems as forceps, a vacuum extractor is a metal cup that is placed over the baby's scalp. A pump then attaches it to the baby's head. The health-care provider can thus manipulate the baby's head to a better position or guide the baby out of the birth canal. Occasionally, there is some bruising under the baby's scalp, which clears up in a few days. However, there may be more excessive bleeding with the formation of a hematoma under the scalp.

JAMIE'S STORY

After almost thirty-five weeks of pregnancy, Jamie was getting used to waking up three or four times a night with a tremendous need to go to the bathroom. On this night, she awoke from a deep sleep with the knowledge that in only five weeks, she'd be awakened not by the pressure on her bladder, but by the call of her baby. No sooner had she climbed back into bed than she felt a trickle of water down her leg. Is incontinence the next indignity of pregnancy?, she thought to herself. The water rushed faster, yet she knew she'd just emptied her bladder. Jumping out of bed with a sudden awareness, she woke her husband with the announcement that her membranes were breaking.

Jamie knew she should call the doctor, but it seemed too soon. Surely she was not about to have the baby. She'd seen the doctor only that morning. Everything appeared normal. Now, over the phone, she heard the urgency in his voice as he advised her to go to the hospital at once.

On the ride over, Jamie insisted that the baby wasn't coming yet. They hadn't finished their Lamaze classes. How would she know what to do during labor?

At the hospital, Jamie was examined by her doctor. The cervix wasn't dilated. Nor was she experiencing contractions yet. At thirty-three weeks, her doctor reassured her, there was every indication that the baby would be born healthy. Yet, there was some concern about the baby's lungs, the doctor explained, since this was the last part of the fetal system to mature. The best plan would be for her to remain in the hospital while labor was forestalled for as long as possible. That way, she could be put on medication which would hasten the baby's lung development.

However, as soon as the doctor left, labor began. When he was called back, Jamie was almost fully dilated. Labor was fast. Within two hours, Jamie's son was born.

At six pounds, seven ounces, the baby appeared healthy. But in a while, it became clear that the baby was having trouble breathing. The pediatrician explained that although this respiratory distress could be a sign of infection contracted after the rupture of the membranes, it was more likely hyaline membrane disease, or incomplete lung development, a common complication of premature birth.

The baby was put in an isolette in the neonatal intensive care unit. The prognosis that he would recover and thrive was reassuring. However, Jamie was frightened and saddened to see her baby lying in an isolette with a tube running out of his mouth and a range of monitors attached.

Jamie's strong feeling was related in part to the sight of her baby in intensive care—although she was comforted by the skill and compassion of the neonatal staff. What she was experiencing—in addition to postpartum exhaustion—also were ordinary and predictable reactions to premature delivery. She had counted on another month in which to ease into motherhood. In many ways, she felt scarcely ready to be finished with her pregnancy, and now, no longer pregnant, she couldn't even hold her baby and begin the process of knowing him.

Her hospital had social workers and a permanent support group to help her, along with other parents in the unit, sort through some of the very complicated and understandable feelings related to premature birth.

Jamie looked around the neonatal unit. There were babies who were very tiny, some who were still fetuslike in so many ways, and some who were terribly ill. She felt lucky that her son looked so hardy. Yet, at the same time, she missed him. In addition, she worried that they had lost the most critical bonding time. Everything she read referred to the importance of the first few hours, the first few days, for parents and child. As her son approached his one-week birthday, she realized that, except for holding him in the first few minutes after his birth, she had only stroked him through the window of his isolette.

On the eighth day after he was born, he was breathing well enough on his own to be taken off the respirator. As Jamie took him in her arms and held him for the first time since his birth, he snuggled right up against her. Then after a short time getting used to the idea, he began to nurse as though he'd been doing it all his life. Jamie and her husband took their son home, ten days after he was born, four weeks before he was due. He showed no health-related effects, and, by the time he was a year old, he resembled children his age in every way.

PREMATURE DELIVERY

Less than one in ten babies in the United States is born before thirty-seven weeks of gestation and is therefore considered preterm or premature. Until recently a baby of five and a half pounds or less was considered premature, but today clinicians are more concerned with the maturity and functional development of the baby than with the baby's weight.

For some of these babies, prematurity reflects a miscalculation of their due date. Others arrive early, but healthy, and ready to go home. Others, however, are born before their fetal development is complete.

These days, advances in neonatal intensive care mean that babies born as early as twenty-five weeks and weighing as little as two pounds have a chance of surviving. With babies this early and this small, though, the risk of serious complications is high. The closer a baby is born to its due date, the higher are his or her chances of survival and full health.

In nearly half of all premature births, the cause is never known. In other instances, prematurity is likely a result of heavy smoking: fetal abnormalities, such placental abnormalities as placenta previa and placental abruption, multiple fetuses, maternal toxemia, infection, and illicit drug use.

Overall, premature labor proceeds much like normal full-term labor. It might be a bit slower because contractions are weaker, or it might progress more rapidly because the baby is smaller.

Almost immediately upon birth, a premature baby's health will be assessed. If it appears that fetal development is not complete, the baby will probably go into the neonatal intensive care unit, where temperature, feeding, and respiration can be monitored and controlled, and where he or she will be protected from infection, to which premature babies are especially susceptible. The smaller and more feeble the baby, the more immediate will be the need for neonatal medical care.

Increasingly, mothers and fathers are encouraged to spend time in neonatal nurseries with their premature baby. Even when they cannot hold their baby, parents can stroke, touch, and talk to him or her. Many hospitals actively encourage mothers to provide breast milk for their baby even when the baby is too frail to nurse. Often, hospitals make breast pumps and nursing rooms available so that new mothers can pump on a regular schedule. This ensures not only that during the baby's stay in the hospital, he or she will get mother's milk, which is rich in colostrum and helps fight infection, but also that the mother's milk comes in and she can later breast-feed her baby, even if she is unable to do so during the first few days or weeks after birth. Many nurseries encourage mothers and fathers to feed their baby with bottles until the baby is strong enough to nurse.

It is not uncommon to find support groups within the hospital to help parents of premature babies deal with their many feelings, apprehensions, and questions. Many parents are not prepared for delivery and find that not only were they caught off guard by the prematurity, but they are also distressed by the fact that, until the baby is well enough to go home, they are deprived of their baby as well.

THE MIDWIFERY OPTION

For centuries, issues around women's and children's health were addressed primarily by other women, and when it was time for a woman to give birth, she was attended by women of the community—neighbors, family members, or simply community wise women. Today, pregnancy and childbirth have drifted some distance from these early woman-centered, woman-attended events. Nevertheless, in the 1960s, as a renewed interest in natural childbirth began to influence birthing customs, midwifery began to reestablish itself as a legitimate and compelling alternative to traditional obstetrics.

At the heart of midwifery is the ideal of childbirth as a holistic, integrated, familiar, and individualized experience that begins with pregnancy, includes labor and birth, and continues after the baby is born. At its best, midwifery offers close, respectful attention to a woman within the context of her family and her pregnancy.

Most midwives in the United States are certified nurse–midwives, that is, nurses educated through graduate programs in normal pregnancy and labor and well-woman care. Most states license professional midwives after they pass a certifying examination that then allows them to practice under state regulations. Certified nurse–midwives practice independently and in private physician-led practices, free-standing birth centers, hospitals, and health clinics. They almost always practice in conjunction with physicians, referring women who have problem pregnancies or bringing doctors into situations and emergencies that require medical care, advice, and/or surgical intervention.

The American College of Obstetricians and Gynecologists officially recognized the midwifery profession in 1971. Since then, the profession has been instrumental in creating out-of-hospital birthing centers and in-hospital alternative maternity-care programs. Because midwife-assisted childbirth can be highly cost-effective, midwives often attend low-income women.

Home birth—delivery in familiar surroundings with family, friends, and other children present—has become almost exclusively the bailiwick of midwives. Some women find that they are better able to relax at home and feel more comfortable with the blood, sweat, and noises of childbirth there.

Childbirth is never a risk-free process. In most situations, it is important to verify that a nurse–midwife has an association with a physician who is available in emergency situations and that arrangements to have emergency transport on call have been made. Otherwise, should something go wrong in the process, the risks to the mother and child can be significant.

The Postpartum Period

CONTENTS

In a rather dramatic way, childbirth marks the end of a pregnancy. After nine months of waiting and wondering, a woman beholds her baby. Suddenly, many questions and speculations are set aside.

Yet, simultaneously, many more questions arise. Childbirth brings new life, not only for the infant, but for the parents as well. In the case of a first child, birth transforms two adult partners into parents. A marriage becomes a family. Even for experienced parents, the birth of a new baby, who will be very different from all other children, brings with it new challenges, new demands, and new experiences.

After each birth, it takes time and careful attention for the mother to acquaint herself with her unique child and to learn just how best to parent this developing individual. At the moment of childbirth, a complex process begins of knowing and forming a mutual relationship with her child, of maturing into motherhood, and becoming part of a new family. Giving birth marks a point of departure for a developmental journey that will continue throughout a woman's life.

A woman who is about to give birth may hear the words, *Having a baby will change your life. It is a big responsibility, and sometimes a big headache. You will love this child in ways you never thought possible.* And she may never stop to contemplate their implications. After childbirth, exhausted and slightly stunned, this same woman may gaze down and marvel at the miracle she has created. So very small, so very helpless, yet this tiny creature brings in its wake momentous changes, the magnitude of which can hardly be imagined in the early days.

Maybe the new mother will catch a glimpse of the significance the first time she feels her baby snuggle up against her heart. Maybe a sense of profound affinity will begin to dawn on her the first time she hears her baby cry and feels her breasts expand. Maybe she will feel it the first time the baby suckles, or on their first night home when the baby's cry wakes her from much needed sleep, or the first time the baby won't be soothed, or during the baby's first illness, or the first time she dreams that she has accidentally left the baby someplace. But sooner or later, usually within the first few months of the baby's life, this mother, like all other mothers before and around her, will begin to feel what it means to be a mother.

Strictly speaking, the postpartum period is the first six weeks after a baby's birth. However, in many ways it stretches out for at least eighteen years—more than enough time to recover from the process, experience the joys, and engage in the challenges introduced at the time of childbirth.

TRINA'S STORY

With considerable pride and joy, after a long but relatively uneventful delivery, Trina and her husband, David, took their healthy, alert son home from the hospital. They weren't home for long, however, before Trina began to respond to the many instances when the baby's needs must supersede her own, not to mention David's. Nor did it take long for her to experience the powerful pull of conflicting needs, both from within and outside her. The baby seemed to have an uncanny sense of when his mother was involved in something. The moment she fell asleep seemed to be the exact moment he insisted on being fed. He fussed to be held whenever he was awake despite Trina's need to attend to her work or to the pot on the stove. He cried whenever she and David started to have a conversation, so that she turned away from her husband to soothe her child.

Even though Trina felt that she was regaining some control over the physical changes affecting her body, she would still look in the mirror and hardly recognize herself. She was eager to lose weight, but she knew that dieting would have to wait until she stopped nursing. She yearned to have the time to read a book, but in the weeks after her son's birth, she could stay awake only for a couple of paragraphs.

David wanted to hold his wife, maybe initiate lovemaking, but every time he tried, the baby started to cry in the next room. He felt a bit selfish making sexual demands, knowing how tired Trina was. Also, her breasts leaked if he touched her. He was embarrassed to admit it, but he was beginning to feel a bit jealous of all the attention the baby was getting.

However much they were coming to love their son, however excited they were by the promises and responsibilities involved in becoming parents, there were many times in the first few weeks of their child's life when both David and Trina looked at each other and asked, Whose life is it, anyway?

MOVING INTO MOTHERHOOD

In the first few days after delivery, a woman's experience is filtered through the emotional, physical, and hormonal impact of giving birth. As her body recovers from the birthing experience, a woman experiences a range of emotions that can be quite bewildering. If the baby is healthy and delivery went smoothly, a woman might feel reassured and exhilarated; or she might feel let down from the emotional peak she experienced during delivery. If, on the other hand, childbirth did not live up to her expectations, or if she encountered unexpected complications, a woman might feel disappointed or depressed, or she might feel relieved and resolute.

Regardless of the actual experience at delivery, most women embrace a full range of feelings just in the first days—including, but not limited to, feelings of wonder, anxiety, tender love, impatience, worry, excitement, exhaustion, uncertainty, sadness, and anticipation.

The newborn period, which follows on the heels of the intense physical drama of childbirth, introduces extraordinary challenges in a woman's life. Women are tired and confronted with a new relationship, the basis of which is one-sided dependency: The baby will need, and the mother will give. It may take considerably longer than she anticipated to feel like a mother. It also takes time to understand the newborn's needs. Each baby is different. Baby-care classes, offered at most hospitals with obstetric services, and hospital nurses can help answer specific questions about caring for the baby. Nevertheless, many women feel particularly alone during the early days of the postpartum period.

Over the next few months, a woman begins to learn what it means to be a parent, gets to know her child, and makes adjustments to life with baby. Usually, by the time the baby is six months old, daily life has become more settled. At this point, most women begin to sort out some of the long-term issues raised by motherhood.

Needless to say, the postpartum experience does not always proceed smoothly and predictably. Many aspects of modern life engender unrealistic expectations in women, especially regarding their feelings and behavior as mothers. Parenting behavior is learned, not instinctive, and our society provides few personal opportunities to learn about infant care before parenthood. Nor does it provide significant supports for parents of young children.

It is not uncommon, as recent studies have shown, for women to assume the role of full-time caregiver, not just to the baby, but to all members of her family. Moreover, it is usually the mother who takes primary responsibility for the household chores, even when she works outside the home. Indeed, many women these days must contend with the strain that results from trying to balance roles as mother, homemaker, worker, and lover.

Each family member has his or her own period of readjustment when the baby arrives. The majority of new parents soon find it necessary to eliminate or cut back on nonfamily needs and interests, but it is important not to relinquish them all. Women who, after a few weeks, return to some outside activity or interest seem to recover sooner from childbirth and adjust more easily to motherhood. Some women find that, if they have just stopped working, they miss not only income, but also the social contacts involved in the job. Additional laundry and caretaking activities may seem overwhelming. The husband and other children may become, or seem to become, more demanding.

In such situations, fathers often feel increased financial pressure as well as stirrings of jealousy. Siblings usually have mixed feelings about the attention paid to the new baby—although they may act otherwise. With time, support, and understanding, the family will reconstitute and stabilize anew to include the new member.

MEETING YOUR BABY

You ache, and worry, and push, and sweat, and yell, and cry, and tear, and hurt—then a tiny new person, a person created from your body, is laid in your arms. The baby is, well, perfect—a bit squished, a bit red, a bit distracted—but perfect. But who exactly, you ask yourself, is this person? And what in the world are you going to do with it? Well, if all the books you've been reading recently are correct, you will bond with this person. But what does that mean and how will it happen?

Simply put, bonding refers to the internal process by which a mother forms a loving relationship with her baby and by which the baby comes to develop a strong internal attachment to the person or people providing care, warmth, protection, and love. It may begin the first time you feel the baby move within you or hear the fetal heartbeat. Or it may begin during or after childbirth.

Although parents want—and may feel outside pressure—to love their new baby right away, in fact, the baby is a stranger. It takes time to get to know the baby, and to develop love. Especially for first-time mothers, it takes a while to feel comfortable and competent in the new role of mother.

People use the term *maternal instinct* to describe a woman's natural desire to nurture and care for her baby. However, rather than being natural capacities, maternal, nurturing, and even loving feelings usually take time to emerge. In most cases, bonding is a natural by-product of the day-to-day exchange between parent and child.

Ordinarily, rudimentary bonding has already taken place by the time a baby is born. From the moment a woman discovers she is going to have a baby, she begins to speculate, form questions, and associate meaning, feelings, and dreams with the developing fetus. She and her partner begin to hatch plans that center on this new member of their family. They try out names and shop for nursery furniture and equipment. During prenatal medical visits, they hear the baby's heartbeat, view computerized images of the baby on the sonogram monitor, perhaps even learn whether the baby is a boy or girl. They feel anxious, excited, apprehensive, protective, hopeful.

At the time of birth, most mothers experience a strong, complicated emotional connection to their infant. Some of the current literature on bonding stresses the first hour after birth as a particularly important time. In many home births, just as in the past when home births were common, the bonding experience may occur naturally, often encompassing the entire family. As voiced in an official endorsement by the American Medical Association, the medical community as a whole promotes the importance of facilitating bonding between the new mother and her newborn baby. Today many hospitals encourage parents to spend the first hour or two after delivery with their newborn. During this time, the infant is active and able to focus on his or her surroundings.

However, when a baby is born prematurely or is seriously ill, circumstances may interfere with this early bonding opportunity. In the event your baby is taken to a neonatology unit, placed in an incubator, and connected to intravenous feeding tubes and machines that monitor vital signs, holding him or her, getting to know your baby, and bonding with your infant will be postponed. It may be possible, and of course, it is preferable, to spend as much time with your newborn as you can. As the baby lies in an isolette, you can stroke your baby, hold his or her fist, soothe his or her cries with your voice. Though this is not ideal, even limited contact is valuable for both you and your baby. Besides, the key is not when bonding occurs but that it does occur. Bonding will take place naturally over time.

The nurturing attachment evolves as the mother acquaints herself with the singular reality of her child. Although it does not always feel as natural or develop as automatically and smoothly as many women had anticipated, once the baby is home, and life takes on qualities of the normal, a relationship between mother and baby will begin to unfold. Newborns sleep much of the time. Nevertheless, the short periods of time during which they are alert can be remarkably social. During this time, the mother can hold, cuddle, coo, and talk to her newborn.

In the days immediately following birth, the baby's personality begins to reveal itself in subtle but distinct ways. The baby is quiet or noisy. The baby responds easily to being held or fusses—sometimes a lot—before settling down. The baby is colicky or cries infrequently. The baby takes the breast or the bottle readily and feeds easily or needs a bit of coaxing or stimulating before eating. The baby enjoys being bathed or startles and cries at the feel of water.

On the other side of the relationship, the mother feels exhausted after the experience of childbirth, or eager to begin. She feels anxious and overwhelmed at the prospect of maternal responsibility, or relaxed and curious about the experience. She feels depressed and detached, or she has friends and family to help her get over the most disturbing times.

The relationship between mother and child grows as they get to know each other. The mother holds, talks to, kisses, touches, and nurses or feeds the baby. She watches her infant respond to caresses. The baby looks up at his mother with something that resembles wonder. All this evokes stirrings of parental love. Even at one month, a baby knows and responds to the voices of family members. Early on, a baby will recognize and engage her mother's face, so that eye contact can be a focus and means of connection. With time, the baby begins to return expressions of attachment and by six weeks may smile back, probably in appreciation.

Though regularly painted in rosy shades, the picture of the bonding process that begins in the postpartum period does not always unfold smoothly or reassuringly. It is not uncommon for a woman to behold her rather funny-looking newborn and wonder whether she could possibly love this creature. Parents of colicky babies face difficult days when the baby cries for hours and will not soothe. Some women find the pull between work and home so conflicting that they discount tender feelings toward their baby. The truth is that many mothers look at their baby, expecting to feel strong, unambivalent love, but feel instead disappointment, indifference, and anxiety. Do not be hard on yourself if you do not immediately feel love for your infant. Parenting is never an easy or predictable process. Even when it seems that you've gotten the knack of it, things change, and new challenges arise. There are times when all parents feel anger, disappointment, regret, impatience, and indifference unexpectedly wash over them.

As with any relationship, love and attachment grow and evolve gradually, often unevenly, over time. The baby, like any new person coming into your life, is actually a stranger—even though there may be physical and personality traits that seem quite familiar. Nevertheless, as the complex threads of emotional investment and commitments that characterize the parent–child relationship continue to weave back and forth between the two of you, as you hold the baby and see the baby's eyes light up in recognition and appreciation when you walk into the room, when the baby smiles for the very first time, love will likely spring up strong and surprising. Where once there was no one, there now exists this small, dependent, demanding stranger, who, for at least the next eighteen years, will hold forth in the center of your life.

CECILIA'S STORY

At first, hearing her baby daughter cry practically sent Cecilia up the wall. What, she wondered, could she possibly be doing wrong? Why did the baby cry so much of the time she was awake?

When her midwife explained to her that crying is the baby's first means of communication, Cecilia could stop taking it so personally and appreciate the effectiveness of crying. She couldn't help but marvel at the ways in which her daughter's cries inevitably induced someone in the house to act in the baby's behalf, whether by picking her up, changing her diaper, or feeding her.

When she began to socialize with other mothers, Cecilia could also appreciate the differences in each baby's cry. She was amazed at how immediately she recognized the sound of her daughter yet hardly noticed when someone else's baby cried. In addition, after a while, she was able to discern differences in her own baby's cries as she communicated different needs: the hungry cry, the "change-me" cry, the fussy cry, and more.

BABIES IN THE NEONATAL INTENSIVE CARE UNIT

As childbirth approached, Vanessa's fantasy about the moments immediately after delivery came into focus. She imagined that her obstetrician would pass the baby over to her as she lay on the birthing table. However exhausted she might be, she and her infant would lie together, perhaps with the baby nursing, and begin the process of getting to know each other. It was quite disappointing, and rather frightening, when, instead of being handed over to her after birth, her son was whisked away to the neonatal intensive care unit (NICU), where he stayed for the next two weeks as a result of a serious infection.

Instead of resting peacefully in his mother's arms, Vanessa's son was placed in an incubator that functioned to conserve his body heat. He was connected to monitors that provided information about heart rate, blood pressure, body temperature, and respiration. Rather than conforming to Vanessa's picture of a peaceful entrance into this world, her baby, and the babies around him, were met in the NICU with bright lights and loud technological noises. Other infants were attached to ventilators through tubes inserted into their windpipe, which facilitated their breathing. Many had feeding tubes running through their nose or connected to intravenous needles.

When babies are born with serious conditions, such as prematurity, major birth defects, severe infections, or respiratory difficulties, they will likely require treatment and monitoring in a neonatal intensive care unit. As upsetting as it is for a new mother to learn that her infant requires intensive care, it is reassuring to note that, as a result of greatly improved health care for sick newborns, the neonatal death rate in the

United States has decreased dramatically in the last forty years. Today most hospitals and maternity centers are equipped to handle all but the most critical neonatal health conditions. Moreover, in most areas, there are designated hospitals that accept sick babies from other sites and provide maximum care and monitoring in their emergency facilities.

As a rule, neonatal intensive care units are staffed by physicians called neonatologists *trained in caring for sick newborns and by neonatal intensive-care nurses. These units have access to pediatric specialists in such related specialties as surgery, as well as twenty-four-hour laboratory services. Most have monitoring equipment to assess all of a baby's vital signs and alarm systems to alert the staff of acute crises, as well as respiratory and resuscitation equipment.*

Though a neonatal intensive care unit is far from an ideal place to begin your relationship with your new baby, it is frequently feasible to spend as much time with your new baby as you can, and most units will encourage you to do so. Although you may not be able to hold your baby, every stroke of the skin, every soft, soothing word uttered, every time you make eye contact paves the way to a loving, caring mother–child relationship.

BREAST-FEEDING OR BOTTLE FEEDING

At its most basic level, the purpose of feeding your newborn is to foster an acceptable rate of growth and to guard against any deficiencies that could lead to health problems by providing adequate nutrition. On another, developmental level, the act of feeding, whether by nursing or bottle, can foster closeness and connection between mother and child.

For newborns, unlike with older babies, a varied diet is not a consideration. An infant will receive all the nutrients he or she needs from breast milk or high-quality formula. The choice of method—whether to breast-feed or bottle feed—often comes down to which is more comfortable or practical for the mother. Although some choose to breast-feed exclusively, others prefer to use bottles. More and more, women today opt for a flexible approach that includes both bottle feeding and breast-feeding to accommodate the many, often conflicting aspects of their demanding lives.

Breast-feeding. Whereas a generation ago, most babies were fed with a bottle, today, many pediatricians, as well as the American Academy of Pediatrics, recommend breast-feeding for at least the first four to six months of an infant's life. Studies in the last two decades show that breast milk is nutritionally superior to manufactured formula or cow's milk. Breast milk provides all the nutrients that the baby needs for the first few months of life.

Breast milk is fresh, free of contaminating bacteria, and readily available. With breast milk, it is not necessary to prepare or carry bottles. Breast milk provides antibodies that help protect infants from infection until they produce their own. A mother who breast-feeds need not worry that her baby will develop an allergic reaction to her milk. Moreover, there are instances in which babies have special nutritional needs; for premature or low-birth-weight babies, for example, breast milk is especially beneficial.

It is becoming an increasingly widespread practice in hospitals and maternity centers to encourage mothers to nurse their newborn immediately after birth. Although mother's milk does not come in until the third day after birth, the nursing infant ingests colostrum, a lemon-colored liquid that provides significant health benefits.

Insofar as it involves skin-on-skin sensation and eye contact between the mother and child, breast-feeding becomes an important means of bonding. Similarly, because she can be so directly involved in satisfying and soothing her child, breast-feeding is thought to foster a sense of competence in a new mother.

Since each baby's needs are different, it is preferable to allow the newborn to set the feeding schedule. Most practitioners these days recommend that you feed your baby on demand unless your own routine requires that you rely on a feeding schedule. Typically, it takes one to two hours for a newborn to empty his or her stomach of breast milk. Most babies naturally regulate themselves to a schedule within a week or so. Because breast milk

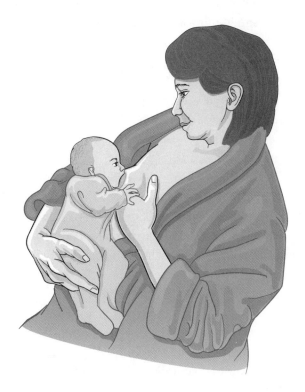

As your baby learns to breast-feed, support the child with one arm while offering the breast with the other hand. Be sure the baby's nose is unobstructed.

is digested more easily than formula, babies who are breast-fed feed more often than those who receive bottles. Your newborn may be content to be fed every four hours, whereas others may demand a feeding every one or two hours. Most infants eat more frequently during the day and less often during the night. As with many other aspects of taking care of your child, even the most dependable schedule will be subject to unannounced changes. You may get used to—and even depend on—nursing every three hours, then suddenly, the baby's needs shift.

The more relaxed a nursing mother feels, the more readily her milk will let down, or fill her milk ducts. While nursing, a woman should either lie down or sit in a comfortable chair with an armrest. Support the baby comfortably with one arm, its face close to the breast. Support and offer the breast with the other hand. Make sure the nipple does not cover the baby's nose. Begin nursing gradually to prevent sore nipples. Five minutes on each side is generally a good start. Alternate breasts and gradually build up to ten minutes on the first breast and twenty minutes on the other. The baby naturally sucks harder on the first breast and will get about 90 percent of the milk he or she needs in the first five or ten minutes. If it's possible, empty at least one breast during each feeding; otherwise it will not be stimulated to refill.

There are a number of ways to prepare for breast-feeding. Start during the last two months of pregnancy. After washing, rub your nipples with a rough terry cloth towel, and periodically massage them between your thumb and forefinger to help toughen them for breast-feeding. It's important to wear a good, supportive nursing bra. Although your breasts most likely will return to their normal size once you wean, they will be quite large and heavy as long as you nurse. Once you begin nursing, breast milk applied after each feeding will help prevent dryness and cracking around the nipple; if you apply breast creams, be sure to apply them after, not before, you nurse. Even before childbirth, your breasts may leak enough fluid to require the use of breast pads.

When you begin nursing, continue eating the same well-balanced diet as you did throughout pregnancy. In general, it is a good idea to increase your intake of fluids to a total of two or three quarts a day. At least one quart (four eight-ounce glasses) should consist of whole or low-fat milk to ensure that you get adequate protein and calcium. Or substitute other dairy products for the milk, such as yogurt, cheese, or ice cream (see *Breast-feeding and Nutrition*, page 346). Lactating takes extra energy, so make an effort to get enough rest. Avoid smoking and excessive alcohol intake. Lactation is not the time to diet; as long as you are nursing, you may not be able to shed much of your pregnancy-related weight. Emotional tension, some of which is unavoidable during the first few months after giving birth, can temporarily decrease milk flow, but it will not affect its quality.

Sometimes, circumstances arise that complicate a woman's intention to breast-feed. With few exceptions, though, women who are determined to breast-feed their infant can and should nurse regardless of such circumstances. For women who deliver by cesarean section, although it may be a bit more difficult to get started, there is no reason not to breast-feed (see page 355). Mothers who give birth to premature infants or to more than one baby can also nurse. For babies who are too small and weak to suck, milk can be expressed and fed through a tube until they are strong enough to nurse. In the event that intensive care treatment of an infant necessitates prolonged separation, mothers can usually make arrangements with the staff to nurse part-time and to express milk at other times.

Many nursing mothers who must take medication are concerned about the effect of the drugs on their milk. Talk to your health-care practitioner to find out whether the drugs you are taking will pass through the milk to the baby, and whether substitution, modification of dosage, or elimination for a specific length of time is possible. In almost all instances, nursing can and should continue.

Frequently, lactation can be restimulated in women who initially choose not to nurse or who stop breast-feeding for some reason. Allow your baby to suckle often. Even though it may be frustrating, with time and patience, milk may well flow again.

La Leche League (9616 Minneapolis Avenue, Franklin Park, Ill. 60131) is an important source of information, advice, literature, and support concerning all aspects of breast-feeding.

Most mothers, even those who embrace fully the experience of breast-feeding, find it necessary to provide a supplemental bottle. In so doing, they are able to leave their infant for an extended time in the care of another. An occasional bottle also gives the father the opportunity to be directly involved in feeding the baby, sometimes allowing him to attend to the middle-of-the-night feeding while the mother sleeps.

Women who choose to supplement breast-feeding with bottles can use a breast pump or can express breast milk by hand. Breast milk can be stored safely in a refrigerator for up to twenty-four hours or in the freezer for up to three months, although frozen milk loses some of its nutritional and immunological value. Formula can also be used. However, if you use formula to supplement more than one or two daily feedings, your milk supply will begin to diminish.

Bottle Feeding. Despite the many advantages to breast-feeding, some women choose to feed their baby formula. For some, the intimacy and exposure of breast-feeding are uncomfortable. For others, breast-feeding requires a degree of availability and flexibility that is not practical in their lives. They like the ease and freedom bottle feeding affords them.

Disposable bottles, bottle liners, and nipples have made bottle feeding easier now than ever before. Today's manufactured formulas are safe and, if used properly, will keep your baby healthy and strong. A particular advantage to bottle use is that anyone can feed, therefore freeing the mother for other activities. Also because it is clear exactly how much formula a baby takes, mothers often feel confident that their baby is getting adequate nutrition.

Formula, which is usually a mixture of water, processed cow's milk, vitamins, and minerals, is available in powdered milk form, concentrated liquid, and ready-to use liquid. All are easily prepared for single bottles. Once formula is in a nursing bottle, it can be stored in the refrigerator for a few hours. Since the milk may not be heated uniformly, never warm bottles in a microwave, to eliminate the risk of scalding the baby. Discard any formula left over from a feeding.

Pediatricians differ in their recommendation concerning how best to clean bottles. Although some recommend that bottles be sterilized for the first three months of the baby's life, most assert that careful washing and rinsing, perhaps boiling the nipples, are sufficient to clean the bottles for formula. Tap water in most communities is safe and bacteria-free. Bottles and nipples can also be run through the dishwasher.

Formula should be warmed to body temperature. Test the temperature by dropping a bit on the inside of your wrist. Warming bottles in a microwave can cause the formula to heat unevenly; though a few drops can feel safe to you, your infant can ingest extremely hot portions of the liquid and be severely burned.

Most bottle-fed babies take their first feeding within six hours of birth. By the end of the first week of life, an infant probably will want between six and nine bottles in a twenty-four-hour period. A bottle feeding can last from five to twenty-five minutes, depending on the baby's eagerness and sucking strength. Hold and cuddle the baby while feeding him or her the bottle; this way, you both benefit from the physical closeness of the feeding experience. Propping up a bottle while the infant lies on his or her back may cause the baby to choke.

Until babies are six months old, they absorb breast milk or formula most efficiently, thereby receiving all the nutrition they need. In most cases, delay introducing solid foods into the baby's diet until he or she is four to six months old. Even then, babies should continue to receive formula or breast milk at least until they are a year old.

The water content of both breast milk and formula is high. So although water is essential for an infant to remain healthy, if the baby is feeding well, the amount of water he or she will ingest through normal feedings will be adequate. However, some babies like to have water from a bottle between feedings.

BREAST-FEEDING AND NUTRITION

There are very few instances when a mother's milk does not suit her baby. In the vast majority of cases, mother's milk is the ideal food, providing all the nutrients and calories needed for healthy development. Nevertheless, since what the mother consumes finds its way into the milk, often affecting its amount, quality, and even taste, women should give some thought to what they themselves ingest.

Women who are nursing need to consume extra calories—between five hundred and eight hundred more than usual—in order to compensate for the calories delivered to the baby as milk. These extra calories guarantee good milk production. Avoid going too long between meals.

Select foods to replenish nutrients otherwise lost in manufacturing milk. Eat foods that ensure additional protein—and consume more meat, cheese, eggs, and addi-

tional calcium—more milk, which also provides vitamin D, and other dairy products. You may be advised to continue taking the calcium and vitamin supplement you took during pregnancy, which will likely include supplemental iron and vitamin D.

It is not a good idea to try to lose weight quickly after the baby is born. If you reduce the number of calories you consume dramatically, it will affect the amount and quality of your milk.

Caffeine passes into the breast and may make the infant irritable and contribute to sleeping problems if the mother's intake is very high. Alcohol also passes into the milk in low concentrations, but occasional, moderate alcohol use by nursing women is not a problem. Most drugs also pass into the milk but rarely are a problem. Review with your health practitioner any prescription or over-the-counter drugs you are currently taking or considering taking (below).

MEDICATION AND BREAST-FEEDING

In most cases, small quantities of any medication a nursing mother takes usually are transmitted to her infant via her breast milk. Thus, it is a wise precaution to mention to both your own health-care provider and your baby's doctor that you are nursing when you are preparing to take any medication, either prescription or over-the-counter.

Barbiturates in high doses, tranquilizers, and sleeping pills can induce drowsiness in the baby, which in turn causes problems in nursing. Laxatives, except for Milk of Magnesia and Ducolax, can induce diarrhea in the baby. Water pills and sulfa drugs can cause jaundice.

A large number of medications, if taken in the recommended dosages, are considered safe when breast-feeding, including antacids; antibiotics like ampicillin, cephalosporin, and erythromycin; mild laxatives and stool softeners; most pain relievers; and vitamins.

Newborns with particular vulnerabilities, such as many premature babies, can accumulate drugs in their bloodstream more readily, and therefore experience side effects. Although rare, it is possible for a newborn to have allergic reactions to medications as they are consumed in breast milk.

PROBLEMS RELATED TO BREAST-FEEDING

Most women experience some breast tenderness during pregnancy, the postpartum period, and breast-feeding. The best way to prevent sore breasts is to wear a supportive bra, twenty-four hours a day if necessary. To prepare your breasts during pregnancy, wash them with soap and water, then dry the nipples briskly with a stiff terry cloth towel. This will help toughen the nipples for lactation.

Engorgement, a condition that can develop a few days after delivery when a woman's milk comes in, causes breasts to become painfully swollen, hard, and sore and makes nursing difficult. Women who nurse regularly according to the baby's demands from birth on often find that engorgement is minimal. For women who do not nurse regularly, engorgement may occur, usually becoming most painful on the second or third day after delivery.

One source of relief is to keep the breasts empty by nursing frequently or by expressing milk manually or with a breast pump for a few days. Applying ice packs, heat from hot showers, warm compresses, and heating pads can also ease the discomfort. Also wearing a bra that offers good support and massaging the breast to promote circulation and letdown will help. In the most severe cases, pain medication can be prescribed by your health-care professional.

For mothers who do not plan to breast-feed, there have been some attempts recently to prevent engorgement with hormonal therapy; this is effective only within seventy-two hours after delivery and is often avoided because of potential medication side effects.

Cracked nipples, which are common among breast-feeding mothers, make nursing painful. If there are soreness and cracking around the nipples, limit nursing time to ten or fifteen minutes on each breast. It is important to keep nipples as dry as possible, since moist nipples tend to chap and crack. Some women find that using a hair dryer to dry them after nursing helps, as does exposure to air. Applying vitamin E oil or other breast creams to cracked nipples after nursing (not before) can help them heal.

Small, hard lumps in your breast can indicate *blocked milk ducts*. Most of the time, these lumps will disappear on their own. If they persist, massage your breast and apply warm compresses. If the lumps do not go away, check with your clinician; there may be a pus-filled abscess that will need to be drained (see page 381).

Breast infection, or *mastitis*, is not uncommon during the postpartum period, when bacteria from the baby's mouth are introduced into the breast, usually through cracks in the nipple. Early symptoms of breast infection are tenderness, redness, and fever. Parts of the breast become hard and hot. Antibiotics, such as penicillin, are commonly prescribed. Continue nursing to empty your breast. The antibiotics will not hurt your infant, although you may notice that the baby's stool will change in color. If the infection fails to clear up in a few days, an abscess can form, which will require surgical drainage.

If you have any of these problems while in the hospital after delivery, the facility may have trained and certified lactation consultants who may be able to offer guidance.

POSTDELIVERY RECUPERATION

Immediately after childbirth, a woman's body begins to undergo tremendous changes as it returns to its prepregnancy state. At delivery, the top of the uterus (*fundus*) can be felt above the bellybutton. For the first few days, it will feel round and solid, a bit like a grapefruit. At the same time, the uterus continues to contract mildly, thus stemming subsequent bleeding.

Throughout this process, called *involution*, the uterus reduces in size and becomes firm.

If a woman delivers in a hospital or birthing center, nurses may press on and massage the abdomen to check the uterus's firmness. You may be encouraged to massage it as well. Breast-feeding stimulates involution by releasing hormones that trigger contractions. It usually takes less than six weeks for the uterus to reach its nonpregnant size, although by the tenth day after birth, you may no longer be able to feel it above the pubic bone.

Common Discomforts. As the uterus continues to shrink, women commonly experience periodic cramping, called *afterpains*. These uterine contractions are more strongly felt during breast-feeding. Some women have found that heating pads applied to the abdomen reduce the sensation.

As the uterine lining sloughs off, it is expelled in a discharge called *lochia*. At first, the discharge resembles heavy menstrual flow. In a few days this vaginal discharge normally turns from red to pink to brown or yellow. However, if bleeding lasts for more than four weeks, is excessively heavy, or smells bad, consult your health-care provider. Infection is uncommon during the early postpartum period.

It may take a while for your bowels to start up again and to become regular after delivery. A bowel movement may not occur for a day or two. Not surprisingly, many women worry that if they strain, they will tear their episiotomy stitches or aggravate hemorrhoids. Also, as internal organs readjust to their normal position, a woman may experience constipation and trouble with urinating. Just relax and let your body do its work. Once you're home, drink liquids to keep bowel movements soft and to guard against urinary tract infections. Eat bran and prunes. Sometimes health-care providers will recommend stool softeners if women are having particular difficulty.

Wash the vaginal area with warm water, usually by using a squeeze bottle, when you urinate or change your sanitary napkin. This helps keep the area clean.

There may be significant discomfort in the perineal area as stitches from an episiotomy heal. This discomfort can last for several weeks. Ice packs applied to the area can reduce swelling and ease pain. Some women find relief with warm sitz baths or heat from a heat lamp starting a day or so after delivery. Also, premoistened gauze pads, held in place by a sanitary napkin, can help, although some find that keeping the area dry works better. If the pain is particularly disconcerting, sitting on an inflatable doughnut-shaped cushion or pillow can lessen direct pressure on the incision.

The abdominal wall muscles remain stretched after childbirth. When a woman first stands up after delivery, these muscles, pushed out by the intestines, fall forward. As a result, a woman may have a still-pregnant appearance. In the next few days, the abdomen will begin to firm up. Usually, a few months will pass before a woman returns to her prepregnancy weight. Meanwhile, Kegel exercises just after delivery, then gentle abdominal exercises and leg lifts, will help restore muscle tone (see *Kegel Exercises*, page 494).

In most cases, women can shower soon after childbirth. Baths can be resumed two or three weeks later. As tissues rid themselves of excess fluid stored during pregnancy, women typically urinate and drink more than usual. The sudden drop in estrogen level can cause night sweats. Some women also experience hot flashes when their milk lets down.

Baby Blues. Pregnancy hormones still present in the postpartum stage can cause mood swings. A women may have unexplained crying spells and fret that she cannot possibly be a good enough mother. A degree of postpartum sadness is normal, especially given the combination of pregnancy hormones still present in the bloodstream, the extreme exhaustion many women experience after childbirth, and the unpredictable sleep patterns that result as mothers get used to having a baby at home and the baby gets used to sleeping outside the womb. If, however, the "baby blues" continue for an extended period or become extreme, they could indicate a serious clinical depression and professional help should be sought (see page 352).

Sex. Couples vary as to when they resume sexual intercourse. Sexual intercourse is usually avoided for four to six weeks after a cesarean section or vaginal delivery. Vaginal discomfort, breast tenderness and engorgement, physical fatigue, and lack of interest due to the new demands and concerns of parenthood may put sex on the back burner for a while.

Women who breast-feed may not menstruate until they wean the baby. Otherwise, menstruation usually begins two or three months after birth. Even before a woman's period returns, it is possible for her to get pregnant. Therefore, it is important that a woman practice some form of birth control during this time unless she wants to conceive again soon. If you have been using a diaphragm, the size of your vagina may have altered as a result of childbirth; check with your health-care provider about having a new one fitted. Use of birth-control pills without estrogen and condom use might also be considered.

Sleep. A woman tends to be extremely tired for the first few hours after delivery. Regardless of how excited she may be after the birth of her baby, it is important that she get as much rest and sleep as she can. This holds true for the early months of the baby's life as well. With a new baby at home whose own sleep schedule may be erratic and unpredictable, and the new demands and concerns of motherhood, it is not unusual for a woman to become overly tired and irritable. Whereas with a first baby, it may be possible to nap when the baby naps, with older children at home, finding time to catch up on sleep becomes more problematic. If possible, ask your partner, family members, and friends to help out with older children so that you can rest. Women who limit visiting during the first few weeks, let some of the household chores go, and listen to their own body in order to set their pace tend to recover quickly and more completely from the physical strain of childbirth.

Work. These days, children are more likely than not to have a working mother. More than half of all women return to work within the first year of their baby's life. Almost half of all married couples of childbearing age are "two-worker" families. So in addition to assuming the role of caregiver, developing a relationship with this new family member, and reorganizing her other important relationships, the mother may also need to find some manageable balance between the needs of her children and the demands of her job. Just as the complex reality of motherhood and of her new baby is beginning to come into focus, the new mother must entertain plans and decisions concerning the time when she will move—both actually and emotionally—between home and workplace. Early on, there is growing pressure for a woman to struggle with the questions of whether, when, and how to return to work.

Planning for child care is now a common part of the childbirth experience. The need for many women to secure high-quality, affordable child care—whether in the form of institutional day-care programs; smaller, family day-care providers; or at-home care by nannies, sitters, and au pairs—may add stress to the mix.

Taking Care of Yourself. No matter how quickly you feel you have recovered from the birth experience, it is important to take things slowly during the early days after giving birth. Resuming strenuous activity too soon can prolong the healing process and leave you feeling exhausted a week or two later.

Keep visitors to a minimum and let other people take care of the household chores and older children. Ask your partner, friends, family, and neighbors to run errands and bring in meals. Perhaps you can hire homemaking and support services for the first couple of weeks. For at least six weeks, set aside extra time for rest and gentle exercise.

As time passes, many women assume, without much thought or a conscious plan, the role of primary caregiver, not only to their infants, but to all members of their family. In addition to providing child care, they take on primary responsibility for household chores and for preparation of meals. In the process, it is not uncommon for women to bury their own needs for adult company, nurturing, and sexuality. Frequently, they neglect their own physical and mental health. However, the time after childbirth is a time that offers new dimensions and new definitions to the concept of caring. It is essential that there be a place, within this new concept of caring, for the mother herself.

VAGINAL DRYNESS

Vaginal dryness may develop during breast-feeding when estrogen production decreases. This can cause the vaginal walls to become thinner and less elastic, resulting in soreness, burning, or itching of the vagina and in bleeding after intercourse. When this condition produces little more than slight daily discomfort, it can make sex a painful and thus problematic experience.

Treatment Options: When this condition develops as a result of breast-feeding, it is almost always temporary. In the meantime, a water-soluble lubricant or estrogen cream can alleviate discomfort during intercourse. Moreover, regular intercourse stimulates circulation in the vaginal area and keeps the tissue pliant. (See also page 506.)

POSTPARTUM BLUES AND DEPRESSION

The prevailing image of the postpartum period—as promoted by popular culture—depicts a woman and her partner as slipping somewhat anxiously but nonetheless smoothly into their new roles as parents. Despite occasional clumsiness around baths and diapers, despite sleep-deprived nights and milk-splattered blouses, the new mother embraces her maternal responsibilities and relishes her maternal feelings— perhaps at the same time as she prepares to return to work and coordinates child care. Mysteriously, but naturally—or so goes the mythology—mother and child develop a loving bond that permits mother to tolerate the most troublesome occurrences in her maternal life happily.

But the reality for many women is that the period following the birth of a child, whether it is the first, second, third, or fourth child, is filled with complicated feelings. Love and bonding tend to evolve erratically, in fits and starts, as do maternal feelings. For most women there are times when they are delighted to be mothers, and other times when they wonder just whose idea this whole thing was.

During the postpartum period, a woman's body goes through abrupt hormonal changes. She experiences sudden changes in both her general life-style and her day-to-day occupations and preoccupations. Furthermore, her own identity, her idea of who she is, undergoes rapid and drastic shifts in order to accommodate her new role as mother. Given all these changes, it is not surprising that so many women experience some sort of "baby blues."

Postpartum blues, the slight depression many women experience after childbirth, may surface in the first few days after the initial excitement of childbirth or weeks later, when the reality of the demands and changes brought on by the birth of a child becomes clearer. Instead of the thrill you thought you'd experience at the birth of your child, you may feel let down or overwhelmed. More often than not, as time passes, and you and your family make adjustments to the baby, your body heals a bit, and you are able to sleep, the blues will pass.

For some 10 to 15 percent of women, however, the postpartum period brings on or exacerbates a severe clinical depression. These women find that the time following childbirth falls under the shadow of dark, helpless feelings. They feel overcome, unmotivated, tired for no special reason, and hopelessly mired. They lack energy and vision to see beyond their immediate situation. In a clinical depression, these feelings do not necessarily subside with time. Often, because women feel embarrassed at their lack of joyous feelings, they do not talk about their depression. Moreover, because clinicians tend to focus on a woman's physical well-being, postpartum depression goes largely undiagnosed and untreated.

Women who have had previous postpartum depressions, depressive episodes, or manic-depressive illnesses are at higher risk for development of serious depression after childbirth. Also, a difficult or prolonged birth, an unwanted pregnancy, or a premature or ill infant predisposes a woman to postpartum depression.

During the postpartum period two very powerful types of stress bear down on the new mother. Physical stress from the dramatic reduction of estrogen and progesterone no doubt plays a role in triggering depression. This hormonal vulnerability is not unlike premenstrual depression in which women are particularly sensitive to mood swings. Some clinicians recommend antidepressive medications to address the chemical implications. Moreover, recent clinical research has indicated that postpartum depression can be addressed chemically, through progesterone therapy. However, there are clearly a number of nonchemical components to postpartum depression that need to be addressed as well.

The second powerful type of stress that a new mother confronts entails changes in her life circumstances. After all the drama surrounding the last weeks of pregnancy, labor, and delivery, a let-down reaction is common. A woman beginning her new life with baby is tired, and, too often, virtually alone. Her natural routine and sleep rhythms shift. For women accustomed to working, staying home entails an enormous adjustment, one that some women make more readily than others. In addition to forgoing extra and independent income, most at-home mothers miss expressing themselves and utilizing their skills in an adult world and having adult conversations that do not revolve around the baby. For women who go back to work soon after their childbirth, the additional exhaustion brought on by work as well as the ambivalence about leaving the baby naturally stir up powerful emotions. Finally, many women are concerned about the way they look and are eager to regain their prepregnancy figure. If they are breast-feeding, they may not be able to lose weight as quickly as they would like.

Studies have shown that the degree to which a woman experiences isolation and loss of control determines in large part her vulnerability to postpartum depression. Factors such as her partner's participation in the process of having and caring for the child, her capacity to stay engaged in or cultivate new interests outside the home, her ability to rely on friends and family for help and advice, and her access to other adults greatly shape a woman's emotional recovery from and response to childbirth.

There are a number of things you can do for yourself to mitigate the blues. First, get as much sleep as possible. Nap when the baby naps. Don't be so concerned with domestic chores that you fail to provide time for yourself. It is sometimes easy for a woman to become so baby-centered that she loses touch with the other people and things that give her pleasure and that challenge her. Stay involved in interests outside the home, even if on a more limited basis.

At the same time, don't forget your partner in all this. A loving and supportive partner can help ease the transition and remind a new mother of the woman she was before the baby was born.

Finally, if the blues continue for more than a few weeks or progress to the point where everything seems dark, if it is hard to get out of bed in the morning, and you find yourself unable to relate to the baby and to others around you, talk to your health-care practitioner. Clinical depression is effectively treated with therapy and medication.

MEAGAN'S STORY

Before the birth of her child, Meagan fully expected that her experience after childbirth would match the picture of motherhood she'd compiled from movies, television, magazine articles, and books. Meagan was more than a little unsettled when her actual experience diverged dramatically from that image.

For weeks, she looked upon her child as a stranger, an intruder, someone who quite suddenly took her away from her work and herself. She was always tired, and without the routine of her work, she found very little reason to get out of bed. Her husband would take the baby in to her before he left for work. She'd nurse the baby, then the two of them would fall back to sleep. Most days, she wouldn't shower and dress until after lunch, and there'd be days when she'd dress only just before her husband came home.

Some days she'd pack up the baby in a front pack and walk down to the playground, but they never stayed long. Other days, Meagan would put the baby in his infant seat and drive to the supermarket. Otherwise, she'd spend days in the house, watching the baby nap, reading magazines, waiting for her husband to get home so she could have adult conversation. At first, her friends and colleagues came by to see the baby, but after a couple of weeks, even that stopped. Luckily, her mother visited often, and together they would take the baby out for walks or to the mall so that they could get some shopping done.

Around the time her baby was three months old, Meagan noticed that when he was awake—which was more of the time—he was much more alert. At the playground, he'd watch the leaves or birds around him or follow the noise of the other children. As they spent more time outside, Meagan met other new mothers and a woman she had met in her childbirth class invited her to join a play group. Once a week, mothers with children the same age got together to talk. As Meagan began to share her experiences with other new mothers, as she began to ask questions about child care and motherhood and to hear that other women had similar experiences, questions, and impressions, her vague depression began to lift.

It wasn't long after this that her mother offered to baby-sit on a regular basis. Meagan could express enough breast milk to allow her to go to an occasional movie during the day, join a book group, and go out to dinner once in a while with her husband. Because the baby was napping on a more predictable schedule, she found time to catch up on her sleep, as well as on a couple of books she'd been meaning to read. By the time her baby began crawling at seven months, Meagan found that she had both the energy and desire to keep up with him.

POST–CESAREAN SECTION RECUPERATION

The average hospital stay for women who have had a cesarean section is between two and three days. After a cesarean, women undergo the usual changes that follow a vaginal birth as well as the physical reactions attendant on a major surgical procedure. Although there is not the perineal pain of an episiotomy, there can be considerable pain from the incision and the stitches under the abdominal scar.

For the first day or so after a cesarean, a woman will feel weak, sick, and sore around the incision. For twenty-four to forty-eight hours, she will probably be hooked up to an intravenous tube for nutrition, and a catheter for draining the bladder for about twenty-four hours. Many women also experience gas pains and constipation; eating light, easily digested foods for the first few days will help.

Most women are able to walk around within a day after a cesarean. Walking may be painful, but it helps the digestive system get going again and prevents blood clots from forming in your leg veins. Also, your health-care provider may be able to recommend certain exercises that promote healing and restore muscle tone.

Occasionally, especially with a midline incision, holding and breast-feeding the baby may be difficult or uncomfortable. Many women worry that the initial feelings of discomfort will impede bonding. In most cases, despite initial feelings of discomfort that follow the surgery, women can successfully nurse after cesarean. Some women find that using supportive pillows or lying on one side helps as they hold and nurse the baby. Also, during the first day or so, if the IV interferes with nursing, ask a health attendant to arrange it in a less obtrusive way.

Women who have undergone a cesarean section will likely need additional support from their partner and additional help when they and their baby return home. Ask your partner, family, and friends to lend a hand or, if finances allow, hire someone experienced to come in for a few days. Avoid heavy lifting and housework for at least the first week or two. Use the muscles in your arms, not your abdomen, to lift the baby, and bend at the knees, not at the waist.

In order to prevent irritating the area around the incision, wear loose clothing. A light dressing on the incision might also lessen irritation. As the area heals, you may experience pulling, twitching, brief pain, and itching. If you are in pain, talk to your health-care provider about taking a mild pain reliever. If the pain becomes persistent, if the area around the incision turns red, or if a discharge oozes from the wound, call your clinician. The incision may have become infected.

Also, talk to your clinician about resuming sexual intercourse after a cesarean. You may be advised to wait four to six weeks before making love.

POSTPARTUM MEDICAL CARE

The Baby. An infant's very first checkup will be performed in the delivery or birthing room. There, and again in the nursery, the baby's general health, physical condition, and newborn reflexes will be assessed. Then, assuming all things are on track, the baby goes home.

Yet parental concern and puzzlement about the newborn's health and well-being do not vanish as they carry the baby over the threshold. As a result, the series of well-baby checkups that most pediatric practitioners recommend for the first year of a baby's life offers parents the opportunity to address many of their natural anxieties. In addition, it provides another occasion through which new parents come to know their new baby.

Each health-care practitioner will have his or her own approach to the well-baby checkups. The way in which the physical examination is organized and the number and types of evaluations performed will vary according to the needs of the individual child. In general, unless there are special considerations—if, for example, the newborn has jaundice, was premature, or has any adjustment problems such as difficulty in establishing breast-feeding, the first well-baby checkup takes place at two weeks of age. If the baby was discharged within the first two days of life, the first checkup may take place within the next two days. Depending on the clinician's approach, subsequent visits may be scheduled each month for the first six months or for the entire first year.

Generally, the health-care provider will ask about the adjustment you, the baby, and the rest of the family are making. Specifically, he or she will be interested in the baby's eating, sleeping, and general progress. The baby's weight, length, and head circumference will be measured, and progress since birth will be charted. Vision and hearing will be assessed. The physical examination will likely include evaluations, either through observation, palpation, or use of stethoscopes and other instruments, of all or most of the following: heart, hips, hands and arms, feet and legs, back and spine, eyes, ears, nose, mouth, throat, neck, thyroid and lymph glands, fontanel (the soft spot on top of the baby's head), respiration and respiratory function, genitalia, anus, and femoral pulse in the groin. The clinician will also examine the skin for color, tone, rashes, lesions, and birthmarks. Overall movement and such behavior as ability to cuddle and to relate to adults will be assessed as well.

Your clinician will offer a general idea of what to expect in the next months in terms of feeding, sleeping, development, and infant safety. He or she might recommend a fluoride supplement if it's needed in your area.

These checkups provide an ideal time to ask more general questions you might have about the baby and baby care. This is also the time to express concerns that have arisen in the period that the baby has been home. It might also be helpful to ask specifically about working with the pediatrician. What, for example, are guidelines for calling when the baby is sick? What would necessitate a call in the middle of the night? Is there a time to call for nonemergency questions? How can the doctor be reached at times other than normal office hours?

The Mother. Unless you have had a cesarean, in which case you will likely see your clinician one to three weeks after childbirth to check on your incision, your practitioner will schedule a checkup around six weeks after delivery. At that visit, your clinician will assess your blood pressure; your weight (which ordinarily will drop twenty pounds after delivery); the size, shape, and location of your uterus; and your cervix, your vagina, the episiotomy or laceration repair site, your breasts, and hemorrhoids or varicose veins. He or she will likely discuss any questions you might have concerning your recovery or general health and your plans for birth control.

BACK TO NORMAL

By the time a woman makes her first postpartum visit to her health-care practitioner, around six weeks after delivery, she will more than likely have begun to get glimpses of her old self. By that time, her baby will have begun to settle into a manageable rhythm, her body will have pretty much recovered from the effects of childbirth, her episiotomy or her cesarean incision will have gone a long way toward healing, and usually she will have had longer stretches of sleep so that sleep deprivation will be less severe.

Within a month, most women can pack their maternity clothes away. It may be a few more months, however, before they can fit into their old jeans. How quickly a woman sheds the remainder of her pregnancy weight and regains her prepregnancy shape depends on how much she gained during pregnancy. Women who gained more than the average twenty-five to thirty-five pounds may have a harder time taking the weight off after the baby is born.

Because they need extra calories as they produce milk, women who breast-feed may find that some of the extra weight will linger until after they wean their baby. It is important that nursing mothers not reduce their caloric intake drastically; this could alter the quality of their breast milk.

There are some ways, however, that the body changes during pregnancy that will likely remain a permanent part of a postpregnant woman's body. The body's structure shifts slightly as the joints, which loosened during pregnancy, now tighten back up. These changes may not be noticeable or they may be significant enough to increase a woman's shoe or dress size. Women may notice that the shape of their abdomen has changed a bit, in a way that not even exercise will fully correct.

CIRCUMCISION

Circumcision is the surgical removal of the foreskin (the *prepuce*), which is the loose skin around the head of the male penis. The prepuce functions to protect the *meatus*, or the opening to the urethra, the tube through which urine passes from the bladder. When the foreskin is removed through circumcision, the bulbous head or *glans* of the penis is exposed.

Up until a generation or so ago, circumcision was considered by many to be a medical necessity. The most commonly cited advantage was that a circumcised penis was easier to clean. As a result, many newborn males were circumcised routinely just after birth. Today, about 70 percent of American males born undergo the procedure.

Although circumcision is no doubt painful, local anesthesia is generally not used since there is a small risk to the infant of a drug reaction. When circumcision is performed by a skilled practitioner, the risk of complications for the baby is minimal. However, in rare occasions, hemorrhage or infections can occur.

In the first few days after circumcision, petroleum jelly is applied when diapers are changed to prevent irritation to the glans. If your baby is not circumcised, do not retract the foreskin in order to clean the glans during baths. Merely wash the uncircumcised penis with a soft washcloth, soap, and water, as you would any other part of your baby's body.

BIRTHMARKS

Birthmarks in newborns are common and generally present little cause for concern. There are a number of different types of birthmarks.

Salmon patches, also called stork bites, are small, flat, pinkish spots that appear most often on the area between the eyebrows, on the eyelids, upper lip, and back of the neck. Comprising a collection of small blood vessels, salmon patches occur in 30 to 50 percent of all newborns. They often become more noticeable when the child flushes in response to a rise in temperature or to a bout of crying. Facial patches generally fade with time; those on the nape of the neck, however, often remain.

Hemangiomas are benign tumors composed of newly formed blood vessels. *Strawberry hemangiomas* appear as bright red, protruding lesions anywhere on the body, most commonly on the chest, face, scalp, and back. As a rule, these lesions initially grow, then remain at a fixed size. Then they fade, usually before a child is five, and almost always before he or she is nine. Approximately 10 percent of children with strawberry hemangioma have slight discoloration or puckering of the skin after the mark is gone.

A *cavernous hemangioma* appears as a red–blue spongy mass. It is made up of blood-filled tissue. Because these are more deeply rooted, the progression is harder to predict than with a strawberry hemangioma. Some disappear without treatment.

A *port-wine stain*, a flat hemangioma, consists of dilated capillaries most often across the face. The size varies; these birthmarks can cover as much as half the body's surface. Though permanent, a port-wine stain can be treated, usually in adolescence and adulthood, with laser therapy.

SLEEPING PROBLEMS

By the time the babies were three months old, the hottest topic at the neighborhood play group was sleep—or lack thereof. No matter how hard Janie tried to keep her son awake, he inevitably fell asleep while nursing. Then the minute she laid him in his crib, his head would pop up and he'd begin to cry. She would have to nurse him before he fell back to sleep, only to have the routine begin again.

Kara's daughter went to sleep easily after being rocked and sung to. But it seemed that the older she got, the more she cried out to be nursed in the middle of the night. Kara was now waking up three times a night to nurse her baby. More often than not, her daughter ate little but lay happily in her mother's arms until she was put back down. Though Kara enjoyed spending the time with her baby, she was finding it harder to fall back to sleep, to the point where she was hardly able to cope with the day. Vivienne couldn't face the middle-of-the night crying, so now, once her son begins to cry, she just takes him into bed with her, where he's able to sleep through the night. The problem now is that she can't sleep because she has become nervous she'll roll over on him. Not to mention that his presence has eliminated any sex life she'd hoped to resume.

Whereas sleep problems are one of the most common complaints for mothers during the first year of a baby's life, they stem largely from well-meaning exhausted parents, who seek easy solutions to their baby's crying and their own sleep disruption. However, their short-term solutions can transmute into entrenched, long-term problems. Once sleep problems take root, they gain a momentum of their own, often rendering parents desperate and resolution inconceivable.

With sleep problems, prevention is generally easier than cure. Parents who, in the first few months, help their babies lull themselves to sleep avoid more intense struggles later. Babies who learn to put themselves to sleep initially can usually return to sleep each time in the night they emerge from deeper sleep.

By the time your baby is two months old, he or she should be out of your bed and in his or her own room. Although it may feel cozy and convenient to have your baby in bed with you, it only sets the stage for problems down the road when having an older child in bed with you may feel crowded and intrusive.

At two months, begin to discourage middle-of-the-night feedings. Do not wake a sleeping baby for late feedings. When your baby calls in the middle of the night, allow a few minutes to pass before going into the nursery. If the baby has not settled back down to sleep, nurse for a slightly shorter period of time than you would during the day. And keep to the business of nursing; avoid playing and making this time too entertaining. When you put the baby back into bed, speak in a soothing and reassuring voice. Let your baby know that you are in the next room but that nighttime is for sleeping.

At four months, few infants actually need a middle-of-the-night feeding. If your baby still cries out for one, it may be force of habit. Or your baby may be accustomed to the sociability of the midnight visit. Instead of offering a feeding or picking the baby up, try rubbing his or her back and speaking in a loving tone.

At six months, when a baby begins to experience anxiety around separation, it might help him sleep if he has a special transitional security object, such as a blanket or stuffed toy. Leaving the door to the room open or leaving a night-light on may help him feel less anxious. Pacifiers may work initially to lull the baby to sleep. All too often, however, problems arise when, after the baby falls off to sleep and drops the pacifier, he or she cries out for you in the middle of the night to retrieve it.

There will always be nights when you have to go into your children's rooms when they cry. If they learn to take comfort from your voice, perhaps as you gently rub their backs, they may internalize sufficient reassurance to be able to fall back to sleep most times on their own.

SIBLING RELATIONSHIPS

Before she got pregnant with her second child, Darlene couldn't imagine that she could love another child as much as she loved her first. As her due date approached, she worried about the ways in which having a baby around the house would affect her son.

After her daughter was born, Darlene looked at her son only to notice how suddenly big and clumsy he seemed. It was all very disconcerting. After all, only a month ago, he was her baby; now he was a three-year-old boy. Then one afternoon, as she lay in bed with her infant daughter and her son sat at her side flipping through a book, she glanced around her and felt deeply fortunate to have these two children. As she thought about it, she knew that they, too, were lucky to have each other.

Although much attention has been focused on feelings of insecurity and hostility that the birth of a brother or sister engenders, sibling relations play a pivotal role in a child's mental and social development. It is often the case that a parent is not able to give a second or third child the same undivided attention she did her first; yet, younger children enjoy the love and attention of persons not so much older than they are. Babies who come into families with children may seldom know what it is to have uninterrupted naps—if it isn't the loud play of the older children waking them up, it's their mother pulling them out of a deep sleep so that she can retrieve the other child from school—but they also will seldom know what it is to be lonely or bored. An infant with an older brother or sister may be subjected to poking and prodding, but at the same time, that infant will be cuddled, held, and generally entertained by an older child. Although parents may have to be especially vigilant in the early months to make sure that small toys and pieces of food don't make their way into the baby's mouth, and that the poking and prodding do not become dangerously rough, the interchange between siblings is delightfully valuable. The infant learns language, self-protection, cooperation, and imagination by watching and interacting with a sibling. At the same time, older siblings cultivate many of the same qualities as well as empathic and nurturing capabilities. Not only do sisters and brothers have a relatively safe arena in which to manage such social feelings as rivalry and jealousy, frustration and anger, but the very nature of their relationship, one rooted in love, shared history, and successful relational negotiations, provides the opportunity to forge a supportive and empathic bond that will continue to develop throughout their lives.

This is not to imply, however, that the relationship between siblings is always a smooth and simple matter. There are times when the exchange between them is extremely contentious and difficult for the parents to tolerate. Around the time a baby is nine months old, the word *rivalry* begins to attach itself naturally to the word *sibling*. At that age, the infant may well become intent on appropriating the older sibling's toys or just on asserting his or her authority.

It is not surprising that the older sibling would be provoked by this sudden intrusion to protest, either loudly or physically. There should be some comfort for parents in the knowledge that this phase will pass or, at least, that the most intense acrimony between brothers and sisters will likely not surface for many years, when parents are better prepared to handle or tolerate it.

TRAVEL WITH BABY

In the days before baby, Michelle gave little thought to traveling. When she had to fly out of town on a last-minute business trip, all she had to do was throw a few garments and toiletries into an overnight bag. And when she and her husband wanted to get away for a weekend, they could and did. Now that baby's here, though, just getting across town is a production, what with the diaper bag, the bottles, the stroller, the pacifier, and the baby's favorite toy, not to mention the need to take the baby's nap and feeding schedule into consideration. The logistics of going to Grandmother's for the weekend—forget someplace more exotic—is enough to exhaust her before she's even begun packing.

No doubt about it, travel takes on a whole new dimension once baby joins in. But with a bit of planning, new parents need not wait until their kids are off at college for their next excursion. Now, though, they may need to allow as much time preparing for a trip as taking one, but there are ways to make the preparation less cumbersome and the trip more pleasurable for all concerned. By the time your children are old enough to pack their own bags, you will have forgotten what it was like to need only a restless spirit to travel. But also, you may well have become an expert in family travel.

First and foremost, be realistic and flexible about your itinerary. It is not possible to keep the same pace you had when you were traveling without a child. Don't overschedule, and don't be overly ambitious. The best way to enjoy any trip with baby is to set a modest agenda and allow for plenty of unscheduled time.

Medical Precautions. If it's been a while since your last well-baby visit, schedule an appointment with your health-care provider to make sure your baby is in good health. At that time, discuss your proposed trip with your clinician. If you've recently been to the office, a telephone consultation may be all that's needed.

If your baby is on medication, be sure you have enough for the trip. You may want to carry a prescription in case the supply is lost or spilled. If the medication needs to be refrigerated, ask your clinician whether substitution is possible. If your baby has a cold, however mild, a stuffy nose may make the baby miserable, interfere with sleep, and cause ear pain during flying; ask the provider for a decongestant. For extended trips, ask for the name of a clinician at your destination.

Introducing Changes. Avoid making any unnecessary changes in the baby's schedule or routine just before a trip. For example, postpone weaning, introducing solids, or breaking the pacifier habit until you return home. Unfamiliar surroundings and routines will be hard enough for the baby without adding other stresses. If the baby is having sleep problems, the period just before a trip is not the time to try to correct them. The baby will probably have trouble sleeping in a new place anyway, and letting the baby cry it out in a hotel room or at Grandma's will only add to the stress of the trip.

Pack Wisely. As the saying goes, mothers don't get a vacation; they only get a change of scenery. Although you may think that you need just about every piece of clothing and equipment from your nursery in order to survive the change, the fact is, an efficient selection will make the scenery seem a bit less cumbersome. Some of the items to include in your baby baggage are small sizes of liquid baby soap, acetaminophen, rash ointment, disposable diapers, wipes, mix-and-match lightweight clothing (that dry fast after rinsing) in bright colors (that hide stains), socks, blankets, toys to amuse and comfort, a night light. It's easy to forget as you pack that unless you're off to a camping trip in the wild, you can usually find whatever it is that you left behind at home.

Air Travel. When scheduling, weigh the time of day or night you will begin your journey against your baby's natural rhythms. Take into consideration how your baby reacts to change and interruptions in his or her sleeping schedule. Sometimes it works to book a flight in the evening if you anticipate that the baby will be able to sleep on the plane. This will likely make the flight easier for you. Many parents prefer to reserve bulkhead seats, which give extra room to move around and allow the baby to sleep or play at your feet. If bulkhead seats are not available, request seats on the aisle, which make it easier to get up and down.

When making reservations, and again when you check in, ask whether it's possible to get a seat with an unoccupied seat next to it. You may have access to empty seats if you fly at off-peak times. If you take along the baby's infant seat, you may be able to buckle it into an empty seat—thus assuring greater safety for the baby as well as an opportunity for you to move around. Flights can seem particularly long when you have a baby in your lap for the entire time. Also, if the plane is not quite full, the baby may be able to crawl around and disturb fewer passengers.

Arrive early enough at the airport to take care of luggage and to preboard the plane. Coordinate feedings with takeoff and landing. Nursing or bottle feeding at these times can relieve some of the baby's ear pressure and pain caused by cabin air pressure changes. Give your baby a lot of fluids during the flight since air travel is dehydrating.

Trains. Board as early as possible to find a good seat. If your ride will be a long one, take plenty of toys in order to distract the baby.

Car Trips. Although driving is slower than other forms of transportation, it can give parents greater control of the trip. It is possible while driving, for example, to set your own pace, to stop where and when you like, and to make detours if they are needed. In order to make road trips as safe, comfortable, and enjoyable as possible, be sure that there are seat belts for all adults and older children, and car seats for the young children. Stop every two hours or so; otherwise the baby may become restless and cranky for long stretches on the road. Do not take the baby out of the car seat to nurse while the car is moving; use rest stops to nurse. Never leave a baby alone in a parked car.

Restaurants. Not long ago, babies were seldom seen in public eating places; many parents today include eating out, with or without baby, in their normal routine. Plan to eat early and quickly. Call ahead to make sure the restaurant is equipped with high chairs. You will be able to tell during this call whether the restaurant will welcome you and your baby. Be sensitive to other diners. If your baby is crying loudly, perhaps it is time to take him outside for a change of scenery. You and your adult companion may have to eat in shifts; one eats while the other strolls with the baby.

Accommodations. Even if you're taking a road trip during off-season, don't leave your accommodations to chance. Make reservations at motels and hotels. Nothing makes for crankier travel than finding one no-vacancy sign after another as night quickly descends. Also, by making reservations, you may be able to arrange for a crib in the room. Whenever possible, look for a hotel or motel that caters to families. You will probably have an uncomfortable stay in places that do not welcome or provide amenities for children.

Confirm both hotel and airline reservations the day before departure.

Finally, it is important to remember whose needs come first during travel. If the baby is happy, chances are the trip will go well.

REDEFINING INDEPENDENCE

Nancy remembers, just after her son was born, the moment that she realized her life and her sense of autonomy were changed forever. The baby was home with her mother-in-law, and Nancy was rushing back from the grocery store. She was walking down a city street, and she stepped out to cross in the middle of the block. She stopped herself. *I can never jaywalk again. What if I get run over? What would happen to the baby?* She walked thoughtfully to the end of the block and crossed at the light.

Indeed, an almost imperceptible yet momentous change occurs for most women when they become a mother. For some, work will never have the same obsessive, absolute hold on them that it did before the baby was born. For others, it becomes easier to miss the hottest movie or to forgo long, leisurely dinners out with friends. Suddenly, conversations focus on or weave in and out of the small details of domestic, maternal life. It now seems inconceivable that there was ever anything in your life called leisure time, or something called spontaneity. Now everything you do requires forethought, planning, and consideration.

Yet ask almost any mother and she will tell you that for every way her life has been circumscribed by children, it has been more than doubly enriched, just by the new dimension that caring for, playing with, holding a baby brings to loving. For women who work outside the home, mothering means struggling to strike a balance, both internal and external, between home and workplace. For women who choose to stay home, mothering means finding ways of reclaiming past interests and seeking out new ones.

Through her baby, through work, through adult relationships, and through personal enrichment, motherhood brings a woman an exquisite opportunity to expand and redefine her life.

Part IV

❧

MEDICAL DISORDERS AND DISEASES OF WOMEN

Even women who practice the good health disciplines discussed in Part I, Maintaining Your Health *(see page 1), do encounter, upon occasion, disorders and diseases. In the chapters that follow, the focus is on the diseases and disorders most common to women.*

In comprehensive fashion, disorders of the breast, urinary tract, vagina, cervix, uterus, and other organ systems are addressed. Other problems for which women are at particular risk are also discussed, including sexually transmitted diseases, endocrine and autoimmune disorders, skin problems, and cardiovascular disease.

CHAPTER 17

⁊

Breast Disorders

CONTENTS

The female breast carries an importance in our society that is both real and symbolic. The breast, along with the ability to breast-feed, distinguishes the female mammal from all other classes of vertebrates in the animal kingdom, representing the high degree of nurture and care that must be offered to her offspring. For humans, though, the female breast is charged with romantic and sexual significance as well.

Indeed, the word *breast* does more than conjure up warm, apple-pie images of motherhood.

Evaluations of mature female beauty put great emphasis on breasts and breast size. Furthermore, unlike a woman's genitalia—the vagina, clitoris, vulva, and uterus, which even today are considered "private parts"—her breasts are very much within the public imagination. Suggestive images bombard us from every direction: Breasts materialize to sell goods ranging from cars to alcohol, they assert themselves on billboards and in advertisements, and they dominate the pages of fashion magazines.

We are a breast-obsessed culture. And although there is no question that a woman's breasts are a central aspect of her sexuality and sexual pleasure, this very functional part of her anatomy has taken on fetishlike qualities almost to the point of becoming a discrete, sexual entity, removed from the context of a woman and her body.

Today, moreover, our feelings about our breasts too often include fear and panic—fear of disease, loss of breasts, loss of life. It seems that we can hardly pick up a newspaper or magazine without reading that the chance we or someone we know will have breast cancer is growing at an alarming rate. Although some of the fluctuation in statistics is associated with testing procedures and calculation, recent numbers indicate that each year breast cancer claims close to 44,000 women's lives in the United States alone.

This complex of social meanings can make it difficult to think about this part of our

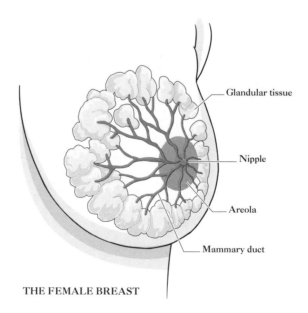

THE FEMALE BREAST

body in health-care terms. Yet, a solid, responsible understanding is necessary to ensure a healthy and enjoyable relationship between a woman and her breasts. There is no reason that every change in the feeling and texture of a woman's breast, every lump or discomfort, should sound an alarm. At the same time, it is imperative that changes be noticed and not be ignored. Lives can be saved—they *are* saved—when a woman is comfortable and familiar with her breasts, practices routine breast self-examination, has regular mammograms, and has regular breast examinations by her health-care provider.

In addition to reviewing those measures that can enhance a woman's breast health, we will discuss the various disorders that can affect the breasts. But, to begin, we will talk about the development and function of these glands we call breasts.

THEY'RE *YOUR* BREASTS

Linda's mother, grandmother, and older sister had large, round breasts. Linda took after her father's side of the family—and throughout her adolescence, her brother called her "flatso." During her teens, she felt inadequate and sometimes humiliated, especially when her mother took her shopping for bras. "Not much there to hold it down, huh, dearie?" one saleswoman once commented. It wasn't until Linda moved away from home in her early twenties that she discarded her padded bra.

Now in her forties, Linda is quite satisfied with the size and shape of her breasts. It wasn't her mother, or a man, or anyone but she who allowed her to accept and be happy with the breasts she had. She got comfortable with herself, as a woman, as a mother, and as a person. And suddenly other people's breasts—or their expectations— just didn't matter anymore.

As she went through puberty, Erika never gave much thought to her breasts—they weren't very big and it wasn't something she worried about. But in early adulthood, she was delighted to discover the intensely pleasurable sensations she felt around her breasts during lovemaking. They may not be the largest or the most perfect, she realized, but her breasts are really something special.

Claire remembers feeling both pleased and self-conscious when her breasts began to develop. She was younger than most of her friends, and pretty soon, much bigger than they in terms of breast size. She was actually buxom by the age of thirteen. She would walk down the halls at school hunched over, clutching her books to her chest, hoping that no one would notice her maturing breasts. But the boys noticed, and pretty soon she couldn't believe how popular she was.

Although Claire instantly liked the social appeal her breasts seemed to offer, it took her a while to put it into perspective. She had boyfriends who had an almost worshipful attitude toward her breasts. At first, she relished this, but later she came to think their attitude a bit silly. It made her angry when some boys (and, later, men) seemed to think her personhood was defined by her chest.

It was only after her daughter was born that Claire arrived at a fuller understanding of her breasts. Her breasts were beautiful to her, too—but for a different reason. They were the source of nutrition and nurture for her beautiful baby.

THE NORMAL BREAST

For all the emphasis placed on the "ideal" breasts, there is a wide range of differences in the size, shape, and feel of the female breast. Despite advertisers' insistence that there are exercises and devices that can alter the dimensions of a woman's breast, the baseline size and shape are determined by her genes. Since something like two thirds of the breast is made up of breast tissue, and about a third is fat surrounding lobules and ducts, the only way to alter breast size is to gain or lose weight. As our weight fluctuates, we gain and lose fat in the breast. Exercise affects breast size only insofar as it affects weight or body fat. Only pregnancy and plastic surgery can have more than a minor impact upon breast size.

Every normal female breast is, in essence, a large fatty gland, containing between twelve and twenty triangular lobes. Each of the lobes, arranged much like the spokes of a wheel around the nipple, has a central duct that opens at the nipple. The nipple is surrounded by a darker area (the color varies according to skin tone) called the *areola*, which contains small lubricating glands that help keep the nipple supple.

A girl's breasts begin to develop between the ages of eight and thirteen, typically one or two years before she begins to menstruate. The process is triggered when the hypothalamus signals the pituitary gland to begin secreting hormones during puberty (see *The Menstrual Cycle*, page 404). The female hormone estrogen is responsible for inducing the growth, division, and elongation of the breast's milk-producing system of glands and ducts, as well as the maturation of the nipples. The nipple begins to grow first, then a mound of tissue appears and develops around the nipple. Progesterone aids in the development of the alveoli, the cavities where milk is produced.

By the time Kailey was fifteen, she'd look at her naked body in the mirror and wonder whether her breasts were okay. They didn't look quite like the ones she'd seen in the bath oil ads in her fashion magazines or like those in the magazines her father kept under the bed. She thought they looked nice, but they weren't quite as round or smooth as she thought they should be.

Most adolescent girls long for perfect breasts. It may be disconcerting when they notice that one breast is larger than the other, or that the areola is larger or smaller, lighter or darker, than they had imagined it should be. These kinds of variations are perfectly normal. In addition, the areola is usually edged in small bumps which may sprout long, fine hairs. These details are often air-brushed out of popular depictions. Whether their breasts are large or small, round or conical, most women accept the shape and size they have by the time they reach their thirties.

Although genetics determines the size and shape, a woman may notice subtle—and sometimes not so subtle—changes in her breasts throughout her life. The texture and overall feel change, for example, as a woman's hormonal levels fluctuate. During the first half of a woman's monthly menstrual cycle, the ovaries release estrogen, causing cells within her breasts to grow and retain fluid. With the second half of her cycle, progesterone is released and, along with continued estrogen infusion, causes a further increase of blood flow to the breasts. As a result of these hormonal changes, some women experience swelling and soreness around their breasts prior to their period. Women with cystic breasts (see page 378) may notice that during this time small lumps swell and become sore as the sacs fill with fluid and semifluid material. Some women who take oral contraceptives have breast tenderness and some swelling. Unless a woman becomes pregnant during a cycle, her body naturally reverses the gland activity, and breast size and tenderness will decrease until her next cycle begins again.

A woman's breasts change again during pregnancy, when hormones from the placenta and pituitary gland cause them to become larger. Each breast may gain as much as a half pound. The duct system expands and branches, the number of glandular cells increases, and the number of cells in the connective tissue or stroma increases as well. As the breast develops according to hormonal signals to produce milk, a woman's nipples grow in size, and the areola enlarges and darkens. As the breast fills with milk during breast-feeding, the breast is further stretched. Breast size decreases once a woman stops nursing (see *Breast-feeding*, page 342).

Breasts change once more in menopause. Premenstrual tenderness that may have bothered a woman will disappear after menstruation ends. For women who suffer from cystic breasts, soreness and lumpiness may diminish or disappear altogether with menopause. However, many women find that some lumps have become permanent and will not shrink even after menopause. Older women may find that their breasts are softer and a bit less firm than they were thirty years before; this is because the proportion of fat in a woman's body increases with age, and stretching of supporting ligaments can cause her breasts to sag.

At the same time, as their bodies cease to produce estrogen, postmenopausal women face an increased risk of breast cancer. Although today there is a raging debate about the impact of estrogen replacement therapy and hormone replacement therapy on the development of breast cancer (see page 390), the best hope in the fight against malignancy is early detection. Thus, it is imperative that, from a very early age, women practice breast self-examination, have her breasts examined by her practitioner, and have periodic mammograms beginning in midlife.

TAKING CARE OF YOUR BREASTS

Now that Andrea is pregnant, she daydreams about what it will be like to be a mother. She thinks about nursing her baby but has questions about what nursing will do to the shape of her breasts. She always liked the way her breasts looked, and these days she is actually busty. She's embarrassed to admit that she's worried that after breast-feeding, she will have sagging breasts.

Beth is delighted with all the weight she's lost; all it took was a new regimen of eating sensibly and exercise. But what, she wonders, has happened to her breasts? They'd always been firm and round, and now they droop. How did that happen?

Although we may well have come to accept and thoroughly enjoy the breasts we have, there is little doubt that certain events in our lives—pregnancy, breast-feeding, and aging among them—take their toll.

Because our breasts are made up of tissue, ligaments, and fat, their size naturally varies with any variation in our weight. Any expansion influences the shape and shapeliness of our breasts. Moreover, during pregnancy and lactation the change is actually localized: The breast can double in size as the mammary ducts expand to produce milk. Whether the increase in size is due to weight gain or pregnancy, the breast acts like a sac that may resemble a deflated balloon once the enlarged ducts and additional fat are gone.

The best way to keep breasts firm is to keep weight as steady as possible. If you have recently experienced substantial weight loss, give your body time to readjust by engaging in a regular exercise program. Eventually your breasts may tighten up.

Your body will also return to a reasonable shape and firmness after pregnancy and lactation. Your choice to breast-feed should not be based on considerations of your breasts, for bottle feeding will not save your figure. Instead, invest in a good nursing bra, and wear it, even at night. Despite claims that cocoa butter and vitamin E will prevent stretch marks, the fact is that they don't.

BLEMISHES AND OTHER SKIN PROBLEMS

Like her facial complexion, the skin on a woman's breasts is not always smooth and clear. Breasts, too, are subject to dermatological eruptions that can be bothersome.

- *Allergies. Red, irritated areas or dry itchy nipples may signal allergy. Suspect your bra. Dye in the material, nickel in the clasp, or the detergent or fabric softener you use may cause contact dermatitis. Switch bras or laundering products. If this doesn't resolve the problem, contact your health-care professional, who may suggest treatment with a gentle cleanser and cortisone-based ointment. In rare instances, redness and localized swelling are caused by inflammatory breast carcinoma (see page 393) or Paget's disease of the nipple, which causes exema-like scaling and weeping (see page 393).*

- *Acne. Gentle cleanser, topical antibiotic, or acne medication will work if breakouts are caused by acne.*

- Cherry angiomas. *These small red masses are actually broken blood vessels and growths. They are harmless, but if you find them disconcerting, a dermatologist can remove them surgically.*
- Hair. *Hair growing from the edge of your areola is perfectly normal. If there is hair on the chest between the breasts, it may indicate hormonal imbalance, in which case a medical practitioner should be consulted.*
- Heat rash. *Sweat glands may become blocked on hot, humid days or during strenuous exercise, causing itchy red bumps to appear on your breasts. Dusting powder or cornstarch should clear up heat rash. If not, consult your health professional.*

BREAST SELF-EXAMINATION

An alarming number of women will have breast cancer at some point during their life. Estimates vary widely, but something like one in every nine women will have breast cancer at some time in her life. Approximately three fourths of these women will die of the disease.

The majority of breast lumps—almost 90 percent—are discovered by women themselves, either accidentally or during systematic self-examination. Generally, lumps found during self-examination tend to be small and in all probability would go undetected otherwise. Although 80 percent of all lumps biopsied are found to be noncancerous, malignancies discovered at this stage are more effectively treated, and it is more likely that a woman's breast and her life can be saved.

In one recent study of two groups of women, those who practiced monthly breast self-examination discovered their cancers at 2.1 centimeters in size, compared to 2.4 centimeters for those who examined themselves haphazardly, and 3.2 centimeters for women who never checked their breasts for lumps. The study was significant especially since the smaller the cancer at diagnosis, the better the prognosis.

Despite widespread evidence of its benefit, an estimated 50 percent of all women do not examine their breasts every month. Ironically, the group most diligent in practicing self-examination are women between the ages of eighteen and thirty-four—the adult age group actually *least* likely to have breast cancer.

Besides being such an effective method of fighting breast cancer, self-examination is free, can be done in the privacy of your home, and is easy to perform once you understand the basics.

No matter what your age, it is not too late (or too early) to start regular breast examination—and it can save your life.

Pick a Time. First, select a regular time each month. The best time for a woman who is still menstruating is a week after her period begins, since her breasts will be less lumpy and tender at that time of her cycle. If a woman has gone through menopause, is pregnant, or does not menstruate, she can pick a day and mark it on her calendar each month, thereby making it easier to incorporate it into her routine.

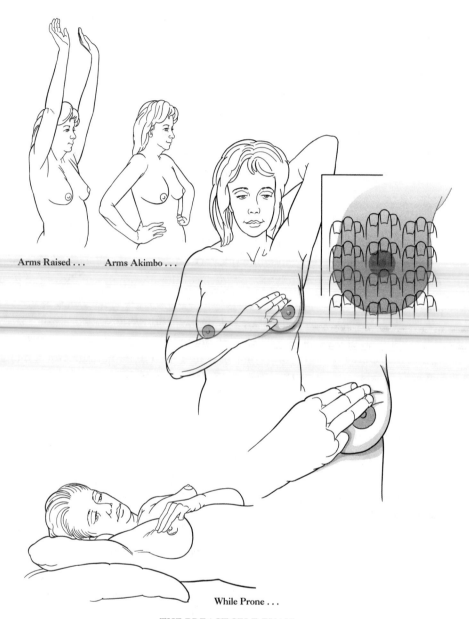

Arms Raised . . .   Arms Akimbo . . .

While Prone . . .

THE BREAST SELF-EXAM

A breast self-exam should consist of a careful, visual examination of the breasts with your arms raised, arms akimbo, and while prone. You are looking in particular for changes. Another key part of the self-exam involves feeling for lumps. With one arm behind your head, move the other hand in a series of rows. If you identify any lumps or changes, contact your health-care provider immediately.

Do It Unclothed. A good breast exam requires both visual and tactile senses. Begin your examination by stripping to the waist and standing in front of a mirror in good light. Notice how your breasts look. Raise your arms and look for new variations in the symmetry of both breasts. Are there any signs of puckering or dimples? Look at your nipples. Are they inverted? Inverted nipples can be normal, but a health-care professional should be consulted if this is a new development. Is there any sign of discharge? Look carefully while holding your arms at your sides, then with your hands on your hips, and finally with your hands held over your head.

Take a Shower. Now, step into the shower and soap your breasts. Picture each breast as a clock, with twelve o'clock at the top and six o'clock at the bottom. Place your left hand behind your head and examine your left breast with your right hand, using the pads of your second, third, and fourth fingers. Press down on your breast, using a small circular motion to feel for lumps as you move your hand from the twelve o'clock position to one o'clock, two o'clock, and downward.

When you return to the original twelve o'clock position, move your fingers closer to the nipple encircling the clock once again. Repeat this procedure, making the circle smaller each time, until you have checked the tissue around the nipple. Again, look for any nipple discharge. The examination of that breast is over after you have felt the adjacent breast area, including under the arm up the collarbone. Then repeat the examination, using your left hand to feel your right breast.

Next, Examine Your Breasts While Prone. After you are dried off, lie on your bed and repeat the examination. To examine your right breast, place a pillow under your right shoulder, with your right hand under your head. For the left breast, the pillow should be under your left shoulder, with your left hand under your head.

Although this process may seem laborious initially, it shouldn't take you long to become adept at self-examination—and the whole process will take a short time each month. Women whose breasts are normally lumpy with benign cysts (see *Fibrocystic Breasts*, page 378) can find self-examination confusing, yet by keeping track of—perhaps even writing down—the number, locations, and approximate size of recurring lumps, they too can develop a fairly accurate feel for their own breast health. Any change in number or size of the lumps will then become apparent.

Breast cancer can occur anywhere in the breast, but it is more likely to strike in certain areas. Forty-one percent of all breast cancers are found in the upper outer quadrant of the breast; 34 percent in the central portion; 14 percent in the upper inner quadrant and but 5 percent in the lower inner quadrant; and 6 percent in the lower outer quadrant.

If you should find a lump when you are examining your breasts, see your clinician immediately—but don't assume the worst. Although it is natural to be frightened at the prospect of cancer, you should know that 80 percent of all breast lumps are benign (noncancerous).

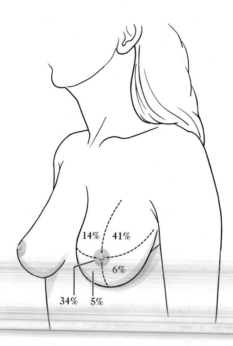

Breast cancer is most likely to occur in the upper portion of the breast, as this graphic of the percentage of cancers in each quadrant suggests.

MAMMOGRAPHY

By examining your breasts regularly for changes or lumps, you can help ensure that if a cancer exists it will be detected early. Even so, by the time most breast cancers are found during self-examination they are the size of a marble and have been growing for many years inside the affected breast.

Currently the best method for detecting the smallest tumors—so small that they may be years away from being felt—is mammography, a special X ray of the breasts and an invaluable cancer screening tool.

A mammogram is performed most often in an outpatient radiology center or, in some cases, at a hospital. Although a mammogram takes only a few moments, the procedure necessitates that the breast be compressed so that its densest areas can be X-rayed. The pressure on the breast can be uncomfortable, so to minimize discomfort schedule the X ray at a time other than just before or during your period, when your breasts may be more tender.

After the procedure, your X ray will be examined by a specially trained radiologist. If you have had a previous mammogram, the earlier X rays will be referred to in order to identify any changes that could indicate a developing problem.

As effective as they are, mammograms do not take the place of either monthly breast self-examination or annual exams by a health professional. Nor is mammography the only radiological technique used in the diagnosis of breast diseases, although to date it is the procedure that combines the highest effectiveness with the least risk. Some of the other methods are discussed next.

Ultrasonography. Ultrasonography is a painless procedure in which high-frequency sound waves are employed to examine body tissue. Often used once a lump is detected to determine its density and nature (when the lump is a solid mass or a cyst), it is not especially effective in detecting small breast cancers.

In one study, mammography detected 97 percent of small cancers, whereas ultrasound's rate of detection was only 57 percent. Moreover, most of the cancers discovered by ultrasound were larger than those found during a mammogram and were, in fact, large enough to be felt by a physician.

Ultrasound can also help guide the physician during needle aspiration, a procedure in which fluid is removed from a cyst in order to resolve or examine it. (For a more detailed discussion, see *Ultrasonography*, page 637.)

Thermography. Thermography is a diagnostic procedure that measures an elevation in skin temperature. The disadvantage of the test is its high rate of both false-positive and false-negative results in the detection of breast cancers.

Magnetic Resonance Imaging (MRI). MRI is a highly sophisticated, expensive, and time-consuming technology (the imaging procedure requires forty-five minutes to one hour). Currently, it is not widely used in the detection of breast cancer, although it does have its place in experimental methods for the diagnosis of breast disease. A magnetic resonance image often works to differentiate between a benign and a malignant tumor. Ultimately this test could reduce the number of breast biopsies done. This imaging technique also eventually might be used to help determine a tumor's stage. (For a more detailed discussion, see *Magnetic Resonance Imaging*, page 636.)

ANNUAL PHYSICAL EXAMINATIONS

Each September, as soon as her kids are settled back into school, Emily schedules her annual physical examination. Although the visit involves a comprehensive health screening and includes all aspects of her health and her body, Emily is especially comforted that her general practitioner spends time and attention examining her breasts. It reassures her to know that, even though she is conscientious about self-examination, her health practitioner provides a professional corroboration of her own findings.

After breast self-examination and mammography, the third line of defense against breast cancer and other breast disorders is an annual physical. With years of training behind them, clinicians often are able to detect a lump that even a diligent self-examiner has missed. In fact, studies have shown that physicians are likely to feel a lump as small as one centimeter; in comparison, the average size lump found by women themselves is twice as large. In one study, 87 percent of clinicians were able to detect a one-centimeter breast mass, and 33 percent of the tested physicians could feel a lump even half that size.

A clinician's examination should resemble your self-examination. Looking at the contour and symmetry of your breasts, he or she will inspect the skin for any signs of irritation, retraction, or swelling. The provider may ask you to raise your arms above your head and then drop them to your hips, thereby causing contractions of the pectoral muscles, which might reveal a lump or other abnormality. As you sit up, the provider will feel the tissue under the arm and around the breast, usually moving the pads of his or her fingers along the breasts in concentric circles or parallel strips. This examination process is called *palpation*. The provider should inspect your nipples as well for signs of retraction, irritation, or discharge.

The physical examination is an ideal time for a clinician to demonstrate, review, or answer questions about self-examination methods.

BREAST CARE AND CONCERNS

Every time Sarah remembers to examine her own breasts, she can feel the panic rise. What if she finds a lump? She'd almost rather not know.

Joy never felt particularly comfortable with the way her body looked—and she is uncomfortable about touching it much, especially her breasts. The thought of examining her own breasts is embarrassing. She just can't do it.

Paula has always considered her breasts her prettiest feature. Having a big chest makes her feel sexy. It's impossible for her to think of her breasts as just another part of her body, and a part that could be sick. No way!

Veronica has cystic breasts. Whenever she checks her breasts there are so many lumps, and their density, number, and location seem to change each month. At first she really worried about them. Since having them checked out by her doctor, she's felt less nervous. Still, self-examination is confusing for her—and a little bit frightening. Besides, she knows she has lumps, so why bother?

There are all sorts of reasons to avoid routine breast self-examination—but there are clearly more compelling reasons to develop a healthy routine and comfort level with your own breasts. Although it is true that there is something about the idea of breast disease that is uniquely frightening, not all breast disorders are as alarming as breast cancer. Some are a bit painful or uncomfortable; some are merely annoying. But because the diagnosis of breast cancer is such a serious and ever-present concern, any kind of breast condition or irregularity should be noted, followed, and discussed with a health-care professional so that cancer can be ruled out. A full range of breast disorders as well as breast cancer are discussed in the following pages.

FIBROCYSTIC BREASTS

The symptoms of fibrocystic breasts include recurring tenderness, pain, or lumpiness in the breasts, typically in the week preceding the onset of your period.

Many women experience breast tenderness or even outright pain at some time during the month—or at different times in their adult life. It is normal to notice swelling, tenderness, lumpiness, and pain as your period approaches. These discomforts are typically associated with natural hormonal changes that cause breast engorgement (the flow and congestion of blood in the breast) and benign (noncancerous) cysts.

Cyclical changes in hormonal levels affect a woman's breasts as well as her reproductive system. Around the time of ovulation and again immediately before menstruation, blood flow to breast cells increases. Development of cysts—small sacs of fluid or semifluid material, which then also expand and retain additional fluid—is not unusual. Cysts may grow in one or both breasts and tend to cluster most often around the armpit. These lumps usually diminish in size or disappear altogether a few days after a woman starts her period. For some women these changes are hardly noticeable and pose no problem; for others the engorgement of their breasts is more extreme, and for these women the pain is most bothersome.

Understanding the Problem. All women undergo some breast changes during their menstrual cycle—but about one in three has an excessive response that causes nonmalignant fluid-filled sacs or cysts to develop. Some cysts are very tiny; others may grow to the size of an egg. Of the women who suffer from fibrocystic breast changes, an estimated 50 percent consult a doctor about breast changes or discomfort.

Fibrocystic breast change (sometimes called chronic cystic mastitis) is most common in women between the ages of fifteen and thirty. Some have the condition with their earliest periods. Others discern lumps later in adulthood. The degree of lumpiness and the discomfort may remain constant, recede, fluctuate, or progress as a woman matures. Except in rare cases, the condition usually disappears after menopause.

The main symptom of cysts is breast pain that tends to worsen with the approach of the menstrual period. The pain may be generalized, or, if a cyst grows abruptly, may be localized to one area. Some women also have pain in the shoulders and upper arms. There may also be slight nipple discharge.

Treatment Options. It is important that a woman with fibrocystic breasts perform regular breast self-examinations and that she see her practitioner periodically. Although there is no connection between cystic breasts and breast cancer, a woman should have any unusual lumps palpated by her clinician.

Treatment for breast pain depends upon its severity. If your breasts are just a little tender prior to your period and you can tolerate the increased sensitivity, you may choose to do nothing. Many women, however, have pain that is impossible to ignore. There are several things you can try to reduce the pain.

Life-style Changes. Although the evidence is inconclusive and somewhat controversial, some studies—as well as much anecdotal material—claim that women with fibrocystic breasts show some improvement after they make adjustments in their consumption habits. In one study of more than one hundred women with fibrocystic breasts, 68 percent showed an absence of symptoms after giving up tobacco and caffeine. Twenty-four percent still had cysts, but the symptoms were less severe than before. Other studies, however, showed no correlation between these substances and breast cysts. At any rate, it may be worth eliminating cigarettes, coffee, tea, cola, and chocolate from your diet.

Some women claim that vitamin E supplements taken by mouth improve the condition, but thus far there are no studies that demonstrate its effectiveness.

A good support bra during the days of discomfort and perhaps at night may relieve some of the feelings of heaviness and tenderness.

Medication. Many women use over-the-counter analgesics such as aspirin or acetaminophen during the most uncomfortable days. Some women, however, require stronger prescription drugs. Danazol is the drug most commonly prescribed for severe breast pain. This drug seems both to reduce symptoms and to improve the condition itself in 90 percent of the women who use it. Moreover, the effect may last for months after the drug is stopped. Danazol, however, is expensive and can cause side effects such as hot flashes, weight gain, migraine headaches, dizziness, fatigue, oily skin, facial hair, and depression. Other medications that may be prescribed include the hormone progesterone and the drug bromocriptine, both of which can reduce breast pain significantly.

Aspiration. Frequently, a health-care professional will drain a lump, first to confirm the diagnosis and rule out malignancy, and second to reduce the size of the cyst. This office procedure, called a needle aspiration, withdraws fluid from the mass by means of a syringe (see also *Benign Lumps*, page 384).

BREAST INFECTIONS

If you have a breast infection, also known as mastitis, you will notice a red, tender, painful swelling or lump in your breast. In some cases, the glands in the armpit also will be swollen. Fever also is common with mastitis.

Breast infections are caused by bacteria that have entered the breast, typically through a crack in the nipple. Most often, mastitis occurs during breast-feeding or immediately after the baby has been weaned. Occasionally a woman who is not nursing will experience mastitis.

Understanding the Problem. If you are nursing and have the associated symptoms, your physician may begin treatment for mastitis without diagnostic tests. If, however, you have these symptoms and have not nursed recently, your health-care provider may run tests to rule out a rare form of cancer that has similar symptoms. These tests may include a mammogram, a needle biopsy, or a surgical biopsy (see *Breast Biopsy*, page 386).

Although you will be uncomfortable for a few days, breast infections generally respond well to treatment.

Treatment Options. Mastitis can often be avoided through conscientious breast care. Nursing mothers should keep nipples as clean and dry as possible between feedings. Clothes that irritate the skin of the breast and nipple should be avoided. When the baby begins nursing, limit the time that the baby sucks on each side. Gradually increase the feeding as your nipples become tougher (see *Breast-feeding or Bottle Feeding*, page 342).

MEDICATION. If you have mastitis, an antibiotic may be prescribed, and your health-care provider may also prescribe medication to relieve the discomfort. These medications will not have adverse effects on your breast milk or your baby; your health-care practitioner may advise you to continue to nurse on the infected side until the problem clears up.

SURGERY. Most of the time mastitis is successfully treated with an antibiotic. Occasionally, however, an abscess (collection of pus) develops, and surgery is necessary to drain the infection. Your physician may make a small incision at the edge of the areola from which the pus can drain. This, in combination with antibiotics, should resolve the problem.

NIPPLE PROBLEMS
Nipple problems can take the form of lumps, discharge, scaling, retraction, or indentation of the nipple itself.

Although the majority of nipple problems are not serious, it is important that you take any change in your nipples seriously and consult your health-care practitioner. Usually nipple problems do not pose a major threat to your health, but in some instances they can be symptoms of breast cancer. In one study of 560 women with nipple discharge, 67 were found to have a malignant tumor.

Breast-feeding mothers commonly are plagued by sore, cracked nipples. Women with fibrocystic breasts (see page 378) sometimes secrete discharge from the nipples. But any woman at any age can have a nipple problem.

Understanding the Problem. The diagnosis depends upon the symptoms. If you have nipple discharge, your health-care provider will examine your breasts and may send a sample of the discharge to a laboratory for analysis. A mammogram is sometimes ordered as well.

KINDS OF NIPPLE PROBLEMS. There are several types of nipple problems, which are identified by their key symptoms.

Discharge. Some women leak a whitish or greenish fluid from their nipples. If the fluid comes from both breasts, it is probably breast milk. It is not uncommon for a woman—even one who is not breast-feeding—to express a few drops of sticky gray, green, or black fluid from a breast. However, if you have any dark-colored discharge from your nipples—especially from one breast only—consult your health-care provider.

Physicians are most concerned when the discharge is persistent and spontaneous (occurs without the nipple's being squeezed). A bloody discharge from the nipple may indicate a benign growth. In both cases, cancer must be ruled out. Scaling and itching may be indications of Paget's disease (see page 393).

Retracted Nipples. Some women normally have inverted or retracted nipples. Although this condition makes it more difficult to breast-feed a baby, retracted nipples are nothing to be concerned about when they occur at puberty. However, if suddenly a nipple retracts, especially if it happens with only one breast, it may indicate breast cancer. Don't delay seeing your clinician.

Cracked Nipples. The problem of cracked nipples often affects nursing mothers, particularly in the first few days of breast-feeding before the nipples have toughened up. The condition is uncomfortable and increases your risk of a breast infection, but does not indicate a serious problem.

Cysts or Boils. A cyst or boil may form in the areola when a blockage occurs in one of the ducts that produce lubricant to keep the nipple supple. A fluid-filled sac then forms in the duct. If the gland becomes infected, the result is a boil.

Treatment Options. Nipple problems such as retraction or discharge usually do not require treatment once the possibility of cancer has been ruled out. If you are nursing and have cracked nipples, keep your nipples clean and dry between feedings. Avoid wearing clothes that irritate the skin. Limit the time the baby sucks on each side, gradually increasing the feeding as your nipples become tougher (see also *Breast-feeding or Bottle Feeding*, page 342). Boils generally are treated by drainage, with or without an antibiotic.

GALACTORRHEA

Galactorrhea is a condition in which the nipples leak milk even though a woman is not nursing. If you have galactorrhea, you will notice a whitish discharge from your nipples, typically from both breasts. Some women with galactorrhea also miss their menstrual period.

Most women produce breast milk only after giving birth (and, in some cases, during pregnancy). When a woman breast-feeds her infant, the breasts are stimulated to produce more milk; if she does not, the milk dries up within a few days. Sometimes, however, the breasts leak milk without the stimulus of birth. A woman (or sometimes even a man) is then said to have galactorrhea.

Derived from the Greek words *galacto* for milk and *rhea* for flow, galactorrhea is a somewhat baffling disorder. In an estimated 50 percent of those with galactorrhea, no cause can be determined. Twenty-five percent of the time there is a benign pituitary tumor called a *prolactinoma* (see page 473) that secretes prolactin, one of the hormones that regulate the production of breast milk. The remainder of galactorrhea cases can be attributed to a variety of other causes, such as hypothyroidism (see page 470) or side effects of some prescription medications.

Understanding the Problem. To determine whether you have galactorrhea, your clinician will examine your breasts and the fluid they are producing. Tests may rule out the possibility that cancer is causing the discharge. Your medical history should indicate whether the problem is a result of a medication you are taking.

In and of itself, galactorrhea does not pose a serious threat to your health. However, if it is the result of a tumor, you will need to have that problem treated.

Treatment Options. The treatment depends upon the cause of the galactorrhea.

MEDICATION. If the cause of the galactorrhea is a small pituitary tumor, your health-care provider may initially treat the condition with bromocriptine, a drug that can shrink the tumor and reduce your prolactin level. This drug also may be used in cases in which no cause for the galactorrhea is determined. If you are diagnosed with hypothyroidism, thyroid hormone drugs such as thyroxine may be prescribed.

SURGERY. In unusual cases when the pituitary tumor is large, surgery may be the best treatment option.

INTRADUCTAL PAPILLOMA
Intraductal papilloma is a tiny, benign tumor that grows in the milk ducts near the nipple. If you have an intraductal papilloma, you may have a watery or bloody spontaneous and intermittent discharge from one nipple. You may also feel a very small lump beneath the affected nipple, although many of these tumors are too small to be felt.

Papillomas are benign (nonmalignant) skin tumors; intraductal papillomas are found in the tissue of the breast, within the ducts that deliver the milk to the nipple. Relatively uncommon, intraductal papilloma is most often found in women around the time of menopause.

Understanding the Problem. Your health-care provider's first task is to ascertain whether your symptoms are the result of intraductal papilloma or a breast cancer (see *Benign Lumps* and *Breast Cancer*, pages 384 and 390). Once it is determined that the problem is an intraductal papilloma, the clinician will try to pinpoint the affected duct by closely examining your breast.

Treatment Options. After an intraductal papilloma is identified, your doctor can surgically remove it. In the event that a tumor isn't found, you will probably be asked to have regular checkups and mammograms so your care health-care provider can closely monitor the condition.

BENIGN LUMPS

Benign lumps are noncancerous cysts or breast tumors that may or may not cause pain or tenderness. In addition to one or more cysts in the breasts, some women with benign lumps in their breasts may experience a greenish or straw-colored discharge from the breast when the nipple is squeezed.

Breast lumps are relatively common. Fortunately, the vast majority are not malignant. Even so, if you discover a lump in your breast, see your health-care provider at once.

There are many conditions other than cancer that can cause a lump to grow in the breast. The vast majority of lumps are cysts that grow in response to a woman's changing hormonal levels. These are particularly bothersome just prior to menstruation, when hormones can cause them to swell rapidly. Less common breast lumps are solid, painless masses.

Understanding the Problem. If you find a lump in your breast, the first step is to determine whether there is a malignancy. If the lump feels like a fluid-containing cyst, your health-care provider may aspirate it. This is a simple procedure that withdraws fluid from the breast with a thin needle. A needle aspiration can be done in the clinician's office without anesthetic.

If fluid can be drawn from the lump, chances are it is a cyst and will disappear. Even so, your health provider may send the fluid to a laboratory to be analyzed for signs of a malignancy. In the event fluid cannot be drawn, or the clinician does not think the lump is a cyst, he or she may want you to have the mass removed (see *Breast Biopsy*, page 386).

Although some types of benign breast lumps can be painful, especially prior to your period, they generally do not pose a health threat. However, a small percentage of women with certain types of benign breast lumps do have a slightly increased risk of development of breast cancer later in life. Moreover, women with lumpy breasts often have a more difficult time detecting a malignant lump, should one later develop.

TYPES OF BENIGN BREAST LUMPS. Noncancerous breast lumps are the result of a variety of causes. The principal ones are as follows:

Fibrocystic Changes. By far the most common benign lump is a saclike fluid-filled cyst, which occurs when breast tissue has an exaggerated response to changes in hormonal levels. An estimated one in three premenopausal women has some degree of fibrocystic changes, although only about half of them are bothered sufficiently to seek medical attention. If you have fibrocystic breasts, you may notice only one lump or you may have many. Some are tiny; some may grow as large as an egg (see also *Fibrocystic Breasts*, page 378).

You may also notice a lump enlarge as your period approaches. This is due to an increase in certain hormones in your body. When you press on the lump, particularly a larger one, it may change shape and move slightly under the skin.

Fibroadenoma. Unlike a cyst, this benign tumor is a firm, rubbery mass usually appearing in the breast of an adolescent girl or woman in her twenties. Because they cause no pain, fibroadenomas are generally discovered accidentally or by routine examination. Fibroadenomas recur in approximately 10 percent of women who have had them removed.

Lipoma is a benign tumor comprised of fatty tissue. It manifests as a single, slow-growing, soft, painless lump. It is most commonly seen in postmenopausal women.

Phylloides Tumor. These are very rare but fast-growing tumors. One in four phylloides tumors is malignant. However, only one in ten malignant phylloides tumors spread beyond the breast to other parts of the body.

Sclerosing Adenosis is a benign enlargement and distortion of the lobular units of the breast. It is usually larger than one centimeter, and may resemble an invasive cancer. It is most commonly seen in women of childbearing and perimenopausal ages.

Treatment Options. Depending upon the variety of breast lump you have, the treatment strategy varies.

MEDICATION. If you are bothered by breast cysts, you may find that taking a mild analgesic such as aspirin relieves the discomfort, particularly during the days just prior to your period. When symptoms are severe, some doctors prescribe oral contraceptives, vitamin E, or the drug danazol. Although very effective, danazol is expensive and may have some unpleasant side effects (see *Fibrocystic Breasts*, page 378).

SURGERY. The most likely surgery is the aspiration of fluid to determine whether the mass disappears. If, however, a cyst is extremely painful, does not improve with medication, or recurs after the fluid has been drawn, it can be removed surgically. The removal of the lump is usually done on an outpatient basis.

When the lump in your breast is solid (not cystic), it should be removed. The procedure can be done under local anesthesia. After removal, the lump is examined to determine whether it is malignant (see page 622).

BREAST BIOPSY

A breast biopsy is a procedure that involves the removal of a lump and/or breast tissue for the purpose of determining whether it is malignant (cancerous). After the lump and a small piece of surrounding tissue are removed, they are analyzed for cancer cells.

The Indications. *If you notice a spontaneous and persistent bloody discharge from your nipple(s), or if a breast lump is detected by you through self-examination, by your clinician, or through mammography, a biopsy may be recommended. In the case of a lump, especially if it feels like a cyst (see* Benign Lumps, *page 384), your clinician may first try to withdraw fluid with a long, thin needle. If fluid can be aspirated, the lump may disappear during the process, generally an indication that it was a cyst. If, however, the lump doesn't feel like a cyst or yields no fluid, its identity can be determined with a biopsy. In addition, women who have sudden nipple retraction or changes in the skin of the breast may be advised to have a breast biopsy to rule out the possibility of cancer.*

The Procedure. *The most common and reliable method of diagnosing a breast cancer is a breast biopsy. Breast biopsies today are done most often on an outpatient basis. A local anesthetic is injected, then the surgeon makes a small incision to remove the lump along with a small amount of surrounding breast tissue. The tissue is examined for the presence of malignancy. If malignancy is found, this small sample of breast tissue also will indicate whether the cancer has estrogen and progesterone receptors, an important factor in determining the best course of treatment (see page 394).*

Although an open breast biopsy is considered the definitive diagnosis for breast cancer, a less invasive form of biopsy called fine-needle aspiration cytology *is gaining some acceptance. This technique involves the insertion of a small needle into the mass. A sampling of cells is removed with the needle and then analyzed for malignancy. In some cases, this technique can diagnose breast cancer, thereby circumventing the necessity of open breast biopsy. However, since this procedure collects individual cells instead of tissue, the diagnostic accuracy of fine-needle aspiration cytology is only between 70 and 90 percent. Moreover, differentiation between an invasive tumor and one that has not yet moved into surrounding tissue is not possible with this test. A larger needle that obtains a core of tissue (called* core-needle biopsy*) can be used to combine the accuracy of open biopsy with the convenience of needle aspiration. This technique is often used for small lumps that are identified on mammography.*

Another variety of biopsy, the stereotactic biopsy, is an image-guided biopsy done under mammography or sonography. Local anesthesia is used. It is especially useful when multiple small suspicious areas in different parts of the breast are viewed.

A needle or wire localization biopsy may be done prior to surgical excision of any mammographic lesion too small to identify by touch. The purpose is to ensure the removal of any clinically tiny lesion with the smallest possible breast deformity. Using mammography, and under local anesthesia, the abnormality is imaged and a needle with a small wire inside is guided to the area. The surgeon then follows the wire to the suspicious area and surgically removes it. The biopsy tissue is then x-rayed to confirm that the abnormality was removed.

If you have a lump or other symptoms that warrant a breast biopsy, it is natural to be frightened at the prospect of a diagnosis of breast cancer. However, it is important to remember that 80 percent of biopsies have negative results; that is, they are nonmalignant. Although the chances that biopsies will show cancer increase as women age, even among all seventy-year-old women biopsied, for example, an estimated 67 percent test negative for cancer.

Nevertheless, a sense of panic lingers around the idea of biopsy. Not many years ago, a woman would undergo a biopsy not knowing whether she would wake up from general anesthesia with her breasts intact. Until recently, it was standard for a woman to remain anesthetized in the operating room while the surgical team waited for word from the pathologist. When the result was negative, the woman was wheeled off to the recovery room with little more than a small bandage on her breast. A diagnosis of cancer, on the other hand, meant hours more of surgery, during which the entire breast and much of the surrounding tissue would be removed.

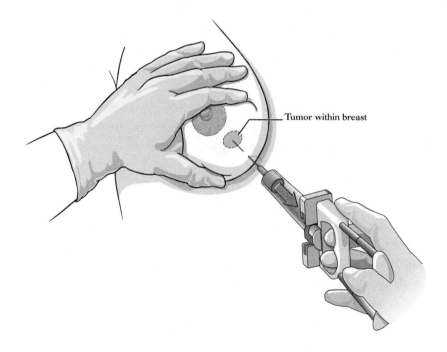

To perform a fine-needle aspiration, the health-care practitioner will insert a small needle into the lump identified in the breast. A sampling of cells can then be withdrawn through the hollow needle for laboratory analysis.

Today, after a woman has a biopsy, she will learn the results and be an active partner in developing a treatment approach. Of course, if the lump is benign, as it is in the majority of cases, there is little else to consider in relation to the condition. If cancer is diagnosed, a woman will have time to explore her options, talk with her family, and address the implications and the complex feelings that arise. Typically, most women who are diagnosed with breast cancer begin their treatment—whether it is surgery, radiation, chemotherapy, or a combination—one to two weeks after the biopsy has confirmed the diagnosis. A delay of a few weeks to explore the options and consult with other professionals will not diminish the effectiveness of treatment, and it will in all likelihood help a woman feel more involved and less helpless during the treatment process.

COMMON QUESTIONS ABOUT BIOPSY

Given the frightening prospect of breast cancer, it is not surprising that many women feel immobilized and bewildered when they hear their doctor recommend biopsy. Nevertheless, it's important to maintain the presence of mind to ask the necessary questions, including the following:

- *What type of biopsy should be done? Would fine-needle aspiration or core biopsy be sufficient?*
- *What type of anesthetic will be used for an open-breast biopsy—local or general?*
- *When will the results be available? Will the clinician contact you or should you call the office?*
- *When will you be able to discuss the results of the biopsy and treatment options with your provider?*

Many women find that being an informed partner in the decision-making process enables them to grapple with the implications of breast disease. Medical and emotional decisions are difficult to separate—and well-informed patients make better decisions.

BREAST CANCER RISK FACTORS

There are several factors that seem to have some relationship to a woman's chance of development of breast cancer. It is important to note, however, that no one can predict who will experience cancer on the basis of these (or any other) factors.

- *As with many diseases and most malignancies, the risk increases with age. Eighty-five percent of all breast cancers are found in women over forty.*
- *A history of breast cancer increases a woman's chances of another primary breast cancer. For women who have had a cancer in one breast, the risk of development of cancer in the remaining breast is 1 percent each year. Those who have had ovarian, endometrial, or colon cancer are two to four times more likely to have breast cancer than the rest of the population.*

• *Women whose mother or sister had breast cancer after menopause seem to have a two to three times greater risk of development of breast cancer. Breast cancer seems to run in families: There may be a genetic predisposition to development of breast cancer when exposed to a combination of other factors, including environmental carcinogens.*

• *Women whose mother had breast cancer before menopause seem to have a six to nine times greater chance than the daughters of mothers who did not.*

• *Women fifty or older who have never given birth to a child may be at an increased risk for breast cancer. There is also evidence that women who gave birth for the first time after the age of thirty-five have a 1.5 times greater risk than those who bore their first child before the age of twenty-six.*

• *Some studies link breast cancer with the length of time a woman's body produces estrogen. Statistics show that girls rarely have breast cancer before menarche (their first menstrual period). Women who have their ovaries removed before the age of thirty-five and do not have estrogen replacement therapy seem to reduce their risk of breast cancer by 70 percent. And women who have an early menopause (before the age of forty-five) are only half as likely to have breast cancer as those who are still menstruating a decade later. One study found that women who menstruated for forty years were twice as likely to have breast cancer as those who had periods for thirty years or less. Some studies have suggested that menopausal estrogen in the form of estrogen replacement therapy increases breast cancer risk—although this conclusion is controversial (see page 90).*

• *Obesity seems to increase the risk of breast cancer after menopause.*

• *Some studies suggest a relationship between dietary fat and breast cancer. They point to the fact that Americans have one of the highest rates of breast cancer in the world and, at the same time, lead the world in consumption of fat. Conversely, in countries where the diets comprise mainly vegetables and grains rather than meat and dairy products, the breast cancer rate is markedly lower. A woman living in the United States, for example, is six times more likely to have breast cancer than a woman in Japan. However, within two generations of emigrating to the United States and of assimilating American eating habits, a Japanese woman's chance will match that of any other American woman.*

• *Women who have been exposed to high doses of radiation are more likely to experience breast, as well as other, cancer. Although there are examples of women who, in the past, received large doses of radiation as treatment for such conditions as breast infection and tuberculosis, the most dramatic illustration of the damage excess radiation can do to the breast is seen in the results of the atomic bombs dropped on the Japanese cities of Hiroshima and Nagasaki at the end of World War II. Female survivors in all age groups had malignancies. The girls who had the highest incidence of breast cancer, however, were teenagers when they were exposed to radiation. Twenty years later, they experienced breast cancer in excessive numbers in a country where the incidence of breast cancer is otherwise extremely low.*

• The incidence of breast cancer is highest in whites. The ethnic groups in the United States with the lowest rates of this disease are Native Americans who live in New Mexico and Filipinos in Hawaii.

THE PROBLEM WITH STATISTICS

It seems that every new study on breast cancer that reaches the popular press quotes another figure for a woman's chance of development of breast cancer in her lifetime. One current figure is one in nine, though one is eight is often cited, as is one in twelve.

This profusion of findings, and much of the fear and confusion provoked by these numbers, result in part from a complicated method of computing the figures which assumes that every woman will live to be 110! There is no question that too many women die of this disease, but actually, the statistics are misleading. The actual risk of getting cancer in your lifetime is not so high. For example, for the average forty-year-old, the chance of breast cancer is 0.1 percent per year, or one in one thousand. For the average fifty-year-old, the number doubles to 0.2 percent. By the time we look at the average 110-year-old, the chance of getting breast cancer is indeed high. So, although it is essential that all women take the risk seriously and assume responsibility for maintaining breast health, it is not necessary to live in fear.

BREAST CANCER

A lump in either breast, a bloody discharge from either nipple, a retraction of the nipple, puckering or other change in the skin of the breast could signal breast cancer and the imperative to consult a health-care provider as soon as possible. The majority of women with breast cancer do not experience pain until the disease has progressed.

Cancer of the breast is a frightening and extremely serious disease—and no woman can afford to ignore the signs. Although much attention has been paid to high-risk factors, only 25 percent of the women identified as high risk ultimately have breast cancer. Statisticians advise us that in actuality, one in every seventeen women who do not fit the high-risk profile nevertheless will have breast cancer. This means that *every* woman has a compelling reason to be alert to the risk of breast cancer. Although men do occasionally get breast cancer, the rate among women is one hundred times greater.

American women are particularly likely to have breast cancer: Our nation has one of the highest breast cancer rates in the world. Breast cancer claims the lives of nearly forty-five thousand American women each year; annually, about four times as many will be diagnosed with the disease. Roughly one in eight American women will have breast cancer in her lifetime. An average woman's chance of development of breast cancer during her life is comparable to a heavy smoker's chance of development of lung cancer.

Despite the alarming statistics—and the alarming reality of the disease—no one knows precisely what prompts cells in a woman's breast to grow abnormally. One recent study at the Strang-Cornell Breast Center in New York, however, found that the varying ways estrogen is processed in breast tissue of different women may be an indicator of risk. Researchers found that noncancerous breast tissue in women with breast cancer had much higher levels of a metabolite of the natural estrogen 17-beta-estradiol than did tissue taken from women without breast cancer. Although this finding has yet to be translated into a means of predicting the degree of risk each woman faces, risk studies such as this one may lead eventually to a test that could determine a woman's vulnerability to the disease.

At present, certain factors have been linked to a woman's risk of the disease. There are data emerging about women with a family history of breast cancer, and there is genetic evidence, too. But even these are not necessarily accurate indicators. Many women who fit the high-risk profile never have cancer. Many other women who appear not to be at risk die of the disease. Although a number of these factors are outside a woman's control, perhaps being aware of them will make a woman more diligent about breast self-examination and annual physical examinations. It might also indicate how often and beginning at what age a woman should have mammograms. On the other hand, being labeled high-risk may lead to unnecessary worries and anxieties, as well as dangerous and expensive procedures and tests.

Understanding the Problem. If your health-care provider suspects a breast malignancy, he or she will want you to have a biopsy, the only definitive method of diagnosing breast cancer. After the lump and some surrounding tissue are surgically removed, the sample will be analyzed for the presence of malignancy (see *Breast Biopsy*, page 386).

The course of breast cancer depends upon several factors, the most important of which is how early the malignancy is found. Breast cancers do not develop suddenly. By the time the lump is large enough to feel, it is probably about two centimeters, about the size of a marble. The average breast mass doubles in volume every one hundred days and in diameter every three hundred days. It is believed that it takes anywhere between six and eight years for a breast cancer to grow to one centimeter, half the size of those typically found during breast self-examination. Throughout this chapter, we have emphasized the importance of early detection. It cannot be overstated: *Early detection is the best weapon against breast cancer.*

A breast tumor itself will not kill you. Instead, breast cancer kills by spreading through the lymph nodes to other organs of the body. Thus, if a tumor is small, the chances that the cancer has spread are lower than if the mass is larger. Even so, breast cancer is a systemic disease that may recur decades after the initial diagnosis. Sadly, an estimated two thirds of all women with breast cancer eventually see their cancer spread. Earlier diagnosis would dramatically reduce this figure.

There are four stages of breast cancer. Treatment is determined by the stage at which the cancer is diagnosed—as are a woman's chances of surviving five years or longer after the initial treatment.

STAGE 0. Pre-invasive cancers that have not broken through the duct or lobe cell membrane are stage 0.

STAGE 1. A stage 1 tumor is smaller than two centimeters. The lymph nodes have not been invaded. Nor has the cancer spread to any other part of the body. An estimated 55 to 70 percent of women with breast cancer in the United States are diagnosed at this early stage. The five-year survival rate for women with stage 1 breast cancer is about 85 percent.

STAGE 2. A stage 2 malignancy can be as large as five centimeters. Some lymph nodes may have been affected at this stage, but there is no sign that the cancer has spread beyond the breast area. Twenty to 25 percent of breast cancer patients have stage 2 tumors. The survival rate after five years is 65 percent.

STAGE 3. The stage 3 tumor is larger than five centimeters, or a tumor of any size that has begun to invade the skin or to attach itself to the chest wall. Cancer can be found in some lymph nodes but is not evident elsewhere. Ten percent of all women diagnosed with breast cancer have stage 3 disease. The five-year survival rate is 40 percent.

STAGE 4. When breast cancer has metastasized or spread beyond the breast and surrounding lymph nodes, it is called stage 4 disease. Unlike some cancers that have a fairly predictable itinerary, the pattern followed by breast cancer is hard to predict. The most common sites for a breast tumor to invade, however, are the lymph nodes, liver, bones, skin, brain, and lungs. Ten percent of breast cancer patients have stage 4 disease at diagnosis. Only about 10 percent of these women survive beyond the five-year period.

In addition to the size of the tumor and the degree to which it has begun to spread to the lymph nodes, an important factor in the treatment of this disease is the presence of receptors for the hormones estrogen and progesterone. The presence of these receptors indicates the likelihood that the tumor will respond to hormonal treatment. Tumors that have receptors generally are less aggressive, do not spread as quickly, and are less likely to recur than those that do not.

Her-2 neu, for example, is a protein that regulates cell growth. Some breast cancers have extra copies of the her-2 neu gene. These cancer cells will produce extra amounts of her-2 protein, causing rapid growth of the tumor. This is a more aggressive tumor, and new treatments are being tailored to this prognostic factor.

Kinds of Breast Cancers. In general, the size of a breast tumor and the degree to which it has spread determine treatment and prognosis. However, identifying the type of breast cancer (malignant tumors) also has an impact.

INTRADUCTAL CARCINOMA. Most cancers originate in the ducts of the breast. Intraductal carcinoma is a disease in which the cancer is confined to the duct itself. These cancers most often are discovered in women after menopause and are also known as *ductal carcinoma in situ*.

INFILTRATING DUCTAL CARCINOMA. This is the most common type of breast malignancy. In this form of breast cancer, malignant cells have invaded the tissue surrounding the duct.

LOBULAR CARCINOMA. An estimated 5 percent of all breast cancers occur in the breast's small end ducts. *Lobular carcinoma in situ* is not a cancer but a marker of increased risk that occurs three out of four times in women who are still menstruating. This type of tumor grows within the lobule and may grow for twenty years before infiltrating surrounding tissue. When the disease is confined to the lobule, it cannot be detected during mammography or a health-care provider's examination of the breast.

MEDULLARY CARCINOMA. Five to seven percent of all breast cancers are found in the interior tissues of the breast. Although these tumors are often large, they are less likely to spread than many other carcinomas, so the prognosis is generally good.

COLLOID CARCINOMA. This is another slow-growing cancer that often becomes quite large. Typically, a colloid carcinoma grows in a part of the breast where it can be felt easily during breast self-examination or examination by a health professional. This malignancy is usually found in women over the age of seventy.

INFLAMMATORY BREAST CARCINOMA. This fast-growing, highly malignant tumor is responsible for 2 percent of all breast cancers. Unlike most breast cancers, inflammatory breast carcinoma appears as an infection in the breast, with redness, local warmth, pain, and swelling.

PAGET'S DISEASE. This rare cancer is found in less than 1 percent of all breast cancer patients. In this form of cancer, an infiltrating carcinoma invades the skin of the breast. Initially, it may appear as a rash such as eczema or dermatitis around the nipple. If left untreated, this nest of tumor cells can colonize the entire breast. The prognosis for women with Paget's is very good.

Treatment Options. In determining the most effective treatment, a woman and her medical team, which usually includes a surgeon, radiologist, and medical oncologist, must take into account not only the size of the tumor and its virulence, but whether it has spread and whether it contains estrogen and progesterone receptors and her-2 neu. Once these factors are considered, treatment options are weighed.

Not very many years ago, treatment meant removing the breast. Today, women with breast cancer have more options. Even with a doctor's recommendation, women can feel overwhelmed by the choices and combinations of treatment procedures. In considering treatment, it may be helpful to keep in mind three clear goals: to remove the tumor, to halt the spread of the cancer and treat any areas already invaded, and to maintain quality of life.

The four general approaches to treating breast cancer are surgery, radiation, hormone therapy, and chemotherapy.

SURGERY. Radical surgery—called a *Halsted radical mastectomy*—was once the treatment of choice for breast cancer. Recent statistics have shown, however, that such surgery does not increase a woman's chance of cure any more than less radical procedures. Today, surgery may involve the removal of more localized breast tissue rather than the entire breast, or only the lump itself (see *Mastectomy and Lumpectomy*, below). Frequently an exploratory procedure, called axillary node dissection, is done in tandem with breast surgery; an incision is made at the armpit and five to fifteen lymph nodes are removed for analysis to determine whether the cancer has spread.

SENTINEL NODE BIOPSY. This is a relatively new procedure intended to spare breast cancer patients more radical surgery. The procedure involves the removal of the nodes to which breast cancer cells first metastasize. If positive, there may be other positive nodes that are then removed. If negative, no further surgery may be required.

MASTECTOMY AND LUMPECTOMY

It wasn't long ago that a diagnosis of breast cancer automatically led to radical surgery. A woman with breast cancer had virtually one option and one option only— the surgical removal of the diseased breast. The common surgery, a Halsted radical mastectomy, was a deforming procedure with a profound emotional impact.

Despite the many drawbacks of a radical mastectomy, many women accepted the disfigurement and discomfort of the surgery so that they could have many more years of life. All too often, however, after enduring the physical and emotional pain of radical surgery, many of these women died eventually of some distant metastasis.

A more comprehensive understanding of breast cancer has evolved over time. Rather than being a localized condition, breast cancer is often a systemic disease, at least by the time it is diagnosed. Thus, removing the breast is often inadequate, for the cancer may have started to invade other parts of the body. In recent years, research has

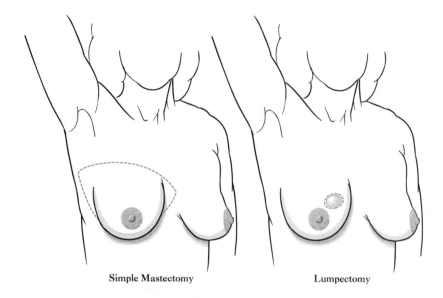

Simple Mastectomy   **Lumpectomy**

When breast cancer is the diagnosis, a range of treatments may be offered. One of the choices may be surgery, and there, too, you and your physician will have options. The choices are to remove surgically more or less tissue, as indicated in these drawings.

shown that in addition to being less mutilating, lumpectomies and modified forms of mastectomy can be equally effective in enhancing life expectancy. So whereas other therapies for breast cancer have become more aggressive, surgical treatment has become more conservative.

The surgical procedures used in the treatment of early breast cancer entail one of several forms of mastectomy or lumpectomy, a procedure in which only the lump and a margin of tissue surrounding it are removed.

Halsted Radical Mastectomy. *After being the treatment mainstay of breast cancer for many years, the Halsted radical mastectomy is now rarely recommended, for the simple reason that such deforming surgery does not have a higher success rate than modified procedures.*

A radical mastectomy removes not only the breast but a layer of chest muscles (the pectorals) and the lymph nodes. A woman who has a radical mastectomy is left with less tissue on what is now a flattened chest, which makes it difficult to fit a prosthesis. Moreover, women who have had radical mastectomies may have some continuing swelling of the arm, which reduces its mobility. Today, a doctor probably would not recommend a radical mastectomy unless the tumor had infiltrated the underlying muscle of the breast.

Modified Radical Mastectomy. *This surgery differs from the radical mastectomy in that the chest muscles are not removed, though the breast and lymph nodes are.*

The modified radical has replaced the radical mastectomy as the most common primary surgical treatment for breast cancer, although many believe this procedure is still too radical.

Simple Mastectomy. *In this procedure, the surgeon removes only the breast, without a sampling of lymph nodes from the armpit. A study by the National Surgical Adjuvant Breast Project found that this operation resulted in comparable survival rates to the radical mastectomy, without the same degree of disfigurement.*

Breast Conservation Therapy (BCT). *A combination approach, BCT consists of a lumpectomy, in which the surgeon removes only the breast lump and some surrounding tissue. In an accompanying procedure called axillary dissection, lymph nodes are then removed from the armpit through a separate incision to ascertain whether the disease has spread. Lumpectomy is usually followed by radiation therapy to kill any cancer cells that may still be within the breast.*

Another treatment for breast cancer, the lumpectomy is also called a tylectomy, wide excision, segmental resection, *or* partial mastectomy.

The aim of lumpectomy is to preserve as much of the breast as possible. In a fairly large-breasted woman, a lumpectomy often does just that. A woman whose breasts are small, however, may have better cosmetic results from a mastectomy followed by breast reconstructive surgery.

The best candidates for lumpectomy are women who have an early-stage cancer, under two centimeters, although some studies have shown positive results for tumors up to four centimeters. The tumor also should be located on the breast's periphery.

The most important factor in weighing BCT against mastectomy is which procedure offers a better chance of survival. Several studies have found that twenty-year disease-free survival rates are similar for BCT and mastectomy in eligible patients. In one study, women with breast cancer of less than two centimeters and with no apparent lymph node involvement were divided into two groups. The women in the first group underwent radical mastectomy. The second group had lumpectomy followed by radiation treatment. Five-year survival rates were identical. Ninety percent of both groups were alive five years later; 83 percent of the mastectomy patients and 84 percent of those who had lumpectomy and radiation remained free of disease. These results were borne out in several other studies. Interestingly, overall survival rate is often slightly higher in the group that has had lumpectomy combined with radiation.

In discussing surgery for breast cancer, it is important to consider the emotional aspects of treatment. Any diagnosis of cancer brings with it myriad feelings, including fear of dying and uncertainty about solutions. Moreover, even when treatment is effective in stemming the disease, the disfigurement that results introduces another difficult issue. It's no surprise, then, that so many women with breast cancer experi-

ence depression long after the doctor has removed the bandages and announced that the prognosis is good.

One study followed 160 women after mastectomy and found that one in four was having marital and sexual problems two years after surgery. It's important to realize that you are not alone in experiencing these problems. There are countless self-help and support groups available through local hospitals and medical centers, churches and synagogues. Another resource is the American Cancer Society's Reach for Recovery program. Call 800-ACS-2345.

There are also surgical options for reconstructive surgery at the time of the mastectomy or at a later time (see Breast Reconstruction, Reduction, and Augmentation, *page 176).*

RADIATION. Radiation therapy is used most commonly in conjunction with a lumpectomy or partial mastectomy. After the tumor is removed, radiation therapy will be prescribed, usually for a period of six weeks, five days a week. Each treatment lasts approximately fifteen minutes, and the goal is to kill any remaining cancer cells within the breast.

In the past, radiation was given to prevent the disease from spreading. Now it appears that although radiation is effective in diminishing the spread of cancer within the breast itself, it does little to stop the disease if it has metastasized throughout the body. Once the cancer has invaded other organs (the bones, for instance), radiation may be used to shrink the tumors and thereby ease the pain. Often, though, the effect is temporary. Radiation will not halt metastatic disease's progression and will likely produce such side effects as fatigue and a slight redness like a sunburn to the breast. Side effects are rarely serious or long-term.

HORMONE THERAPY. This form of treatment typically involves the use of certain antiestrogen drugs. In the past, surgical removal of the ovaries was common in an attempt to block estrogen production. However, the advent of such antiestrogen agents as tamoxifen has markedly decreased the use of surgical hormonal manipulation.

Hormone therapy is increasingly used for all breast cancers. It is generally most effective when a tumor is found to have estrogen and/or progesterone receptors, that is, proteins within the tumor that bind these hormones. If a biopsy determines that a tumor has estrogen receptors, there is a 60 percent chance that hormone therapy will help stall the progression of the disease; if the tumor has both estrogen and progesterone receptors, the response rate increases to 80 percent. Conversely, fewer than 10 percent of tumors without hormone receptors respond to hormone therapy. As a group, the women who respond best to hormone therapy have gone through menopause, were disease-free at least two years between their diagnosis and the cancer's recurrence or spread, or have metastases confined to the bone or soft tissue such as skin or lymph nodes.

Hormone therapy can stop a tumor from growing and may cause it to shrink. Women given hormone therapy may see their disease go into partial or even full remission (disappearance of the signs and symptoms). Hormone therapy may be used in conjunction with chemotherapy.

Side effects from hormone therapy include mild nausea, vomiting, and, in some women, hot flashes and vaginal dryness. There may be an increased risk of uterine cancer with some hormones, such as tamoxifen, so special monitoring is required with this kind of treatment.

Hormonal therapy has been used in the treatment of advanced disease, and some women whose cancer has not yet spread are now having adjuvant hormone therapy in an attempt to prevent the cancer from spreading. Studies have shown that adjuvant hormone therapy appears to increase the survival rate considerably in some women with early cancers.

CHEMOTHERAPY. In the past, chemotherapy—the use of highly potent drugs to kill cancer cells—was medicine's heavy artillery, a weapon that was reserved for the last fight and recruited only when nothing else worked. Today, chemotherapy still is very much a top gun against this disease. But more and more doctors have become convinced that this powerful weapon may, in fact, have an important role to play not only in advanced breast cancer but in early-stage disease as well. Such recent discoveries as taxol, a drug derived from the bark of a tree, and herceptin, a monoclonal antibody designed to attack specific cancer cells, offer new hope of effective treatment and cure. Bone marrow transplants—in which marrow is removed before chemotherapy and returned after—is also proving an effective therapy.

There is little doubt that chemotherapy can prolong the life of many women whose breast cancer has spread beyond the breast. The women most likely to respond to chemotherapy are those menstruating or just beginning menopause. Moreover, chemotherapy is more effective at killing some cancers than others. A breast cancer that has spread to the skin or lymph nodes is more likely to respond to chemotherapy than one that has spread to the bones, although chemotherapy may help reduce pain in the latter case.

Medical oncologists have a wide array of cancer-fighting drugs from which to choose. But over the years doctors have determined that a combination of several of these drugs is generally more powerful than a single agent.

Because these powerful drugs don't discriminate between cancer cells and healthy cells, they attack both. As a result, a woman's immune system is suppressed, rendering her especially vulnerable to infection. Moreover, she may feel unusually tired and have no appetite. Nausea, vomiting, and diarrhea are common side effects, as is the temporary loss of hair.

Despite these side effects, many women consider the potential gain worth the price. Numerous studies have shown response rates of anywhere between 50 and 75 percent in women with advanced breast cancer. This means that these women's tumor responded—in some cases shrinking, sometimes even disappearing. It is estimated that of all the women given chemotherapy for advanced breast cancer, 10 to 20 percent have a complete remission and the disease's symptoms disappear. In the majority of cases, however, this remission is temporary, on average eighteen months. When the return of the disease signals the end of a remission, a second round of chemotherapy can be tried, but generally the response is not as good since some of the cells have become resistant to the drugs.

Thirty percent of women who have early breast cancer eventually go on to have metastatic breast disease. As a result, some doctors advise their patients with early disease to follow surgery with several cycles of chemotherapy. This additional therapy, termed *adjuvant chemotherapy*, in fact can reduce the rate of cancer recurrences in some women with early-stage disease. The next logical step facing breast cancer researchers is to determine which women are at high risk for development of metastatic disease so that low-risk women can weigh clearly the benefits and the costs of this treatment.

A RISKY HERITAGE

Sue is in her early thirties and unmarried. Her mother contracted breast cancer before menopause and subsequently died from it after a long and valiant fight. An aunt and a cousin also had breast cancer; one had a mastectomy and seems to be cancer-free; the other died after the disease metastasized to her bones.

Although Sue tries not to dwell on her prospects of getting breast cancer, still it's like the sword of Damocles hanging over her head: Will she be lucky and live a long and healthy life? Or will she, too, become yet another sad statistic in the war against breast cancer? She knows the odds are not good, but to what lengths is she prepared to go to better those odds?

Certainly she does what she can to improve them: Through a strict regimen of diet and exercise Sue has lost a considerable amount of weight and continues to exercise regularly and vigorously to maintain her weight loss. She stays away from fatty foods, and she eats lots of vegetables and little animal protein. But in the end will that be enough? Right now it's anybody's guess, including Sue's.

She has been following closely news reports about genetic testing for breast cancer. She has also noticed articles and television features about women at high risk of development of the disease who have had their breasts removed prophylactically to ensure that they won't contract breast cancer as so many of their relatives did. Is Sue willing to go that far?

"I think about it, certainly," she says. "I keep up with the latest research on genetic testing for the breast cancer marker. Right now the results of the test aren't applicable to enough women for me to take such a drastic step. But if I did have the tests, and if the test proved that in all likelihood I will, indeed, contract breast cancer, I would have my breasts removed."

For Sue the choice is obvious and simple.

"We live in such a breast-fixated society that it's easy to forget what's important. But I'd much rather go through life with no breasts than to have breasts and not go through life. When it comes right down to it, there's no contest, is there?"

ONE WOMAN'S STORY

Rita's family history made her very conscientious about doing monthly breast self-examinations and having yearly mammograms. Her mother's twin sister had contracted breast cancer, as had another sister (both had had a mastectomy, one some fifty years earlier). A female cousin had also died of breast cancer.

It was during one such monthly exam some ten years ago that Rita felt a painful lump in her breast and immediately called her doctor. On palpating it himself, the doctor wasn't terribly concerned and was quite sure it was nothing to be worried about since breast tumors are predominantly painless, but of course a mammogram was done. It turned out that the painful lump was nothing to worry about—but the small spot that the mammogram detected was another story. A biopsy proved the spot to be malignant.

Needless to say, Rita's diagnosis was frightening, but given her family history, it came as no surprise to her. What was a surprise—to her and to everyone who knew her, including her husband and her doctor—was how calmly she dealt with it. Her basic attitude was "Okay, I have cancer. Let's go take care of it."

Fortunately the lump was so small and had been detected so early that only a lumpectomy—removal of the mass itself and nearby lymph nodes to determine whether the cancer had spread—was necessary, plus follow-up radiation treatment. In fact, the radiation treatments proved to be hardest of all on Rita, necessitating hospital visits five days a week for six weeks, and the resultant fatigue lingered for almost nine months after they were stopped.

The radiation treatments finally did end, as did her visits to the radiotherapist at six-month intervals. After that Rita just had yearly checkups with her oncologist plus her usual yearly mammogram, and, of course, she performed her monthly self-exams religiously. Her ninth yearly postoperative exam was strictly routine and, just as routinely, brought her yet another clean bill of health. Four weeks later, while examining her breasts during her monthly self-exam, Rita found a lump, and, as if confirming the disquieting discovery, her nipple had suddenly retracted. Her oncologist saw her that day and was stunned by the rapidity of the tumor's growth. A biopsy showed the mass to be malignant, and a modified mastectomy was immediately performed.

Later, Rita consulted a plastic surgeon. He explained that breast reconstruction options are dictated by a woman's body shape, size, and general muscle tone. Rita was not in good physical condition. Therefore, because reconstruction is major surgery, and all surgeries carry some risk, Rita chose not to have reconstruction. Her position was "I am not any less of a woman without my breast." If her husband had felt strongly about her having reconstruction, she probably would have done so, but he supported her decision wholeheartedly. Rita purchased a breast form instead.

But Rita's cancer was fast-moving and aggressive. Just two months later a biopsy done in the left breast found malignant cells in it, too, necessitating removal of the breast.

Several months have passed since the one–two punch of Rita's mastectomies, yet her optimism continues unabated. Although she misses the sensation of having breasts during lovemaking, it's a minor regret and, at age forty-eight, no more so than losing other aspects of her youth.

The surgery wasn't easy—in fact, it was, in her words, "a big, scary deal." But having a loving, supportive husband certainly makes it easier for her, and being prepared, being strong, and refusing to be a victim are Rita's most powerful weapons in her fight against the cancer that has invaded her body and her life.

MAKING INFORMED DECISIONS

In order to develop a thorough understanding of treatment options, a woman should consult one or more health professionals as well as other women who have undergone cancer therapy. Local libraries and bookstores will offer a range of titles that address most of the important questions you have, and you can find the most up-to-date information through the American Cancer Society, the National Cancer Institute, the Susan G. Komen Breast Cancer Foundation, the Y-ME National Breast Cancer Organization, or the National Alliance of Breast Cancer Organizations.

The American Cancer Society's Cancer Response System will answer questions about standard treatments for any form of cancer. In addition, they will be able to refer you to local divisions of the society that can provide you with a list of specialists in your area of the country. Call 800-ACS-2345.

The Cancer Information Service of the National Cancer Institute will answer questions about new and promising treatments as well as the more conventional approaches. If you are interested in experimental therapies, they will refer you to doctors conducting clinical trials. Call 800-4-CANCER.

The other organizations may be contacted at:
Susan G. Komen Breast Cancer Foundation
Occidental Tower
5005 LBJ Freeway
Suite 370
Dallas, TX 75244
972-855-1600

Y-ME National Breast Cancer Organization
212 W. Van Buren Street
Chicago, IL 60607
312-986-8228, or toll-free hotline 800-221-2141 (9:00 A.M.–5:00 P.M. CST)

National Alliance of Breast Cancer Organizations (NABCO)
9 East 37th Street
10th Floor
New York, NY 10016
212-889-0606, or information services 800-719-9154

CHAPTER 18

The Menstrual Cycle
and Related Conditions

CONTENTS

Menarche—which is marked by a girl's first menstrual period—heralds the reproductive phase of a woman's life. Usually it begins around the age of thirteen. The menstrual cycle—which begins on the first day of one period and ends with the onset of the next—lasts an average of twenty-eight days. Individual cycles can span several days more or less and still be normal.

During each menstrual cycle, the body's balance of hormones rises and falls to create an optimal environment for the release of an egg. Should the meeting of a sperm and the egg produce conception, the developing embryo will find a blood-enriched home.

Every female is born with a complete supply of eggs (ova); she will not produce more. In fact, the number of eggs actually decreases before a girl is born. At six months' gestation, the female fetus holds close to seven million eggs in her ovaries. By the time that girl child is born, most of her eggs have been absorbed, though a million or two remain. When the eggs are finally summoned by hormonal signals at menarche, there are about 400,000 left in the ovaries. By menopause—which signals the conclusion of a woman's reproductive phase—only a few hundred are still to be found in the ovaries.

During her reproductive years, every woman experiences—on both physical and emotional levels and with varying degrees of awareness—the continual and successive progression of her cycle.

THE MENSTRUAL CYCLE

A woman's cycle is regulated by a series of complex and overlapping interactions among hormones and organs. An intricate dialogue among hormones governs the release of an egg from the ovary (ovulation), the preparation of the endometrium (uterine lining) for pregnancy, and the shedding of endometrial tissue when no pregnancy is begun (menstruation).

Menstrual cycles vary in length from woman to woman—and in some women, they vary considerably from month to month. Ranging between twenty-three and thirty-five days in length, the average cycle is twenty-eight days, counting from day one of a menstrual period up to but not including day one of the next period.

Each cycle includes three phases: the menstrual phase, the proliferative phase, and the secretory phase. In the average twenty-eight-day cycle, the menstrual phase ranges from the first day of menstrual bleeding to about day five; the proliferative phase ranges from around day five to day thirteen; and the secretory phase ranges from around day fourteen to day twenty-eight. Ovulation takes place at midcycle, between the proliferative and secretory phases, on or about day fourteen. To determine somewhat predictably, for example, when ovulation last took place, a woman whose cycle spans twenty-eight days can count back fourteen days from the first day of menstrual flow. However, given the fundamental variability of women's cycles—emotional or physical stress can slow or hasten menstrual rhythm, as can such life-cycle events as pregnancy, breast-feeding, or the approach of menopause—it is not always possible to specify the exact day of ovulation or the precise length of each phase.

CHARTING YOUR OWN CYCLE

Many women find it helpful to chart their characteristic cycle in order to have a good baseline understanding of what is usual and normal. Such knowledge can prove useful during gynecological consultations, especially when there are persistent or worrisome changes, and in planning for pregnancy.

Start by noting the first and last days of menstrual flow on a calendar. Over the course of the month, note changes in breast tenderness as well as any changes in cervical discharge. Look for changes in cervical mucus: There is more of it, and it is clear and watery, during ovulation.

Body temperature is another predictor of ovulation. Your temperature should rise immediately after ovulation, but the most fertile days are just before *that increase. If your cycles are regular, you can anticipate ovulation from one cycle to the next by monitoring temperature changes. To do so, take your temperature each morning with a special thermometer before getting out of bed. Start the last day of your period and record the readings. For most women, the temperature rise occurs at about day fourteen of the cycle, but over a period of months you can establish your usual pattern.*

Note, too, variations in your general physical, emotional, and sexual feelings. Record distinct deviations or discernible rhythms at particular times during your cycle that repeat from month to month.

A clear understanding of your characteristic cycle can be used to help prevent or achieve pregnancy. It can also provide you with the tools to be a more active partner in medical consultations and decision making.

Menstrual flow, which is the shedding of endometrial (uterine) lining, is initiated by declining levels of the hormone *progesterone* toward the end of the previous cycle's secretory phase. These low hormone levels activate a regulatory center in the brain called the *hypothalamus* as well as the pituitary gland at the base of the brain. The hypothalamus produces *gonadotropin-releasing hormone* (GnRH), which in turn acts on the *pituitary* gland, at the base of the brain, causing it to secrete *follicle-stimulating hormone* (FSH) and *luteinizing hormone* (LH). FSH stimulates the growth of several egg-containing follicles in the ovaries. These follicles begin to produce their own estrogen as one becomes dominant (the *Graafian follicle*) and the others recede.

As the follicles in the ovaries secrete estrogen, the activities of the proliferative phase, which starts with the end of menstrual flow and ends with ovulation, are triggered. Estrogen levels continue to increase, all follicles other than the Graafian follicle atrophy, and the endometrium thickens in preparation for implantation of a fertilized egg. Increased estrogen levels inhibit the pituitary and FSH levels decline. At midcycle, the peak level of estrogen signals the pituitary to release a surge of LH, which ripens the Graafian follicle. Once it reaches maturity, it bursts open and the egg is released. For some women, the release of the egg may cause a brief, sharp pain on one side (see *Mittelschmerz*, page 424). For others, there may be noticeable discharge of vaginal mucus or slight spotting around the time of ovulation.

After ovulation, the empty follicle changes into the *corpus luteum*, which secretes both estrogen and progesterone. These changing levels of hormones are responsible for many premenstrual discomforts. The released egg passes into the fallopian tube, usually the one on the side where ovulation has occurred, and proceeds on its six-day journey to the uterus.

Ovulation marks the conclusion of the proliferative phase. At this point, estrogen is replaced by progesterone as the dominant influence on the sequence. In the next phase, the secretory phase, progesterone is secreted, along with estrogen, by the corpus luteum, which terminates the thickening of the endometrium. If the egg is fertilized, the secretions from the corpus luteum come under the control of a different hormone, human chorionic gonadotropin (hCG), and the process of pregnancy begins (see *Pregnancy and Childbirth*, page 237).

If conception does not take place, the unfertilized egg begins to disintegrate and will shortly be expelled along with menstrual blood. The higher levels of estrogen and progesterone now exert an inhibiting influence on the production of LH and FSH. The corpus luteum starts to die and production of estrogen and progesterone also diminishes. The thick endometrium can no longer be sustained, and it is therefore shed, along with blood and mucus, in the form of menstrual flow. The lowered hormone level again triggers the hypothalamus and pituitary, which increases pituitary production of LH and FSH, and the entire cycle begins again.

Changes During Each Cycle. With the wax and wane of the body's hormones, most women notice cyclical changes that correspond to their menstrual cycle. During ovulation, a woman's temperature may fall slightly in anticipation of the egg's release, and she may notice a watery discharge of mucus. If she has intercourse now, sperm can easily swim up through the cervix, into the uterus, and on down the fallopian tubes. After ovulation, the mucus thickens as the progesterone level rises with the approach of menstruation, and her vagina may feel drier. Some women describe a twinge of pain on one side when the egg is released.

On the days prior to and during menstruation, many women experience symptoms that stem from hormonal changes, such as breast tenderness, bloating and temporary weight gain, abdominal cramps, depression, and mood swings (see *Menstrual Concerns*, page 409).

Menstruation spans, on the average, thirty-eight years, and ends with menopause (see *Menopause and the Climacteric*, page 87). During this time, menstrual cycles fluctuate considerably, not only among women, but for each woman at different times throughout her reproductive life. Although the average cycle is twenty-eight days, the average period itself lasts between four and six days, although some women have periods as short as two days or as long as ten.

At different points in their life, most women find that their periods are more variable—during the first two years after menarche, for example, and in the years prior to menopause. As a woman ages, changes in her cycle are normal. She may skip a period from time to time without significance, or her cycle may be longer or shorter than usual, her flow heavier or lighter. Stress, too, can have a profound influence on a woman's menstrual cycle; the hypothalamus, which plays such a vital role in regulating and directing hormonal signals, is sensitive to illness and to physical and mental stress.

THE COMMONSENSE APPROACH TO MENSTRUAL PROBLEMS

Most women experience occasional or regular problems around their cycles, ranging from mild discomfort to acute pain. It's important to recognize these discomforts as a part of one's life and make reasonable accommodations for them. For women who are healthy, it becomes a matter of taking simple measures or making small life-style adjustments.

Get Adequate Rest. *Be aware of your needs and rhythms during your cycle. If you find you need more sleep at certain times of the month, try arranging your schedule so that it is less demanding at the times when your body needs more rest.*

Pay Attention to Your Diet. *Some women find that they can alleviate many symptoms by maintaining a healthier diet, consuming more whole grains and breads, beans, vegetables, and fruit and reducing their intake of salt, sugar, alcohol, and caffeine. It is usual for a woman's appetite to increase just before and during menstruation; eating more frequent, smaller meals instead of three large meals can help to counteract feelings of being bloated.*

Stay Active. *Exercise is an important aspect of a healthy life-style and most women can maintain their usual level of physical activity during any part of their cycle. Exercise can also ease cramps and lessen premenstrual syndrome. Unless you experience excessive bleeding, there is little reason to avoid most activities during menstruation, though many women find milder forms of exercise including yoga, swimming, fast walking, and moderate cycling preferable to more strenuous aerobic exercises during menstruation.*

There is a related caution, though: Excessively rigorous exercise, such as that undertaken by professional athletes and dancers, can interfere with regular menstruation. This is due to the concentrated effort, length of workout, amount of fat loss, and emotional stress. If menstruation stops as a result of any or a combination of these factors, try cutting back on your workouts. If menstruation does not resume after a more moderate regimen is established, consult your health-care provider. (For further discussion on exercise-related problems, see page 420.)

Look to the Obvious. *If you're continually tired or pale, ask your health-care provider to check for anemia. If you have occasional or periodic aches and pains in the course of your cycle, try nonprescription pain relievers such as aspirin, acetamino-phen, or ibuprofen.*

Listen to Your Body. *Above all, know yourself, your symptoms, and what works for you.*

EASING MENSTRUAL DISCOMFORT AT HOME

For generations, women have been treating their premenstrual and menstrual symp-toms through a series of home and herbal remedies. More recently, women have begun to turn to vitamin supplements in an effort to relieve their discomfort and pain.

For cramps and backaches, many women swear by herbal teas, especially rasp-berry leaf, evening primrose, and black cohosh teas. Others take calcium and magne-sium supplements. Still others simply apply heat to their stomach to relieve cramps or to their back to soothe aches.

Zinc; copper; vitamins A, E, and B$_6$; various amino acids; and enzymes have been used to ease premenstrual symptoms. An increase in potassium and a decrease in sodium are sometimes recommended during menstruation to address a string of symp-toms, from depression to tension, from moodiness to bloated feelings. Some women take vitamin C and bioflavins in response to heavy or irregular flow.

Medical research has not shown herbal remedies and vitamin supplements to have an effect on menstrual symptoms. It is a good idea to consult your health practitioner, a nutritional counselor, or a holistic practitioner before treating any physical symp-toms with alternative methods. Each woman, along with her symptoms, is different; how she responds to each remedy will be different. It is, therefore, essential that every woman know herself and assess her response to each remedy she tries. If there is any question about or dramatic side effect of any remedy, consult a health-care profes-sional.

To locate a doctor or health professional who includes alternative treatments, con-tact the following:

National PMS Society
P.O. Box 11467
Durham, N.C. 27703

Premenstrual Syndrome Action
P.O. Box 9326
Madison, Wis. 53715

Premenstrual Syndrome Program
40 Salem St.
Lynnfield, Mass. 01940

MENSTRUAL CONCERNS

Most women experience some type of menstrual irregularity from time to time. Take, for example, Elaine. She had been spending unusually long hours at the office, eating out of vending machines, and getting little sleep. She was too busy to notice that the day she should have started her period had come and gone. Then a week later she realized she was more than late; she had missed a period. There was little chance she could be pregnant. Was something wrong? Should she consult a health professional?

Then there's Deborah. She is routinely miserable during her periods. Her stomach aches, she feels nauseated, and the simple act of rising from bed seems beyond her capabilities. Is it normal to feel this awful every month?

Suddenly, your periods, once scant and short in duration, are heavy and long-lasting. Should you be concerned?

Although it is normal for the menstrual cycle to change throughout a woman's reproductive life, certain changes might indicate problems. In this section, we will explore the most common changes and problems associated with the menstrual cycle. After reading the section, you should have an idea about what problems require your health-care provider's expertise, as well as those that probably are nothing to worry about.

A BRIEF GUIDE TO
TESTS AND PROCEDURES

If you are consulting a health-care professional about a possible menstrual problem, you may undergo one or more diagnostic or treatment procedures. The following are the most common:

Pap Smear: *During a pelvic examination, your clinician will swipe a plastic or wooden spatula or a Q-tip over the cervical surface, to remove sample cells from the tip of the cervix; using a brush or Q-tip, he or she will also remove sample cells from the endocervical canal (see page 634).*

Hysterosalpingogram: *By capturing an image of a dye injected into the uterus, this gynecological X ray allows the clinician to visualize the interior of the uterus and fallopian tubes (see page 630).*

Hysteroscopy: *The hysteroscope consists of a lighted telescopelike instrument which is inserted into the uterus through the cervical canal. The procedure can be done in the office or in an outpatient operating room (see page 632).*

Sonogram: *Also called ultrasound, this procedure uses sound waves, which are sent into the body to create a picture on a TV screen (see page 637).*

Computed Axial Tomography (CT) Scan: *This X-ray machine produces a series of highly detailed images. CT scans are commonly used to look at the pituitary or adrenal glands (see page 635).*

Magnetic Resonance Imaging (MRI): *A patient lies within a tunnel-shaped metal core while this sophisticated device uses both magnetic fields and radio waves to create exact images. MRI is used to image the brain and pituitary, among other organs (see page 636).*

Laparoscopy: *In this procedure, the clinician inserts a telescopelike device (the laparoscope) through a small abdominal incision in order to allow a direct view of the pelvic or abdominal cavity (see page 632).*

Dilation and Curettage (D & C): *In this procedure, a health-care professional dilates the cervix and scrapes the uterine lining in order to remove endometrial tissue (see page 633).*

Hysterectomy: *In this surgical procedure, the uterus is removed. The operation is necessary for some women who have cancer of the reproductive tract and may also be used for women who have excessive bleeding, fibroids, endometriosis, and menstrual or pelvic pain (see page 542).*

Progestin-Withdrawal Test: *If a woman has not had a period and is not pregnant, her practitioner may give her oral progestin, which when stopped should cause her uterus to slough its lining. This test indicates estrogen production and pituitary function.*

Myomectomy: *This surgical procedure involves removing fibroid tumors from the uterus (see page 543).*

PREMENSTRUAL SYNDROME (PMS)

PMS is a predictable pattern of both physical and behavioral symptoms that occurs in the second half of the menstrual cycle. The physical symptoms may include bloating, fluid retention, weight gain, sore breasts, abdominal swelling, aching and swollen hands and feet, fatigue, nausea, vomiting, constipation, headaches, skin problems, and respiratory ailments. Behavioral symptoms include depression, irritability, anxiety, tension, mood swings, difficulty in attending to tasks, and lethargy.

Many woman experience some degree of discomfort before their periods. Current estimates hold that 40 percent of women have significant bouts of PMS at some point in their reproductive life. A small segment of menstruating women—between 2 and 3 percent—have symptoms so severe that they interfere with work and relationships.

By definition, the symptoms of PMS develop before menstruation begins and disappear soon after it starts.

Thus far, no one knows what causes PMS, although there are many theories. Some researchers link it to altered levels of neurotransmitters (chemical messengers) in the brain. Clearly, it is in some way related to cyclic changes in hormone levels because symptoms disappear during pregnancy and after menopause.

PMS is not simply "all in her head." Although there is no question that psychological and psychiatric problems can manifest in PMS patterns, there is always a danger in ready psychogenic explanations. Besides often being simplistic and blaming, these kinds of answers at times can discourage women from seeking help and therefore delay diagnosis and treatment of underlying conditions.

Understanding the Problem. When a woman experiences premenstrual problems, her health-care professional should conduct a thorough history to discover a predictable pattern that indicates PMS. He or she may ask that the woman keep a record of her symptoms for several menstrual cycles. The health-care professional also will want to rule out any underlying problems, such as clinical depression, panic disorder, infections, fibroids, and endometriosis, that may contribute to the symptoms.

The symptoms of PMS can make life difficult each month, but there is seldom an underlying cause that will jeopardize a woman's health. Most women find that as they age, the symptoms of PMS abate. The more disconcerting symptoms can often be easily treated or modified.

Treatment Options. Treatment aims at eliminating symptoms and is determined by identifying which symptoms are most bothersome.

Vitamin E supplements have been used to reduce tenderness around the breast. Some women alleviate discomforts by making simple dietary changes—avoiding salt, for example, which can exacerbate water retention, and giving up caffeine, which can induce palpitations and feelings of anxiety. Some believe that a diet rich in nutritional sources of vitamin B_6, which is commonly found in meat, poultry, fish, shellfish, green and leafy vegetables, whole grains, and legumes, may ease discomfort.

Exercise may be helpful as well. Many health-care professionals believe that exercise can help lift mood and ease physical discomfort by releasing endorphins, chemicals produced by the brain that influence the body's perception of pain.

MEDICATION. Over-the-counter pain relievers can reduce aches and cramping, and there are preparations to address fluid retention and swelling. Pharmacological treatment for more severe cases of PMS has long been a subject of debate. Progesterone, once touted as a cure for PMS, may be no more effective than a placebo. Birth control pills, prescribed in low dosages, can modify some of the symptoms by overriding the body's natural hormonal signals and leveling out hormonal levels.

Although progesterone may not work better than a placebo, some practitioners have had success in treating PMS with supplemental estrogen. Low-dose estrogen replacement therapy can also help women approaching menopause.

When the symptoms are severe, some doctors will consider drugs that block signals from the pituitary gland to the ovaries. These GnRH agonists prevent the pituitary from making FSH and LH. Without these chemical signals, the ovaries do not make estrogen and progesterone. After a trial of six to twelve months, the drug is discontinued and normal menstruation resumes within a few months, sometimes without a return of the severe PMS symptoms.

During use, GnRH agonists can cause side effects typical of menopause, including hot flashes, moodiness, and sleep difficulties. However, use of hormone replacements can correct these symptoms.

DYSMENORRHEA

Dysmenorrhea *is the medical term for painful periods. Many women suffer from painful periods, characterized by severe cramping in the lower abdomen prior to and during menstruation. Women with dysmenorrhea also may experience sweating, headaches, nausea, vomiting, and diarrhea during their periods.*

The numbers vary, depending upon age and other factors, but the statistics consistently suggest that dysmenorrhea affects a large number of women. In one study of college students, more than 72 percent indicated they suffered to some degree from dysmenorrhea: Of these, 34 percent classified their symptoms as mild; 22 percent said they had moderate pain that required medication from time to time; and 15 percent said they experienced severe cramping that significantly interfered with their ability to work and that rarely responded to usual pain medication.

Dysmenorrhea is classified as either primary or secondary. *Primary dysmenorrhea* is menstrual pain that is not linked to any other condition or disease; its cause remains unknown. Typically, it begins in adolescence, usually shortly after regular menstruation is established. Roughly half of women who suffer from primary dysmenorrhea experience symptoms within a year after having their first period.

Primary dysmenorrhea appears to be an exaggeration of normal processes. In recent years, studies have looked at prostaglandins, a group of fatty acid derivatives found in human tissue that are capable of stimulating uterine contractions, and have suggested that excess levels of prostaglandin may be responsible for cramping and other body aches and spasms during menstruation.

The term *secondary dysmenorrhea* describes a condition in which severe cramps are caused by some associated disease. Unlike primary dysmenorrhea, secondary dysmenorrhea can occur at any point in a woman's reproductive life. There are many factors or conditions that can induce severe menstrual pain, including endometriosis (see page 545), fibroids (page 543), scar tissue from surgery or previous infections, or, less commonly, the use of an intrauterine device (IUD).

Sometimes the cervical canal is abnormally narrow or blocked as a consequence of congenital blockage or injury. Menstrual flow is therefore impeded, and the pressure exerted in the uterus results in considerable pain. This condition is called *cervical stenosis.*

Endometriosis, a disease in which endometrial tissue escapes the uterus and implants elsewhere in the pelvic cavity, is often responsible for secondary dysmenorrhea. This misplaced tissue still responds to hormonal cycles, even though it is no longer in the uterus. If it is on the ovary, for example, cysts that contain blood accumulated over many cycles can form. This tissue can cause pain as it grows and causes delicate pelvic structures to stick to each other, impeding their function and potentially impairing fertility.

Women who use oral contraceptives, which suppress ovulation and decrease the amount of menstrual flow, tend to experience less pain around their periods than women who use other forms of contraception. Also, primary dysmenorrhea is typically less severe in women who are over twenty-five and in women who have delivered babies vaginally.

Understanding the Problem. If a woman has pain during her periods, her health-care provider will first want to rule out underlying factors. He or she will ask about birth control, do a pelvic examination to look for signs of endometriosis or fibroids, and perhaps take a sample of cervical secretions to rule out infection.

Depending upon the initial findings, more extensive diagnostic procedures may be warranted. For example, if there is scarring of the cervix, the clinician may suspect cervical stenosis, a condition that can be treated with an office dilation (in which the cervical opening is enlarged). In some cases, an ultrasound—pictures of internal organs taken by high-frequency sound waves—may be ordered to look for cysts, fibroids, or other tumors.

If a condition such as endometriosis is suspected, a health-care professional may perform a laparoscopy, a procedure in which a lighted instrument is inserted through a tiny incision in the abdomen, allowing the clinician to check for abnormalities on the uterus, fallopian tubes, and ovaries.

Although primary dysmenorrhea can be extremely uncomfortable and distracting, it is seldom a cause for serious concern. Many women find that menstrual cramping decreases with age. Unless secondary dysmenorrhea is a consequence of endometriosis, which is the leading cause of infertility, it rarely prompts serious concern, and most disorders that cause pain during menstruation can be addressed effectively.

Treatment Options. If you have primary dysmenorrhea, your health-care provider may recommend an analgesic drug that blocks prostaglandins and therefore eases cramping. Natural or home remedies, such as hot baths, heating pads, yoga, pelvic exercises, deep breathing, and massages, may ease some of the discomfort.

The treatment of secondary dysmenorrhea depends upon the underlying cause, but, in some cases, surgery may be required to remove fibroids, endometriosis, or scar tissue.

MEDICATION. Prostaglandin-synthetase inhibitors, drugs that reduce uterine contractions, are the treatment of choice for primary dysmenorrhea. Studies evaluating the success of such prostaglandin-synthetase inhibitors as ibuprofen, naproxen, and mefenamic acid have shown that more than 72 percent of primary dysmenorrhea sufferers who take these medications get significant pain relief.

Birth control pills, which suppress ovulation, are often effective in relieving symptoms and may be prescribed if a woman needs a contraceptive method as well.

SURGERY. Some of the disorders that cause secondary dysmenorrhea may require surgical intervention to correct the problem. Endometriosis and fibroids may be treated with surgery or with drug therapy (see page 405 for a discussion of GnRH agonists).

If a woman is diagnosed with cervical stenosis, her clinician will dilate her cervix, although the stenosis may recur later. A longer-lasting therapy for this problem actually is pregnancy with vaginal delivery.

CHANGES DURING MENOPAUSE

Though menopause is a natural and universal passage for women, many of its symptoms, including hot flashes, vaginal dryness, depression, irritability, and insomnia, cause considerable discomfort. These symptoms range from mild to severe; in most women they are transitory and simply signal the natural cessation of the reproductive phase of their lives.

Menopause occurs when a woman stops ovulating and her ovaries no longer produce enough estrogen to stimulate the lining of the uterus. Many people use the word *menopause* or the phrase *change of life* to describe the climacteric, a gradual process that takes place over many months or years. The terms are not technically interchangeable, as *menopause* itself means only the cessation of menses (for a more detailed discussion, see Chapter 5, *Menopause and the Climacteric*, page 87).

Once a woman has passed the age of forty, her periods tend to become more variable, signifying the approach of menopause. Some women menstruate more often than usual, others less often. Some skip periods altogether. Menstrual flow may be heavier or lighter than it used to be. This increased variability can occur for years before menstruation actually stops.

Menopause is a normal stage in every woman's development. It generally occurs between the ages of forty-five and fifty-five, with the average age around fifty-one years. If a woman smokes, she may have an earlier menopause than a nonsmoker.

Understanding the Problem. As your periods begin to change at this stage, it is not necessary to consult a health-care provider unless you have heavy, prolonged, or persistent bleeding or bleeding between periods. Take note of any particular change and extreme or sudden variations in menstrual patterns.

While menopause is a normal process, some symptoms may strike you as severe or abnormal. Trust your own judgment and have them checked out. If, for example, your menstrual bleeding is alarmingly heavy or gushing, if your periods occur more frequently than every twenty-one days, if you have bleeding between periods, or if bleeding starts again a year after your last period, consult your health-care provider.

Two conditions—*osteoporosis* (loss in bone density) and *atherosclerosis* (hardening of the arteries)—occur with greater frequency once a woman stops menstruating, and these may require treatment (see pages 598 and 563).

Treatment Options. The advantages of estrogen replacement therapy (ERT) and hormone replacement therapy (HRT), which uses both estrogen and a progestin, continues to be debated both within the medical community and in the general media. Although many questions and concerns remain, many health professionals recommend hormone therapy for women during and after menopause. Estrogen not only relieves such symptoms as hot flashes, vaginal thinning, and dryness but can decrease the chances of osteoporosis and atherosclerosis. However, the newer drugs Edista and Fosamax have rapidly been gaining acceptance as safe and effective treatments, especially for beneficial effects on bones and, in the case of Edista, in helping prevent heart disease.

Lubricants like Astroglide, Transi-Lube, and Replens can be beneficial if reduced vaginal lubrication is resulting in painful sex.

Some women find that vitamin supplements resolve some of the discomforts of menopause, but to date there is no scientific proof that vitamin supplements are effective (again, see *Menopause and the Climacteric*, page 87).

CLAUDIA'S MARATHON

Claudia's father had been a runner; until he broke his hip in an automobile accident, he had been an excellent over-forty racer. Claudia had never been interested as a young woman, though she had inherited her father's slender build and long legs. As a teen, she'd been more interested in social things.

After the birth of her first child, however, Claudia had some trouble taking off the extra pounds she had put on. At the suggestion of a friend, she took up jogging—and discovered almost overnight why her father had loved it so. Claudia quickly worked up to five miles a day; within six months she was running ten and fifteen miles a day on weekends.

As a lifelong New Hampshire resident, Claudia had heard about the Boston Marathon all her life. She made running in it her goal and trained for it. She almost didn't notice when her periods stopped. When she realized it had been almost two months since her last period, she worried she might be pregnant again, but the over-the-counter pregnancy test she took reassured her. She just put it out of her mind for a couple of months, so focused was she on her running.

After she had missed three consecutive periods, she went to see her gynecologist. He examined her, did another pregnancy test, then sat her down for a life-style conversation. He remarked on her weight loss and the tone of her muscles. Was she on an exer-

cise regimen? he asked. She had known him for many years, and he knew her family. He asked her more questions about her running, how many miles a week, about her diet, and her overall health.

She realized from the relaxed look on his face that she didn't have a life-threatening problem. "You're not pregnant, Claudia," he said.

"I don't have cancer, either, right?"

"Of course not. You have what we call exercise amenorrhea, a kind of secondary amenorrhea. It means you've stopped menstruating because of your rigorous exercise routine."

He explained that secondary amenorrhea means the cessation of menstrual bleeding after regular menses has begun. It can be caused by pregnancy—which the tests they'd done ruled out—by extreme weight gain or loss, hormonal malfunction, or emotional stress—or by the kind of extreme athletic activity she had embarked upon.

Claudia suddenly felt panicky—she was counting on running the marathon. She confided in her doctor that it was really important to her. He told her, in turn, that long-term amenorrhea could be harmful but that, since the race was only two months off, she didn't have to abandon her dream. He recommended she take it a little easier—and then after the marathon, that she cut back some more.

Claudia followed his advice. She ran her race and was proud to clock a time of less than three and a half hours. She then settled on a pattern of three to five miles a day and no more than ten on a weekend. Her periods returned within two months. Her doctor told her that the next time they stopped, it would probably be because she was pregnant if she limited her exercise exertions. She looked forward to being pregnant—and to the half marathons that she had decided to run in occasionally: just to satisfy those competition instincts that she hadn't realized she had inherited from her dad.

AMENORRHEA

Amenorrhea, *a medical term meaning without menstruation, may be either primary or secondary. If a girl has reached the age of sixteen without beginning to menstruate, she has* primary amenorrhea. *If an adult woman who has menstruated does not have a period for an extended length of time, she has* secondary amenorrhea.

Although the absence of menstruation in itself does not harm a woman's body, it is unusual and may be indicative of a serious condition and should be corrected. There is an elevated incidence of endometrial cancer when the uterine lining is not shed regularly in women whose body is making estrogen. Women whose periods stop because of low estrogen level have an increased risk of bone thinning (osteoporosis). Moreover, amenorrhea makes getting pregnant less likely. For this reason, the absence of periods in a woman of reproductive age should be a source of concern.

Primary amenorrhea is, simply put, delayed menarche. Although most girls begin menstruation by the age of fourteen, the failure to menstruate by the age of sixteen or even eighteen is not necessarily cause for panic. Girls who are athletic or unusually thin often mature later than average; more often than not, they will eventually reach menarche without treatment.

That does not mean, however, that the problem should be ignored. A small percentage of girls have underlying hormonal or anatomical abnormalities. If, for example, a girl's breasts have not yet begun to develop by her midteens, she may have an undiagnosed chromosomal disorder that impedes ovary development and therefore ovulation. Ovarian failure is the most common cause of primary amenorrhea.

Rarely, when a girl's breasts develop but menstruation does not, an examination will reveal the congenital absence of a uterus, which occurs in one out of every four thousand to five thousand female births. About one third of girls who fail to menstruate appear normal in every other way. They have developed breasts and other female secondary sex characteristics, and their reproductive organs appear normal.

In many cases, primary amenorrhea is due to hormonal problems. In about one quarter of the cases, there is a benign pituitary gland tumor (prolactinoma) or other source of excess prolactin that interferes with the production of follicle-stimulating hormone (FSH) and luteinizing hormone (LH). Prolactin is a pituitary hormone that normally induces the production of breast milk in new mothers. Excess prolactin affects the hormonal balance.

Swimmers, dancers, gymnasts, runners, and other athletes who engage in strenuous routines are more likely to start menstruating later than average, although most start before it becomes a concern. Girls who suffer from anorexia nervosa, an eating disorder, or who are abnormally thin are more likely to have primary amenorrhea.

Secondary amenorrhea is the diagnosis when a woman stops having periods. In the absence of pregnancy, there can be a number of explanations for secondary amenorrhea. Stepping up an exercise regimen can disrupt menstruation because hormone changes in the brain prevent the hypothalamus from working properly to stimulate pituitary gonadotropins.

Because the hypothalamus is responsive to a host of internal and external signals, stress can trigger hormonal disturbance and, consequently, secondary amenorrhea.

As a woman nears the age of menopause, her periods may naturally become less frequent and then stop altogether.

Medications and drugs can interfere with predictable and regular menstruation. Women who use oral contraceptives frequently skip menses. It is not unusual for women to miss a few periods initially when they discontinue using birth control pills. Drugs used to treat some psychiatric disturbances and hypertension may interfere with hypothalamic functions, and therefore disrupt menstrual cycles.

Sometimes, however, the cause of secondary amenorrhea is more complicated and more serious. Scarring inside the uterus can prevent menses. Occasionally, adhesions form after certain medical procedures including dilation and curettage (D & C), which is commonly used for abortion and diagnostic purposes (see page 539). Rarely, lesions develop in the hypothalamus and interfere with the release of gonadotropin-releasing hormone (GnRH), the chemical signal that governs the menstrual cycle.

Amenorrhea can also be a symptom of *Sheehan's syndrome*. Associated with shock and extreme blood loss during childbirth or with postpartum infection, Sheehan's syndrome results from pituitary damage. Symptoms, including amenorrhea, inability to produce breast milk, vaginal dryness, and loss of body hair, may not appear for many years after the trauma.

Ovarian problems that increase or decrease the normal secretion of estrogen and progesterone can disrupt menstruation. Suspect conditions include ovarian tumors (see page 549) and rare chromosomal abnormalities such as Turner's syndrome (page 472), hermaphroditism (in which an individual has both male testicular tissue and female ovarian tissue), or testicular feminization, when an individual appears to be female but is genetically male (see also *Primary Ovarian Failure*, page 422).

Understanding the Problem. If primary or secondary amenorrhea is suspected, the first diagnostic step is a pregnancy test. If you are not pregnant, schedule a pelvic examination. Your health-care provider will check your vaginal walls for moisture and a sample of cervical mucus will be analyzed to determine whether there is adequate estrogen production.

When girls have never menstruated, the provider will look for indications of adequate growth and other pubertal development.

A thorough medical history will include questions about diabetes, thyroid disease, infections, medication, abortions, D&C, heavy bleeding associated with childbirth, rapid weight gain or loss, and eating and exercise habits.

The initial findings will determine the next step. A simple test in cases of amenorrhea is the *progestin-withdrawal test* in which progestin (a synthetic progesteronelike hormone) is given orally for five to fourteen days. When it is discontinued, the level of progesterone falls. If the uterus has been previously exposed to adequate levels of estrogen, the uterine lining will break down and shed. Bleeding also suggests at least some pituitary function.

Women with polycystic ovarian syndrome (see page 551) or those whose amenorrhea is due to moderate stress or weight loss generally will have bleeding after taking the progestin. If there is no bleeding in spite of the progestin, the conclusion is that production of estrogen is insufficient. Women experiencing severe stress or weight loss or anorexia nervosa, or those who have pituitary tumors, ovarian failure, or hypothalamic lesions typically do not bleed even with progestin. In such cases, estrogen is given to determine whether the uterus can respond to hormonal stimulation by building up and shedding its lining. Depending upon the probable cause of the problem, further testing may be needed.

If the health-care provider suspects a pelvic tumor or other lesion, a sonogram may be scheduled. If a brain, pituitary, or adrenal problem is suspected, a computed tomographic (CT) scan or magnetic resonance imaging (MRI) may be ordered.

Treatment Options. Treatment for amenorrhea is initiated only after a complete diagnostic workup. In most instances, the root of the problem is not serious; nevertheless, amenorrhea causes many women great concern. More often than not, appropriate treatment results in the timely resumption of menstruation.

Medication. If a woman is trying to get pregnant, her health-care provider may prescribe various hormones to induce ovulation. If not, to reduce any risk of endometrial cancer, she may be asked to take a progestin or oral contraceptive so that her uterine lining is shed regularly. Also, if estrogen levels are habitually insufficient, hormone therapy will contribute to keeping bones strong and the cardiovascular system healthy.

Hyperprolactinemia or small pituitary tumors can be treated with a medication called *bromocriptine*, which works to inhibit prolactin secretion. However, the medication may produce side effects such as fainting, dizziness, and nausea if the dose is raised too rapidly.

Surgery. If a large tumor is discovered in the pituitary gland, it should be evaluated by a neurosurgeon or neurologist. Intrauterine adhesions can often be removed by a hysteroscopy, a surgical approach using a lighted, telescopelike instrument inserted into the uterus through the cervical canal.

Self-help and Alternative Remedies. When amenorrhea is due to extreme or precipitant weight loss, the best way to resume menstruation is through weight gain. Similarly, if a woman's periods have stopped as a result of strenuous exercise, it is best to modify the regimen. Proper nutrition and stress reduction can have curative effects.

Anorexia Nervosa and Amenorrhea

Most often appearing in teenage girls and women in their early twenties, anorexia nervosa is an eating disorder in which a woman experiences an intense aversion to food and, as a result, eats very little. Serious weight loss occurs and malnutrition develops. It is not uncommon for an anorectic woman also to have hypothalamic amenorrhea, a condition in which she either fails to begin menstruating, if prepubescent, or ceases menstruating if menses has commenced. The failure to menstruate is caused by brain hormone changes associated with the combination of dramatic weight loss and malnutrition.

Anorexia is a psychiatric disturbance alarmingly common in adolescent girls. In addition, it often occurs concurrently with bulimia. Bulimia is characterized by self-destructive eating patterns that typically involve compulsive overeating (binge eating) and purging through inducing vomiting or using laxatives. Bulimia profoundly disrupts the body's delicate nutritional balances and damages internal organs. Like anorexia, it can interfere with a woman's menstrual cycle.

A comprehensive assessment process for amenorrhea associated with eating disor-

ders should include, in addition to psychiatric and psychological consultations, an assessment of hypothalamic function (see Eating Disorders, *page 70).*

THE FEMALE ATHLETE AND MENSTRUATION

Although the benefits of an exercise program for most people are indisputable, many women have menstrual problems associated with strenuous physical training.

The female athlete, dancer, or gymnast may find that she is menstruating less often than before and she may stop menstruating altogether.

On average, prepubescent female athletes and dancers start menstruating about two years later than girls who are less physically active. As a rule, the onset of the first period is delayed five months for each year of athletic training.

How does something as healthful as exercise interfere with a woman's ability to menstruate? Researchers believe that amenorrhea associated with strenuous exercise results from the perception of stress by the brain. Studies show that strenuous and regular exercise stimulates hormonal secretions that suppress the release of GnRH, the hormone necessary to run the menstrual cycle.

Most female athletes resume menstruating once they ease up on their training schedule. If, after a more moderate exercise schedule is established, a woman still fails to menstruate, her health-care provider may prescribe estrogen supplements, because this hormone can be suppressed in a particularly athletic woman. Estrogen supplements also help guard against osteoporosis; studies have shown that when young women fail to have regular menstruation or to menstruate at all, there is a marked decrease in their bone density, which predisposes them to osteoporosis, a serious bone disorder most common in women whose body produces insufficient estrogen (see page 598).

Keep in mind that even when a woman is not menstruating, she may still ovulate; contraception is necessary to guard against unwanted pregnancy. Birth control pills are frequently a convenient way to replace estrogen and, at the same time, prevent unwanted pregnancy.

AMENORRHEA AND PREGNANCY

Amanda is a dancer. As a result of her strenuous training, it is not unusual for her to miss a period or two. Ilana is breast-feeding her six-month-old son and has not resumed menstruating after her pregnancy. Anne at forty-nine is nearing menopause and is never quite sure whether she will menstruate in any given month. Barbara has lost a great deal of weight in the last two months and hardly notices that she isn't menstruating. Sue Ellen is not quite sure why she has missed her period: She assumes, with all the new pressures at work, that it's stress-related. She's waiting a couple of months before consulting her doctor.

How many of these women are at risk of becoming pregnant if they fail to use proper contraception?

All of them. Even though it appears that a woman's body has shut down reproductive operations, it is possible to ovulate at any time and become pregnant as a result of unprotected intercourse. It is necessary, therefore, to take precautions to prevent against unplanned pregnancies (see Birth Control, *page 101).*

OLIGOMENORRHEA

If a woman has infrequent menstrual periods occurring in intervals of anywhere between thirty-five days and six months, she has oligomenorrhea.

Most women of reproductive age have monthly periods, with the average menstrual cycle being twenty-eight days. Some women, though, for a variety of reasons, ovulate and menstruate less frequently.

As a woman approaches menopause, it is normal for ovulation and menstruation to become less frequent. Some women throughout their adult life have infrequent periods, simply because this pattern is normal for them.

Sometimes a woman who is not nearing menopause and who has previously had regular periods will begin to menstruate less frequently. When this is accompanied by an outbreak of acne and the development of hair on the face and body, it may be a sign of excessive levels of male hormones, which can result from an adrenal gland disorder or an ovarian tumor.

Infrequent periods may also be caused by certain abnormalities of the hypothalamus or pituitary glands.

Understanding the Problem. Identifying the cause of infrequent periods may require a physical examination, blood tests to measure hormonal levels, and possibly a sonogram to look for ovarian cysts.

Assuming that oligomenorrhea is not a symptom of glandular abnormalities or ovarian tumors, it is not considered a dangerous condition. If a woman wants to become pregnant, however, infrequent ovulation and menstruation may present a problem.

Treatment Options. If tests reveal that the cause of oligomenorrhea is inadequate estrogen, a doctor may prescribe an estrogen and progestin supplement to restore the natural hormonal balance. Not only should this hormonal regulation restore normal menstruation, but it can help prevent osteoporosis, a serious degenerative bone disease that sometimes occurs when the ovaries reduce their production of estrogen. The need for supplemental hormones may be lifelong.

If oligomenorrhea is the result of excessive amounts of male hormones (androgens), a health-care provider may order further tests to uncover the source—which can range from ovarian or adrenal tumors to glandular disorders. Treatment will be tailored to the test results (see *Endocrine and Autoimmune Diseases*, page 460).

PRIMARY OVARIAN FAILURE

If a girl is sixteen or older, has not begun to menstruate, and has a delay in the development of breast and pubic hair, she may have a form of primary ovarian failure. Often primary ovarian failure is rooted in congenital defects that result from chromosomal abnormalities.

Most girls who reach the age of sixteen without menstruating are simply late in maturing or, as a result of vigorous exercise, delayed. Some girls, however, have congenital abnormalities that interfere with pubertal development. In some cases, these chromosomal defects are evident at birth; in other cases, there is no indication anything is amiss until the girl fails to menstruate.

One third of the girls who do not menstruate have *gonadal dysgenesis*, or abnormal ovaries. There are several types of this disorder, but the most common is Turner's syndrome, which occurs in 1 out of 2,500 female births (see page 472). Turner's syndrome varies in severity and may be diagnosed at birth or not until puberty. Girls with this disorder are born with undeveloped ovaries that do not contain follicles or eggs. Adolescents with Turner's syndrome are typically short, with a childlike body that shows little evidence of pubertal development.

Another chromosomal abnormality that can cause primary ovarian failure is testicular feminization, which is usually diagnosed at puberty when a girl fails to start menstruating. Such girls have breast development but scanty pubic and underarm hair. Although external genitals appear normal, upon examination a health-care provider will discover that the vagina is short and there is no cervix. A girl with this disorder lacks female internal reproductive organs. In place of uterus, ovaries, and fallopian tubes, she has undescended testes within the abdomen or groin. This condition carries an increased risk of gonadal cancer.

Understanding the Problem. The first step in diagnosing primary ovarian failure is a physical exam. If a health-care provider has reason to believe that delayed development may be due to a congenital problem, he or she may order a chromosomal study and blood tests to measure hormone levels.

Reaching a diagnosis may involve a progestin-withdrawal test. The hormone progestin is given for a time and then stopped. If the ovaries are producing estrogen, the progestin therapy will cause withdrawal bleeding (that is, bleeding that occurs when progestin stops). If there is no bleeding in spite of the progestin, the conclusion is that production of estrogen is insufficient.

The diagnosis of primary ovarian failure sometimes can be serious. On the other hand, a girl with primary ovarian failure may have enough normal ovarian tissue so that occasional menstruation and even conception are possible. However, most women with this problem never menstruate and are unable to conceive.

Treatment Options. The optimal time for diagnosing and treating primary ovarian failure is around the age of puberty. At that time, estrogen replacement therapy can be prescribed to stimulate the development of secondary sex characteristics.

MEDICATION. Estrogen and progestin replacement therapy in various combinations will enable breasts and other secondary sex characteristics to develop. Therapy will protect her from development of osteoporosis, a bone disease more likely to occur when estrogen levels are low. Estrogen and progestin can be used throughout a woman's life or can be stopped at the usual time of menopause.

SURGERY. If a woman has testicular feminization, her health professional may recommend surgery to remove any testicular tissue in order to diminish the risk of cancer.

Often, surgery is also recommended for girls whose genitals are sexually ambiguous or for girls who lack a functioning vagina. Surgery can create a vagina capable of intercourse but not reproduction.

MENSTRUAL CARE

Women today have several options when it comes to sanitary protection. Most use commercially available, disposable sanitary napkins and tampons. Recently reusable devices such as menstrual sponges and rubber menstrual caps have offered environmentally friendly alternatives.

Tampons. *Directions are included in the package. Refer to the degree of absorbency on the tampon box and match it to your flow; use the lowest absorbency you can. If your vagina feels dry, if it's hard to pull a tampon out, or if it shreds as you remove it, it's too absorbent. If you experience irritation, soreness, or itching, reduce the level of absorbency or the brand, or don't use tampons.*

Menstrual Sponges and Menstrual Caps. *Because the FDA has not approved either of these devices, they are not widely available in pharmacies and convenience stores. However, they may be found in alternative and health stores. Both the sponge and the cap can be reused, offering advantages in terms of cost, convenience, and environmental considerations. On the other hand, because they lack FDA approval, they do not have to meet the same stringent health and sanitation standards that regulate pad and tampon production, and that may mean potential problems for the consumer.*

Menstrual sponges are produced from natural (not cellulose) sponges. Soft, damp, and pliable, sponges assume the shape of the vagina when inserted. This device often eliminates irritation and dryness associated with tampon use. Typically, a woman dampens the sponge before inserting. To remove it, she pulls it out with her finger. It needs to be rinsed out with cool water, then squeezed to expel excess water before reinsertion. Rinsing it in water and vinegar will control any odor that might develop.

Similar in appearance to the diaphragm, the rubber menstrual cap is worn near the vaginal opening, where it is held in place by suction to catch and hold menstrual flow. In fact, some women use their diaphragm in much the same way. Both hold more fluid than a sponge or tampon and are easily removed and cleaned for reinsertion.

Since the development of internal sanitary protection devices, many women have replaced sanitary pads with tampons and, to a lesser degree, the menstrual sponge. A few years ago, however, numerous cases of toxic shock syndrome, a potentially fatal disease, were associated with tampon use, particularly in women who used superabsorbent tampons. The tampon brand associated with the initial toxic shock scare was taken off the market and the number of cases has since declined. Although you need not give up your tampon or sponge, most health-care providers recommend you use these products with care to lessen your risk of development of toxic shock syndrome. Many recommend using regular absorbency tampons in place of the superabsorbent product. Women also are advised to change the tampon at least every four hours and to substitute a pad at night.

Many women are concerned about odor during menstruation. Menstrual fluid itself is odorless, but odors can develop when fluid comes into contact with bacteria and air. The key to feeling clean and fresh during your period is to bathe or shower daily and change sanitary protection frequently.

The vagina has a natural cleansing process, even during menstruation. Frequent douching is, therefore, unnecessary. It removes the vagina's normal secretions and, in so doing, encourages infection.

Some sanitary napkins and tampons are scented or deodorized. Although some women can use these products without any problem, others have allergic reactions to various chemicals. If your vagina or vulva becomes irritated or begins to itch during your period, it may be wise to use an unscented product. If symptoms continue, the tampon may be too absorbent for the amount of menstrual flow, causing your vagina or vulva to feel dry. In this case, a less absorbent sanitary product would be advisable.

From a health perspective, there is nothing wrong with sexual activity during menstruation. A diaphragm will temporarily block menstrual flow during intercourse, if that is a concern.

MITTELSCHMERZ

The symptom of mittelschmerz is pain in the lower abdomen during ovulation, sometimes accompanied by spotting or slight bleeding.

Mittelschmerz is a German word meaning "middle pain." It is used to describe the pain some women feel in the middle of their menstrual cycle during ovulation. The pain, typically a dull ache, may last for only a few minutes or for several days.

Although the cause of this midcycle pain is unknown, there are theories as to its origins. One theory holds that when the egg is released from the ovarian follicle, fluid from the ruptured follicle leaks into the abdominal cavity and causes irritation. The bleeding that some women experience with mittelschmerz may be due to the drop in estrogen level that takes place when they ovulate.

Understanding the Problem. Usually the timing and location of symptoms are adequate to confirm the diagnosis of mittelschmerz, although in rare cases, the pain may be so severe as to be confused with the pain of appendicitis.

Mittelschmerz is not a serious problem. Although it may be uncomfortable and disconcerting, the pain is rarely severe or incapacitating.

Treatment Options. A mild analgesic—aspirin or a nonsteroidal anti-inflammatory drug such as ibuprofen—may be taken in the middle of the menstrual cycle to ease discomfort. If a woman is in enough discomfort that her health-care provider believes additional treatment appropriate, oral contraceptives may be recommended since the pill prevents ovulation and therefore can mitigate mittelschmerz pain.

MENOMETRORRHAGIA

If you have unusually heavy periods you have menorrhagia. Metrorrhagia, *meaning bleeding between periods, may accompany menorrhagia, in which case the words are often combined as* menometrorrhagia.

An estimated 9 to 14 percent of healthy women have menorrhagia. Most of these women do not have unusually long periods—the average woman's lasts four days—but have excessively heavy blood loss, most of which occurs during the first two days of menstruation.

Excessive menstrual bleeding can be due to many physical factors. Girls who have recently begun to menstruate and who are not ovulating regularly often have heavy bleeding. At the other end of the reproductive spectrum, women approaching menopause may also notice their periods becoming heavier.

Although some women seem to have consistently heavy periods, others may suddenly notice excessive bleeding. Systemic diseases such as thyroid disorders (see page 468) and disorders of blood coagulation may be underlying causes. An intrauterine device (IUD) also may cause unusually heavy flow. Fibroids (see page 543), pelvic infections, and, sometimes, adenomyosis (endometrial tissue implanted into the muscle wall of the uterus, see page 545) can significantly increase the amount of blood a woman loses each month.

Unusually heavy bleeding among women of reproductive age may be related to miscarriage. Typically in miscarriage, a woman bleeds heavily after missing a period. If she suspects a miscarriage, she should see her health-care provider immediately to be certain that it was complete and that all the products of conception were expelled.

If all these organic causes are ruled out, the cause may have been anovulatory bleeding, sometimes called *dysfunctional uterine bleeding* (DUB). This is vaginal bleeding without the release of an egg. Women who have anovulatory bleeding have continual estrogen production, but, because there is no ovulation, a corpus luteum does not form, nor is progesterone produced. With the normal hormonal feedback system interrupted, the steady stream of estrogen causes the endometrium to grow continuously. The built-up lining is eventually shed, but not at a predictable rate. Menstruation becomes irregular, ceases altogether, or may turn into heavy, long-lasting periods. Anovulatory bleeding is relatively common during the first two years following menarche and again with approaching menopause. One risk is that excessive and irregular bleeding often leads to anemia.

Understanding the Problem. If you have an isolated case of abnormal bleeding, are not menopausal, and have no possibility of being pregnant, there is little reason to consult your health professional. If the bleeding has not subsided within twenty-four hours, however, call your clinician. In the event that pregnancy is possible or that you have several heavy periods, an examination is also warranted.

Your health professional will take a thorough history that should include questions about the frequency, duration, amount of bleeding, and changes in your menstrual pattern. You may be given a calendar on which to chart the days you bleed. It is difficult to ascertain precisely how much blood a woman loses each month, and determining the quantity of your menstrual flow is, to a large degree, subjective. It may seem heavy when, in fact, your blood loss is normal.

Rather than attempting to measure the amount of blood you lose, most clinicians concerned with excessive blood loss will do a blood test to determine whether your hemoglobin level is low, a finding that should reflect whether you have become anemic through excessive blood loss.

Your health-care provider also will do a pelvic examination to check for uterine fibroids and ovarian cysts that might be responsible for heavy or irregular bleeding.

If you are not ovulating, tests may be done to rule out endometrial cancer and other uterine problems. These tests may include an office biopsy or a hysteroscopy, a procedure in which a lighted instrument is inserted into the uterus (see page 632).

Treatment Options. The treatment approach varies, depending upon a woman's age and the persistence of the problem. Except when it is a symptom of endometrial cancer, menorrhagia in itself is seldom serious. In most cases, there is a related risk of anemia.

MEDICATION. If your uterus is healthy, your health-care practitioner may prescribe oral contraceptives to reduce your bleeding. If you are diagnosed with anovulatory bleeding, progestins or oral contraceptives may be prescribed to regulate bleeding. For women wishing to become pregnant, clomiphene citrate often is prescribed. Administered for approximately five days around the time of the menstrual period, the drug works on the pituitary to increase the level of FSH, which causes eggs in the ovary to ripen and be released at ovulation.

For those women with menorrhagia who are ovulating, the treatment may involve the use of antiprostaglandins, which inhibit uterine contractions; oral contraceptives; or progestins. In cases of menorrhagia in which the bleeding is severe, hospitalization, bed rest, and hormone injections may be necessary.

If tests determine you are anemic, you may need an iron supplement.

SURGERY. If you have an episode of dangerously heavy bleeding, your health professional may recommend dilation and curettage (D & C), a procedure in which the uterine lining is scraped (see page 539). Though done less often than in the past for excessive bleeding, this procedure may enable the doctor to identify the source of your problem by providing tissue for examination. Even when a cause is not found, the procedure may temporarily stop the abnormal bleeding, although for most women with recurrent menorrhagia, a D & C usually does not cure the problem.

Another surgical option for women with dysfunctional uterine bleeding that does not respond to medication is endometrial ablation, a procedure in which a laser or electrocautery device is inserted through a hysteroscope into the uterus. The hysteroscope allows the clinician to see into the uterine cavity, to locate and cauterize the uterine lining. Another, newer method employs a heating device and doesn't require hysterectomy. Endometrial ablation is more often the treatment of choice for older women who might otherwise need a hysterectomy. This is not an option, however, for women who want to protect their capability to have children, since infertility may result from the procedure.

Another common surgical procedure is myomectomy when the diagnosis for menorrhagia reveals submucus fibroids that protrude from the uterine wall. A myomectomy involves removing the fibroids and leaving the uterus intact.

Before the development of these techniques, women were frequently offered only one surgical option—a hysterectomy, or removal of the entire uterus. Though used today less frequently to treat menorrhagia than in the past, hysterectomy may still be the best choice when the underlying cause cannot be treated medically and childbearing is no longer desired. Hysterectomy might also be recommended for older women whose excessive bleeding does not respond to medication.

HYPOMENORRHEA
When a woman has regular menstrual cycles but the flow is unusually light or she simply has spotting, she has hypomenorrhea.

Seldom a cause for concern, hypomenorrhea can be caused by medications, such as oral contraceptives, or can result from an obstruction of the uterus.

Women who have had dilation and curettage (D & C) may, on rare occasions, have intrauterine adhesions, or bands of fibrous tissue that have bound together to obstruct the endometrial cavity, thus leading to hypomenorrhea. This condition is called *Asherman's syndrome.*

Understanding the Problem. If your health-care provider believes the symptom warrants investigation, he or she will examine your uterus for signs of an abnormality. To do this, a special procedure called a hysteroscopy (see page 632) may be performed. Routinely done in the office or in an outpatient operating room, this test uses a lighted instrument called a hysteroscope to examine the uterus.

Treatment Options. In the event that birth control pills are causing scanty periods, no action needs to be taken. Treatment is seldom necessary unless intrauterine adhesions are present.

If a woman who has been diagnosed with Asherman's syndrome wishes to become pregnant, treatment involves breaking up the scar tissue with the use of small scissorlike instruments inserted through the hysteroscope. An intrauterine device (IUD) may be inserted for a few months to keep the wall open and to prevent further adhesions from forming while endometrial tissue heals. Estrogen is also prescribed for a short time (about sixty days) to speed tissue repair. Over a period of months, normal menstruation will resume and the IUD will be removed.

TOXIC SHOCK SYNDROME (TSS)

The symptoms of toxic shock syndrome include a sudden fever of 102 degrees Fahrenheit or higher, vomiting, diarrhea, dizziness, weakness, fainting, disorientation, and a peeling rash that resembles a sunburn, especially when it occurs on the palms of your hands or the soles of your feet.

Few people had heard of toxic shock syndrome (TSS) until the early 1980s, when a small but highly publicized epidemic broke out among previously healthy young women. Not coincidentally, most of these women used superabsorbent tampons.

Subsequently, researchers found that a toxin produced by *Staphylococcus aureus* caused TSS. This type of bacterium is normally found, without adverse consequences, in the vagina of many menstruating women. Although it is not known precisely how superabsorbent tampons induced TSS, it is known that their prolonged use in the vagina increases the growth of these bacteria and encourages the production of the toxin. It may be that these tampons also produce minute ulcerations in the vagina that allow dangerous toxins to enter the bloodstream. The brand of tampons associated with these early cases of TSS was taken off the market, but most tampons available today still contain some superabsorbent fiber.

In the 1980s more than 95 percent of women with TSS were menstruating. Now, only about 50 percent of all TSS cases involve young menstruating women. The remainder of cases occur in men, nonmenstruating women, and children, typically after surgery.

Understanding the Problem. If you have the symptoms of TSS, especially if you are menstruating and using tampons, call your health professional immediately. Usually the symptoms are a good indication of the disease, although your health-care provider may also take a sample of your vaginal discharge to see whether it contains the *S. aureus* bacterium.

Both the severity of TSS and its symptoms vary, depending upon which organs have been affected. Most menstruating women who have TSS first notice the symptoms between the second and fourth days of their period. The initial sign may be a high temperature with a headache, sore throat, vomiting, and diarrhea. Blood pressure may fall abnormally low, resulting in faintness or dizziness. Within the first forty-eight hours, a skin rash that looks like a severe sunburn develops. Later in the illness—between twelve and fifteen days—the skin on the face and body begins to peel.

TSS is a serious illness that should not be ignored. Although the majority of individuals with TSS recover, the disease can be life-threatening. TSS also can recur, especially if a woman's vagina is colonized with *S. aureus* and she continues to use tampons. Up to 30 percent of women who have had TSS have recurrences, although subsequent bouts tend to be milder.

Treatment Options. TSS requires treatment with antibiotics for ten to fourteen days. In some cases, hospitalization is necessary to prevent shock and to treat kidney or lung failure.

PREVENTION. The best way to reduce the risk of TSS is to avoid using tampons, especially if you have had TSS in the past. If going back to using sanitary pads seems a bit extreme, try alternating pads with tampons. And by all means, wear the pads at night. If you do use tampons, use light or regular absorbency tampons and change them every four hours.

When is a tampon too absorbent? Unfortunately, one brand's "regular" may be stronger than another brand's "super." A good rule to follow is that if a tampon leaves your vagina feeling dry or is difficult to pull out, it is too absorbent.

ENDOCRINE ABNORMALITIES

Hormones are chemical substances carried in the bloodstream that regulate bodily functions. They are part of the endocrine system, which, along with the nervous system, oversees the body's responses to both the usual and the unusual. Think of a hormone as a chemical messenger whose message can be understood only by certain organs (target organs) or tissues. Generally, the greater the amount of a particular hormone in your bloodstream, the greater the activity of its target organ.

Hormones are produced in several glands housed throughout the body. The endocrine

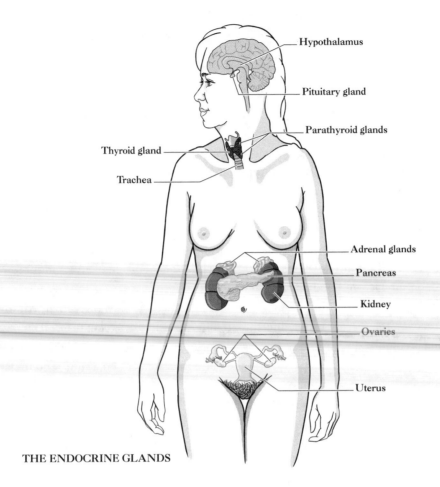

THE ENDOCRINE GLANDS

system consists of the hypothalamus, the pituitary, the thyroid and parathyroid glands, the pancreas, the adrenal glands, and the ovaries (testes in a male).

As we have seen in previous sections in this chapter, the regulation of the menstrual cycle is a complex process with many components. In addition to healthy reproductive organs, normal menstruation requires that hormones be released both in adequate amounts and in proper sequence.

In a healthy woman, the hormonal events that produce menstruation occur in the following order: The hypothalamus, which sits atop the brain stem, sends chemicals called releasing factors directly to the pituitary gland, which is located at the base of the brain. The pituitary, in turn, sends out gonadotropins, which travel through the bloodstream to the ovaries, where they stimulate the ovarian follicles to produce estrogen and progesterone. In turn, these hormones prepare the uterus for pregnancy.

As you can see, each organ that secretes hormones involved in the process of reproduction is dependent on others. A failure in any one part of this vast and complicated hormonal system can adversely affect another hormone, impairing the body's ability to respond and function normally. Faulty hormonal communications often manifest in problems with the menstrual cycle.

Many health problems—some alarming, others relatively minor—occur when any one of these glands fails to function properly. Probably the best-known endocrine failure is diabetes, which occurs when the pancreas produces little or no insulin, a hormone necessary for the body to process glucose.

Although some illnesses associated with endocrine problems do not affect the menstrual cycle, many of them do. It is the disorders of the pituitary, thyroid, and adrenal glands with which we will be concerned in this part of the chapter. In Chapter 20, *Endocrine and Autoimmune Diseases*, we will address other glandular problems (see page 460).

Pituitary Gland Tumors. The pituitary gland, which is roughly the size and shape of the last two segments of your little finger, is the most important of all endocrine glands. Located at the base of the brain behind the nasal passages, this gland functions as the body's control center, regulating growth, the daily functioning of the body, and the ability to reproduce.

The pituitary gland is divided into two parts, the front (anterior) lobe and the rear (posterior) lobe. Six distinct hormones are produced within the front lobe of the pituitary, including prolactin, which stimulates the production of breast milk, and growth hormone, which regulates growth throughout the body. The other hormones in this section of the gland influence various parts of the endocrine system such as the ovaries in the female, testes in the male, and adrenal and thyroid glands. The rear lobe produces oxytocin, a hormone that stimulates the breasts to release milk during breast-feeding and triggers contractions during labor. The posterior pituitary also releases antidiuretic hormone, which helps control the kidneys' output of urine.

Tumors of the pituitary gland account for 10 percent of all tumors found in the skull. There are two main types of pituitary gland tumors. Pituitary adenomas are typically benign tumors and, as such, do not spread. But because they grow in a confined space, they are capable of damaging the optic nerves and may cause headaches and, sometimes, serious brain problems. About half of all pituitary adenomas secrete the hormone prolactin, which can cause menstrual and other problems that we will discuss later in this section.

The other pituitary type of tumor is a craniopharyngioma. This tumor grows progressively larger in time, and, although it does not cause the overproduction of hormones, it can exert pressure on the gland, resulting in a host of serious disorders including hypopituitarism, the failure of the gland to secrete adequate levels of necessary hormones. Hypopituitarism often results in the absence of periods (amenorrhea) and infertility.

Thyroid Disorders. Shaped like a bow tie, the thyroid gland is housed at the base of the neck and wraps around the trachea or windpipe.

This gland is responsible for setting the rate at which the body functions. Prompted by

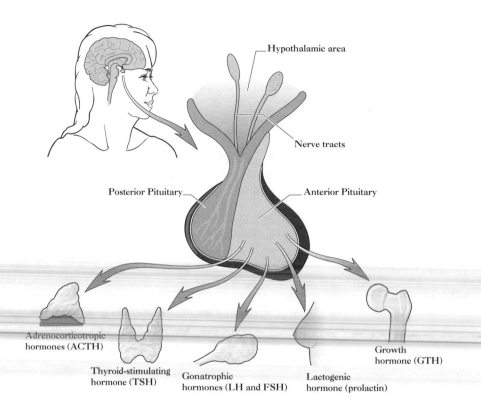

*The pituitary gland produces a range of hormones that, in turn, produce a variety of effects
on the body, by stimulating other glands (ACTH, TSH, FSH and LH), the breasts (prolactin), or
muscle and bone growth (GTH).*

chemical signals from the pituitary, the thyroid secretes the hormone thyroxine, which controls the body's pace of chemical activity. The pace varies: The more thyroxine in the bloodstream, the faster chemical reactions occur. The parathyroid also produces calcitonin, a hormone that affects the quantity of calcium in blood.

Either an excess of or a deficiency in the amount of thyroxine produced can result in disorders that may, along with other effects, alter menstruation.

Adrenal Gland. The two adrenal glands are located on top of each kidney. Each gland contains an inner core or medulla and a cortex, the outer layer of the gland.

The medulla produces hormones under the control of the brain that affect bodily functions such as heart rate and blood pressure. The adrenal cortex produces a group of hormones known as steroids. There are three kinds of steroids: Glucocorticoids regulate energy utilization; mineralocorticoids control the body's use of sodium and potassium; the sex hormones are androgens, which play a role in a woman's sex drive, and the estrogens, which are responsible for the development of secondary sexual characteristics and the regulation of the menstrual cycle.

PROLACTINOMA

A prolactinoma is a pituitary tumor that secretes excessive amounts of the hormone prolactin. This usually leads to irregular periods or interrupts menstruation altogether. Galactorrhea, the production of milk in a woman who is not pregnant or has not given birth recently, is another symptom of prolactinoma. Infertility is often associated with this type of tumor as well. A small percentage of women with prolactinomas have headaches during pregnancy. Furthermore, these tumors, when large, can alter a woman's field of vision.

A pituitary tumor called a *prolactinoma* is associated with hyperprolactinemia, which is the excess production of prolactin, the hormone that stimulates the production of milk.

In healthy women, many factors can trigger the pituitary gland to increase its secretion of prolactin. After a meal or a vigorous workout, a woman's prolactin level usually becomes elevated. Stress commonly causes a slight rise in prolactin levels, so it shouldn't be alarming when hormone levels fluctuate to some degree.

Sometimes, however, a person's prolactin level becomes abnormally high, resulting in menstrual irregularities as well as other symptoms. Frequently, drugs such as some tranquilizers, narcotics, and oral contraceptives cause abnormally high prolactin levels and the accompanying symptoms.

Prolactinomas are found in about half of all women with hyperprolactinemia. The tumor is relatively common, occurring in perhaps one of ten or twenty persons, yet many women never have symptoms. In general, the larger the tumor, the more prolactin it produces. Tumors smaller than one centimeter in diameter are called *microadenomas.*

Prolactinomas often develop during pregnancy; 15 percent of women with prolactinomas are diagnosed soon after giving birth.

Understanding the Problem. If a prolactinoma is suspected, a clinician will take a thorough history, perform a physical exam, and order special blood and urine tests to measure hormone levels. When prolactin levels are high, a computer tomography (CT) scan (see page 635) or magnetic resonance imaging (MRI) (see page 636) may be recommended to see whether there is a tumor.

Studies of patients with microadenomas have shown that most of these tumors do not grow; some actually shrink over time. Menstrual problems resolve without treatment in about one fourth of all women with microadenomas. Even so, a medication called bromocriptine may be recommended. A woman who wishes to get pregnant will likely have difficulties conceiving without bromocriptine treatments to reduce prolactin levels that otherwise inhibit estrogen production.

Treatment Options. Bromocriptine inhibits prolactin production. When doctors prescribe it, the medication is usually taken at least twice a day with food to lower the risk of nausea. Other side effects include faintness, headaches, nasal congestion, fatigue, constipation, and diarrhea. In most cases, these reactions are mild and short-lived.

About 10 percent of women cannot tolerate bromocriptine at first; in this case, the drug can be started at lower doses and increased gradually.

If a woman becomes pregnant while taking this medication, as a precaution, her doctor will probably take her off bromocriptine. There is no evidence, though, that the drug will harm the fetus or hinder the pregnancy.

Bromocriptine is often successful in restoring normal prolactin levels in women with microadenomas. Although in most instances it will shrink the size of larger tumors, surgery also may be necessary to remove them altogether.

SURGERY. If medication fails to alleviate symptoms, a health professional may recommend removal of the tumor. Some of these tumors recur, however, within a few years after the surgery.

RADIATION. If a large tumor cannot be completely removed, radiation therapy sometimes may be used after surgery in an attempt to reduce its size further.

HYPOPITUITARISM

The symptoms of hypopituitarism, a deficiency of the pituitary hormones, are varied. A child's failure to grow and mature sexually may be an indication of a deficiency of growth hormone, whereas the same hormonal deficiency in an adult will be more subtle, often producing a pronounced fine wrinkling around the mouth and eyes as if the person were aging prematurely. If a woman has a deficiency of gonadotropins, the hormones that in women stimulate the ovaries, a cessation of menstruation and infertility are not uncommon. Fatigue, lack of appetite, weight loss, and inability to produce milk after the birth of a child are other symptoms associated with a pituitary hormone deficiency.

Some people are born with a pituitary hormone deficiency; others experience the problem later in life, sometimes for reasons that never become apparent. Often, however, the cause of hypopituitarism can be identified. A serious head injury, a pituitary gland tumor, trauma from surgery, or irradiation of the gland all can cause hypopituitarism. Some women experience a pituitary hormone deficiency after childbirth. This rare occurrence, known as Sheehan's syndrome (see page 418), happens when the pituitary gland, which normally increases in size during pregnancy, loses its blood supply as a result of excessive hemorrhage and shock during delivery. When this happens, a part—sometimes all—of the gland is destroyed.

Because the pituitary produces hormones that activate other glands, a deficiency here can also result in symptoms more often related to other glands, among them thyroid and adrenal gland disorders.

Understanding the Problem. When a health-care provider suspects hypopituitarism, he or she will perform blood tests that measure hormone concentrations. To determine whether a patient has a deficiency of growth hormone, the clinician may inject her with insulin to induce hypoglycemia or low blood sugar, a condition that stimulates the pituitary gland to produce growth hormone, which then can be measured.

If the tests indicate hypopituitarism, further studies will be done to determine the underlying cause.

If untreated, hypopituitarism can be life-threatening because, in the absence of necessary hormones, the adrenal gland may be unable to respond to stress or infection.

Treatment Options. The treatment of hypopituitarism consists of replacing or supplementing the hormones that are deficient. Growth hormones may be necessary, and perhaps adrenal and thyroid hormones as well. If tests show that the adrenal glands are not functioning properly, the natural hormone cortisol will be replaced by a steroid drug such as prednisone or hydrocortisone.

To guard against possible infection or undue vulnerability to the system, these synthetic steroids may be given in larger amounts if a patient needs to undergo surgery or is under particular stress. Estrogen and progestin therapy may be necessary. And, if a woman is trying to get pregnant, her physician may prescribe gonadotropins in an attempt to induce ovulation (see also *Endocrine and Autoimmune Diseases,* page 460*).*

Hyperthyroidism

If a woman has hyperthyroidism, she may begin to lose weight even though her appetite increases. Nervousness and sweating, muscle weakness, a swelling at the base of the neck called a goiter, *increase in the frequency of bowel movements, and infrequent (or, in some cases, absence of) periods are all symptoms associated with this endocrine disorder. In one form of hyperthyroidism, Graves' disease, her eyes may protrude, her eyelids widen, and she may have excessive tearing and redness, and sometimes double vision.*

Hyperthyroidism occurs when the thyroid gland produces an excess of the thyroid hormone, thyroxine. Different types of hyperthyroidism have different roots. There are two major types of hyperthyroidism: Graves' disease (also called *toxic diffuse goiter*) and hyperfunctioning nodular goiter, which is sometimes referred to as *thyroiditis* or *Plummer's disease.*

Graves' disease is the result of an autoimmune disorder in which an abnormal antibody stimulates the thyroid gland. Graves' disease is more likely to occur in women, generally during the third and fourth decades of life, and tends to run in families.

Thyroiditis, or hyperfunctioning nodules, occurs when masses in the thyroid become overdeveloped, the result of which is the formation of an adenoma. The adenoma then produces an excessive amount of thyroxine.

Understanding the Problem. In addition to taking a medical history, a health-care provider will carefully question a woman about any recent changes in bowel habits and in sensitivity to temperature changes. A physical examination will be performed. A blood test will likely be done to measure blood levels of thyroxine. If a nodule is suspected, a thyroid scan can help identify the source of the problem.

Treatment Options. In some people, a brief course of treatment is all that is necessary to cure the problem; others require lengthy therapy. Left untreated, hyperthyroidism is potentially fatal. In most cases, however, appropriate treatment restores normal health.

MEDICATION. The most common treatment for hyperthyroidism is oral administration of radioactive iodine liquid. The iodine finds its way to the thyroid gland, causing the gland to decrease production of thyroxine. Two or three months after treatment, the clinician will follow up with a blood test. If the condition has stabilized, periodic reassessments are usually recommended.

Other medications used include prophylthioyracil and methimazole, which are given for a longer period of time.

SURGERY. Hyperfunctioning thyroid nodules may require surgery to remove a portion of the gland.

HYPOTHYROIDISM

The symptoms of hypothyroidism, a condition in which the thyroid gland is not producing an adequate amount of thyroxine, are lethargy, a marked decrease in physical and mental prowess, intolerance to cold, constipation, dry skin and hair, a slowed heart rate, heavy and prolonged menstrual periods, and a decrease in libido. Some people with this disorder also will have a goiter.

Hypothyroidism generally develops slowly over a period of months or years. The changes can be so gradual that you may not notice them, although it is likely that someone who has not seen you for a while will notice them immediately.

The most common cause of hypothyroidism is the gland's gradual destruction by an abnormal antibody. Sometimes, however, the pituitary gland fails to produce thyroid-stimulating hormone. In other cases, the deficiency may have been precipitated by treatment for the opposite condition, hyperthyroidism (see page 435). In some people with hypothyroidism, the cause remains undiscovered.

Hypothyroidism occurs most often in middle-aged women, although this condition can turn up in men or women of all ages.

Understanding the Problem. If you have symptoms of hypothyroidism, your health-care professional will perform a history, physical examination, and blood studies to analyze your body's hormone concentrations.

Hypothyroidism is usually chronic, but, in most cases, it is easily managed through treatment. Because thyroid hormones are crucial to development, it is especially important that infants and young children with this disorder receive treatment to prevent mental retardation or dwarfism. On rare occasions, a condition known as myxedema coma sets in, and hypothyroidism can become life-threatening. This usually happens only in cases in which the hypothyroidism progresses untreated for an extended length of time.

Treatment Options. People with hypothyroidism typically take thyroid hormone daily to compensate for their body's deficiency. In general, symptoms improve noticeably within a week or so and may disappear within a few months. Medication, however, will be needed for the rest of their lives.

CUSHING'S SYNDROME

A person with Cushing's syndrome has a humplike pad of fat between and above the shoulder blades and red lines called striae on the lower trunk. Over a period of months or years, her face becomes rounded and redder. Water retention, high blood pressure, susceptibility to bruising, and mood swings are common. Some women with this syndrome begin to have excessive hair growth on places where most women have little hair (hirsutism). Menstrual problems, usually in the form of amenorrhea (cessation of menstruation), are common.

Cushing's syndrome occurs when there is an excess amount of glucocorticoid hormone in the bloodstream. This hormone, produced by the adrenal glands, normally transforms protein and fat into blood sugar. In some cases, the adrenal gland simply produces too much glucocorticoid hormone. However, tumors of the adrenal or pituitary gland also can cause the syndrome, as can the prolonged use of high doses of steroid drugs. In rare instances, a malignant tumor of the lung or of another organ can cause this disorder.

Women are three times more likely than men to have Cushing's syndrome, which is more likely to appear when a person is in her twenties or thirties.

Understanding the Problem. Beginning with a thorough history and a careful examination, a clinician should also ask questions about the use of steroids. If there is no steroid use, further tests may be indicated, including blood analyses to check for greater than normal amounts of steroid hormones and a CT scan (see page 635) to search for possible tumors of the pituitary and adrenal glands.

Treatment Options. Untreated, Cushing's syndrome can lead to death. If the disorder is a result of steroid use, the doctor will likely recommend that the dosage be gradually reduced or another drug be substituted. It is important, though, not to stop taking the drug abruptly since the original condition may worsen.

SURGERY. When the cause is a benign tumor, removal generally results in a full recovery. A tumor of an adrenal gland often requires the removal of the entire gland, though such tumors are sometimes treated with radiation.

Excess Adrenal Androgen

When the adrenal glands produce excessive amounts of androgens (male hormones), symptoms include the development of excessive hair (hirsutism), irregular menstrual periods, acne, and the development of male characteristics, such as balding, an increase in muscle mass, clitoral enlargement, and deepening of the voice.

Whether male or female, the body produces both male and female hormones in varying amounts. Naturally, men produce more male hormones (androgens) and women produce more estrogens. However, sometimes a woman's body produces a disproportionate amount of male hormone. When this happens, she begins to take on physical traits usually associated with males and loses some of her feminine traits.

Adrenal tumors—both benign and malignant—can cause these symptoms in women (conversely, in men feminization occurs when an excess of estrogen is produced). Androgen-producing tumors of the ovary itself also produce androgen.

Another cause is *congenital adrenal hyperplasia*, a gland disorder caused by an enzyme defect occurring in infants and children. Congenital adrenal hyperplasia is an inherited disorder that occurs worldwide in 1 of 14,500 births. Female infants born with this disorder may have ambiguous external genitals and fail to thrive during the first few months of life.

The adult form of this disorder is *late-onset adrenal hyperplasia*, a partial enzyme deficiency that results in menstrual irregularities and hirsutism, or excessive body hair (see page 472). Also inherited, this disorder usually appears in girls in their teens or early twenties. The highest incidence is found among Ashkenazi Jews, who have an incidence of 3.7 percent.

Understanding the Problem. When a woman has symptoms of androgen excess, her health-care provider will do a careful history, a physical examination, and blood tests to determine whether it is the adrenal glands or the ovaries that are producing the excess hormone. If the clinician suspects an ovarian or adrenal tumor, he or she will order a sonogram, CT scan, or MRI. The diagnosis of late-onset adrenal hyperplasia can be established with special blood tests.

Treatment Options. Except when the condition is the result of malignant ovarian or adrenal tumors, in which case treatment is surgical, an androgen excess disorder usually responds successfully to medical treatment.

Medication. The treatment for late onset adrenal hyperplasia is a daily dose of such glucocorticoids as hydrocortisone, prednisone, or dexamethasone to decrease androgen production. Usually ovulation begins within a few weeks of initiating treatment, and other symptoms abate within a few months.

SURGERY. Most adrenal and ovarian tumors, whether benign or malignant, require surgery. Because ovarian surgery most often involves only one ovary, fertility may not be significantly compromised.

Malignant adrenal tumors, however, have often spread to the liver by the time they are detected, so even with chemotherapy, the prognosis for this relatively rare form of cancer is not generally good.

After surgery, most symptoms of excess androgen resolve, but any excess hair, although finer and slower-growing, does not disappear on its own; cosmetic approaches such as electrolysis may be used.

CHAPTER 19

Sexually Transmitted Diseases and Other Infections

CONTENTS

Avariety of microorganisms can cause infection when introduced into the body. These disease agents (or pathogens) are broadly categorized as bacteria, viruses, and parasites. Some are transmitted primarily through sexual contact, and the resulting conditions are commonly known as venereal diseases. Among these are gonorrhea and syphilis, afflictions that have plagued humankind for centuries. Other, more recently identified diseases include AIDS and herpes.

In the pages that follow we will discuss sexually transmitted diseases or STDs, as physicians now refer to them. We will also consider at length the subject of safe sex—what it means, how to do it, and when abstinence really *is* the wisest course.

CONTRACEPTION OR DISEASE PREVENTION?

Until recently, most people regarded contraception as a way to prevent pregnancy, nothing more. That was before the current epidemic of sexually transmitted diseases (STDs) produced a counterrevolution in sexual mores and practices. Today, in addition to helping prevent pregnancy, contraceptive devices such as condoms and spermicides can also protect users from a variety of STDs.

Previous generations, of course, knew about diseases that were spread through sexual contact. And as embarrassing as it might have been for our parents' generation to contract a disease such as gonorrhea, a "magic bullet" in antibiotic form was as close as the nearest doctor's office. Although most STDs still can be cured with the right medicines, some strains are resistant to the drugs traditionally used to treat them. In addition, some STDs more commonly seen now—genital herpes, for instance, and, of course, human immunodeficiency virus (HIV)—have so far resisted all efforts to find a cure.

Because the stakes are so much higher now, everyone, from the government to the medical establishment to school officials, is preaching the doctrine of "safe sex" (see page 442). The practice of safe sex requires extremely careful selection of sexual partners and the use of a barrier method of contraception during sex. Condoms, especially when used properly and with a spermicide, offer particularly good protection against STDs, including acquired immunodeficiency syndrome (AIDS).

VAGINITIS

Vaginitis *is the general term given to a variety of commonplace infections of the vagina, some of which are sexually transmitted. If you have vaginitis you usually know it; its symptoms are not subtle. You may notice an unusual odor or profuse discharge, the vulvar area may be itchy and irritated, and intercourse may be painful.*

Most gynecologists commonly see three varieties of vaginitis among their patients: trichomoniasis, caused by a parasite that inhabits the vagina and lower urinary tract; bacterial vaginosis, caused by various organisms including Gardnerella vaginalis; *and candidiasis or yeast infections, caused by a fungus.*

Trichomoniasis *affects women primarily during their reproductive years and without question is transmitted sexually. Women with multiple sex partners are at greater risk for both trichomoniasis and bacterial vaginosis. Symptoms include heavy, frothy greenish yellow discharge; itching and painful urination may also be present. Sexual partners of women with trichomoniasis, whether or not they show symptoms, should be treated at the same time to prevent reinfection.*

Bacterial vaginosis *is marked by an unpleasant vaginal odor and pale, watery vaginal discharge, although some women with this condition are asymptomatic (without symptoms). Although it is not transmitted via sexual intercourse, it is more prevalent among sexually active women. Sexual partners need not be treated.*

Candidiasis or yeast infections *are produced by an overgrowth of fungi. Symptoms include discharge that resembles cottage cheese, severe vulvar itching, and irritation.*

For a full discussion of vaginitis—symptoms, causes, links to sexual activity, and prevention—see page 501.

What Is Safe Sex?

The consensus among health-care professionals suggests that, when it comes to avoiding sexually transmitted diseases, you have three viable choices. One is abstention from sexual relations: No sexual contact equals no risk. Another choice is a mutually monogamous relationship with a person who is not infected. The third is the proper use of condoms during intercourse.

You are probably aware that numerous studies have found that condoms help prevent the transmission of viruses such as herpes, HIV (the cause of AIDS), and Chlamydia trachomatis, *the organism responsible for some cases of pelvic inflammatory disease in women. (For further information about each of these, see pages (454, 451, and 444, respectively.)*

What you may not know is that not all condoms are equally effective. *For protection against disease, use a latex condom, rather than one of the so-called natural prophylactics (generally lambskin). The porous material with which the latter are made is more likely to allow passage of a virus or bacteria from your partner's ejaculate through the membrane and into your vagina. A polyurethane or "plastic" condom is now on the market for those allergic to latex (although its efficacy against STDs has not been fully tested).*

Equally important, the condom must be used correctly. *Before your partner puts it on, examine it for cracks, tears, or other signs of damage. Make sure he puts the condom on his erect penis* before *there is any genital contact and that he does not remove it until the sexual act is completed. Also make sure the vagina is well lubricated, either naturally or with a water-based lubricant, because the condom may tear if the vagina is dry. To prevent sperm leakage into the vagina, your partner should with-draw immediately after ejaculation, while the penis is still erect. Otherwise the condom may slip off. Never reuse a condom.*

Use a spermicide, too. *In conjunction with the condom, you should insert a spermicide such as nonoxynol-9 into your vagina. Studies have shown that the use of a spermicide with a condom will decrease your risk of gonorrhea and chlamydia.*

The diaphragm won't protect you. *Don't assume that the other popular bar-rier method of contraception, the diaphragm, will perform the same protective services a properly used condom will. A diaphragm, with or without spermicide, will* not *nec-essarily protect you against AIDS or herpes.*

The female condom, *the newest over-the-counter contraceptive device, is a soft, prelubricated, loose-fitting sheath that is inserted into the vagina. The exterior portion rests between the woman's labia and the base of the man's penis during intercourse. Although initial tests have found that viruses do not penetrate the sheath, further stud-ies are needed to determine fully the female condom's effectiveness against STDs.*

BACTERIAL INFECTIONS

Among the various genital tract diseases are a number of ailments that are caused by microorganisms classified as bacteria. Not all bacteria cause disease—many are essential to good health—but among those that do are such familiar ones as streptococcus (strep), which causes sore throats, and staphylococcus (staph), the cause of toxic shock syndrome, among other ailments. Sexually transmitted diseases caused by bacteria include chancroid, chlamydia, gonorrhea, granuloma inguinale, and syphilis.

The incidence of some STDs caused by bacteria has fallen over the last several years, largely because of successful campaigns to educate the public on prevention and treatment. Bacterial STDs, unlike their viral counterparts, are eminently curable with antibiotics.

CHANCROID

Chancroid is an ulcerative disease of the vulva characterized by one or more small lesions near the clitoris or on the vulva. In rare cases the lesions may appear on the vagina or cervix.

Within forty-eight to seventy-two hours after it appears, the lesion fills with pus and becomes ulcerated and foul-smelling. Unlike the hard, painless chancre (sore) associated with syphilis (see page 447), the chancroid chancre is soft and painful.

Until relatively recently, chancroid was a disease commonly found only in the Third World. Since the 1980s, however, a growing number of cases have been reported in the United States.

Chancroid is caused by a contagious bacterium called *Hemophilus ducreyi*. If you have intercourse with a person who has chancroid, you run the risk of development of the disease within three to six days. Not everyone who is exposed contracts the disease, however, as

H. ducreyi cannot invade normal, healthy skin. The vulvar tissue must be irritated or cracked in order for the bacteria to gain entrance.

The incidence of chancroid is five to ten times higher in men than in women. As with many sexually transmitted diseases, chancroid often occurs simultaneously with another STD. An estimated 18 percent of people in large cities who have chancroid are also infected with HIV, the virus responsible for AIDS.

Understanding the Problem. If you have chancroid symptoms, your physician will perform a pelvic exam and obtain a sample of cells from the chancre. In some cases he or she may want to do a biopsy—that is, remove a small piece of tissue for laboratory analysis.

If you are diagnosed with chancroid, both you and your sexual partner(s) should be treated. Although treatment is generally successful, approximately 10 percent of women whose ulcer heals have a recurrence of the disease at the same site. Moreover, chancroid in women who are also infected with HIV is often resistant to the standard treatment and may require a different medical approach.

Treatment Options. The most commonly prescribed treatment for chancroid is a seven-day course of oral antibiotics. Symptoms should begin to disappear five to seven days after beginning treatment. If the infection proves resistant to the prescribed medication, prolonged treatment or switching to a different drug may be necessary.

CHLAMYDIA

The symptoms of chlamydia include painful or frequent urination, watery vaginal discharge, vague lower abdominal discomfort, and pelvic pain during intercourse. A majority of infected women show no symptoms at all.

Chlamydia is an especially insidious sexually transmitted disease because it often produces no symptoms until it has invaded a woman's upper reproductive organs and produced what can be irreparable damage. It is a highly infectious disease that can spread from the genitals to other parts of the body. If, for example, you are infected and rub your eyes after touching your genitals, a serious eye infection may develop. Chlamydia is, in fact, a leading cause of blindness worldwide. Moreover, an expectant mother can pass the infection to her infant during delivery, causing eye infections or even chlamydial pneumonia in the newborn. Chlamydia is very common in teenagers and college students.

Caused by the bacterium *Chlamydia trachomatis*, the disease is transmitted by vaginal, anal, or oral sex, and the symptoms described typically surface one to three weeks after exposure—in the women who show symptoms. If the disease is undetected or left untreated, the bacteria can migrate upward into the fallopian tubes. Chlamydia is thought to be involved in at least 40 percent of hospitalizations in this country for pelvic inflammatory disease (PID), a serious infection of the uterus, fallopian tubes, and ovaries that can lead to ectopic (tubal) pregnancy and infertility (see *Pelvic Inflammatory Disease*, page 449).

Understanding the Problem. Many health professionals routinely test women for chlamydia. If you have symptoms and your doctor suspects chlamydia, he or she will test for it and possibly for other STDs such as gonorrhea or HIV infection, because women at risk for chlamydia are more likely to have another STD as well. In addition to a pelvic exam, your doctor will obtain a sample of cervical secretions for laboratory analysis. Throat and rectal cultures may also be taken if necessary.

Treatment Options. Both you and your sexual partner(s) must be treated to prevent the disease from passing back and forth or to other partners. Typically one to two weeks' therapy with an antibiotic such as doxycycline is sufficient for a complete cure—provided the drug is taken for the full prescribed term—although newer regimens using single doses of certain antibiotics are also effective. Because chlamydia is so contagious, sexual contact should be avoided until both partners are confirmed by the clinician to be disease-free.

Lymphogranuloma Venereum (LGV)

Lymphogranuloma venereum (LGV) is a chronic infection of the vulva characterized by a single painless ulcer. After the ulcer heals, severe swelling of the vulvar lymph nodes follows, producing pain and, in some cases, headache, fever, and general malaise.

In women this highly contagious infection primarily affects the vulva but may also involve the urethra, rectum, or cervix. It is uncommon in the United States, occurring mainly in tropical countries, and is five times more likely to be found in males than females.

Understanding the Problem. Typically, a woman with LGV notices a painless sore, usually on the labia, that heals on its own. The second phase of the disease occurs one to four weeks later, when the lymph nodes in the groin become swollen and painful. This is when most women see their health-care provider, who diagnoses the condition by administering a Frei test—injecting the forearm with a diagnostic substance and observing skin reaction—or by obtaining a laboratory culture of pus from the inflamed lymph node.

If LGV is not treated, the lymph nodes enlarge, grow together, and form grooves in the skin. Within a week or two the nodes rupture into painful sores that take a long time to heal and may form cavities in the skin. Ultimately, the tissue is destroyed.

Treatment Options. LGV is generally treated with a three- to six-week regimen of oral antibiotics. In more serious cases, surgical reconstruction of the damaged tissue is necessary. Sexual partners must be treated as well.

Gonorrhea

The majority of women with gonorrhea exhibit few or no symptoms in the early stages of the disease. Those who do may notice a thick, puslike discharge from the vagina or urethra; frequent and painful urination; and pelvic pain during intercourse. Left untreated, gonorrhea can cause serious health problems.

In the United States alone, almost three million cases of gonorrhea ("the clap") are reported annually. The disease, caused by the bacterium *Neisseria gonorrhoeae*, is usually transmitted via sexual contact—vaginal, anal, or oral—but may also be passed by a pregnant woman to her baby during childbirth. It is often spread by carriers who either ignore their symptoms or have none.

Symptoms generally appear in men two days to two weeks after sex with an infected person; for women the incubation period is one to three weeks. Typically, however, the early symptoms, if they appear at all, are so mild—perhaps a slight increase in vaginal discharge and some inflammation—that most women have no inkling of the problem.

Although the genitals and reproductive organs are most commonly affected, they are not the only parts of the body vulnerable to this infection. Anal sex with an infected partner may lead to such symptoms as unusual discharge and discomfort in the rectal area. Similarly, some people contract pharyngeal gonorrhea after oral sex with an infected person, the symptoms of which may be a sore throat and painful swallowing. Gonorrhea may also spread to the eyes. Even infection in these areas, however, does not always produce symptoms. For many women, the first indication they might have gonorrhea comes when male sex partners inform them that they have contracted the disease and—very likely—transmitted it.

The disease is most frequently found in men and women between the ages of fifteen and twenty-nine, particularly those with multiple sex partners. Newborn babies today often have ointment placed in their eyes after birth to protect against undiagnosed gonorrhea or chlamydia in the mother.

Understanding the Problem. If your health professional suspects you have gonorrhea, he or she will take a specimen of vaginal discharge. Similar samples of throat and rectal secretions may also be necessary. Many women with gonorrhea are found to be infected with chlamydia or other STDs, which will also require treatment, as well.

If gonorrhea is left untreated or does not respond to treatment, the bacteria can spread to the uterus and fallopian tubes, causing a condition called pelvic inflammatory disease (see page 449), the result of which can be abdominal pain, ectopic pregnancy, or infertility. Gonorrhea can also spread via the bloodstream to other parts of the body, causing joint diseases, skin lesions, and, in rare instances, meningitis and endocarditis, inflammations of the covering of the brain and heart, respectively.

Treatment Options. Gonorrhea is treated with antibiotics, either by mouth or by injection. To be fully effective, the antibiotic must be taken for the full term prescribed by the clinician, and all sexual partners must be identified and treated as well. The infection generally clears up in a week or so.

If you are diagnosed with gonorrhea, it is crucial that you abstain from sexual intercourse until treatment is completed. Gonorrhea is highly contagious, and reinfection is common. Your clinician will advise you when it is safe to resume activity.

GRANULOMA INGUINALE

The first symptom of the rare disease granuloma inguinale, which may be transmitted sexually or through close nonsexual contact, is the appearance of painless red bumps, usually on the vulva but occasionally in the vagina, cervix, or anal area, that eventually ulcerate and become itchy and painful.

Granuloma inguinale, also known as donovanosis, is most commonly found in tropical areas, usually in island countries. Fewer than one hundred cases are reported in the United States each year; most of these are in the southeastern states and involve homosexual men.

The infection is not as contagious as most sexually transmitted diseases; it is found in 10 to 50 percent of the sexual partners of infected people. Repeated exposure is generally necessary for the infection to spread. The incubation period varies from one to twelve weeks, with most lesions occurring within thirty days after exposure.

Understanding the Problem. In areas where granuloma inguinale is more common, the diagnosis is typically made on the basis of the symptoms. In this country, however, where it is rarely seen, it may initially be mistaken for other diseases such as syphilis or even cancer. Thus it is important that your health-care provider take a sample of cells from the ulcerated area to be analyzed for signs of the disease.

Treatment Options. Persons who are or may be infected with granuloma inguinale are often tested for syphilis as well, as the two diseases often occur together. Granuloma inguinale can usually be cured with antibiotics—tetracycline, erythromycin, or ampicillin—taken for a minimum of two to three weeks. After a week on antibiotic therapy, most patients show some improvement, although it may take three to five weeks for the ulcers to heal completely.

SYPHILIS

The earliest symptom of syphilis is a hard, painless sore called a chancre that develops generally on the vulva, vagina, cervix, or, less commonly, the mouth, anus, or nipple. If undetected or untreated, syphilis progresses to a secondary and possibly a tertiary stage, both marked by more serious symptoms that involve the rest of the body.

The first clear description of syphilis was recorded at the end of the fifteenth century, when an epidemic known as the pox spread over Europe and Asia. Although syphilis is not as prevalent today as many other sexually transmitted diseases, it nevertheless remains a serious public health threat because of the potentially devastating consequences when the infection is not treated.

The Centers for Disease Control and Prevention estimated in 1990 that annually there are more than 100,000 new cases of primary and secondary syphilis in this country, although epidemiologists believe that only one in four new cases is reported.

Syphilis is most likely to develop in those between the ages of fifteen and thirty-four. There are more than twice as many infected men as women.

Syphilis is caused by *Treponema pallidum*, a spirochete bacterium that penetrates skin and mucous membranes. It is spread by vaginal, oral, or anal intercourse; having multiple partners increases the risk. A pregnant woman may pass on syphilis to the fetus in utero or to the infant during childbirth, causing deformities and even death.

The first stage of the disease, called *primary syphilis*, is characterized by the sore described, which usually heals without treatment in two to six weeks. If the chancre is undetected or treatment is not sought, the disease spreads throughout the body, typically six weeks to six months (the average is nine weeks) after the chancre disappears. The symptoms of this stage—secondary syphilis—may include a red rash over the palms of the hands and the soles of the feet, hair loss, and large grayish white sores on the vulva, mouth, throat, lips, or anus. Flulike symptoms such as headache, mild fever, and joint and bone pain may develop as well. Most women with syphilis are diagnosed during this secondary phase, but, if left untreated, the disease then goes into a latent stage with few or no symptoms that can last from two years to a lifetime.

The final stage—tertiary syphilis—develops in 35 percent of patients who either have been untreated or have been unsuccessfully treated during the earlier stages. The bacteria assault the central nervous, cardiovascular, and musculoskeletal systems, causing a variety of debilitating symptoms such as paralysis, blindness, and dementia and eventually leading to death.

Compared to many STDs, syphilis is only moderately contagious. An estimated 10 percent of persons who contract the infection do so after only one sexual encounter with an infected person; 30 percent of those who are exposed for a month to an infected partner contract the disease. The incubation period—the time between exposure and development of the initial-stage chancre—ranges from ten to ninety days, with an average of three weeks.

Understanding the Problem. If you have any of the symptoms of syphilis or suspect you have had sex with an infected person, see your health professional at once. If you have an open sore, he or she will take a sample scraping for analysis. Blood tests for the presence of certain antibodies are also used for diagnosis. Conditions such as pregnancy, hepatitis, malaria, intravenous drug use, and autoimmune disease can cause false-positive readings in a small percentage of these tests, so your clinician may repeat the tests or try another procedure.

When diagnosed early, syphilis can be completely cured without irreparable damage to the body. Often, however, the diagnosis is not made for many years, after the infection has spread throughout the system, potentially causing damage to the brain, heart, and other vital organs.

Treatment Options. If you are diagnosed with syphilis, you will be instructed not to have sex until you have been fully treated. All sexual partners must also be notified and treated, and many states require that diagnosed cases of syphilis be reported to local health departments.

Both the primary and secondary stages of syphilis are cured by antibiotics, typically penicillin. If you are allergic to penicillin, another drug can be substituted. Blood tests will be ordered every three months for the first year after your diagnosis to make sure the antibiotic has successfully eliminated the syphilis organisms from your system.

Antibiotics may not be effective during the final, tertiary stage of syphilis. Early detection and treatment are therefore critical; sensible preventive measures such as safe sex and mutual monogamy are also prudent behaviors.

PELVIC INFLAMMATORY DISEASE (PID)

Pelvic inflammatory disease (PID) is characterized by fever and constant and dull pain in the lower abdomen and pelvis. Some women with PID also complain of foul-smelling vaginal discharge; 40 percent have abnormal vaginal bleeding. Heavy periods and pain during intercourse are common. Nausea and vomiting may occur late in the course of the infection.

The term *pelvic inflammatory disease* refers to an infection of the upper genital tract, which includes the uterus, the ovaries, and the fallopian tubes. Infection of the tubes is also referred to as *salpingitis*, which results in scarring that obstructs the passage of the egg down the tube.

The common symptoms have been cited; however, perhaps the most disturbing characteristic of PID is that there may be no symptoms—until a woman tries to get pregnant and discovers her fallopian tubes are obstructed as a result of infection. About half of women who are infertile because of obstructed tubes do not recall having ever had the symptoms of PID.

PID is caused by a variety of bacteria that travel from the vagina and cervix upward into the reproductive organs and later the pelvic cavity. Some of these bacteria are transmitted sexually. The infections most commonly responsible for causing PID include chlamydia and gonorrhea (see pages 444 and 445), but PID can also be traced to bacteria that enter the reproductive tract during childbirth or gynecological surgery, after miscarriage, or even during use of an intrauterine device (IUD).

PID is typically found in sexually active young women; 75 percent of cases occur in women under the age of twenty-five. Women with multiple sex partners increase their risk of PID fivefold.

Of all the preventable causes of infertility in the United States, PID is the most common. In one survey of women who did not use contraception, 15 percent considered themselves sterile as a result of PID. Those women are more likely to have an ectopic (tubal) pregnancy than women whose tubes have not been scarred. Ectopic pregnancy can be life-threatening and may require surgery.

Other dangerous consequences of PID include the formation of an abscess within the fallopian tube or ovary, which requires emergency surgery if it ruptures. PID can also lead to peritonitis, an inflammation of the membrane that lines the abdominal cavity. Chronic pelvic pain and recurrent infection, which occur in 15 to 25 percent of women, are other risks.

With the current epidemic of sexually transmitted diseases, PID has become a major health concern. An estimated one million cases occur in the United States each year and are responsible for between 250,000 and 300,000 inpatient hospitalizations annually.

Understanding the Problem. During a pelvic examination, the health-care provider obtains for analysis a sample of cervical secretions to determine whether gonorrhea or chlamydia is present. If there is any doubt about the diagnosis or about the extent of the pelvic infection, the provider may want to perform a laparoscopy, a minor surgical procedure generally done on an outpatient basis at the hospital. During this procedure, the doctor inserts a tiny lighted instrument through a small incision in the abdomen in order to inspect the pelvic organs and ascertain the extent of the problem.

Treatment Options. PID is difficult to diagnose because it resembles other pelvic diseases, but if it is caught in its early stages, antibiotics usually eliminate the infection. In more advanced cases or cases that do not respond to outpatient therapy, hospitalization may be recommended.

MEDICATION. Upon diagnosing PID, your health-care professional will prescribe an antibiotic regimen. A follow-up examination will likely be required, and your doctor may advise hospitalization for more intensive therapy.

SURGERY. PID is usually not treated with surgery except when the infection is life-threatening or an abscess develops. Surgical attempts to repair tubal damage from PID may be made in infertile women who want to become pregnant.

PREVENTION. You can help lower the risk of PID by practicing safe sex. Have your partner wear a condom during sexual intercourse (see *What Is Safe Sex?*, page 442). Douching increases the risk of PID and should be avoided.

VIRAL INFECTIONS

Viruses are parasitic microorganisms that depend on other cells for their survival. They are so small—much smaller than bacteria—they cannot be seen except through electron microscopes.

Like bacteria, not all viruses are harmful to humans. However, more than two hundred are known to cause a variety of ailments, ranging from the common cold and most childhood diseases to cancer. A number of viruses are responsible for sexually transmitted diseases, including AIDS, genital warts, hepatitis, and molluscum contagiosum.

Viral STDs are not as easily cured as STDs caused by bacteria, and therefore pose the greater public-health threat. Genital herpes, for instance, is so widespread one expert estimates that up to a quarter of all Americans are infected by the age of thirty-five. The presence of virtually any STD may render the carrier more susceptible to infection by the AIDS virus, which enters the body through tiny lesions in the genital tract.

Because viral and other STDs are so easy to contract and have potentially serious—sometimes fatal—consequences, the doctrine of safe sex cannot be preached too loudly or too often, particularly among the young.

"IT CAN'T HAPPEN TO ME!"

Julie's a senior at a women's college in Massachusetts. She's a straight-A student, editor of the literary magazine, soccer star—and she's got venereal warts. "How can this be happening to me?" she wailed to her doctor. "I'm not one of those people!"

Her doctor told her that STDs do not discriminate in their choice of victims: Some experts estimate that half the U.S. population will contract a sexually transmitted disease by the age of thirty. Genital herpes alone will be "shared" by about one fourth of all Americans by the age of thirty-five.

Julie admitted to her doctor that she'd had a brief affair some weeks earlier with a graduate student at an Ivy League school. "Law school!" she howled. Unfortunately, law school—or getting straight A's—doesn't mean someone's necessarily smart enough to practice smart sex. The package may look great on the outside—good bones, good genes, good school—but you simply never know where that package has been. Anyone can be infected with an STD or be an unknowing carrier.

Fortunately for Julie, her warts were not particularly large or plentiful, and the doctor readily removed them.

Julie's come out of the experience a lot smarter. Instead of feeling betrayed by Mr. Law School ("I'm a good girl—how could he do this to me?"), she's taken a little graduate course on her own: on safe sex. Now she realizes that STDs are not something for other *people to worry about. Safe sex is everyone's business.*

It can *happen to you.*

ACQUIRED IMMUNODEFICIENCY SYNDROME (AIDS)

Initial infection by the human immunodeficiency virus (HIV) may be asymptomatic (without symptoms). However, well over half of all persons who acquire HIV infection have such symptoms as fever, pain in the joints, and night sweats. Less common symptoms are oral thrush (white patches and ulcers in the mouth), sore throat, and skin rash. These symptoms may last only a few weeks, and although the patient is still contagious, other symptoms may not develop for up to ten years.

Left untreated, the virus will gain a foothold and the body will become vulnerable to opportunistic infections and tumors, with symptoms that include swollen lymph nodes, diarrhea, dry cough, and a persistent low-grade fever.

Later, as the virus continues to destroy the body's immune system, the individual exhibits the more serious symptoms of full-blown AIDS: persistent infection, purplish or discolored lesions on the skin (Kaposi's sarcoma), shortness of breath, severe and persistent diarrhea, weight loss, thrush, night sweats, pneumonia, confusion, and dementia. With the immune system so badly compromised, coma and finally death result.

HIV infection has been called the most important epidemic of the twentieth century. First described in 1981, AIDS has since claimed hundreds of thousands of victims from virtually all walks of life. The news from the World Health Organization is grim: By the year 2000, it estimates there will be more than one million cases of AIDS worldwide and twenty to thirty million people who are HIV-positive.

HIV is generally transmitted by the exchange of body fluids in one of three ways: sexual contact with an infected person, use of contaminated needles or blood products, and transmission in utero from mother to fetus. Unlike many sexually transmitted diseases, HIV infection is not highly contagious. During sexual intercourse, for example, the virus must find a route into the bloodstream through tiny abrasions or cuts in the mucous membranes. Homosexual men who practice anal intercourse are at elevated risk for HIV infection because of the possibility of injury to delicate anal tissue during sexual activity, injury that allows the virus entry into the bloodstream.

A healthy person's immune system produces white blood cells, called T-cell lymphocytes, that orchestrate the attack of infectious agents that enter the body. HIV, however, invades and damages these protective T cells, then goes on to multiply and ultimately destroy the body's ability to defend itself.

Anyone can become infected with HIV. Some groups, however, are at higher risk: homosexual men, intravenous drug users and their sex partners, and hemophiliacs, who, because of their disease, require blood products (although since 1985, when health officials began to test the nation's blood supply for the AIDS virus, the risk of getting the infection from blood products has been markedly reduced). In the United States, the vast majority of AIDS victims are men, though in some countries, up to half the victims are female. More women are being infected with HIV and this trend seems likely to increase.

Understanding the Problem. If you are in a high-risk group for HIV infection, have symptoms, or believe you may have been exposed to the virus, ask your health-care provider or clinic to give you a blood test, which will determine whether your body is producing HIV antibodies, a sign you have the infection. The most common test is the enzyme-linked immunosorbent assay (ELISA), which, however, is not foolproof; it sometimes does not detect infection in the earliest stages and occasionally registers false-positive results (meaning the test results indicate the presence of the virus when it is not actually present). A positive ELISA test result is confirmed by a more accurate test called a western blot.

To date, there is no cure for AIDS, although with new drug therapies many people with HIV are living longer, healthier lives. After infection with the virus, an individual may have no symptoms or suffer from illness similar to mononucleosis, with fever, sore throat, and malaise. Within four to six weeks the body produces adequate antibody levels and the patient generally feels better. He or she is still contagious, however. Then follows a latent period that may last ten years or more. Although there may be times during this period when flulike symptoms return, for the most part the patient is able to function normally. In time, however, the disease progresses as the number and quality of lymphocytes are destroyed.

Treatment Options. Although there is currently no cure for AIDS, many new drugs have been developed for use in treating both people with AIDS and those who are HIV-infected but do not yet have AIDS. Powerful new combinations of medications ("drug cocktails") have been found to cut the death rate even among people with a severely compromised immune system by as much as 75 percent.

MEDICATION. HIV is one of several retroviruses that cause human disease. The strategic approach to treating HIV infections has been to develop drugs that interrupt the multiplication of virus particles at different stages of their normal life cycle. The drugs developed to date that are in clinical use are called *antiretrovirals*. The drugs block enzymes that are essential to viral multiplication.

There are three classes of antiretrovirals currently prescribed by clinicians. There are *nucleoside reverse transcriptase (enzyme) inhibitors*. These include zidovudine (AZT), didanosine (ddI), zalcitabine (ddC), stavudine (d4T), and lamividine (3TC). The second class is the *nonnucleoside reverse transcriptase inhibitors*, which include nevirapine (Viramune) and delcivirdine (Rescriptor). The third class consists of the *protease inhibitors* indiriavir (Crixivan), ritouavir (Norvir), saquinavir (Duvirael and Fortauace), and nelfinavir (Viracept).

Current recommendations for the treatment of symptomatic HIV-infected individuals or those asymptomatic persons who reveal laboratory evidence that the disease is progressing were released by the Centers for Disease Control (CDC) in 1998. At least one protease inhibitor and two reverse transcriptase inhibitors are recommended for initial therapy and have been shown to slow the disease progress and to prolong life. More information about antiretroviral therapy is becoming available; it will help determine the best time to initiate therapy, the best time to alter it, and the most effective dosages and *combinations* to use.

Other agents that improve the immunological function in people with HIV may also prove to be of significant benefit when used with antiretroviral drugs.

PREVENTION. The only truly effective preventive measure is abstinence or a mutually exclusive sexual relationship with an uninfected partner. But if you do have HIV or AIDS or are sexually intimate with someone who does, it is crucial that you practice safe sex to prevent spreading the infection. Avoid anal sex and sex with multiple sex partners. Always have your partner use a condom during sex, and remember that latex condoms offer more protection than "natural membrane" prophylactics. Spermicides such as nonoxynol-9 further increase the protection, but they are *not* guaranteed to prevent infection (see *What Is Safe Sex?*, page 442). When receiving care in a hospital, clinic, or health-care provider's office, one must also be cautious of contamination with blood or body fluids. Needles should never be reused, and health-care providers should wear gloves when drawing blood or administering medications.

Keep in mind that HIV is *not* tramsmitted by hugging, kissing, shaking hands, or sharing a glass with an infected person.

The use of antiretroviral drugs in pregnant women with HIV infection both for maternal health benefits and for reduction or prevention of transmission to the unborn child has been recommended by the CDC (cesarean section has also been suggested to reduce transmission). Similar recommendations have been made for occupational exposure in healthcare workers. Vaccines to prevent HIV infection are currently being tested and preliminary results are somewhat encouraging for the development of an effective human HIV vaccine in the future.

The overall advances in the treatment and prevention of HIV infection as well as the treatment of the numerous opportunistic infections which occur in the advanced stages of HIV infection (AIDS) are extremely encouraging and directed toward the eventual control of this infection.

GENITAL HERPES (HSV)

The most noticeable symptom of genital herpes are small red blisters on the vulva and sometimes in the vagina and cervix as well. Prior to the formation of these blisters, you may feel tingling or itching at the site (called prodrome*); some women feel pain along the buttocks and the backs of the legs. A few days after the blisters appear, they open up to become ulcers that ooze or bleed. During this time it may be excruciatingly painful to urinate. About 70 percent of women during their first (primary) bout with herpes have flulike symptoms such as fever and fatigue.*

Herpes is a highly contagious and recurrent viral infection that is transmitted sexually; about 75 percent of sexual partners of infected persons contract the disease. In recent years the number of people with herpes has reached epidemic proportions. An estimated half million to two million new cases of herpes occur each year in the United States; up to sixty million Americans carry the herpes virus.

The effects of herpes are not only physical. Women (and men) often suffer psychologically as well. Because the disease is contagious and recurrent, many sufferers are reluctant to enter into a sexual relationship for fear of infecting their partner. But, although herpes can be considered a chronic disease, the vast majority of infected people lead normal lives, with only occasional mild outbreaks that restrict sexual activity.

Herpes is caused by the same family of viruses that cause chicken pox and mononucleosis. There are two types of herpes simplex virus. Type I usually infects the lips or the inside of the mouth; the lesions are commonly called cold sores or fever blisters. Type II is the culprit in most cases of genital infection, although type I is responsible for up to one third of cases. Once the virus enters the body—by penetrating the skin—it never leaves but instead retreats to nerve cells near the spine and remains dormant ("latent") until something triggers a flare-up. Type II infections are four times more likely to recur than type I.

Symptoms of initial herpes outbreaks usually appear three to seven days after exposure, but some infected people are asymptomatic (without symptoms) for years. Studies have shown that one in two hundred women who show no symptoms nevertheless carries the herpes virus, which she can transmit to sexual partners.

Understanding the Problem. Typically, women experiencing their first infection have painful enough symptoms that they see a health professional, who can usually diagnose the disease simply by looking at the sores. To confirm the diagnosis, however, the clinician may culture some cells from the blisters or ulcers. He or she also will want to rule out the possibility of other STDs.

Although herpes does not cause serious or permanent complications, there is no cure or vaccine for it at this time. If you are experiencing your first infection, you can expect to be bothered by multiple crops of blisters for up to two weeks if untreated. Generally the symptoms are severe during this period; then you begin to feel better. After the initial infection the virus remains dormant in the body but is periodically reactivated, often during times of stress, both physical and emotional, or even during menstrual periods. Fifty percent of women have their first recurrence within six months of the initial infection; the average woman with type II virus can expect four recurrences the first year. The good news is that recurrences tend to be less painful and shorter in duration than the initial attack.

If you have herpes and are pregnant, there is the danger that the virus will be passed to the infant during delivery. A newborn who contracts herpes in the birth canal may suffer brain damage, blindness, mental retardation, or even death. So make sure your obstetrician or midwife knows your history so you can be monitored for the presence of active lesions—both on the vulva and on the vagina and cervix—prior to delivery and, if necessary, recommended for cesarean section to protect the baby. Herpes during pregnancy will not harm the baby except at the time of delivery.

Some researchers hypothesize that the ulcers associated with herpes may increase the risk of contracting HIV during sex with an infected person, but this has not been proved.

Treatment Options. Left untreated, the lesions dry up spontaneously within a week or two. Aspirin or acetaminophen may be taken to relieve pain. Keeping the genital area clean and dry and wearing loose-fitting cotton underwear aid in healing, and sound health practices—plenty of rest, proper diet, good stress management techniques—help strengthen the body's defenses.

The prescription medication most frequently used to relieve herpes symptoms is the antiviral drug acyclovir. Although it does not cure the infection, oral doses taken during the primary outbreak will help speed up healing and reduce discomfort. If you have frequent recurrences, your health-care provider may prescribe acyclovir for several months or years to suppress the virus. Valacyclovir and famciclovir are equally or more effective.

PREVENTION. Herpes is contagious when you exhibit any of the symptoms. Thus it is important that you abstain from sex at the first sign of an outbreak, whether that be the pain and tingling of the prodrome stage or the actual appearance of sores. Wait to resume sexual activity until all the sores have dried up and scabs have disappeared. For partners who don't already have the virus, condoms may reduce the risk of transmission but are not a foolproof measure; abstinence is the more reliable practice. Frequent handwashing is recommended, as in special care to avoid contaminating contact lenses and causing eye infection. A mutually exclusive sexual relationship with an uninfected person, of course, is the best preventive measure.

If you do get herpes, keep in mind that it is largely an annoying inconvenience, not a serious disease, and you can expect to lead a normal life in spite of it. A positive attitude, open communication with your partner, and a healthy life-style are all helpful in coping with herpes and keeping it under control. (And it may help to know that several vaccines for genital herpes are being tested and may be on the market in a few years.)

HERPES: RECURRING NIGHTMARE?

Since the sexual revolution of the sixties, millions of men and women have been afflicted with the herpes virus. Although its symptoms are sometimes painful and demoralizing, they are not debilitating. What is frustrating about herpes is that it cannot be cured, only driven into latency until the next flare-up.

The notion of a latent period in the life of a virus has given rise to confusion, mistrust, and misunderstanding among couples. Karen and Spencer, for example, had been married six years when Karen was diagnosed with a bad case of herpes. She explained to her husband that, like a lot of her friends, she'd had herpes in college, many years earlier. She insisted she had never been unfaithful to him. But Spencer refused to believe that the virus could return after such a long time. He himself had managed to stay uninfected in the freewheeling years before his marriage, and now he was at risk for a sexually transmitted disease! Angry and confused, he accused his wife of infidelity. The impasse was resolved only when Karen's gynecologist assured Spencer that latency—of a few months or many years—is typical of the herpes virus.

After the initial outbreak, the herpes virus retreats into other cells in the body, where it remains quiet and inactive until some event lowers the body's immune defenses and the virus attacks again. The event may be quite minor, like a cold or a menstrual period, or it may be the run-down state a women finds herself in after a series of late nights, too many meals on the run, deadlines at work, and lots of stress at home.

Once you have the virus, it's impossible to predict when or even whether it will strike again, but you may be able to reduce the frequency of recurrence by cultivating life-style habits that bolster the immune system. It's also important to be honest with your partner, to educate him or her on the disease and its subversive ways, and to enlist his or her emotional support.

VENEREAL WARTS (HPV)

Small, fleshy warts on the genitals or around the anus are the characteristic symptom of infection with human papillomavirus (HPV). The growths may appear alone or in clusters resembling cauliflower.

HPV infection, also known as venereal warts, is a widespread viral STD. The number of new cases has increased by 700 percent over the past twenty years, and as many as forty million Americans are estimated to have it.

There are more than sixty types of human papillomavirus, and a few varieties are associated with cancer. Women with cervical cancer typically have been infected with one of three types of HPV, but most women with ordinary warts have not been exposed to those three.

Venereal warts are infectious; 25 to 65 percent of partners of infected persons become infected themselves. The average incubation period after exposure is around three months, although the warts may remain invisible for years. The disease is most prevalent among sexually active young people and those with multiple sex partners. Pregnant women, diabetics, and people with an impaired immune system are also more susceptible.

Understanding the Problem. HPV can be diagnosed during a pelvic examination, during which the health-care provider examines the warts and possibly performs a biopsy. Sometimes the first indication of an HPV infection is an abnormal Pap smear finding.

Treatment Options. Although venereal warts sometimes clear up spontaneously, most people choose to have them removed because they are bothersome, unsightly, and, of course, contagious. If you are diagnosed with HPV, both you and your sexual partner(s) should seek medical treatment to prevent reinfecting each other. Warts are removed by the application of caustic topical solutions, cryotherapy (freezing), electrocautery, or laser surgery (for more detailed information, see *Venereal Warts*, page 508).

HEPATITIS B

The initial symptoms of hepatitis often resemble those of flu: nausea and vomiting, loss of appetite, head and body aches, and fatigue. Urine the color of very strong tea and whitish-colored stools are also common. All these symptoms may occur one to two weeks prior to the onset of jaundice, a yellowing of the skin and eyes, the symptom most laypeople associate with hepatitis.

Hepatitis is not a disease most people associate with STDs. But one strain, hepatitis B, is transmitted sexually—at the rate of up to 100,000 new infections a year—as well as in other ways. About five thousand people a year die of acute hepatitis infection, and another five thousand die of the chronic hepatitis that can result if the disease does not get better.

Hepatitis is an inflammation of the liver that is usually caused by a virus but sometimes may be the result of certain medications or toxic substances. The infected liver is unable to filter bilirubin (the yellowish pigment found in bile) from the blood, and jaundiced skin and the excretion of bile in the urine result. Five types of viral hepatitis currently identified are hepatitis A, B, C, D, and E. Viruses such as cytomegalovirus and Epstein-Barr virus can also cause the disease.

Hepatitis is transmitted in various ways, according to the particular type of virus involved. Hepatitis A, for example, is generally transmitted through a fecal–oral route: eating or drinking contaminated food or water or having direct or indirect contact with an infected person's feces. Hepatitis B is acquired through contact with infected blood or during sexual intercourse and is found most often among homosexual men, the spouses or sexual partners of infected persons, intravenous drug users who share contaminated needles, and health-care workers who are exposed to blood. An infected pregnant woman may pass the virus to her baby during childbirth.

Hepatitis C in the United States is most often transmitted via blood transfusion; however, new blood-screening techniques are now used to test for this. Hepatitis D is generally confined to drug addicts and hemophiliacs.

Understanding the Problem. If your symptoms suggest hepatitis B, your doctor will question you about your sexual history, medications you may be taking, and any recent blood transfusions. A blood test can detect most forms of hepatitis.

The majority of patients with hepatitis B recover in three to four months, but 10 percent go on to have chronic hepatitis, a progressive disease that is associated with cirrhosis of the liver and liver cancer.

Treatment Options. There is no specific treatment for hepatitis, whatever its type. If you are diagnosed with hepatitis and feel well enough, you need not stay in bed, although it is best to take it easy. Your health-care provider may advise you to avoid alcohol and eat a high-calorie diet. Many people with hepatitis suffer nausea late in the day, so it is advisable to ingest the bulk of your nutritional requirements in the morning and early afternoon. Hospitalization generally isn't called for unless symptoms are severe.

Although it is not necessary to isolate a person with hepatitis from the rest of the family, the entire household should observe the strictest rules of hygiene to prevent spreading the disease. These include thorough hand washing after using the bathroom and certainly whenever one has contact with the infected person's feces, blood, or body fluids.

PREVENTION. Hepatitis B vaccine, though it is not effective as a vaccine against other forms of hepatitis, provides extremely effective protection against the hepatitis B virus. Many pediatricians today recommend that their patients be vaccinated soon after birth to prevent them from contracting hepatitis B later, but certainly adolescents, sexually active young adults, and health-care workers would benefit from vaccination as well. Immunoglobin may be used to reduce the risk of infection in people recently exposed.

If you have sexual intercourse with an infected person, be sure to use condoms, or avoid sexual contact altogether until you are told you are no longer infectious.

MOLLUSCUM CONTAGIOSUM

Molluscum contagiosum is characterized in adult women by one or more small pearl-like, painless nodules, usually on the vulva but sometimes also on the lower abdomen and inner thigh. Each nodule has a small white dot at its peak.

Molluscum contagiosum, caused by a mildly contagious virus, is a relatively common infection that is transmitted sexually but may also be spread through close nonsexual contact. It affects men and women with an impaired immune system, as well as children, in whom the growths may appear anywhere on the body. It typically surfaces two to eight weeks after exposure.

Understanding the Problem. Often your health-care provider need do nothing more than examine the lesions to make the diagnosis. If left untreated, they disappear spontaneously within two months to a year, although often the virus sheds and new crops of nodules appear.

Treatment Options. Molluscum contagiosum is not a debilitating condition, and a woman may choose to allow the disease to run its course. Proper diet, plenty of rest, and meticulous care of the genital area—keeping it clean and dry—are all sensible measures that will help build up the immune system and aid in healing.

If your health professional recommends removal of the growths, the procedure he or she will most likely perform is freezing (cryotherapy), surgical scraping, or squeezing out of the core material.

PARASITIC INFECTIONS

Sexually transmitted parasitic infections affect the genitals as well as other parts of the body. Depending upon the particular parasite, symptoms may include vaginitis and constant itching.

Pediculosis pubis, infestation by crab lice, is the most contagious STD. It is usually confined to the hair of the vulva but occasionally may be found elsewhere on the body. Scabies, caused by the itch mite, can occur anywhere on the body and is characterized by intense itching. Trichomoniasis is caused by a sexually transmitted protozoan parasite that is responsible for one in four cases of vaginitis.

For more information, see Infestations (Pubic Lice and Scabies), *page 510, and* Trichomoniasis, *page 503.*

CHAPTER 20

❧

Endocrine and Autoimmune Diseases

CONTENTS

Your endocrine system, a complex system of interrelated glands, acts as the body's control system and coordinator, regulating the responses and activities of many of the body's processes. The endocrine system's primary mechanism is the hormone, varying types of which (with an array of vital functions) are secreted by each gland directly into the bloodstream, delivering instructions to targeted organs and tissues.

Stress or fear or even exercise might, for example, signal the adrenal glands to produce the hormone epinephrine (also called adrenaline), which prompts a change in heart rate that in turn increases blood flow to the muscles while decreasing it to the gastrointestinal tract. This temporarily gives more blood to the muscles, where the need is suddenly greater. Hormones also control metabolic and growth rates as well as secondary sex characteristics such as breast development.

The Endocrine Glands. The glands that make up the endocrine system are the pituitary, the thyroid and parathyroid, the pancreas, the adrenal glands, and the ovaries (the testes in the male). Each gland has a specialized role in the body's complex processes.

PITUITARY GLAND. Though only two thirds the length of your little finger, the pituitary gland, located beneath the base of the brain behind the nasal passages, is sometimes called the master gland, since it controls the functions of other endocrine glands. The front (anterior) lobe of the pituitary secretes growth hormone, which regulates the body's overall growth, and prolactin, which stimulates the mammary glands to secrete breast milk. The anterior lobe also produces hormones that influence the thyroid gland, the adrenal cortex, the ovaries, and the testes—that is to say, your daily functioning, long-term growth, and reproductive ability.

The back (posterior) lobe of the pituitary secretes oxytocin that stimulates contractions during labor, and vasopressin that regulates the kidneys' urine output.

ADRENAL GLANDS. The two adrenal glands, each situated on top of a kidney and about the size of the end of your thumb, are vital to the body's fluid balance, reproduction, and stress reaction. The two parts of the adrenal glands are the outer layer (the cortex), which secretes corticosteroid hormones that regulate a number of the body's processes, and the inner core (the medulla), which secretes epinephrine (adrenaline) and norepinephrine (noradrenaline), hormones that increase your heart rate, blood pressure, and level of usable glucose (sugar) to cope with a variety of stressors.

PANCREAS. Located in the abdominal cavity, below the stomach, this organ resembles a turkey drumstick in size and shape. It produces the three hormones—insulin, glucagon, and somatostatin—that balance your blood sugar level. It also produces enzymes essential to food digestion.

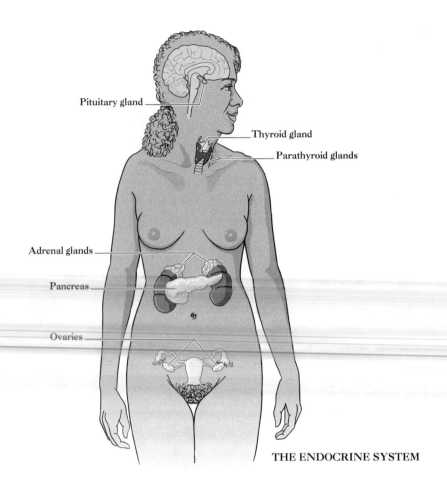

Pituitary gland

Thyroid gland

Parathyroid glands

Adrenal glands

Pancreas

Ovaries

THE ENDOCRINE SYSTEM

THYROID GLAND. The primary function of this bow tie–shaped gland at the base of your neck, which has two main lobes connected by a narrow band of tissue called the *isthmus*, is setting your body's metabolic rate. It responds to instructions from the pituitary by secreting the hormone thyroxine. The more thyroxine in your bloodstream, the faster your metabolism.

PARATHYROID GLANDS. These four rice grain–sized glands located on the corners of each lobe of the thyroid produce parathyroid hormone, which regulates the amount of calcium in the blood.

OVARIES. The production of estrogen and progesterone is the responsibility of the ovaries. These hormones govern monthly ovulation and a woman's secondary sex characteristics such as breast development.

On page 475, you will find a discussion of autoimmune disorders, in which the body mistakenly attacks itself.

ENDOCRINE DISEASES

When the endocrine system is working properly, the flow of your body's hormones is smooth and efficient and goes virtually unnoticed by you. But the system sometimes malfunctions, and many problems—both major and minor—can result. Some disorders, such as diabetes, can be controlled but not cured and require constant monitoring; others can be corrected with medication or surgery.

In the pages that follow, we will discuss the most common endocrine diseases, their causes, and their treatment.

DIABETES MELLITUS

Diabetes mellitus produces an increase in both thirst and output and frequency of urination (as often as every hour or so). You are likely to have an increased, even voracious appetite yet be losing weight. Fatigue, nausea, vomiting, vaginitis, skin infections, blurred vision, and frequent bladder infections also are commonly reported symptoms.

However, some diabetics with a mild form of the disease are asymptomatic.

Emergency Symptoms

DIABETIC KETOACIDOSIS (DKA). This life-threatening condition will likely occur when a diabetic misses a dose of insulin or when the body is stressed by infection or illness. Symptoms are dry mouth, dry and flushed skin, nausea, labored and more rapid breathing, sweet- or fruity-smelling breath, and abdominal pain with or without extreme thirst and excessive urination, leading to a gradual loss of consciousness.

HYPOGLYCEMIC COMA. This life-threatening reaction to too much insulin (and too little blood sugar) produces trembling, weakness, or drowsiness, followed by headache, confusion, dizziness, double vision, and a lack of coordination (making the diabetic appear intoxicated), possibly resulting in convulsions and loss of consciousness.

HYPEROSMOLAR COMA. Caused by an extremely high blood sugar level, this life-threatening condition usually occurs in older, non-insulin-dependent diabetics in conjunction with another serious underlying illness (such as a stroke) and is characterized by extreme thirst, lethargy, weakness, and mental confusion, leading to loss of consciousness.

Contrary to what your mother may have told you, eating loads of candy does not cause diabetes. It's a disease caused by the body itself.

The pancreas produces insulin, a hormone that stimulates our muscles and fat cells to absorb glucose from the blood. This blood sugar, derived from the food you eat, is an energy source. But when insulin production is impaired (either partially or completely), the body's cells and the liver (which stores glucose) cannot absorb what they need, and the glucose level in the bloodstream becomes abnormally high. Diabetes is the result.

More than ten million Americans have been diagnosed as diabetics; another five million are thought to have the disorder but are unaware of it. Before the discovery of insulin in 1921, a diagnosis of diabetes was generally a death sentence. Though there's still no cure for this disease, most diabetics who monitor their glucose level regularly, control their diet and medications carefully, and exercise routinely can lead a relatively normal life. An example of this is pregnancy: Today diabetic women give birth to healthy babies, an event that even a generation ago was rare.

Kinds of Diabetes. The two common forms are type 1 diabetes (insulin-dependent diabetes) and type 2 diabetes (non-insulin-dependent diabetes).

Type 1 Diabetes. Type 1 diabetes can occur at any age but generally surfaces before age thirty, with the average onset between twelve and fourteen. An estimated one in ten diabetics has this form of the disease. It begins suddenly as a result of the immune system's mistakenly attacking healthy insulin-producing cells in the pancreas. Insulin production halts completely. The body then seeks to convert fats and proteins into energy. This drain of nutrients causes rapid weight loss, and, without prompt treatment, coma and even death can occur.

Heredity appears to play a role in the development of type 1 diabetes; two of every three insulin-dependent diabetics have a family history of the disease. People with insulin-dependent disease produce little or no insulin of their own and require daily insulin injections. (Insulin must be injected rather than taken orally because digestive juices would destroy it.)

Type 2 Diabetes. Nine out of ten diabetics have type 2 diabetes. These diabetics generally produce sufficient insulin, but their body is resistant to it and so greater amounts are needed to maintain a normal blood glucose level. People with type 2 diabetes are predominantly over forty and overweight or obese (in some five million Americans diabetes has developed in the past decade, and increasing obesity is a major component). Genetic factors also predispose people to type 2 diabetes (African Americans, Hispanic Americans, and Native Americans are more likely to contract type 2 diabetes than other ethnic groups), as does the use of certain drugs, such as corticosteroids. Pregnant women may experience gestational diabetes; it may disappear after childbirth, but it increases a woman's chance of being diagnosed with type 2 diabetes within ten years.

Although some people with this form of diabetes require insulin injections to keep their blood sugar level in check and others may need other medications, most can stay healthy by observing a strict diet and exercise program.

You can dramatically decrease your risk of adult-onset diabetes by maintaining the weight you had when you were young or reducing it. A recent study found that women who had gained from eleven to twenty-four pounds since age eighteen were about twice as likely to become diabetic as women who had gained less. Women who lost more than eleven pounds from their eighteen-year-old weight had less than half the risk of women with more stable weight.

Understanding the Problem. If the symptoms of diabetes are present, your doctor will test your blood for an abnormally high glucose concentration. (If results are ambiguous, a glucose tolerance test may be administered; it involves fasting for two hours, then drinking a glucose mixture. Blood sugar level is measured thereafter.) The doctor may also order a blood test for glyco-hemoglobin, an excellent indication of your average blood sugar over several weeks time. Treatment will depend upon the form of diabetes mellitus.

Diabetics have both short-term and long-term disease risks. The two most frequent short-term dangers are those posed by adverse reactions to insulin (very low concentrations of glucose in the blood), a problem usually resolved by modifying the dose. Diabetic ketoacidosis, or DKA (discussed on page 463), is the cause of some one in ten deaths in diabetics, although DKA is most likely to occur in undiagnosed diabetics or in individuals whose diabetes is not under control. Injury, infection, and severe fluid loss from diarrhea or vomiting also pose significant risk for DKA. When ill, insulin-dependent diabetes mellitus (IDDM) patients should test their blood sugar level every four to six hours.

Longer-term complications develop slowly, with few initial symptoms. When glucose blood level isn't properly controlled, blood vessels are damaged; stroke, heart attack, and gangrene in the feet can result. Blindness and kidney disease due to deteriorated small blood vessels also are potential long-term problems, as is nerve damage (diabetic neuropathy), particularly in the legs and sometimes the hands.

Treatment Options. Taking responsibility for your wellness is the most important element of managing this disease properly. This means monitoring your blood sugar level with self-administered blood or urine tests, giving yourself insulin injections, and maintaining a stringent diet and exercise regime (see *The Diabetic Diet*, page 466).

MEDICATION. Depending on your form of diabetes, you may need to take insulin. People with insulin-dependent diabetes mellitus (type 1) must, as the name implies, receive daily injections of insulin to control the blood glucose level.

Many diabetics with non-insulin-dependent diabetes (type 2) are able to maintain the correct blood sugar level with diet and exercise alone. Those who cannot, however, can take an oral hypoglycemic agent that stimulates the pancreas to increase its insulin output. Insulin injections may be necessary for more severe cases of type 2 diabetes or for a type 2 patient who contracts an additional illness.

EXERCISE. Whereas exercise is important for everyone, for the diabetic it's critical to maintaining good health. A regular exercise program not only helps lose weight and maintain overall good health, but it also may improve your circulation and keep your heart and blood vessels functioning well. Because muscles use glucose during vigorous exercise, the diabetic's blood glucose concentration is decreased after a workout. Moreover, exercise makes your cells more sensitive to insulin, enabling them to use any available insulin more efficiently.

If you are diabetic, be sure to check with your health-care practitioner before embarking on an exercise regimen. Both insulin and exercise lower the glucose level, meaning injections must be timed so that they don't inadvertently cause hypoglycemia, a dangerous drop in blood sugar level (see *Hypoglycemia*, page 467). A light carbohydrate snack and a glass of milk thirty minutes before your workout prevent hypoglycemia. Again, discuss your routine with your health-care practitioner.

DIET. A strict diet is crucial for the diabetic, in terms of both what's eaten and when. As a diabetic you should be mainly concerned with eating foods that help control your body's concentration of glucose, preferably those high in complex carbohydrates but low in fat. Since obesity increases your need for insulin (which you have in short supply or lack altogether), your diet must be tailored toward helping you reach and maintain a weight normal for your height and body build. For people with type 2 diabetes, in many cases the pancreas produces an adequate amount of insulin once normal weight is reached.

THE DIABETIC DIET

If you are diagnosed as having diabetes, your health-care practitioner or a dietitian will recommend a diet that meets your special needs, employing the right foods and the right amount at the right times. Eating right and at the right time will help control your blood sugar level and lower your risk for certain complications.

Your diet needs to be individualized to suit your particular needs, but in general the bulk of your food should come from starches and complex carbohydrates such as those in whole-grain bread, cereals, and rice; potatoes; and pasta. High-fiber and natural-sugar foods are also important. Choose fresh fruits and vegetables over canned or frozen and whole-grain breads over white, and stay away from foods rich in simple sugars like candy and other sweets. This doesn't mean forgoing an occasional treat, as many desserts are now made with the diabetic in mind.

Working with your dietitian, you need to establish a plan for reaching an ideal weight. Basic guidelines for the diabetic diet have been issued by the American Diabetes Association. These recommendations focus on restricting fats in the diet and consuming ample quantities of complex carbohydrates such as those in breads, cereals, and fruits and vegetables. Reducing your intake of animal fats will make for healthier arteries. Although protein builds and repairs body tissue and provides energy, you need only small amounts of meat or other proteins daily.

Avoid alcohol, as it's high in calories. And eat less salt. Diabetics are more likely to have high blood pressure—and high blood pressure and diabetes are a dangerous combination. Use less salt when you cook, remove the salt shaker from the table, and buy fewer frozen meals, canned soups, and other prepared foods with high sodium content.

HYPOGLYCEMIA

Although symptoms vary considerably among individuals, hypoglycemia often begins with the sensation of feeling hot. You then may break into a sweat and feel dizzy, weak, hungry, and unsteady. Other symptoms include trembling, blurred vision, slurred speech, headache, and tingling in the lips or hands. To a casual observer you may appear intoxicated. In extreme instances you can suffer seizures or lose consciousness.

Hypoglycemia occurs when the concentration of glucose in the blood is below normal, causing the body's cells to become starved for energy (in a sense, then, it's the opposite of diabetes). Contrary to popular belief, hypoglycemia is a relatively rare condition, most often occurring in diabetics because of an insulin overdose, a skipped meal, or excessive exercise. When hypoglycemia occurs in a nondiabetic, it's often the result of too much alcohol and too little food. Certain tumors also can produce hypoglycemia.

Understanding the Problem. If you're diabetic, you must learn to recognize the onset of an attack of hypoglycemia. Most attacks are treated before they progress and become serious. But if nothing is done and the condition is allowed to worsen, unconsciousness can result.

Treatment Options. At the first sign of a hypoglycemic attack, stop all activity (if you're driving, for example, immediately pull off the road) and eat one portion of a fast-acting carbohydrate: four ounces of fruit juice, milk, some hard candies, or glucose in any form. Don't eat chocolate, though; the fat will slow absorption of sugar into the bloodstream. If the symptoms don't disappear within a few minutes, eat a second helping.

Try to avoid being alone when you're experiencing a hypoglycemic attack in case severe symptoms that require immediate medical attention develop.

If your symptoms don't improve, see your health-care practitioner promptly. If you're taking insulin or a drug that sometimes triggers hypoglycemia in susceptible individuals, your medication may need to be adjusted. You may also be given, and taught how to use, a glucapon injection. Glucapon raises blood sugar and is sometimes used in diabetics who are unusually hard to control.

PRECAUTIONARY TIPS FOR THE DIABETIC

Diabetics usually can tell when their blood sugar level is falling too low, but sometimes the symptoms are subtle. Hypoglycemia generally occurs if you take too much insulin, eat meals or snacks at the wrong time, skip or don't finish meals and snacks, and/or get more exercise than usual.

If you are diabetic and any one of the following symptom occurs, your body may be warning you that your blood sugar level is too low:

- *You feel shaky.*
- *You become sweaty.*
- *You feel suddenly overtired.*
- *You are suddenly hungry.*
- *You become grouchy or confused.*
- *You experience rapid heartbeat.*
- *Your vision becomes blurred or you get a sudden headache.*
- *You sense numbness or tingling in your mouth and lips.*

These indicators of low blood sugar are variable, so not everyone will experience all of them. But if you feel different from your normal self, low blood sugar may be the cause, and you should do a blood sugar test. Since a severe drop in your blood sugar level can cause you to pass out or be unable to speak, get into the habit of taking some precautionary measures.

Carry around a small box of raisins. a handful of hard candies, or several small sugar cubes. If you feel your blood sugar level is low but can't test it, eat something sugary. It's safer to eat the extra sugar than to risk having a bad low blood sugar reaction.

Carry diabetes identification with you: a medical necklace or a bracelet, and a wallet card that lists your name, phone number, and health-care practitioner's name and number.

Keep a glucagon emergency kit on hand and instruct your friends, family, and coworkers beforehand *on what to do if an emergency arises.*

HYPERTHYROIDISM

If your body has too much thyroid hormone, the disease is termed *hyperthyroidism*. An overactive thyroid causes weight loss despite increased appetite, increased heart rate and blood pressure, anxiety, and sleep disturbances. You may sweat profusely and be intolerant to heat (or, conversely, be insensitive to cold). More frequent bowel movements, even diarrhea, may occur. Muscle weakness and fatigue or tremors in the fingers or tongue may occur. The eyes may bulge or be watery and feel gritty and may be sensitive to light. A goiter—a swelling in the neck at the thyroid gland—may develop.

Excess thyroxine speeds up the metabolism and may cause many or all of the symptoms described. Hyperthyroidism is easily treatable, though if left untreated severe cases can be fatal. The disorder usually strikes people between thirty and forty years old and is five times more likely to affect women than men.

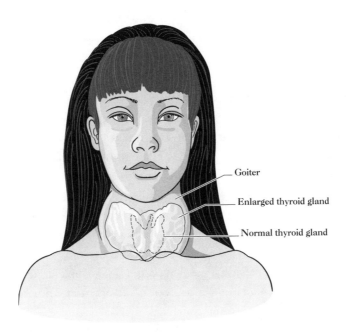

Goiter

Enlarged thyroid gland

Normal thyroid gland

One symptom of an overactive thyroid is a swelling in the gland itself.

Forms of Hyperthyroidism. An overactive thyroid produces an excess of the thyroid hormone thyroxine. Most often this is caused by *Graves' disease*, an autoimmune disorder. Graves' disease occurs when the thyroid gland is excessively stimulated by an abnormal antibody. It is characterized by bulging eyes with a widening of the lids and excessive tearing and redness.

More rarely, overproduction of thyroxine is caused by a thyroid nodule, a mass of cells growing abnormally within the thyroid gland. These are called hyperfunctioning thyroid nodules. They can also be cysts, fluid-filled cavities, or swellings. These are not cancerous and usually will not interfere with your health if treated. Occasionally, however, thyroid nodules are so large that they press on other structures in the neck.

In some cases treatment of an overactive thyroid produces an underactive gland. This occurs when a part of the thyroid gland has been destroyed or when the pituitary gland fails to produce thyroid-stimulating hormone (TSH) (see *Hypothyroidism*, page 470).

Treatment Options. The most common treatment for hyperthyroidism is orally administered radioactive iodine. Since iodine is absorbed by the thyroid, the radiation it contains destroys part of the gland, resulting in decreased production of thyroid hormone. Your health-care practitioner will want to see you every six to twelve weeks to check your thyroid function. One risk of radioactive iodine treatment is that ultimately the thyroid produces too little hormone, necessitating lifelong replacement therapy.

HYPOTHYROIDISM

If your body has too little thyroid hormone, the disease is termed *hypothyroidism*. The signs and symptoms of an underactive thyroid are fatigue and lethargy (characterized by a slowing of mental and physical acuity) as well as a slowed heart rate; intolerance to cold; constipation; dry, flaky, thickened skin; and dry, lifeless hair or hair loss. Some people have a goiter. Menstrual irregularity and a lack of interest in sex may also occur, as may a deepened voice, muscle cramps and weakness, and puffiness around the eyes. The number and severity of symptoms vary with the duration and degree of thyroid hormone deficiency.

An underactive thyroid does not produce enough thyroid hormone, thyroxine. Hypothyroidism is frequently due to an autoimmune disorder called Hashimoto's Thyroiditis (below). It may also occur when the pituitary gland fails to produce sufficient quantities of the hormone that regulates the thyroid gland, after surgical removal of the thyroid gland or after previous treatment for an overactive thyroid gland.

Over five million Americans have hypothyroidism, and some degree of thyroxine deficiency may affect as many as 10 percent of all women. Individuals at greatest risk of hypothyroidism are over fifty and female.

Hypothyroidism is easily treatable and is neither chronic nor progressive. But if left untreated, symptoms usually worsen. Treatment is especially crucial for infants, who may have dwarfism and mental retardation if not treated, and people with severe hormone deficiencies.

Hashimoto's Thyroiditis. The signs and symptoms of Hashimoto's thyroiditis are much the same as those for hypothyroidism. Hashimoto's disease is a chronic inflammation of the thyroid gland which occurs most often in middle-aged women. This autoimmune disease causes the thyroid to lose its function, preventing the gland from producing adequate amounts of its hormone, a condition called *hypothyroidism*.

Understanding the Problem. If you have symptoms of an underactive thyroid or a swelling in your neck indicates a possible goiter, see your health-care practitioner. If a thyroid problem is suspected, a blood test will be done to check your level of thyroid hormone and an antibody that causes the disease. A needle biopsy may also be done.

If your problem is hypothyroidism, your health-care practitioner will prescribe a daily dose of thyroid hormone replacement. Dosage needs to be reevaluated and adjusted monthly until the proper dosage is established. After that, it should be reevaluated annually. A slight response to the drug therapy will be noticed within a couple of weeks, but full metabolic response may take about a month. You must continue treatment for the rest of your life.

It's particularly important for patients with heart disease to have the correct dosage of thyroid hormone because even a slight excess may increase the risk for heart attack or worsen angina. New research indicates that excessive thyroid hormone may also cause excessive bone mineral loss, increasing the risk for osteoporosis, making annual reevaluation even more important.

SURGERY. Patients with extreme thyroid enlargement may need surgery to remove a portion of the gland. Often as an adjunct to surgery you will need to take radioactive iodine or antithyroid drugs described earlier.

THYROID PROBLEMS AND PREGNANCY

Since most thyroid conditions are more common in women and often affect younger women, it's possible that one of them will occur right before, during, or soon after a pregnancy.

Hypothyroidism (underactive thyroid gland) can be hard to detect during pregnancy because some of its symptoms—like tiredness and weight gain—are also common to pregnancy. Blood tests measuring the level of thyroid-stimulating hormone (TSH) can easily determine whether a pregnant woman's problems are due to hypothyroidism or not.

Hypothyroidism in the mother does not cause problems for the baby. The fetus's thyroid gland develops normally even if the mother's thyroid is underactive, and thyroid medications are just like those made naturally by the body, so as long as the proper dose is taken, there are no side effects for either mother or baby.

Hyperthyroidism (overactive thyroid gland) can also be difficult to detect during pregnancy because some of its symptoms, too—nervousness, insomnia, and nausea—mimic those of pregnancy. But hyperthyroidism makes it harder for women to become pregnant. Radioactive iodine, the most widely recommended permanent treatment, should not be taken during pregnancy because it can damage the fetus's thyroid gland. Therefore, it's best to have your thyroid condition resolved before becoming pregnant. Apart from radioactive iodine, other antithyroid medications can be used during pregnancy.

Occasionally, a woman experiences postpartum thyroiditis *(thyroid inflammation) a few months after delivering. Though this form of thyroid disorder is painless and causes little or no gland enlargement, the condition interferes with the even production of thyroid hormone, causing either an excess or a deficiency. Postpartum thyroiditis disappears by itself after one to four months, but while it's active, women often benefit from thyroid treatment.*

DELAYED PUBERTY

The age at which girls' sexual characteristics begin to develop and the rate of these physical changes vary markedly among individuals. One girl may start menstruating at eleven and her best friend not begin until fourteen or fifteen. One is slightly early in her development; the other on the late side. But both are within the normal range.

When does a teen's development cross the line between normal and delayed? When should she and her parents become concerned that something may be wrong?

If you're thirteen and have yet to develop breasts or pubic hair, or if more than four years has passed since your breast development began and you haven't yet menstruated, it would be prudent to see your health-care provider.

Many things can slow development. Some children are simply slow developers. Being very thin can also contribute to the delay. Your health professional may want to test for conditions such as diabetes, hypothyroidism, or inflammatory bowel disease, all of which can contribute to delayed puberty. Rarely, development is delayed because of a hormonal deficiency, which can be corrected once diagnosed. A blood test can determine hormone level.

A very small percentage of girls fail to mature as a result of genetic abnormalities. However, in some cases the abnormalities are apparent at birth.

TURNER'S SYNDROME

An estimated one in three thousand girls is born with Turner's syndrome, a genetic abnormality in which the child has one rather than two X chromosomes.

Girls with Turner's syndrome are born without functioning ovaries. Typically, they are abnormally short and have a webbed neck, a low hairline, a high arched palate, a broad chest with widely spaced nipples, and cardiovascular abnormalities. They do not grow and sexually mature as other girls do.

Years ago Turner's syndrome usually went unrecognized until the girl reached the age of puberty and did not develop. But now doctors are much more aware of the initial symptoms, so most girls with this syndrome are diagnosed at birth.

Treatment of this rare condition usually involves estrogen, which will stimulate the development of secondary sexual characteristics and prevent bone loss. Often birth control pills are also prescribed, permitting regular monthly bleeding and a sense of normalcy, although pregnancy remains impossible.

HIRSUTISM

Hirsutism *is the term used to describe excessive hair growth in women in areas not normally hairy (for example, the face, breasts, and abdomen). The hair may be soft and fine or coarse, and if the onset is sudden, it may be cause for concern.*

There are many causes of hirsutism but usually it is due to a hormonal imbalance. In some cases, certain drugs—Dilantin, a medication used to treat epilepsy, is one—are responsible. Tumors as well as disorders of the ovaries (such as ovarian cysts and enlarged ovaries) and adrenal glands also may cause hirsutism. Hirsutism is seen in women with Cushing's syndrome (which involves an excess of corticosteroids in the bloodstream).

Often no cause is found. This idiopathic hirsutism is thought to be mainly due to a slight increase in sensitivity to the male hormone (androgen) normally produced by all women. Women with idiopathic hirsutism have normal reproductive organs and a normal menstrual cycle.

Understanding the Problem. If you have hirsutism, your health-care practitioner will do a thorough history and examination in search of a cause. You will be asked about medications you're taking and about your menstrual history. Blood tests will be done to determine hormone levels.

Hirsutism can be symptomatic of an underlying problem requiring treatment. If no underlying cause can be found, your hirsutism poses no health risk, though it may be a nuisance from a cosmetic standpoint.

Treatment Options. If a medication is the suspected culprit, your doctor will likely suggest you discontinue taking it. In the event an ovarian or adrenal tumor is found, the problem will require treatment.

Drugs such as spironolactone, oral contraceptives, and corticosteroids (depending on the underlying disorder) will suppress androgen levels, thereby curtailing hirsutism. However, thus far no drug has been specifically approved for this purpose. It will be months before you notice any results in the growth of new hair.

Medications will not affect established hair so cosmetic removal of the hair that has already grown will be required. Available methods include waxing and electrolysis.

PROLACTINOMA

Prolactinoma, a tumor of the pituitary gland, causes irregular periods or absence of periods. Some women also have galactorrhea, a condition in which the breasts secrete milk without a recent pregnancy. Some women with this tumor have no symptoms.

A prolactinoma is a tumor that causes the pituitary gland to overproduce the hormone prolactin, resulting in the symptoms described. An estimated one in ten persons has a prolactinoma, and many of them have no symptoms.

Understanding the Problem. If you have the symptoms of a prolactinoma, your health-care practitioner will order magnetic resonance imaging (MRI) or a computed tomography (CT) scan.

In many cases, a prolactinoma doesn't require treatment, especially if you don't want to conceive. But you should have your prolactin level measured yearly. Osteoporosis is also a risk among women with a high prolactin level whose estrogen level is low.

Treatment Options. The first line of treatment for a prolactinoma usually is bromocriptine, a drug that reduces the overproduction of prolactin and in most cases the tumor mass as well. Side effects of this drug include lowered blood pressure, nausea, and vomiting.

SURGERY. Removal of the tumor is recommended when medical treatment fails to alleviate the symptoms. In about 20 percent of cases, however, the tumor recurs.

HYPOPARATHYROIDISM

Most commonly, numbness or muscle spasm in the feet, hands, and throat is symptomatic of hypoparathyroidism.

The parathyroid glands maintain your body's level of calcium. When parathyroid tissue is accidentally removed during thyroid or other neck surgery or destroyed as a result of an autoimmune disorder, hypoparathyroidism may occur, resulting in too low a level of calcium in your blood.

Understanding the Problem. If your symptoms suggest hypoparathyroidism, your physician will do a blood test to determine whether your blood calcium level is abnormally low.

Hypoparathyroidism can be successfully treated. But if you ignore the problem, convulsions and death may eventually occur.

Treatment Options. The treatment for this disease involves taking calcium supplements and large amounts of vitamin D for the rest of your life. When symptoms are severe, you may need a calcium injection to provide immediate relief. Severe muscle spasms or convulsions may require hospitalization for intravenous infusions of calcium. Periodic monitoring of your calcium level is vital.

ADDISON'S DISEASE

Early symptoms produced by Addison's disease, a disorder of the adrenal glands, include weakness, lethargy, and faintness upon standing suddenly. Increased skin pigmentation gives an all-over-the-body "tan," and often black freckles on the forehead, face, and shoulders; white patches on the skin (vitiligo) may also appear. Later symptoms include anemia, weight loss and decreased appetite, low blood pressure, hypoglycemia, abdominal pains, nausea, vomiting, and diarrhea as well as lack of sexual interest. A decrease in body and pubic hair also may occur.

Addison's disease is a result of the adrenal glands' failure to produce adequate amounts of steroid hormones. The cause of the disease can seldom be pinpointed, though it seems that most cases are due to autoimmune destruction of the adrenal cortex—that is, the body produces antibodies that act against its own tissues. Less frequently Addison's is the result of a complication of certain infections such as tuberculosis.

Understanding the Problem. If your symptoms suggest Addison's disease, your health-care practitioner will perform blood and urine tests to determine your steroid level.

When diagnosed early, people with Addison's disease can lead normal lives. However, if it is ignored and acute adrenal failure occurs, emergency hospitalization is required for this potentially life-threatening condition.

Treatment Options. Basic treatment for Addison's disease is with replacement hormones, usually cortisone. A second drug, fludrocortisone, helps control your sodium and potassium levels so that the low blood pressure of severe Addison's disease can be prevented.

Continual medical supervision will prevent emergencies caused by situations in which the body has increased need for hormones, such as infection, injury, dental extractions, pregnancy, surgery, or other severe stresses. If infection develops, it must be treated aggressively and hormone levels monitored.

People with Addison's disease should always carry an identification card or medical bracelet describing their condition and their need for cortisone.

AUTOIMMUNE DISEASES

Under normal circumstances, the human body marshals a vast network of defense (the immune system) against foreign invaders (antigens) whose mission is to make you sick. In some cases, however, the immune system gets confused.

When this occurs, antibodies are formed and begin attacking the body itself, resulting in inflammation that damages the organs. Though autoimmune disorders frequently affect the joints, they can impair numerous other organ systems as well.

Many of these disorders seem to have a genetic component. The number of autoimmune cases is steadily rising, at least in part because of improved diagnostic techniques and fewer misdiagnoses.

In this section, we'll look at some of the more common autoimmune disorders.

RHEUMATOID ARTHRITIS

Rheumatoid arthritis causes red, painful, swollen joints of your hands, wrists, elbows, feet, ankles, knees, shoulders, neck, or hips. Symptoms generally occur symmetrically, affecting, for example, both hands or both knees. Joints may be warm to the touch and over time may become gnarled and bent. Other symptoms may include low-grade fever, fatigue and weakness, and loss of appetite.

Of the several forms of arthritis, the most common is osteoarthritis, the result of cumulative wear and tear on joints and a normal part of aging (see *Osteoarthritis*, page 597). Rheumatoid arthritis, however, is an autoimmune disease, perhaps triggered by a virus, whereby the immune system attacks the body's own cartilage. Genetic factors may play a role. A children's form of the disease, juvenile rheumatoid arthritis, is similar to rheumatoid arthritis in adults.

Understanding the Problem. If you have symptoms of rheumatoid arthritis, your healthcare practitioner will do a thorough examination. A blood test to check for the antibody

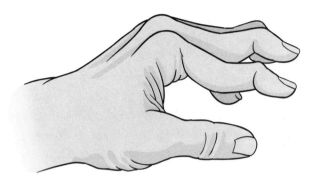

In severe cases of rheumatoid arthritis, the joints can, over time, sustain substantial damage. For example, some people develop what is known as the swan-hand deformity pictured here.

called rheumatoid factor may be indicated (four out of five people with rheumatoid arthritis have this antibody). An X ray of the joint may be helpful in establishing a diagnosis of rheumatoid arthritis.

Rheumatoid arthritis can be very debilitating, often deforming the joints and thereby impairing mobility. In some cases other organ systems—including the heart, lungs, and eyes—may also be affected.

The disease is often chronic. Some people with rheumatoid arthritis have lengthy episodes of disease ("flare-ups")—even as long as a year or two—followed by periods of remission. Although there's no cure for rheumatoid arthritis, with proper treatment most people with this disease can lead a relatively normal life.

Rheumatoid arthritis can strike anytime, but it typically develops between the ages of twenty and fifty, and its prevalence increases with age. Women are affected about three times as often as men.

Treatment Options. Your clinician may prescribe large doses of aspirin or another nonsteroidal anti-inflammatory drug such as ibuprofen to reduce both fever and pain. A wide range of other drugs may be prescribed as the disease progresses. Gold salts, either taken orally or injected, may be prescribed to reduce inflammation and pain; if symptoms persist, immunosuppressants may be recommended.

Also potentially beneficial are the "slow-acting antirheumatic drugs" (SAARDs), which include hydroxychloroquine, D-penicillamine, methotrexate, and azathioprine. There is a new form of treatment now available for rheumatoid arthritis called Etanercept, which represents a major advance in managing this disease.

EXERCISE AND REST. During flare-ups, people with rheumatoid arthritis are at risk of joint damage if they exercise too vigorously. For this reason, they are advised to limit the use of the affected joint. However, regular, gentle exercise is necessary to maintain range of motion of the joints and prevent muscle atrophy. Sometimes a splint is recommended to relieve pain by immobilizing the joint.

People with rheumatoid arthritis often need ten hours of sleep daily—either all at night or eight hours at night with a two-hour nap during the day—and sometimes more during severe flare-ups.

SURGERY. When a joint has become so badly damaged or deformed that function is greatly impaired, joint-replacement surgery may be recommended. Hip and knee joints are most frequently replaced with mechanical counterparts, but joints in the elbows, hands, feet, and shoulders can also be replaced.

SYSTEMIC LUPUS ERYTHEMATOSUS

The symptoms of systemic lupus erythematosus include fever and fatigue, loss of appetite and weight loss, abdominal pain, nausea and vomiting, and joint pain and swelling, usually in the fingers and wrists. A rash, most commonly across the nose and cheeks, develops, as do small ulcers in the mucus membranes of the nose and mouth. Chest pain and accompanying cough are also symptoms, as is unusual bruising or bleeding.

This chronic autoimmune disorder affects the *synovium*, the membrane that lines individual joints, producing pain and inflammation. The symptoms of this disease tend to be episodic, triggered by sun exposure, infection, childbirth, or stress.

Systemic lupus erythematosus (SLE) typically affects women between the ages of fifteen and thirty-five, with an increased incidence among Native Americans and people of Asian and African descent. SLE affects women eight to ten times more often than men, and hereditary factors and sex hormones are believed to play a role.

Understanding the Problem. If lupus is suspected, your health-care practitioner will want to test for the presence of particular antibodies commonly found in people with SLE. Blood tests will determine autoimmune antibodies, anemia, and decreased white blood cells and platelets. A kidney biopsy may be performed, as may a spinal tap, CT scan, or MRI.

There is no cure for lupus. But many people with lupus have no major problems as a result of the disease, and those with mild symptoms may need no treatment at all. For others, lupus is a serious disease that can produce major health problems such as kidney disease, depression, and joint damage.

Treatment Options. Depending upon the severity of your disease, your doctor may prescribe corticosteroids to reduce inflammation or immunosuppressants to subdue the immune system.

CHANGE OF LIFE-STYLE. If you have lupus, you'll need to adjust your life-style to stay as healthy as possible. Avoid stressful situations whenever you can, get adequate rest (as much as ten hours during flare-ups), and avoid exposure to excessive sunlight, which can aggravate the disease.

SCLERODERMA

This disorder of the connective tissue causes a thickening and tightening of the skin, particularly on the arms, face, or hands, making the skin appear shiny or waxy. Constriction of blood vessels may occur in response to cold. Hands, face, and arms may be puffy, and there may be changes in pigmentation. Joint pain and stiffness may be present as well as difficulty in swallowing. Fatigue, weakness, and a persistent slight fever may be evident, along with heartburn, especially when bending or lying down.

We don't know precisely what causes scleroderma—a disease in which excessive collagen is spontaneously produced—though it seems to be an autoimmune disorder. In severe cases it may affect more than the skin, possibly interfering with circulation through the buildup of dense tissue and even affecting internal organs.

Women are four times more likely than men to have scleroderma, which typically occurs between the ages of twenty and fifty.

Understanding the Problem. If you have the symptoms of this disease, your health-care practitioner will do a careful physical examination of the skin of your hands, face, feet, and arms. A tissue biopsy may also be done.

Most people with scleroderma notice the affected skin hardening and thickening for about two years, after which the symptoms don't usually progress and may even lessen to some degree. Rarely, a person's hands become crippled from scleroderma.

In a minority of cases, fibrous tissue slowly infiltrates internal organs (usually the lungs, heart, or kidneys); its presence may lead to life-threatening conditions such as kidney failure. Others may experience hypertension and intestinal disorders that can lead to malnutrition.

Treatment Options. There is no known treatment for scleroderma, but some of the symptoms and complications can be treated. Aspirin can reduce joint pain. Skin lotions can help soften the skin. If your blood pressure is high, hypertensive drugs may be prescribed.

If you smoke, it's important to quit: Nicotine causes the blood vessels to contract, exacerbating circulation problems. In the cold, protect your hands with warm gloves.

Exercise keeps the affected area supple and helps maintain blood flow.

SJÖGREN'S SYNDROME

The symptoms of Sjögren's syndrome are dry, red, painful eyes (as though grit were in the eye); dry, painful mouth; swallowing difficulty; frequent cavities; reduction in ability to distinguish tastes and smells; hoarseness and a dry cough; dry skin and vaginal dryness; joint pain; and fatigue.

This autoimmune disorder, in which the body's defense system mistakenly attacks cells in the salivary and tear glands and, in some cases, glands such as those producing vaginal lubrication, can occur by itself or in conjunction with other autoimmune disorders like rheumatoid arthritis, lupus, or scleroderma. Sjögren's syndrome usually attacks people in their thirties and forties and is ten times more likely to affect women than men.

Understanding the Problem. Your health-care provider will take a medical history and do a physical examination, along with a biopsy of the salivary gland or lip, and conduct blood tests for autoimmune factors.

The prognosis for most patients is good. In some cases, though, corneal infections can develop, and vascular and kidney problems may arise. Lymph glands are often enlarged, and those with Sjögren's syndrome have a higher incidence of lymphoma.

Treatment Options. There is no cure for Sjögren's syndrome. Treatment is geared toward alleviating symptoms. Artificial tears relieve eye dryness, and hard candies or gum will stimulate salivation. Increased water intake is recommended, but avoid alcohol and caffeinated coffee, which are diuretics. Prudent dental hygiene measures must be taken to prevent cavities. Corticosteroids may be prescribed if the disease has affected your kidneys.

POLYMYOSITIS AND DERMATOMYOSITIS

The symptoms of polymyositis and dermatomyositis are a weakness in the hip or shoulder muscles; pain; swelling, redness, and heat in the small joints; a red, itchy rash across the bridge of the nose and the cheeks; a rash on the knuckles, elbows, knees, and ankles; purple discoloration and swelling of the eyelids, particularly on awakening; cold hands and feet; difficulty swallowing or speaking; nausea and weight loss; and fever.

Polymyositis is a rare autoimmune disease in which the muscles become inflamed. When it is accompanied by inflammation of the skin, you have dermatomyositis.

Two thirds of those affected by these disorders are women. Though dermatomyositis and polymyositis can strike at any age, the typical patient is a child between the ages of five and fifteen or an adult between thirty and sixty.

Understanding the Problem. If you have the symptoms described, your doctor will conduct a thorough examination. Blood tests are carried out to seek certain muscle enzymes and rheumatoid factor (see *Rheumatoid Arthritis*, page 475). Electromyography, which measures the electrical patterns in your muscles, may be performed. A biopsy of muscle tissue may also be done.

The onset of symptoms may be either gradual or sudden. In some cases, polymyositis and dermatomyositis disappear shortly after they develop, but some people go on to have lung problems.

These diseases are potentially life-threatening when they affect vital organs such as the heart muscle and the involuntary muscles that control swallowing. But the survival rate is now about 75 percent, and most patients improve with treatment.

Treatment Options. If you have these disorders, your doctor will prescribe a corticosteroid medication such as prednisone to reduce inflammation. Immunosuppressant drugs may also be used.

RAYNAUD'S PHENOMENON

Raynaud's phenomenon is a consequence of other ailments such as scleroderma (see page 478) or exposure to certain chemicals or vibrating tools like pneumatic drills or jackhammers.

Raynaud's phenomenon results from changes in the circulation of the hands or feet. When you're exposed to cold, it's normal for the blood vessels in your extremities to constrict. With Raynaud's, this normal response is exaggerated. Fingers or toes will turn white and then blue as blood vessels constrict when exposed to cold. As circulation returns to the affected digits when they are warmed, the skin turns red and often stings or burns. The diagnosis of Raynaud's phenomenon is done with a thorough history and physical examination.

In most cases, Raynaud's, although uncomfortable, doesn't pose a serious threat to your health. But in rare cases gangrene or ulcers of the fingertips will develop.

You may be able to prevent some attacks by protecting yourself against the cold. Wear gloves when outside or when opening your freezer. Don't smoke, since nicotine constricts blood vessels. Use insulated glasses for cold drinks.

If you have Raynaud's, avoid over-the-counter cold medications that contain the drug phenylpropanolamine. If the problem is severe, your doctor may prescribe medication to prevent the blood vessel spasms that lead to the symptoms.

In extreme cases and only when all else has failed, your doctor may recommend surgery to cut the nerves that control the blood vessels. However, this surgery isn't always successful.

SARCOIDOSIS

Symptoms of this disease are fatigue, aching muscles and shortness of breath (especially after exercise), fever, swollen lymph nodes, difficulty breathing, dry cough and wheezing, loss of appetite, painful joints, reddish skin bumps on the legs. Some people with sarcoidosis have no symptoms.

Sarcoidosis, which is thought to be an autoimmune disorder, is an accumulation of a protein material called *sarcoid* in bodily tissues, most often in the lungs, lymph nodes, eyes, and skin. When this occurs in the lungs, as it typically does, the walls of its small air sacs, the bronchial tubes, and the blood vessels become distorted, and diffusion of oxygen into blood is altered.

Sarcoidosis typically affects African Americans more than Caucasians, usually between the ages of twenty and forty, and women more than men.

Understanding the Problem. Sarcoidosis, especially in its early stages, is often discovered by accident during a routine chest X ray. To confirm the diagnosis, a biopsy of your lung tissue may be obtained by a bronchoscopy, a procedure involving the insertion into the lung of an instrument that allows both visual examination and removal of tissue. If other tissue is involved, that will be biopsied, as well.

Though sarcoidosis is a potentially serious disease, most cases subside spontaneously within two or three years. An estimated 50 percent of people with this ailment recover completely or with only minor effects, often without treatment; about 10 percent have chronic or long-term sarcoidosis; 5 to 10 percent eventually die of the disease, usually after many years.

Treatment Options. If your symptoms don't resolve spontaneously within a few months, your doctor may recommend corticosteroids. The drugs are often prescribed for months or even years and then gradually tapered off. If the symptoms reappear, a second course of drugs may be given, though generally the second course of treatment isn't as successful as the first.

CHAPTER 21

Lower Urinary Tract Disorders

CONTENTS

The bladder and urinary tract are parts of the body's filtration system, which collects and then eliminates the waste products and excess water produced by the kidneys.

Urine flows down two long, narrow tubes, called *ureters,* into the bladder, a muscular sac situated between the pubic bone and the uterus. As urine flows into the bladder and collects, its walls expand; with urination, the walls contract, squeezing the urine into the urethra, a narrow, one-and-a-half-inch-long tube located between the clitoris and vagina.

The female urinary tract can be the site of a variety of problems, including infection, incontinence, and elimination difficulties.

Infection is probably the most common ailment, a result of bacteria that invade the urinary tract.

Incontinence—the leaking of urine—can result if the muscles, tendons, and ligaments that support the bladder and reproductive organs are weakened by childbirth, trauma, decreased estrogen level, or advancing age.

The postmenopausal years can give rise to significant changes in the urinary tissue as the body stops producing estrogen, often inducing painful urination, increased frequency and urgency of urination, and incontinence.

These conditions are usually not cause for alarm, and fortunately many can be alleviated or even prevented altogether with better daily habits, pelvic floor muscle exercises, and estrogen replacement therapy (see *Hormone Replacement Therapy,* page 90).

In this chapter we will discuss the various disorders of the lower urinary tract most frequently encountered by women.

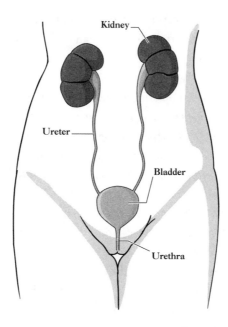

Kidney

Ureter

Bladder

Urethra

Urinary Tract Infections

As many as one third of all women will have a urinary tract infection at some point in their life, and half of them will have a repeat infection within a year. Many women suffer with chronic urinary infections. Ten percent of women over the age of seventy are plagued with frequent infections.

A number of factors make women vulnerable to these infections.

The opening of the urethra, which is the entry point to the urinary system, is close to both the vagina and the anus, areas of the body that normally harbor bacteria with no ill effect. But improper wiping and otherwise poor hygiene can easily introduce bacteria into the urethra, from which it is only a short trip to the bladder.

A link between sexual intercourse and urinary tract infections has been established. The physical movements involved during sex may irritate the opening of the urethra, setting the stage for the infection. And using a diaphragm increases the risk of urinary tract infections two- to threefold.

During pregnancy, the urinary tract may drain less efficiently, and anywhere from 2 to 8 percent of pregnant women experience urinary tract infections. Untreated bacteria in the bladder during pregnancy may lead to kidney infection or premature labor. Women catheterized after surgery or for other reasons also are more likely to have these infections.

Finally, the tissue changes that result from a loss of estrogen after menopause often can make a woman more prone to urinary infection.

The most common urinary tract infections involve the bladder, urethra, or both. In many cases the symptoms are the same, and often it is difficult to distinguish one from the other.

A clear understanding of the various lower urinary tract infections, their causes, and the most effective treatments is important for a woman to maintain her health.

Cystitis

The symptoms of cystitis may include a feeling of pressure and an urgency to urinate, frequent voiding with only small amounts of urine passed, lack of urinary control, need to urinate in the middle of the night, and a burning sensation during voiding. You may also notice blood in your urine, although blood without pain may indicate a more serious problem such as a tumor or kidney stone. If your urine develops an unusually strong odor, it may occasionally be a sign of an infected bladder. Other possible symptoms include a low-grade fever (under 102 degrees Fahrenheit), pain in the lower abdomen or the lower back, and painful sexual intercourse.

Alison was worried: Simple urination had become painful. She also noticed her urine had a cloudy appearance. Worse yet, it hurt when she and husband had intercourse. And here she was on her honeymoon. She sought the help of the hotel doctor and he reassured her it was nothing to worry about. "Honeymoon cystitis," he called it.

Technically, cystitis is an inflammation of the bladder. However, the term is also used to denote a bladder infection, the most common urinary tract infection.

Because of the proximity of the shorter female urethra to the vagina and anus, a woman is particularly susceptible to such infections. More than 80 percent of all cases of cystitis are caused by bacteria that commonly inhabit the rectum and vagina. Most of the time these bacteria are rinsed out of the body with urination; urine itself has antibacterial properties that inhibit the growth of these invaders. Sometimes, however, certain conditions make it easier for bacteria to become established in the urinary tract and then develop into a full-blown infection.

Sexual intercourse is a common trigger for cystitis—so much so that this condition is often referred to as "honeymoon cystitis"—although any sexually active woman, not only a honeymooner like Alison, is susceptible. The forceful movements during intercourse can irritate the opening of the urethra and push bacteria farther up into the urethra, from which they make their way to the bladder. Sexual activity can also bruise the urethra, causing swelling that obstructs bladder emptying or making urination painful and thereby hampering complete elimination. Diaphragm users are more often afflicted with cystitis because the diaphragm's rim presses against the urethra and the bladder, and pressure may interfere with elimination by obstructing the flow of urine.

Although most women with cystitis are sexually active and between the ages of twenty and fifty, it isn't uncommon for even little girls to have lower urinary tract infections. Some older women as they age have symptoms of cystitis that is due to the loss of estrogen rather than a bacterial infection.

Understanding the Problem. If you have symptoms of cystitis, your health-care provider will want a "clean-catch" urine sample to check for signs of infection. You will be asked to wash the vaginal area with a cleansing solution or towelette, then void a small amount of urine into the toilet before collecting a sample in a sterile cup. This ensures that a midstream portion of urine, the most accurate for determining whether you have a bladder infection, is collected.

The urine will be analyzed for signs of inflammatory cells and bacteria. If this urinalysis shows infection, a urine culture is then done to determine the specific bacterium responsible so that the appropriate antibiotic can be started.

If you have recurrent urinary tract infections, your clinician may advise having a complete evaluation of your urinary tract to determine whether a structural abnormality is causing the problem.

Treatment Options. Cystitis, although uncomfortable and even painful at times, is usually not a serious health threat; some infections even resolve themselves without treatment. However, if the infection travels upward into the kidneys, the consequences can be serious. Thus, if the result of your urine test indicates an infection, your health professional will want to treat the problem.

MEDICATION. Your doctor will prescribe the drug best suited to kill the specific organism causing your infection. Common types of antibiotics used in the treatment of cystitis include nitrofurantoin, sulfa drugs, penicillin, cephalosporin, and quinolones.

Treatment regimens vary from a single dose of medication to medication taken for three to as long as fourteen days. Even though your symptoms will probably disappear within a day or two after initiating treatment, the prescribed medication must be taken for the recommended number of days or the infection may recur.

If you have frequent bouts of cystitis, your health professional may prescribe low doses for prolonged periods to prevent infection or even low doses of antibiotics to take after sexual intercourse.

PREVENTION. Although it isn't always possible to prevent cystitis, the risk can be minimized. Proper hygiene is especially important. To prevent introducing vaginal or anal bacteria into your urinary tract, wipe from front to back after using the toilet. Wash the genital and anal areas every day with a mild soap, and avoid douches, bath oils, feminine hygiene sprays, scented toilet paper, and bubble baths, all of which can irritate the urethra. To lessen the risk of infection after sex, make a point of emptying your bladder immediately after intercourse. Unromantic as it may seem, the practice will flush any bacteria introduced into the urethra—and it is certainly preferable to suffering with cystitis.

SIMPLE PREVENTIVE MEASURES

Studies show that women prone to recurrent cystitis often don't urinate frequently enough. If you don't urinate every three to four hours while awake, the bladder, like a stagnant pool, promotes bacterial growth. By emptying the bladder regularly during the day when you get the urge and by urinating within fifteen minutes after intercourse, infection can usually be prevented.

One of the most highly recommended preventive measures also ensures good general health: Drink plenty of fluids (especially water), at least eight to ten glasses a day.

Cranberry or mandelamine tablets increase the acidity of the urine, making it difficult for bacteria to thrive. They also hasten a cure since some medications are more effective with a more acidic urine. Also, avoid caffeine and alcohol, which may irritate the bladder.

If you are sexually active, try side-by-side and rear entry positions, which may decrease friction on the urethral opening. However, avoid anal intercourse, which can contaminate your vagina and urethral opening with bacteria from the rectum. And stop having sex if you begin to feel sore or tender.

PAINFUL URINATION

Painful urination, or dysuria, is a frequent complaint associated with cystitis and often is accompanied by an increase in the frequency and urgency of urination. But not every woman who has burning or stinging when she urinates has an infected bladder.

Painful urination may also indicate an inflamed or infected urethra, at times caused by chlamydia, gonorrhea, or other sexually transmitted organisms (see pages 444 and 445). Some women experience painful urination when the urethra is bruised during sexual intercourse or as a result of irritation from bath oils or feminine hygiene sprays. And postmenopausal women often complain of painful urination, not due to a bacterial infection, but to the urinary tract's adverse reaction to a lack of estrogen. Rarer causes of bladder pain include structural urethral problems, urethral spasms, trauma to the urinary tract, interstitial cystitis, and psychological or neurological damage.

Although painful urination is usually a symptom of a urinary disorder, some gynecological problems also can produce dysuria. Cervicitis, an inflammation of the cervix, may make urinating painful, as can vulvovaginitis (see pages 536 and 501). Women who have outbreaks of genital herpes often find urination excruciatingly painful (see page 454).

In evaluating the cause of your symptoms, your health-care provider will question you about the location of the pain. With vulvovaginitis, for example, the pain is more likely to be external rather than the deeper pain typically found with cystitis, and will tend to occur near the end of urination.

Your clinician may perform a pelvic examination to determine whether a vaginal or cervical infection is responsible for the pain. A urinalysis may be done, and a culture can also detect whether bacteria are growing in the urine.

In most cases these simple tests can identify the problem. However, when a cause for your pain can't be found or you have recurring infections, your doctor may recommend more extensive tests such as cystourethroscopy (see page 631).

DIAGNOSING BLADDER PROBLEMS

If you have symptoms that indicate a urinary problem, your doctor may recommend cystourethroscopy, a procedure that allows for the direct examination of the inside of your urethra and bladder.

During a cystourethroscopy, a narrow tube (the cystourethroscope) is inserted through your urethra and into your bladder. With its special lens and fiber-optic lighting system, the cystoscope enables the doctor not only to see the lower urinary tract but even to remove tissue samples to diagnose cancer or other diseases. Small bladder stones also can be removed with this technique. During this procedure the urethra is also evaluated for signs of inflammation or other abnormalities.

Cystourethroscopy is most often used to evaluate urinary problems such as recurrent infection, blood in the urine, and unexplained pain during urination. It is also an important diagnostic tool in the detection of bladder cancer.

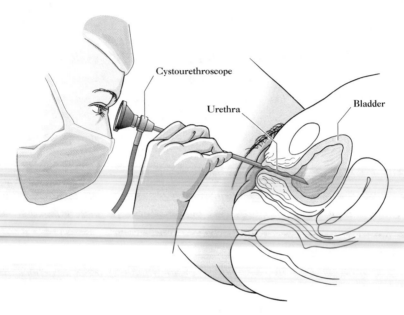

The cystourethroscope is an optical instrument that enables your physician to examine visually the urethra and bladder for abnormalities.

URETHRITIS

The main symptoms of urethritis are frequent urination that is accompanied by a burning sensation, symptoms often associated with other lower urinary tract disorders. However, unlike in other infections such as cystitis, the urethra itself may be tender to the touch, and there may also be some yellowish, puslike discharge. Other symptoms may include blood in the urine, lower-abdominal pain, and painful sexual intercourse.

Urethritis is a recurrent inflammation of the urethra, the tube that carries urine from the bladder out of the body. Urethritis may persist over many weeks, months, or even years. It may be caused by bruising or irritation to the urethra during intercourse; by an adverse reaction to soaps, bath oils, or feminine hygiene sprays; or, more commonly, infection by sexually transmitted bacterial organisms such as chlamydia and gonorrhea and the herpes virus.

Understanding the Problem. The usual way to differentiate between urethritis and cystitis is through urinalysis. Approximately 30 percent of women who have painful and frequent urination do not have significant amounts of bacteria in their urine, an indication that the problem may be in the urethra. Your clinician also may try to express some discharge from your urethra for analysis.

Treatment Options. Never ignore urethritis, even though the symptoms may seem to disappear. Some cases are caused by sexually transmitted diseases, which, if left untreated, can ultimately lead to serious problems such as pelvic inflammatory disease (PID), a serious abdominal condition and a major cause of infertility (see page 449).

MEDICATION. If a precise organism is identified as the cause of your urethritis, your healthcare provider will prescribe the appropriate medication. If no specific bacterium is found, you may be given a broad-spectrum antibiotic. (For sexually transmitted urethritis, only one partner may exhibit symptoms, but it is likely that the symptomless partner is also infected; therefore, both partners must be treated to prevent a continual cycle of reinfection.) Antibiotics should be taken for the full course of treatment, since stopping the medication too soon may result in a rebound infection, which is more difficult to treat.

Sometimes no evidence of infection is present. If the urethra is repeatedly inflamed, glands around it may also become chronically inflamed or infected. In this situation, your doctor may recommend sitz baths and anti-inflammatory medication.

INTERSTITIAL CYSTITIS

A chronic inflammation of the bladder wall, interstitial cystitis produces an urgent and frequent need to urinate and, in some women, pain in the urethra and lower abdomen, and vaginal discomfort after intercourse. Women with interstitial cystitis frequently say they feel as though they have a constant bladder infection.

Madeline had what she believed was a simple bladder infection—the symptoms were identical, after all, and when she described them over the phone to her gynecologist, he prescribed a short course of antibiotics. But instead of improving, the symptoms worsened. She then consulted a urologist, who looked into the bladder with a cystoscope and then diagnosed interstitial cystitis. Unfortunately, Madeline had taken medication intended for an entirely different ailment, and she may also have exacerbated her condition by drinking cranberry juice to help clear up a bladder infection. An increase in bladder acidity is usually desirable for common cystitis but further aggravates an already irritated bladder lining when interstitial cystitis is the problem.

For this reason, if you have interstitial cystitis, some experts believe you should avoid drinking coffee and tea and eating very acidic or spicy foods.

Though an estimated 450,000 women suffer from interstitial cystitis—a condition in which portions of the surface of the bladder are inflamed and occasionally ulcerated—it is a poorly understood bladder disease. Its cause remains unclear. An inflamed bladder may be the result of infection, a defect in the bladder's lining, or an autoimmune reaction. The condition is found primarily in women.

Understanding the Problem. The typical patient with interstitial cystitis sees four to six physicians before the diagnosis is made and, even worse, has often been told that her symptoms are "all in her head." If you repeatedly experience the symptoms discussed here, consult a urologist or gynecologist who has an interest in this disease.

The diagnosis of interstitial cystitis is made by ruling out other conditions with similar symptoms, such as bacterial infection or even cancer. To this end, it is imperative that a sample of your urine be cultured.

To get a precise assessment of the condition, your doctor will most likely perform a cystourethroscopy, a procedure that involves threading a small scope into the bladder to examine its lining (see page 631).

Treatment Options. There is no cure for interstitial cystitis, although treatment can help most patients. Treatment may involve several components, including a special diet, medications to relieve pain, antibiotics, anti-inflammatory drugs, and medications that synthetically replace the damaged bladder surface. Another option is hydrodistention—pumping fluid into the bladder under pressure while the patient is under anesthesia—which stretches the organ and brings some temporary relief in about 60 percent of cases.

UNSTABLE BLADDER

The primary symptom of unstable bladder (often called irritable bladder) is the sudden, urgent, and sometimes uncontrollable need to urinate—so urgent, in fact, that at times you may not make it to the bathroom. Having an irritable bladder frequently means getting up several times during the night to urinate.

Unstable bladder is a term given to any persistent condition that triggers involuntary contraction of the bladder muscles, resulting in a powerful need to urinate immediately. Unstable bladder sometimes occurs along with stress incontinence (see page 492), prolapse of the uterus or vagina (page 496), urinary infection (page 484), pregnancy, estrogen deficiency, some neurological disorders of the bladder, or obstruction of the flow of urine due to a tumor. In many cases the cause is unknown. Although an irritable bladder may be chronically inflamed, the reason why is often unclear.

Understanding the Problem. Your health-care professional will first want to do a urinalysis and urine culture to determine whether an infection is causing your symptoms. Other diagnostic tools that may be indicated are a cystometrogram, which measures bladder pressure (abnormally high pressure indicates sudden, uncontrollable bladder contractions), and cystourethroscopy (see page 631), a procedure in which a lighted instrument is inserted through the urethra and into the bladder, permitting a direct view into this muscular sac. In certain instances catheterization of the bladder will be recommended to measure the amount of urine remaining in the bladder after voiding and to observe the effects of filling the bladder with fluid through the catheter.

Treatment Options. Although an unstable bladder can be uncomfortable and embarrassing, it is not a dangerous condition.

MEDICATION. When irritable bladder is due to an infection, your health-care provider will prescribe the appropriate antibiotic. Your clinician may also prescribe an antispasmodic to relax the bladder muscles or drugs that inhibit the nerves that control contractions.

SELF-HELP. Many women have found that it is possible to "retrain" their bladder (see *Taking Control*, below).

TAKING CONTROL

Some people have regained or improved their bladder control by utilizing a technique known as bladder retraining, which is simply practicing urination on a schedule. To begin with, urinate every two hours, whether the need is there or not. Gradually increase the interval by a half hour at a time, aiming for a goal of four hours between toilet visits. Often the bladder will adapt to this routine and incontinence will be eliminated.

Despite advertisements extolling the virtues of adult diapers, these pads are not recommended except for short-term use unless your doctor advises otherwise.

INCONTINENCE

If you have a urinary incontinence problem, you may leak urine when exercising, laughing, sneezing, or coughing; when lifting something; or when performing other activities that put pressure on the bladder. Incontinence is involuntary and unpredictable urination that causes women to wet themselves. An inability to stop the urine stream is another symptom.

Incontinence—the term simply means the loss of urinary control—occurs for many different reasons, although it is more common among the elderly and more common among women than men.

The bladder stores urine and the urethra allows urine to pass out of the body. Most female incontinence occurs when the pelvic muscles that support the bladder and the urethra weaken and bladder pressure overcomes urethral resistance.

An estimated 30 percent of all women suffer from some degree of incontinence during their lifetime. The occasional involuntary loss of a few drops of urine is common under certain circumstances, and even a healthy young woman may experience a urine leak if her bladder is very full and she forcefully coughs or sneezes. However, prolonged or regular incontinence should be evaluated and its cause determined.

Women who have had children tend to have weakened muscles of the pelvic floor. Postmenopausal women who don't take estrogen are also more likely to have incontinence problems, which are due to a wasting of the tissues of the urethra resulting from decreased estrogen production. Although urinary incontinence is a very common condition in older women—twice as common as in older men—it is not an inevitable consequence of aging.

Incontinence can also occur when the bladder wall muscle is overactive (see *Unstable Bladder*, page 490). Other possible causes are a urinary tract infection and overflow from an overfull bladder that has sustained nerve damage as a consequence of diabetes. Certain birth defects, spinal cord injuries, surgery or radiation therapy of the pelvic area, urethral stricture, and stroke can also be responsible. Many drugs, including some diuretics, sleeping pills, antidepressants, tranquilizers, and medications used for heart problems or gastrointestinal spasm, can cause incontinence. In some cases, more than one cause contributes to the development of this condition.

Understanding the Problem. Incontinence is a serious problem: Fifteen to 30 percent of people over sixty who live at home and at least half of the 1.5 million Americans who reside in nursing homes are affected. Indeed, incontinence may be a crucial factor in determining whether someone is put into a nursing home. In the majority of cases, however, the problem can be successfully treated.

If you are having problems holding your urine, your health-care provider may first do a urinalysis or culture to rule out a bacterial infection. To determine whether your bladder is emptying adequately, either bladder ultrasound is done or a catheter is inserted into your bladder after urination to measure the amount of urine that is left. The bladder may also be filled with fluid through the catheter to determine how much liquid it takes to produce the sensation of a need to void.

If these relatively simple tests fail to reveal the cause of the incontinence, your clinician may recommend a more sophisticated (and expensive) urodynamic evaluation that uses special equipment to view your urinary system as it functions.

Kinds of Incontinence. Five different types of incontinence have been distinguished:

STRESS INCONTINENCE. This is a common form of female incontinence. With stress incontinence, a small amount of urine will leak when some activity—exercising or sneezing, coughing, or laughing—temporarily increases the pressure on the bladder. The incontinence is due to a weakening of pelvic support muscles and ligaments, as well as possible urethral weakness. It is especially common among postmenopausal women.

URGE INCONTINENCE. Often produced by an unstable bladder (see page 490), this usually chronic condition involves the loss of a large amount of urine. Typically, a woman with urge incontinence has to urinate often and with such urgency that she can't make it to the bathroom. Women with urge incontinence may be up several times during the night or even wet the bed. Many women with this form of incontinence suffer from detrusor instability, an abnormality of the muscle that contracts to force urine out of the bladder. Urine release is due to the sudden stimulation of nerve receptors in the bladder wall, which can be caused by emotional problems, chronic irritation of the bladder, or estrogen deficiency. In some cases women have other diseases that affect the bladder and contribute to incontinence. Some women have both stress and urge incontinence.

OVERFLOW INCONTINENCE. This unusual disorder occurs when the bladder, unable to empty itself completely, becomes overdistended. Women with overflow incontinence may leak small amounts of urine throughout the day and night, though they may not feel there is urine in their bladder. Overflow incontinence can be caused by a partial obstruction of the urethra or by a neurological disorder that interferes with the bladder's normal reflexes such as multiple sclerosis, diabetic neuropathy, or tumor of the central nervous system.

MIXED INCONTINENCE. This is a combination of stress and urge incontinence.

URETHRAL WEAKNESS. Incontinence due to more severe forms of urethral weakness is most common in women who have had incontinence surgery that failed or surgery that interfered with the nerves to the urethra, such as some pelvic cancer operations.

Treatment Options. The embarrassment and frustration of incontinence are often emotionally devastating and may even lead to social isolation and depression. Don't be ashamed to discuss the problem with your health-care provider as soon as possible.

MEDICATION If incontinence is due to a bacterial infection, the appropriate antibiotic should clear up the problem. In some postmenopausal women, estrogen replacement will strengthen the urethra and the muscles of the pelvic wall and improve urinary control, lessening or even alleviating the incontinence. Anticholinergic drugs (which block the neurotransmitter acetylcholine) also are sometimes helpful in treating urge incontinence.

EXERCISE. Often the first approach in treating stress incontinence is to strengthen the pelvic muscles with Kegel exercises (see *Kegel Exercises*, page 494). Women with urge incontinence often benefit from bladder retraining (see *Taking Control*, page 491), which teaches the patient to lengthen progressively the time between urinations. Retraining is sometimes combined with biofeedback to increase a patient's awareness and control of her bladder muscles.

VAGINAL DEVICES. A pessary, which is essentially an oversized diaphragm, or a new device marketed under the name Introl, may be placed in the vagina. Both provide support to the urethra and should improve symptoms.

SURGERY. When other methods fail, women with stress incontinence may choose to have surgery to tighten the pelvic floor muscles and restore the bladder and urethra to their normal positions. A sling of firm connective tissue or synthetic material to compress the urethra may be implanted, or collagen may be injected around the urethra. Such procedures are effective in 90 to 95 percent of the women who undergo surgery for stress incontinence. However, surgery is often a last resort in treating women with the muscular abnormality detrusor instability, so a preoperative evaluation will likely be done to predict whether you will benefit from surgery.

KEGEL EXERCISES

Many women with incontinence problems can improve their condition by incorporating a simple isometric exercise into their daily routine. Kegel exercises strengthen the muscles that control the urethra, which often weaken with age.

In the late 1940s, Dr. Arnold M. Kegel suggested to a patient having incontinence problems that she begin exercising the pubococcygeal muscle, which surrounds the anus and vagina. Repeatedly contracting her anal sphincter as if trying to prevent a bowel movement significantly improved her urinary problem.

Since then, Dr. Kegel's exercises have been used by countless women. If you are having problems with stress incontinence—or if you don't yet have a problem and want to keep it that way—you may want to begin this strengthening technique. It will help you maintain better bladder control and often improves sexual sensations as well.

The Exercises. Kegel exercises can be done while urinating: Try to stop and then restart your urine stream—or imagine you're trying to grip a slipping tampon. Next, squeeze the muscles firmly for a three count, then relax. Finally, squeeze and relax the muscles five times as fast as you can.

The squeeze/relax exercises can be done almost anywhere at any time—sitting at your desk, waiting in line, making dinner, driving. Begin with five to ten repetitions of each set, holding each squeeze for five to ten seconds, and gradually increase to at least two hundred repetitions a day.

Several studies have shown that women who spend twenty minutes a day Kegeling have a good chance of regaining control over their urination. In one study, 67 percent of women after three months of Kegel exercises either had complete control or showed significant improvement in their ability to hold their urine. Women who have been incontinent for a year or less experience the greatest improvement, so it probably pays to start Kegeling before you have a significant problem.

Avoid Alcohol and Caffeine. *Alcohol and caffeine are notorious diuretics (agents that increase the excretion of urine). Sources of alcohol include beer, wine, and spirits; caffeine is found in coffee, tea, and many soft drinks. Both alcohol and caffeine are also found in many medications. Limit or eliminate consumption of all of them.*

Avoid Grapefruit Juice. *This is yet another popular diuretic. Drink cranberry juice instead. It will also increase the acidity of your urine, which is beneficial to the bladder.*

Do Not Smoke. *Nicotine irritates the bladder surface and is also likely to stimulate cough—which can cause leakage if you have stress incontinence.*

Empty Your Bladder Regularly. *Holding urine in too long may lead to a bladder infection. And always empty your bladder after intercourse and just before going to sleep.*

Cross Your Legs. *When you feel a cough or sneeze coming on, cross your legs—a simple solution that works—whether you're sitting or standing. You may also prevent an accident by squeezing your sphincter muscle in advance of a cough or sneeze.*

PELVIC FLOOR RELAXATION

Pelvic floor relaxation is a term for vaginal and uterine prolapse, cystocele, and rectocele.

Normally, strong muscles hold your reproductive and abdominal organs in position. But with pelvic floor relaxation (also called pelvic relaxation), the underlying muscles on the floor of your pelvis and the ligaments at the base of your abdomen that should support the bladder, rectum, and uterus have weakened. A variety of factors, including childbirth, trauma to the pelvis, heavy lifting, and aging, can weaken these muscles and ligaments.

CYSTOCELE

If you have a cystocele—which occurs when the bladder drops into the vaginal canal—you may have a sensation of pressure and fullness. Some women say it feels as if their lower organs are going to fall out of their vagina. Incontinence, especially when you exercise or laugh or sneeze, may accompany this condition. Sometimes women with a cystocele can actually feel or see a bulge in the vagina.

A cystocele is a bulging of the bladder against the roof of the vagina. Women with cystoceles, as with other pelvic support disorders, are more likely to have had children. In fact, many women who delivered vaginally have some degree of cystocele although they may not have any symptoms. The problem is more often found in older women.

Understanding the Problem. Your health-care provider will first do a pelvic examination, during which you will be asked to bear down as though you were having a bowel movement.

Treatment Options. Many women with cystocele have no symptoms and do not require treatment. However, if symptoms are present, they can be very uncomfortable. In addition, urine may become trapped in the bladder, making you susceptible to cystitis (see page 484).

NONSURGICAL. Your health-care provider may recommend Kegel exercises (see page 494) to strengthen the muscles and ligaments, which may relieve some of the uncomfortable pressure. He or she may also recommend a pessary, a small rubber, plastic, or silicone ring inserted into your vagina to move the bladder back into place. If you are postmenopausal and are not already taking estrogen, hormone replacement therapy (HRT) may be prescribed (see page 90). HRT has been shown to improve and maintain muscle and ligament elasticity.

SURGERY. Sometimes surgical repair of a cystocele is necessary. This procedure involves putting the bladder back into its proper position, then tightening the muscles and ligaments of the pelvic floor. If you opt for surgery, you may spend a day or two in the hospital. A catheter may also be required temporarily to empty your bladder even after you return home.

UTERINE PROLAPSE

One common symptom of uterine prolapse, a condition in which the uterus and cervix sag into the vagina, is a sensation that your organs are "falling out." In severe cases, women can actually see their cervix protruding from the vagina, especially when they strain. The cervix may ulcerate, causing pain and bleeding. There may also be lower-back pain, anal pain, and pain during sexual intercourse. Accompanying infections sometimes occur, producing a vaginal discharge.

Uterine prolapse results from injury to or weakening of the pelvic muscles and supporting ligaments that hold the uterus in place. It is often accompanied by a rectocele (the rectum pushes against the back wall of the vagina), a cystocele (the bladder bulges against the roof of the vagina), or an enterocele (the small intestine pushes against the upper part of the vagina).

Although most women with this condition have had several children, congenital damage to the pelvic floor can cause uterine prolapse even in young women who have never given birth. Respiratory diseases such as chronic bronchitis and asthma as well as smoking can also increase your risk. Heavy lifting or straining may promote the condition when pelvic muscles are already weakened.

Understanding the Problem. Uterine prolapse is diagnosed during a pelvic examination.

Treatment Options. The decision regarding treatment depends upon the severity of the prolapse.

NONSURGICAL. As with a cystocele, your clinician may recommend Kegel exercises to strengthen the muscles and ligaments (see *Kegel Exercises*, page 494). This may relieve some of the uncomfortable pressure you feel. For a mild prolapse, a pessary may be recommended to provide support. This ring made of rubber, plastic, or silicone is inserted into the vagina and positioned against the cervix to hold the prolapsed organ in place. If you are post-menopausal and are not already taking estrogen, your doctor may prescribe hormone replacement therapy (HRT; see page 90), which has been shown to prevent and even improve the loss of elasticity in the pelvic muscles and ligaments.

SURGERY. For a severely prolapsed uterus, the most common surgery is a vaginal hysterectomy, the removal of the uterus through the vagina. However, if you have had endometriosis, a cesarian section, or pelvic inflammatory disease (PID), your physician may advise you undergo an abdominal or laparoscopically assisted vaginal hysterectomy instead. For women who want to retain their ability to get pregnant, the uterus may be surgically attached to supporting ligaments in the pelvis, although prolapse may occur again.

RECTOCELE

A rectocele, or bulging of the rectum against the back wall of the vagina, will produce the sensation that something is about to fall out of the vagina. Women with this problem are often constipated and may even have to push the fingers against the wall of the vagina in order to have a bowel movement. Even after the bowels are empty, they may still feel full.

Rectocele and cystocele often coincide. As with other pelvic support disorders, rectoceles are more frequently found in women who have had children and in elderly women.

Understanding the Problem. Your health professional will be able to determine whether you have a rectocele by doing a rectal and pelvic examination.

Treatment Options. The course of treatment will depend on the severity of the problem.

NONSURGICAL. Your clinician may recommend Kegel exercises to strengthen the muscles and ligaments (see *Kegel Exercises*, page 494). This may relieve some of the uncomfortable pressure. A pessary may also be recommended. This rubber, plastic, or silicone ring is inserted into your vagina and positioned to hold the bulging organ in place. If you are post-menopausal and are not already taking estrogen, your clinician may prescribe hormone replacement therapy to improve and maintain muscle and ligament elasticity.

SURGERY. Most of the time, women who need surgery for a rectocele also require other pelvic support repairs. Surgery involves repositioning the prolapsed organs and tightening the surrounding support structures.

SELF-HELP. Some women with rectocele find that a high-fiber diet, bulking agents such as Metamucil or Fibercon, or stool softeners relieve the symptoms because they make it easier to have a bowel movement without straining.

ENTEROCELE

The most noticeable symptom of an enterocele is a feeling of heaviness deep in the pelvis, although the problem is often without symptoms.

An enterocele is a hernia of the small intestine in which the intestine exerts pressure down onto the top of the vagina. This condition is often without symptoms.

Enterocele is more likely to occur in women who have had a hysterectomy.

Understanding the Problem. Your health-care professional will diagnose an enterocele during a pelvic and rectal examination, although the problem is sometimes difficult to differentiate from a rectocele.

Treatment Options. Surgery to repair the hernia is the recommended treatment for an enterocele. A pessary placed into the vagina to support the vagina may also improve symptoms.

Vaginal and Vulvar Disorders

CONTENTS

The vagina is a muscular, elastic passageway, four to five inches long, that connects the uterus to the vulva, or external genitals. At the upper end of the vagina is the cervix, the neck of the uterus. Normally the vagina is collapsed so its walls touch, but any woman who has had a child knows that it has a tremendous capacity for expansion. The vagina's elasticity allows it to lengthen during sexual intercourse, and its resilience enables it to heal well and resume its normal shape and functioning after childbirth or even severe infection. *Vulva* is the term used to describe the many parts that make up your external genitals, including the mons pubis, labia, clitoris, urethral opening, and various glands.

In the following pages, we will discuss the most common problems that affect the vagina and the vulva.

VAGINAL DISORDERS

The lining of the vagina produces fluids that keep the vagina moist, flush out dead cells and other debris, and lubricate the vagina prior to intercourse. The amount and consistency of normal vaginal and cervical secretions vary at different points in the menstrual cycle. At times, however, this moist environment becomes the host for infectious organisms.

This can happen as a result of a change in the delicate ecosystem of the vagina, which

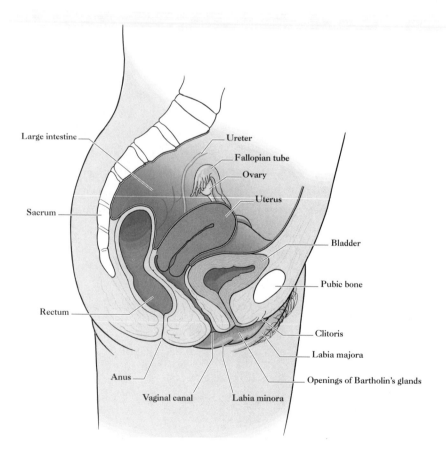

is inhabited by a number of normally beneficial organisms; or infection may be introduced during intercourse with an infected partner. Sometimes vaginal infections travel to other parts of the reproductive system, but more often they remain in the vagina, causing such symptoms as itching, burning, and discharge with an unpleasant odor.

With the exception of cancer, the majority of vaginal problems are not serious, but they can be uncomfortable. Fortunately, treatment in most cases is straightforward and effective.

VAGINITIS

Vaginitis is inflammation of the vagina and is often associated with vulvitis, inflammation of the external genitals. Symptoms include profuse, often foul-smelling discharge; burning and itching of the vulva; and pain during urination and intercourse.

Rare indeed is the woman who has never had some form of vaginitis. This ubiquitous ailment sends about five million women a year to their health-care provider; the average gynecologist sees between two and four patients a day with one variety or another of vaginitis.

The fact that vaginitis is so common is small consolation to those in the middle of an outbreak. Take Erica. For years she suffered three or four yeast infections a year, in spite of all the suppositories, vinegar-and-water douches, and stress reduction exercises her clinician and friends recommended. One day, a coworker aware of her complaint casually asked her whether she'd tried switching to cotton underpants. Erica had heard that advice before and always scoffed at it. Now, in desperation, she threw out her beloved lacy nylon panties and replaced them with ordinary cotton ones. That one small change did the trick: She's had one yeast infection in the eight years since then.

Vaginal health is something most women take for granted—until something goes wrong. The vaginal tract has a delicate ecosystem with a pH level (acid–alkaline balance) typically between 3.8 and 4.2. A variety of hormonal and biological factors work together to maintain a healthy acidic pH level, which in turn helps control the growth of potentially infectious organisms. Although some of these organisms are normally found in healthy vaginas, they are harmless until some alteration in the environment allows them to multiply unchecked and produce the symptoms of vaginitis.

The three most common varieties of vaginitis are candidiasis or yeast infection, trichomoniasis, and bacterial vaginosis. Each has its own distinct set of symptoms (see pages 505, 503, and 502 for detailed descriptions). A medical examination is usually necessary for an accurate diagnosis.

In the past, the most frequently occurring form of vaginitis was inaccurately labeled "nonspecific vaginitis." Now called *bacterial vaginosis*, the condition is caused by an overgrowth of certain bacteria, *Gardnerella vaginalis* and a number of others. Trichomoniasis, on the other hand, is a sexually transmitted disease caused by a parasite, a one-celled protozoan that infects the vagina and lower urinary tract. Candidiasis, more commonly referred to as "yeast infection," is caused by an overgrowth of fungus that may be normally present in the vagina. Yeast infections are most likely to occur when a woman is at a certain point in her hormonal cycle or when her immune system is suppressed. For example, she is more susceptible during pregnancy and immediately before and after her menstrual period. Women who have diabetes, are obese, have AIDS, or take corticosteroid medications or antibiotics are also at higher risk for yeast infections.

Understanding the Problem. Vaginitis symptoms are fairly easy to recognize, but discovering the cause may involve consulting your health-care provider so that he or she can perform a pelvic examination, during which a sample of discharge is obtained for analysis. With appropriate treatment, symptoms should clear up within a few days, but it is not uncommon for symptoms to recur.

Treatment Options. The treatment of vaginitis depends upon which organism is the culprit. All the disorders described can be treated with oral medication, and some also respond to vaginal suppositories or creams. Often, vaginitis symptoms are not due to infection at all but to sensitivity to soap, perfumed toilet paper, or other products that come in contact with the skin. In these instances, identifying and eliminating the source of the irritation are all that is needed to solve the problem.

BACTERIAL VAGINOSIS

The most common symptom of bacterial vaginosis is a thin, grayish white, sometimes frothy discharge with an unpleasant, fishy odor that frequently worsens after intercourse. Pain on urination and during intercourse is usually not present.

Bacterial vaginosis (which was at one time called "nonspecific vaginitis"), although not a true infection, is the most common form of vaginitis, affecting 50 percent of all women with vaginal complaints. Bacterial vaginosis is caused by an overgrowth of several different organisms that normally inhabit the vagina, often, but not always, including *Gardnerella vaginalis*. This particular bacterium is normally present in the vagina of 30 to 40 percent of women without symptoms (see also the discussion of *Vaginitis*, page 501).

Although bacterial vaginosis is not usually transmitted via sexual contact, it is more common among sexually active women, suggesting that sexual activity may play a role in increasing a woman's risk of development of the disease.

Understanding the Problem. If you have the symptoms of bacterial vaginosis, your health-care provider will perform a pelvic exam to obtain a sample of the discharge. The sample will be analyzed to determine the cause so that the appropriate treatment can be prescribed.

Treatment Options. Although not dangerous to a woman's general health, it is an annoying and often recurrent problem in pregnant women, and it may be associated with preterm labor. However, with proper treatment, the overgrowth can usually be cured within a week.

The most commonly prescribed medication is metronidazole (Flagyl, Metryl, Protostat, and Satric), an oral antibiotic. The usual dosage for a bacterial infection is twice a day for seven days. In one study, eighty of eighty-one women showed no signs of bacterial vaginosis after one week on metronidazole. Side effects of this medication may include nausea and a metallic taste in the mouth. Also, alcohol must be avoided during metronidazole therapy and for twenty-four hours thereafter.

Clindamycin is another effective treatment. This medication works by killing the bacteria that cause certain vaginal infections. (It does not, however, work for vaginal fungus or yeast infections.) In rare cases, this medicine can cause dizziness.

Both metronidazole and clindamycin are available as vaginal preparations, which tend to be more expensive than the pills and not as effective during pregnancy.

Your symptoms should improve within a few days of beginning use of any of these antibiotic agents; if this is not the case, or if symptoms become worse, check with your health-care professional. Also, your health-care professional will probably schedule a follow-up appointment after treatment is completed to make sure the problem has cleared up.

If a woman has signs of bacterial vaginosis present in the vagina, but experiences none of the distressing symptoms, many health professionals opt not to prescribe medication. However, many health-care professionals may treat the condition, regardless of symptoms, in pregnant women to prevent premature labor.

TRICHOMONIASIS

Trichomonal vaginitis is characterized by vulvar irritation, redness, pain, and profuse discharge that may be white, gray, yellow, or green. In some instances, this discharge is frothy and foul-smelling. Itching and painful urination may also occur. However, many women have the infection and experience no symptoms at all.

In the United States, up to three million women each year have vaginitis as a result of a trichomonal infection. *Trichomonas vaginalis*, a one-celled protozoan parasite, is responsible for 25 percent of all diagnosed cases of vaginitis (see also the discussion of *Vaginitis*, page 501). And because this parasite has two or three tails that can whip air into vaginal mucus, the discharge associated with this type of vaginitis can have a distinct, frothy quality.

The trichomonas parasite is spread through sexual intercourse, and it is common for both partners to be infected. In fact, trichomoniasis is the most common nonviral sexually transmitted disease found in women. In one study, 85 percent of women who had sex with infected men became infected themselves.

Symptoms typically appear between four and twenty-eight days after infection, but the condition may remain asymptomatic for many years. Some women are unaware of infection until it shows up on a routine Pap smear result.

Understanding the Problem. A diagnosis of trichomoniasis is made by analyzing a sample of vaginal discharge. The cervix may also be examined for petechiae, small red spots caused by the trichomonas protozoa.

Usually the infection is cured after one course of treatment. Women who suffer recurrent bouts either have become reinfected or have not taken their medication as recommended. Occasionally, though, a woman may harbor a strain of trichomoniasis that is resistant to the usual therapy.

Treatment Options. If trichomonas are found in your vaginal discharge—whether or not you exhibit the other symptoms—many health professionals will recommend treatment to prevent the disease from spreading. To prevent reinfection, your sex partners must be treated at the same time. The most effective drug for trichomoniasis is metronidazole (Flagyl, Metryl, Protostat, and Satric), the same medication used most often in the treatment of bacterial vaginosis. In most cases, metronidazole is prescribed in tablet form, although for cases that resist the usual treatment, the drug may be administered through injection.

Your clinician will probably prescribe a one-day dose of metronidazole, although some physicians still prefer a twice-daily course of medication for seven days. Both regimens have a very high cure rate, but many health-care providers prefer the one-day regimen because it is less expensive, has fewer side effects, and has a greater patient compliance rate than the longer regimen.

There are some minor side effects associated with metronidazole, including nausea and a metallic taste in the mouth. Alcohol should be completely avoided during metronidazole therapy and for twenty-four hours afterward.

WATASHA'S STORY

Almost every woman has a yeast infection at one time or another in her life, but Watasha felt she had had way more than her share. She'd get rid of one and another would ensue to take its place. They made her uncomfortable and interfered with her sex life. The cheesy discharge was unpleasant; the inflamed flesh around her genital area was constantly itchy.

When she changed HMOs, she consulted a new health-care provider. This clinician talked Watasha through her history of infections, explaining that many things can alter the vagina's ecosystem, permitting certain fungi to proliferate.

Watasha confided that she had tried everything to get rid of her Candida infections. The pill fluconazole worked for a while. So did the cream, but only in the short term.

"The thing that works best is the douching," Watasha concluded. "I do it almost every day."

Inferring that it was constant douching that had upset the natural balance in Watasha's vagina, making it ripe for yeast infections, her clinician responded immediately, "That could be your problem. You could be confusing the cure with the cause!" The practitioner suggested a standard regimen—keeping the vulva clean and dry, wearing cotton panties, wiping from front to back, and not wearing pants that are tight around the genitals. But most important, she recommended that Watasha stop douching. "No more. Never again. Stop. Forget about douching. Period."

The stratagem worked. Watasha had only one yeast infection in the last ten months. She's happy. And she doesn't miss the douching at all.

YEAST INFECTIONS

Candida (or Monilia*) vaginitis, more familiarly known as yeast infection, is characterized by a distinctive white or yellowish discharge that resembles cottage cheese. The amount of discharge varies; some women may show only a trace and others have more copious amounts. The discharge often has no odor, or it may have a mild and "yeasty" smell. Another common symptom is severe itching in the genital area that becomes more intense with scratching. The skin may become red and raw-looking, and intercourse may be extremely painful.*

A yeast infection is not a sexually transmitted disease, although 10 percent of the male partners of women with yeast infections exhibit irritation of the skin of the penis from contact with the vaginal secretions (see also the discussion of *Vaginitis*, page 501).

Yeast infections occur as a result of the overgrowth of one of a number of fungi. *Candida albicans* is responsible for the vast majority of cases, although *Candida glabrata* and *Candida tropicalis* also are culprits in some instances.

An estimated 25 percent of all healthy women have the fungus present in their vagina. As long as the vaginal environment remains in balance, the fungus is harmless. But hormonal changes, antibiotics, or an impaired immune system can alter the vagina's ecosystem, lowering the pH level enough that the fungus proliferates, eventually causing the uncomfortable symptoms of a yeast infection.

Like other types of vaginitis, yeast infections most often occur in women of reproductive age. Treatment with antibiotics, regular use of birth control pills, and pregnancy all increase the risk. Diabetes, AIDS, extreme overweight, and corticosteroid therapy are other risk factors. Tight clothing like form-fitting jeans or panty hose, which tend to keep the genital area moist, can create an ideal environment for yeast overgrowth.

Understanding the Problem. The local symptoms of a *Candida* infection are fairly easy for a woman to recognize. Itchiness around the genital area is usually the first sign. With the help of a mirror you can examine your genitals, and if you see a red, swollen vulva and a whitish discharge from the vagina, you can be reasonably certain you have a yeast infection.

Your health professional will confirm the diagnosis by taking a sample of your vaginal secretions for analysis. Although yeast infections are not dangerous to your overall health, they can make you feel miserable, and they do require treatment to alleviate symptoms. A small number of women suffer recurring yeast infections, which may call for a slightly different course of treatment.

Treatment Options. These infections can be treated either by one or several topical treatments such as Monistat, Mycelex, Terazol, or Femstat, which are available in suppositories or creams that are inserted directly into the vagina; or by fluconazole, a pill taken by mouth one time with a 90 percent cure rate. Some of the topical treatments are available over the counter at drugstores and supermarkets without a prescription.

It is common for yeast infections to recur. Some strains of *Candida* are especially resistant to the usual topical treatments. In such instances, your clinician may recommend oral fluconazole. You may want to consider longer-term treatments with topical medications—for example, a seven- to fourteen-day initial treatment followed by monthly one- or two-day treatments—as a preventive measure.

COMMONSENSE MEASURES FOR VAGINAL HEALTH

There are several things a woman can do to restore and maintain normal vaginal balance. Sound health practices are crucial both to overall well-being and to genital health.

Keeping the vulva clean and dry, wearing cotton panties, wiping from front to back, and not wearing panty hose and tight pants are all good habits. Also avoid deodorant pads and tampons. Douche only when recommended by your clinician. Don't use petroleum-based lubricants such as Vaseline for intercourse. Water-soluble lubricants are less irritating and easier to cleanse from the vagina. Spermicides, which contain nonoxynol-9, although known to protect against HIV, irritate the vulvar tissue in some women.

Some women have found that yogurt made with live lactobacillus culture, taken orally or inserted into the vagina, prevents or mitigates yeast infections. Although there is no scientific evidence that yogurt actually prevents infections, advocates suggest that supplementing the lactobacillus bacteria that are already present in the vagina helps restore, to some degree, normal flora and acid balance. Lactobacillus is also available in capsule form under the name acidophilus.

DYSPAREUNIA AND VAGINISMUS

Dyspareunia—painful sexual intercourse—and vaginismus—involuntary spasm of the muscles around the vagina—are disorders that may be of physical or psychological origin. Vaginismus can make intercourse painful and routine gynecological procedures or the insertion of a tampon difficult.

Painful intercourse—vaginismus and dyspareunia—can result from physical abnormalities, including prolapsed uterus, vaginal scarring from childbirth, vaginitis, endometriosis, fibroid tumors, vaginal dryness, or the loss of vaginal elasticity that sometimes accompanies menopause.

However, for many women, the source of vaginismus is a fear of or aversion to sex. Many women who find it difficult to have and enjoy sexual intercourse were either sexually abused as children or raised in homes in which sex was viewed as shameful, evil, or painful. Other contributing factors include the aftereffects of rape, anxiety about pregnancy, or feelings of aversion to one's partner.

Left untreated, dyspareunia can take a toll on a woman's self-esteem and sexual relationships; fortunately, the various possible causes generally respond well to treatment.

Understanding the Problem. A description of your symptoms, along with a pelvic examination, may be sufficient for your clinician to make a diagnosis, but often a more thorough examination may be necessary to determine the underlying cause.

Treatment Options. If your health-care professional finds a physical cause at the root of your sexual difficulties, that will be addressed. If vaginitis is present, for example, it will be treated with medications. Hormone replacement can help with irritation of vaginal tissues in postmenopausal women or postmenopausal vaginal dryness. Water-soluble lubricants may also make intercourse easier and more pleasurable in these situations. However, should the sexual difficulty result from a prolapsed uterus, scarring, endometriosis, or fibroids, your health-care provider will discuss appropriate treatment options with you.

Vaginismus, the involuntary spasm of the vaginal muscles, can usually be treated by vaginal manipulation with dilators. These are available in graduating sizes, and the woman inserts them herself, beginning with the smallest size and gradually moving on to the next until a penis-size dilator can be inserted without pain or spasm. This therapy should take as long as the woman needs to allow her body and particularly her vaginal muscles to relax.

If the problem is emotionally based, improved sexual response and enjoyment are often achieved with the help of therapy with a mental health professional or sex therapist. Counseling may be recommended for both the woman and her partner, since sexual problems tend to create stresses in the relationship.

VULVAR VESTIBULITIS

Distinct tenderness and redness in the vestibule (or vaginal opening) is known as vulvar vestibulitis. This condition may be present from weeks to several years and can be incapacitating. Painful or impossible intercourse is the most common complaint. Stinging or rawness at the vaginal opening can also be experienced with moderate exercise or in more severe cases with no movement.

While early studies implicated human papilloma virus as the cause, this has not been established. Some women relate the beginning of their symptoms to an infection, trauma, or an obstetrical or gynecologic event. It is not believed to be a sexually transmitted disease and cannot be passed on to a sexual partner. Vulvar vestibulitis is not associated with cancer. It is also not associated with poor hygiene; in fact, strong soaps can worsen the condition.

Understanding the Problem. Usually a woman visits her practitioner after weeks or months have passed and a number of over-the-counter topical preparations have failed or worsened the condition. On examination the diagnosis is made by identifying distinct areas of tenderness to touch at the vestibule (vaginal opening) with or without associated redness.

Treatment Options. Treatment of this condition is complicated by the fact that the cause is unknown in most situations. Topical agents such as antifungal medications, steroids, and antibiotics are not typically effective. Topical anesthetic agents such as Viscous Lidocaine Gel can help with temporary symptomatic relief. Certain oral medications such as anticonvulsants or tricyclic antidepressant agents have been successful in some women complaining of chronic pain. The action of these medications may be to interfere at some level with pain messages being transmitted to or processed by the brain.

Dietary changes may produce an improvement in symptoms. In particular, avoiding oxalic-rich foods (such as green beans, celery, various berries, tea, and even chocolate) may be helpful. National support groups and centers have also been organized to help address the needs and issues associated with vulvar vestibulitis.

Surgical excision is a consideration if more conservative methods have failed. The surgery can be disfiguring, however, and is best performed in the hands of those with considerable experience with the procedure.

VENEREAL WARTS (HPV)

The most obvious symptom of Condylomata acuminata, *more commonly known as venereal warts, is the presence of small pink, red, white, or gray swellings on the genitals. Warts may appear smooth, round, raised, or flat. They can occur as single or multiple growths. The warts, which start out the size of a pinhead, grow quickly and sometimes cluster together in large masses that resemble cauliflower. The most visible warts grow around the labia, vaginal opening, and rectum, but upon examination, a health-care provider may find them around the cervix and urethra as well.*

Venereal warts may cause itching, burning, or mild pain, depending on the area infected. Some people have no symptoms. But since these warts are fragile, the slightest trauma may cause them to bleed. Should they become infected, they can cause pain and an unpleasant odor. Because they thrive in a moist environment, warts tend to grow more rapidly when there is another vaginal infection that produces discharge.

Venereal warts are caused by the human papillomavirus (HPV), which is transmitted sexually. In one study, 60 percent of the adults who had intercourse with someone infected with HPV went on to have venereal warts. In the past twenty years, the incidence of venereal warts has increased by *700 percent.* As with other sexually transmitted diseases, the age group at highest risk for development of venereal warts is between fifteen and twenty-five.

The incubation period for HPV is one to eight months after exposure; the average is three months. In some cases, though, warts do not appear for many years after exposure to the virus. Symptoms can flare when a women is pregnant, if she has diabetes, or if her immune system is suppressed by disease or medications.

Understanding the Problem. Generally a health professional makes the diagnosis by physical examination. However, other sexually transmitted diseases such as gonorrhea may occur with HPV, and your clinician may want to take a specimen of vaginal or cervical discharge or even a biopsy to rule out the possibility of a more dangerous disease. In any case, a thorough examination is necessary to locate all infected sites, especially in the cervix.

There are more than sixty kinds of HPV, some of which predispose the sufferer to cervical cancer. These warts are chiefly a nuisance rather than a genuine health threat. If left untreated, they can disappear spontaneously, but they are more likely to multiply and spread. They are fairly easily treated, although they tend to recur.

Treatment Options. Because venereal warts are contagious, it is a good idea to seek treatment promptly. Treatment will depend on a number of factors, including the location of the warts, their size and number, and whether you are pregnant. Your sexual partner should be evaluated and, if infected, treated at the same time to prevent reinfecting you.

MEDICATION. For small warts, your health provider may recommend a caustic solution that is applied like paint to the infected area. Two such solutions, Condylox and Aldera, are safe enough for you to administer yourself. Others are podophyllin and bichloroacetic or trichloroacetic acid, which turn the warts white and may cause some discomfort for a few minutes. Because these chemicals can be irritating to the skin, they should be applied with care to the surface of the warts only.

SURGERY. If the medication does not work or if the warts are excessively large or located inside the vagina or cervix, cryosurgery (freezing), electrocautery (burning), or laser surgery may be suggested. If warts persist in growing back, a biopsy may be recommended to make sure that they are not cancerous. And because some strains of the virus have been associated with an increased risk of cancer of the cervix and vulva, your health-care professional may recommend that you have frequent Pap smears.

DOUCHING

If television and magazine advertising is to be believed, a woman just isn't clean and fresh if she doesn't douche and use a feminine hygiene spray. In fact, douching, the infusion of liquid into the vagina, has been credited with everything from preventing pregnancy to making a woman more confident socially. Douching, of course, does not prevent pregnancy, nor will it turn an introvert into the life of the party.

In truth, douching is unnecessary for most women and may be harmful.

Under most circumstances, the vagina cleanses itself naturally. The vaginal walls produce a fluid that carries dead cells and other debris out of the body. In the absence of infection, normal vaginal secretions are clear or milky, turning slightly yellow as they dry. They have a mild but not unpleasant odor. Still, women have been made to feel that any vaginal odor indicates a lack of cleanliness. Hence the popularity of douching.

Most clinicians recommend against douching. Some commercial douches contain harsh chemicals that alter the vagina's pH balance and irritate delicate tissues, leaving the vagina at increased risk for infection. If you douche more than once a week, you also run an increased risk of pelvic inflammatory disease (PID; see page 449).

If you feel you must douche, some guidelines may be helpful. Douche no more than once a month. Use plain water and keep the water pressure as gentle as possible. Do not douche if you think you have an infection and do not douche within three days of a pelvic exam. And remember: Douching is not a reliable method of birth control.

INFESTATIONS (PUBIC LICE AND SCABIES)

Severe itching is often the first sign of infestation by a parasite—either solely in the pubic area or, in the case of scabies, anywhere on the body that is affected. Sometimes the parasites are visible as pin-head-size grayish insects or tiny white particles (the eggs) clinging to the pubic hair. Scabies, tiny burrowing mites, leave thin lines along the surface of the skin.

Marian, a college student, was taking summer classes at her school. To save money, she lived off-campus for six weeks in a rented room in a house run by other students. Her first night there, she slept in bedding left by the previous occupant, then laundered it the next day. A couple of weeks later, she started scratching. And scratching. When she finally took a good look at her pubic area, to her horror she found it inhabited by a thriving colony of crab lice, courtesy of some anonymous fellow student who'd left them behind in the bed sheets.

The crab louse and the itch mite are the most common pubic parasites, and together they account for the most contagious of all sexually transmitted diseases. It is possible to pick up these parasites from infected clothing, bedding, soap, and toilet seats. However, they are most commonly transmitted through sexual intercourse. Ninety percent of those who have intercourse with an infested person contract lice after only one exposure.

Understanding the Problem. A close examination of your pubic area is usually all your health provider needs to make a diagnosis of crab louse infestation. If scabies is a possibility, the clinician will examine you for characteristic bumps, sores from itching, and thin, wavy lines that indicate where the mites have burrowed under the skin.

Although not serious, infestations are extremely uncomfortable, and often embarrassing. Early diagnosis and treatment are important to controlling the infestation. Nevertheless, because many women associate parasitic infestation with being unclean, they often delay treatment until their symptoms become intolerable.

PUBIC LICE. Crab lice, also called crabs or *Pediculosis pubis*, are related to the insect that typically infests the head and other parts of the body. However, this particular tiny, blood-sucking insect thrives in the hairy areas of the vulva and rectum, though it may occasionally be transmitted to the eyelids or some other part of the body.

The louse's life can be divided into three stages: egg or nit, nymph, and adult. After sexual contact with an infested person, during which the parasite travels from one partner to the other, it deposits its eggs, or nits, at the base of pubic hair follicles. Within ten days or so, the nits become adults the size of a pinhead and are a grayish color when not engorged with the host's blood.

ITCH MITE. The itch mite is the parasite that causes scabies, a condition characterized by severe itching, especially at night, when the skin is warmer and the mites are more active. Scabies is common among schoolchildren and can travel through a family very quickly. Unlike pubic lice, itch mites do not confine themselves to the genitals. Instead, they burrow under the skin between the fingers, in the armpits, on the insides of the wrists, on the soles of the feet, and elsewhere. Once the female mite has made a home under the skin, she begins to lay eggs.

Treatment Options. Treatment for both parasites requires killing both the adult parasites and the eggs. Your health provider may recommend an over-the-counter solution such as Nix Cream, which you apply to the skin for ten minutes and follow up with a second application ten days later to kill any recently hatched eggs. Or your clinician may prescribe Kwell, a 1 percent solution of the potent pesticide lindane in the form of cream, lotion, or shampoo. This solution may cause allergic reactions in some individuals and should not be used by pregnant women or children under ten. None of these preparations should be used on the eyelashes or eyebrows; special ophthalmic ointments are available by prescription.

If you have scabies, your health-care provider may also recommend an antihistamine to relieve the itchiness that can persist for several days after treatment.

With either infestation, it is crucial that your sex partner be treated at the same time you are. In the case of scabies, family members and any others living in the same home should also be treated. To prevent reinfestation, bed linens, blankets, towels, and recently worn clothing should be laundered in hot water, and combs and brushes washed in Kwell shampoo.

ATROPHIC VAGINITIS

After menopause, some women experience frequent soreness, burning, or itching in the genital area. The vulva may become swollen or unusually red and irritated and may even have tiny sores or cracks. The vaginal muscles lose some of their elasticity and lubricating capacity. This condition, called vaginal atrophy, *does not signal the end of a woman's sexual functioning, only the need for changes in her methods of arousal and intercourse.*

Elsewhere in this book, we have discussed the physical changes that occur when a woman's body produces smaller amounts of the hormone estrogen (see Chapter 5, *Menopause and the Climacteric*, page 87). Areas that are particularly affected by the decrease in estrogen are the vagina and vulva. The vaginal walls gradually become thinner and less elastic, and the decrease in lubrication can lead to irritation and injury during intercourse. In fact, atrophic vaginitis is the leading cause of vaginal bleeding among postmenopausal women.

Understanding the Problem. If you suffer the symptoms described, with or without the loss of bladder control that sometimes accompanies them, your health-care provider will conduct a thorough pelvic examination. In cases of a vaginal infection, treatment is necessary.

Treatment Options. If you have had an infection as a result of irritated vaginal tissues, your health professional will prescribe an antibiotic. He or she may also recommend that you use a water-soluble lubricant such as K-Y Jelly, Replens, Lubrin, or Gynemoistrin to make intercourse easier and more enjoyable.

The only medical treatment for the source of the problem is estrogen. Initially your health-care professional may prescribe an estrogen cream to apply locally to the vagina. However, to minimize your risk of osteoporosis and heart disease, your clinician may recommend estrogen replacement therapy (ERT) (see *Hormone Replacement Therapy*, page 90).

SELF-HELP. Whether or not you choose ERT, it is worth exploring different ways in which you and your partner can minimize the discomfort of intercourse. An extended period of foreplay and arousal can increase lubrication. New positions and techniques may be helpful. Kegel exercises (see page 494), which strengthen vaginal and anal muscles (as well as enhancing bladder control), may help also. Strong muscles in this area are important in facilitating arousal and orgasm.

PRECANCEROUS CHANGES IN THE VAGINA
A woman who has precancerous changes in the vagina generally has no symptoms.

Although cancer that originates in the vagina is rare—accounting for less than 2 percent of gynecological malignancies—any precancerous changes in the vaginal tissues must be taken very seriously.

Precancerous cell changes in the vagina occur more frequently in women who also have had precancerous changes in the cervix (see Chapter 23, page 529). Both vaginal and cervical precancerous changes are associated with certain types of human papillomavirus (HPV), although not usually the types that cause venereal warts.

Understanding the Problem. Precancerous vaginal tissue changes are generally detected through a routine Pap smear. If your Pap test result raises concerns, your clinician will examine the cervix and vagina with a magnifying instrument called a colposcope and remove a small piece of vaginal or cervical tissue for laboratory analysis (biopsy).

Treatment Options. If the lesions are small, your health-care professional may be able to destroy them surgically with a surgical laser, a procedure that can be done on an out-patient basis under local anesthesia. General anesthesia may be necessary if the lesions are widespread. After laser surgery, you can expect some vaginal discharge for a few weeks.

A medication used when the precancerous lesions are widespread is 5-fluorouracil cream. Inserted into the vagina for seven days, the cream can be irritating to the external genitals. Therefore, zinc oxide or some other protective ointment is usually first applied to the vulva. If the initial treatment does not take care of the problem, it is repeated.

VAGINAL CANCER

The most common initial symptoms of vaginal cancer are abnormal bleeding and/or discharge. The bleeding, which is not associated with the menstrual cycle, may occur after intercourse or a pelvic examination. Most women with vaginal cancer do not experience much pain unless the disease is well advanced. In some early forms of cancer, though, women can experience discomfort in the pelvis, back, or legs, as well as leg swelling (edema).

Although cancer frequently spreads to the vagina from other reproductive organs, a malignancy that originates in the vagina is rare, accounting for less than 2 percent of all gynecological malignancies. For this reason, most women do not recognize the warning signs of vaginal cancer, and the problem often goes undiagnosed in its earliest stages. As with most malignancies, the longer you wait to begin treatment, the more dangerous the condition becomes.

The most common type of vaginal cancer develops in the surface (squamous) cells lining the vagina. About 90 percent of vaginal cancers are squamous cell carcinomas. These tumors occur most frequently in women over the age of fifty, although they are seen occasionally in younger women.

About 5 percent of all vaginal cancers develop in the glandular tissues. These clear cell adenocarcinomas are particularly common in young women whose mother was exposed to diethylstilbestrol (DES) during pregnancy and usually affect young women during their reproductive years. However, as DES was taken off the market in 1971, the incidence of these cancers is dropping.

Rarer types of vaginal cancer include melanoma, sarcoma, and endodermal sinus tumor.

Understanding the Problem. Most vaginal cancers are discovered during a routine pelvic examination and Pap smear. Other times, abnormal bleeding or discharge may lead to the diagnosis. Women who have certain risk factors are usually followed more carefully with twice-yearly pelvic examinations. For example, women who have a history of genital warts or cancer of the cervix or vulva, and associated radiation therapy, are at higher risk for development of squamous cell tumors.

In addition to the pelvic examination and vaginal Pap smear, screenings for malignancies of the vagina include Pap smears of the cervix and vaginal wall and colposcopic (magnification) examination of the vagina.

If your health-care provider detects a tumor, he or she will perform a rectal examination to assess the local spread of the cancer. Blood tests will be conducted, and a biopsy, by which a piece of tissue will be removed and analyzed, will help identify the particular type of cancer. Depending on the degree to which the cancer has advanced, chest X ray and imaging procedures (CT scan of the pelvis and abdomen and MRI of the pelvis) may be recommended.

Vaginal cancer is staged to determine whether it has spread beyond the pelvis. When this cancer is diagnosed early before the tumor has grown large and spread, the chances that treatment will be successful are quite high. When, for example, squamous cell carcinoma or adenocarcinoma is detected and treated in stage 1, when the cancer is limited to the vaginal wall, the five-year survival rate is 70 to 80 percent. In stage 2, when the carcinoma involves the adjacent vaginal tissue but has not extended to the pelvic wall, the five-year survival rate is about 50 percent.

Treatment Options. There are a number of factors involved in choosing the most appropriate way to manage vaginal cancer. These include the age of the woman; the type of cell; the stage, location, and size of the tumor; the presence or absence of the uterus; and whether the woman has had previous radiation to the pelvis. Early carcinomas are generally treated with surgery and radiation therapy. Surgery may involve removing the uterus (hysterectomy) and the vagina (vaginectomy). In some cases, plastic surgery can reconstruct the vagina. In young women, it may be possible to leave the ovaries intact so they continue to receive the benefits of their body's own estrogen. Occasionally, a very small tumor can be removed in such a way as to preserve a woman's chances of getting pregnant later. However, when the cancer has spread or when it recurs after radiation treatment, more radical surgery that involves the removal of the bladder and rectum may be necessary.

Advanced cancers are treated with radiation therapy alone with or without chemotherapy.

VULVAR DISORDERS

The parts of the vulva are the mons pubis, a fatty pad of tissue at the base of the abdomen that in the adult female is covered with hair; the labia majora, liplike folds of tissue; the labia minora, two small pink folds between the labia majora and the vaginal opening; the clitoris, a small organ that swells during sexual arousal and is the female counterpart to the penis; the urethral opening, just below the clitoris, through which urine flows from the body; and various glands.

The moist environment of the vulva makes it susceptible to many ailments, most of which are not a threat to general health. Minor skin irritations and infections—similar to pimples found elsewhere on the body—are common vulvar complaints, as are allergic reac-

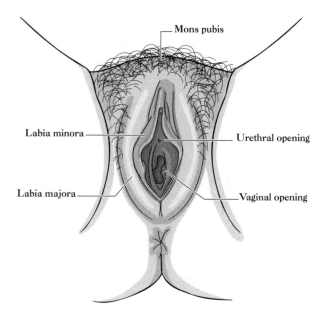

tions. However, cysts and abscesses may also develop, especially in the Bartholin's glands (please note that Chapter 19, *Sexually Transmitted Diseases and Other Infections*, includes a detailed discussion of another common ailment that has as its key symptoms vulvar blisters and ulcers; see *Genital Herpes [HSV]*, page 454).

VULVITIS

Swelling of the vulva, with redness, itching, and blisters that may ooze or form a crust, defines the condition known as vulvitis. In chronic or long-term vulvitis, the skin of the vulva may thicken and turn white.

Vulvitis—the inflammation of the external genitals—has many causes. Vulvar skin is quite sensitive, particularly after menopause. An allergic reaction to a feminine hygiene spray, scented toilet paper, lubricant, or a new detergent used in washing underwear may be responsible for the irritation. Often vulvitis is the first sign of a vaginal infection, but it also can be a symptom of vulvar cancer. Another cause of the disorder is herpes, a sexually transmitted viral infection (see page 454).

Even in the absence of infection or an allergic reaction, just the dampness around a woman's vulva produced by urine and vaginal and cervical secretions can produce inflammation. In particular, women who regularly wear tight-fitting underwear, panty hose, and jeans are likely to experience recurrent vulvitus.

Vulvitis can occur at any age, even during childhood.

Understanding the Problem. Your health professional will ask you a series of questions regarding your use of soaps, feminine sprays, spermicides, or any other product that might be causing your symptoms. During a pelvic examination, he or she will probably take a sample of your vaginal secretions to check for the presence of infection such as *Candida* vaginitis (see *Yeast Infections*, page 505) or a sexually transmitted disease. Vulvitis usually responds well to treatment. If the condition does not clear up with treatment, your health-care professional may want to do a biopsy to check for viral infection or precancerous changes.

Treatment Options. Cortisone cream applied to the area will usually relieve the itch. It is important that you keep the area clean and dry. Wear loose-fitting cotton underpants and avoid panty hose and the use of sprays, perfumes, or deodorants on your vulva.

If an underlying infection is involved, your health professional will prescribe the appropriate medication.

PRURITUS VULVAE

Pruritus *means itching and can be a symptom of many vaginal and vulvar disorders. An itch–scratch cycle can develop, resulting in an increasingly irritated and painful vulva. The skin burns, stings, and becomes raw-looking. This condition can become chronic.*

A wide range of diseases—some serious, most not—can cause pruritus vulvae. Vaginal infections, skin infections such as contact dermatitis, sexually transmitted diseases, allergies to medications, vitamin deficiencies, lice or mite infestations, diabetes, lichen sclerosis, leukemia, and premalignant and malignant vulvar diseases all can cause unrelenting itching. Prepubescent girls and postmenopausal women frequently complain of vulvar itch. In some women, no physical cause can be found.

Understanding the Problem. Pruritus vulvae by itself is not dangerous, but a few of the conditions that cause it can be threatening to your health. Before prescribing treatment, your clinician will perform a pelvic examination and take a sample of vaginal discharge to test for infection.

Treatment Options. Depending on the cause, a number of treatment approaches may be used.

SELF-HELP. Many times, mild itching will stop in a few days. In the meantime, stop using feminine sprays or any other product on the area. Wear cotton underpants, avoid panty hose, and bathe once a day with a mild, unscented soap. However, if the itching is severe and there is an abnormal discharge, contact your clinician.

MEDICATION. Your health professional can prescribe a corticosteroid cream to break the itch–scratch cycle. Any underlying condition will require treatment with the appropriate medication.

SURGERY. If tests indicate your itching is caused by human papillomavirus, medical or surgical treatments may be employed to destroy the infected tissue (see *Venereal Warts*, page 508).

VULVAR CYSTS

Vulvar cysts typically do not produce any symptoms and are often discovered during a gynecological examination. Sometimes a particularly large cyst will protrude from the vaginal opening. Symptoms occasionally associated with vulvar cysts include painful intercourse, general vaginal pain, urinary problems, infection, and difficulty in using tampons.

Sometimes cysts, small closed, filled sacs, develop along the wall of vulva. The two main types of vulvar cysts are inclusion cysts and Bartholin's cysts.

Often found in women who have had children, inclusion cysts can result from trauma during childbirth. They can also develop if the vaginal walls do not heal completely after an episiotomy or another type of gynecological surgery.

Bartholin's and other vestibular cysts occur when glands around the opening of the vagina become blocked or infected.

Understanding the Problem. Vulvar cysts are usually discovered during a routine pelvic examination. If the cyst is not causing you problems, your health-care provider may elect not to treat it, but instead to examine you periodically to make sure it isn't enlarging. If the clinician suspects cancer, which is extremely rare, he or she will remove the cyst to analyze it for the presence of cancer cells.

Treatment Options. If the cyst is causing pain or other problems, you may have it surgically removed. In cases in which the cyst is small, your health-care provider may be able to remove it in the office under local anesthesia.

BARTHOLIN'S GLAND ABSCESS

The symptoms of a Bartholin's gland abscess are vulvar pain, painful intercourse, and pain when walking. The vulva is likely to be red, swollen, and hot to the touch.

Bartholin's glands—named for the Danish anatomist Casper Bartholin—are two pea-sized structures located on the sides of the vaginal opening and deep within the perineum that provide vaginal lubrication. Normally, the glands are too small to be felt even by the practiced hand of a gynecologist. In about 2 percent of adult women, however, the glands become enlarged, usually because of a cyst (see *Vulvar Cysts*, above). Other causes of enlarged Bartholin's glands are abscesses and, rarely, cancers.

The majority of women with Bartholin's gland cysts do not have symptoms other than a slightly enlarged gland. Sometimes, though, the gland becomes infected, and an abscess results.

It was once believed that gonorrhea was always the cause of an enlarged Bartholin's gland. We now know that in many cases it is not caused by a sexually transmitted disease. More than 85 percent of women with enlarged Bartholin's glands are of childbearing age.

Understanding the Problem. Bartholin's gland abscess is readily diagnosed during a physical examination. The abscess itself usually is cured with drainage. Even without treatment, most abscesses rupture and heal by the third or fourth day. However, because drainage is often incomplete, the abscess tends to recur.

Treatment Options. Your clinician may prescribe oral antibiotics for the infection and may also recommend sitting in a hot bath to induce rupturing of the abscess.

Often the treatment for a painful cyst or abscess involves a minor surgical incision to complete drainage of the abscess. Usually done under local anesthesia in your health-care provider's office, this procedure provides the greatest relief and the fastest recovery.

However, since the recurrence rate for Bartholin's gland abscesses is fairly high, simply draining them is usually not sufficient. One highly successful procedure, called *marsupialization*, involves creating a large opening that allows the gland to drain constantly into the vagina. Another successful procedure involves incising the abscess and inserting a small balloon-tipped catheter. This allows for a drainage tract to form. The catheter is tolerated and is removed after one to two weeks.

In cases of recurrent abscesses or persistent infection, removal of the entire Bartholin's gland is sometimes warranted.

LICHEN SCLEROSIS (ATROPHIC VULVAR DYSTROPHY)

Patches of dry, itchy, and inflamed skin in the vulva are characteristic of lichen sclerosis (formerly called atrophic vulvar dystrophy). These same areas may turn white, thicken, and contract. Eventually the skin may become shiny or paper-thin, and the clitoris and vaginal opening may shrink. Intercourse may be painful.

Lichen sclerosis relates to the gradual degeneration of the vulva, although the skin around the rectum may also be affected. The exact cause is unknown. The condition occurs most commonly in postmenopausal women, although it can occur in women of any age.

Understanding the Problem. To make sure that the whitened areas on your vulva are not malignant, your health-care provider may do a vulvar biopsy, a procedure in which a small piece of tissue is removed and analyzed by a pathologist. This can often be done under local anesthetic in the health-care professional's office. He or she may also want to check for signs of an underlying infection.

Lichen sclerosis itself is not a precancerous condition and does not increase your risk of later development of vulvar cancer. In one study of 107 patients with this condition, only 1 went on to have vulvar cancer over the period of the next twelve years. Lichen sclerosis can be persistent, however, and does tend to recur.

Treatment Options. Because the cause of lichen sclerosis has not been determined, no genuine cure is available. But the symptoms can be managed.

Relieving the itch is usually one of the first treatment goals, so corticosteroid cream may be prescribed. A cream containing testosterone may also be recommended to help alleviate symptoms. To prevent further irritation, it may be advisable to avoid using harsh soaps on the genital area and to wear cotton rather than synthetic underwear.

CANCER OF THE VULVA
The main symptom of cancer of the vulva is a small, hard, itchy lump in the skin. As the disease advances, a "sore" may develop that just won't heal and that bleeds or leaks fluid.

Cancer of the vulva is relatively rare, accounting for only 4 percent of cancers in the female reproductive organs. Most vulvar cancers are squamous cell carcinomas, although melanomas and sarcomas can also occur.

Vulvar cancers usually begin as premalignant tissue changes associated with certain kinds of papillomavirus, but in many women who have this form of cancer no such changes are ever noted. Vulvar cancer appears with increasing frequency in women who have had squamous cell carcinoma of the vagina or cervix, both of which are associated with the high-risk types of papillomavirus.

Vulvar cancer occurs most commonly in older women; one study found that only 15 percent of new cases occurred in women under the age of forty, and more than half were diagnosed in women between the ages of sixty and seventy-nine.

Even though this is primarily a disease of older women, health-care professionals are seeing an increasing number of premalignant vulvar changes in women in their twenties and thirties. The increase may be due to an increase in certain strains of sexually transmitted papillomavirus infection.

Understanding the Problem. If you have a lesion that might be vulvar cancer, your health-care provider will remove a small piece of tissue for analysis. The outlook for a woman who has cancer of the vulva depends on the size of the tumor and the extent to which the disease has infiltrated surrounding tissue or spread to lymph nodes. For a tumor that is less than two centimeters and confined to the vulva (stage 1), the worldwide five-year survival rate is about 69 percent.

BARTHOLIN'S GLAND CARCINOMA. This rare cancer, an adenocarcinoma, occurs in the Bartholin's glands, which are located at the entrance to the vagina. It is more likely to occur in postmenopausal women. When the disease is diagnosed before it has spread to the lymph nodes, the prognosis is good.

BASAL CELL CARCINOMA. This is the skin cancer so frequently found in fair-skinned people and inveterate sun worshipers. Although basal cell cancer is usually limited to parts of the body exposed to the sun, some women experience it on the vulva. Treatment generally involves removal of the lesion, which almost always effects a complete cure.

MELANOMA. This is the most frequent non–squamous cell malignancy of the vulva, accounting for about 6 percent of vulvar cancers. The average age at diagnosis is fifty, although the cancer is known to occur in older teenagers. Like melanomas elsewhere on the body, this vulvar malignancy arises from a mole. An especially virulent malignancy, it appears as a brown, black, or blue-black mass on the vulva. The outcome depends on how deeply the cancer has invaded. The overall five-year survival rate is 50 percent. Younger women, who tend to be diagnosed before the melanoma has spread, have a much better prognosis.

VERRUCOUS CARCINOMA. Another rare vulvar cancer, this is a variant of the more common squamous cell carcinoma. This slow-growing cancer appears as a large wart on the vulva and usually does not metastasize (spread).

Treatment Options. Most vulvar cancer is treated with surgery to remove the tumor, surrounding skin, and lymph nodes in the groin (vulvectomy). If the lymph nodes are cancerous, radiation therapy is also recommended. In cases in which vulvar cancer recurs after treatment, a combination of radiation and chemotherapy may be used.

CHAPTER 23

Cervical, Uterine, Fallopian Tube, and Ovarian Problems

CONTENTS

When it comes to the reproductive system, Leah is like a lot of women. As long as her female parts—her vulva, vagina, cervix, uterus, fallopian tubes, and ovaries—are functioning properly, she doesn't spend much time thinking about them. Yet when something, however small, goes awry, she becomes acutely aware that all those parts tucked away between her legs and hidden under the skin of her abdomen constitute an elaborate, dynamic system. For Leah, as for so many women, her sexual and reproductive organs are the site of immense pleasure, occasional pain, and a certain amount of ambivalence—as well as the source of at least part of her identity as a woman.

It's difficult for most women to think of their own reproductive system in the same cold clinical terms that they might use to talk about their gallbladder, for instance. Although no one wants to undergo surgery, if your gallbladder is hurting and surgery is the best alternative, you will probably opt for the operation. For most people, it's a pretty straightforward choice.

The distinction between an ailing gallbladder and a problem with the female reproductive organs, however, goes beyond function. People are seldom emotionally attached to a gallbladder. However, most women have complex and often conflicting feelings about their genitals and reproductive organs. The first time a young girl notices discharge in her panties, she and her mother might overlook it, or they might wonder whether it's a sign that something is wrong, or they might regard it as dirty. When a girl begins menarche, she and her mother may celebrate the beginning of womanhood and discuss all the responsibilities of reproductive maturity. Or they may view menstruation as a burden, a curse. For some women, sexual relations are a source of pleasure and satisfaction; for others, they are a source of discomfort and conflict. For many women, sexual relations bring a bit of both. Pregnancy prompts all sort of changes in a woman's body and stirs up all sorts of feelings, some of which may well surprise her. Years later, when a doctor confirms a woman's suspicion that she is entering menopause, she may recall the day she started menstruating, her early sexual relationships, and her first pregnancy, and wonder whether the woman she knows herself to be is soon to be a memory.

In much the same way, when sensations, signs, and changes are related not to normal developmental milestones, but rather to disease of the reproductive system, a woman's reactions will likely include considerable and complicated distress. A diseased uterus, after all, is not the same as a diseased gallbladder. A woman facing a hysterectomy for endometrial cancer is dealing not only with a frightening diagnosis, but with the impending loss of a part of her body that may embody her femininity. The sense of loss may be even more painful for young women who have not yet borne children.

Most women have a relatively healthy reproductive system. Whatever problems they experience are likely to be minor and transient. Most times, the concerns a woman has about this part of her body involve pregnancy, menstrual disorders, and natural hormonal changes. In some instances, sexually contracted infections can also cause disorders of the reproductive system. Occasionally, problems arise from birth defects. And then there are

THE FEMALE REPRODUCTIVE ORGANS

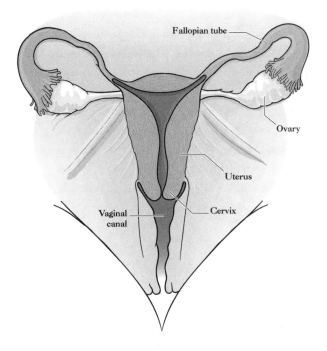

potentially more serious disorders that seemingly appear out of nowhere—fibroids, cysts, cancers. All these types of problems and disorders will be explored in this chapter.

Keep in mind as you read through this chapter that the majority of problems of the reproductive system are diagnosed during routine pelvic examinations. It is therefore essential that you visit your health-care professional each year. That way, you increase the odds that your reproductive system will remain healthy, and any problems that arise will be discovered—and treated—early.

KAREN'S STORY

Karen was sixteen and had not yet begun to menstruate. At fourteen, no one gave it much thought. At fifteen, Karen was pretty sure she was the only girl in her class who hadn't yet had her period. A few days after her sixteenth birthday, she experienced severe abdominal cramping but still no period. This was enough to dispel the notion that Karen's only problem was that she was a late bloomer.

Her mother immediately made an appointment with their health-care professional. Upon examination, the gynecologist discovered a condition called an imperforate hymen, meaning that Karen had no vaginal opening through which vaginal secretions—and monthly menstrual flow—could leave the body. Before she reached puberty, it hadn't mattered, but now it did.

In most girls with an imperforate hymen, the vagina expands to accommodate the monthly flow, and only a minor procedure is needed. Once the hymen is punctured, blood gushes from the vagina. But Karen's problem was more severe. She appeared to have been menstruating for some time, and her menstrual flow had backed up through her fallopian tubes into her pelvis. Bits of uterine tissue had accumulated in the lining of the pelvic cavity and on the ovaries (see Endometriosis and Adenomyosis, *page 545).*

Karen required surgery to open the hymen and remove the tissue that had attached itself in various places within the pelvic cavity. Her surgeon used a laparoscope, a long, narrow tube inserted through a small incision into her abdomen. The lighted tube allowed the surgeon to view the interior organs, locate the unwanted tissue, and destroy the tissue with electrocautery.

Today, Karen is menstruating normally. Her clinician continues to monitor her to make sure all the misplaced tissue is gone. Yet, in every respect, Karen is a healthy, normal teenage girl.

CONGENITAL ABNORMALITIES

A woman's reproductive system is formed during the first half of fetal life. It is a complicated process that begins at the moment of conception. When the sperm that happens to be carrying an X sex chromosome fuses in the mother's fallopian tube with an ovum (which always carries an X sex chromosome), a female is created. She begins as a single cell that instantaneously starts to divide millions and million of times. Every cell in the evolving female fetus has the same forty-six chromosomes—forty-four plus two X sex chromosomes—that carry the genetic code. In all cells except those few designated "reproductive," the first forty-four chromosomes dominate. But in those special reproductive cells, the two sex chromosomes dominate all others.

For the first eight weeks of fetal development, it is impossible to distinguish a girl embryo from a boy embryo. Slowly, a rather indistinct outline forms as reproductive cells begin to sort themselves out. External genitals appear from a small groove near the fetal tail. In a girl, the upper portion develops into the clitoris; in a boy, it becomes the tip of the penis. Later, two cords of cells move down toward the pelvic floor. In a girl, the lower stems fuse and hollow out to become the vagina and uterus, while the upper segments become the fallopian tubes. In a boy, these cords disappear.

As a female fetus grows, other reproductive cell groups cluster into specific tissue. The possibility of error is easy to imagine when we consider that every fragment of the human body, every limb and eyelash, comes from a single fused cell. Yet, only rarely do mistakes occur. Instead, in the majority of cases, a baby girl is born with a perfectly intact vagina, cervix, uterus, fallopian tubes, and two ovaries.

Occasionally, however, something does go wrong. Genetic error, the use of certain drugs such as diethylstilbestrol (DES) by the mother during pregnancy (see *DES-Related Disorders*, page

547), and maternal or fetal disease can conspire to alter the normal process of fetal development.

Congenital abnormalities—those conditions that a person is born with—range from ambiguous external genitals, to the rare absence of the cervix and uterus, to a completely duplicated uterus and vagina. Most defects are minor, but even these can impair a woman's ability to conceive or have a healthy full-term pregnancy.

Defects of the external genitals are noticeable at birth. An abnormality of the internal reproductive organs may not be discovered until a woman reaches puberty or has difficulty conceiving or carrying a fetus to term. Some researchers estimate that as many as 15 to 25 percent of women who have repeated miscarriages actually have some type of uterine abnormality.

For your health-care provider to diagnose the problem, he or she will take different approaches, depending upon the symptoms and the suspected defect. Pelvic imaging studies, chromosomal analysis, and studies that measure hormone levels may be needed. A procedure called a *hysterosalpingogram*, in which a special dye is injected into the uterus, allows the interior of the uterus to be x rayed (see page 630). Another commonly used test is a hysteroscopy, a procedure in which a lighted instrument is used to see the inside of the uterus (see page 632).

Unlike some congenital abnormalities of vital organs, a defect in the reproductive system is usually not life-threatening, although some may make it impossible for a woman to become pregnant. Even if pregnancy is achieved, the uterus may be unable to support the fetus.

Among the variety of abnormalities that occur in the female reproductive system are the following:

Ambiguous Genitals. When most babies are born, the sex is usually readily apparent to anyone examining the organs. Such is not the case in a newborn with ambiguous genitalia, an extremely rare congenital abnormality in which it is not obvious whether the infant is a boy or girl.

This condition can manifest itself in several ways. A female who was exposed to high levels of male hormones in utero may have an enlarged clitoris and the vaginal lips may be fused, forming something that resembles a penis and scrotum. Yet, the vagina, uterus, and ovaries are intact. This condition is called *female pseudohermaphroditism*. Rarely, children are born with both ovaries and testicles, and their genital tracts are neither totally female nor totally male; this is called *true hermaphroditism*.

A child born with ambiguous genitals usually requires more than a physical exam before the proper sex can be assigned. Chromosomal analysis, hormonal measurements, and pelvic imaging may be employed.

Labial Fusion. Sometimes, during the formation of the fetal sexual organs, the adrenal gland makes an excessive amount of male hormone, causing the lips of the vagina to fuse and the clitoris to be enlarged. This treatable condition is called *congenital adrenal hyperplasia*.

Imperforate Hymen. The hymen is a membrane that partially covers the opening to the vagina. A woman with an imperforate hymen does not have any opening through which vaginal secretions can leave the body. An imperforated hymen is generally diagnosed at puberty when a girl fails to menstruate, even though she may have cramping and other symptoms associated with menstruation.

Absent Vagina (Vaginal Agenesis). The vast majority of girls born without a vagina and uterus have Rokitansky–Kuster–Hauser syndrome, a developmental deviation in which ovaries and sex hormone production are nonetheless normal. Women with this syndrome frequently have disorders of the urinary system as well because the duct from which the genitals is formed is located beside the duct from which the urinary tract is formed. Many also have skeletal disorders for some unknown reason. A functioning vagina can usually be created through either surgery or the use of progressively larger vaginal dilators over a period of several weeks or months. However, a uterus cannot be constructed and menstruation and childbearing will not occur.

Absence of Cervix and Uterus. Rarely, a woman is born with a vagina but her cervix and uterus are missing. Women with this birth defect frequently have urinary abnormalities as well.

DES-Related Disorders. Women whose mothers took the synthetic estrogen DES during pregnancy are more likely to have an abnormal cervix or a T-shaped uterine cavity instead of the normal triangular shape. Because of this birth defect, these women are more likely to suffer miscarriages in the middle part of pregnancy because the uterine cavity does not expand to meet the needs of the growing fetus.

Unicornuate Uterus. Normally, one horn-shaped fallopian tube branches off each side of the uterus. In women with a unicornuate uterus, one tube is absent. Sometimes a kidney and ureter are also missing. In most cases, a woman with a unicornuate uterus can have children, although occasionally the uterus cannot expand enough to accommodate the pregnancy.

Duplication of the Vagina, Cervix, and Uterus. A partial or total duplication of these reproductive organs may not be discovered until a girl begins to menstruate and tries to use a tampon. The tampon does not absorb her menstrual flow because it obstructs only one vagina. Menstrual blood from the second uterus continues to flow through the vagina.

Accessory Ovary and Supernumerary Ovary. An accessory ovary occurs when a woman is born with extra ovarian tissue connected to one of her ovaries. A supernumerary ovary is a separate, third ovary. Either condition is rare; the reported incidence is 1 in 93,000 patients. A woman with a third ovary still has only two fallopian tubes. She can, however, ovulate from that extra ovary. The ovum is then picked up by one of the other ovary's tubes.

Treatment Options. In cases of ambiguous genitals, reconstructive surgery may be necessary.

Abnormalities in which there is no obstruction often require no treatment unless the defect is causing infertility or pregnancy-related problems.

Sometimes surgery is used to correct a cervix that is unable to support a pregnancy to term. This procedure, called a *cerclage*, is considered when a woman has a history of painless midpregnancy miscarriage (see page 302).

THE PELVIC EXAM

When Anna was a child, she was constantly in and out of doctors' offices because of severe ear infections. To the frightened child, men and women in the medical profession represented needle pricks and vile-tasting medicine. Luckily, the adult Anna has never been so ill that she needed to consult a doctor.

Now that she is about to turn thirty, Anna has begun to wonder whether avoiding medical checkups is such a good idea. Perhaps she should take a more active role in maintaining her own health, rather than relying on luck. She called a local women's health clinic and scheduled her first gynecological exam.

For Elizabeth, the benefits of a yearly pelvic exam are underscored every time she holds her nine-month-old daughter. Two years earlier, a routine Pap smear revealed the earliest stage of a small cervical cancer. Because the cancer was detected so early, only a small section of Elizabeth's cervix was removed, enabling her later to conceive her daughter.

When was the last time you had a pelvic exam? According to the American College of Obstetricians and Gynecologists, every woman should have a yearly pelvic examination once she turns eighteen—even earlier if she is sexually active. Nevertheless, many healthy women forget or avoid regular examinations. For some women, gynecological checkups are time-consuming. Other women don't think of seeing their health-care professional unless they are sick. And for many women, the exam itself is awkward, uncomfortable, and embarrassing.

For any woman, the first step is to find a health-care practitioner with whom she feels at ease. Because of the intimate nature of a pelvic examination, some women will be more comfortable with a female gynecologist. Male or female, the clinician's ability to relate to you in a caring, nonjudgmental manner is the most important factor.

Many women entrust their gynecological care to a family physician or internist with whom they have an ongoing professional relationship. Conversely, other women choose a gynecologist as their primary care physician. Many gynecologists today are trained to treat not only problems of the reproductive organs but also their patients' bronchitis, rashes, depression, and the like.

No matter whom you choose to do the exam, most routine pelvic examinations start out with the health-care provider or nurse questioning you about the date of your last menstrual period, past pregnancies, surgeries, and current contraceptive method.

Your health-care practitioner also may ask you whether you are currently sexually active, and whether you smoke or use drugs or alcohol. If the clinician is not familiar with your general state of health, he or she may ask about your family's health history and ask for the date of your last general physical. You also will be weighed and have your blood pressure tested. Most clinicians will request a urine sample, especially if you have not recently had a physical examination.

The pelvic exam itself is a relatively simple procedure. You are asked to disrobe and wear an open gown. You will lie on an examining table, with your knees bent and your heels in metal supports or stirrups.

It is routine for the health-care provider to begin with a general physical, including a breast exam (see page 377). The external genitals are inspected for any evidence of sores, swellings, or discolorations that could indicate an infection or other problems.

The clinician then inserts an instrument called a speculum *into your vagina to hold the vaginal walls apart. After inspecting the vagina and cervix for lesions, inflammation, or suspicious discharge, the clinician gently brushes a swab across the cervix. This is the Papanicolaou (Pap) smear (see page 531). The cervical cells contained on the swab are then sent to a laboratory and analyzed for the presence of cancer or precancerous changes.*

Some women are curious about how their reproductive organs look. If at any time during the exam, you have the urge to see what's going on, ask your health-care practitioner for a mirror. After the Pap smear your clinician will palpate your internal reproductive organs by inserting one or two lubricated, gloved fingers into your vagina and, pressing down on your abdomen with the other hand, locating and feeling the uterus and ovaries. Your health-care provider determines whether your organs are the correct size and shape and in the proper position. If you have a tumor or cyst, your clinician may be able to feel it during the exam.

To feel your organs from a different angle, the health-care provider may also insert a finger into your rectum. Many times, the stool that is on the glove is tested for blood, a sign of a possible colon cancer.

Although a pelvic exam can be a bit uncomfortable, it is seldom painful. The more you can relax your muscles, though, the less uncomfortable the exam will be. If you do feel pain, tell your examiner immediately; this could be an indication of a problem.

CERVICAL DISORDERS

The cervix is the narrow lower portion of the uterus that extends down into the vagina. Normally, the cervical opening is so narrow that even a tampon cannot fit through it. But like the rest of the uterus, the cervix is capable of enormous expansion to accommodate the head of a newborn as it makes its way down the birth canal.

The cervix is frequently the site of disorders, some serious and some that may require no treatment other than observation. The most serious disorder of the cervix is cancer, but thanks to widespread screening with the Pap smear, precancerous changes can be discovered when they are completely curable.

In this section, we will examine the most common cervical problems.

CERVICAL POLYPS

Cervical polyps are benign grapelike growths that usually protrude from the opening of the cervix. Many women with the condition have no symptoms, and the polyps are first discovered during a routine pelvic examination. Those who do have symptoms usually notice unexpected vaginal bleeding, often after intercourse, between periods, or after menopause. Cramps and heavy, watery, bloody discharge also may occur with cervical polyps.

A polyp grows on a stalk of tissue. Unlike a cyst, which is fluid-filled, a polyp is solid. Cervical polyps are relatively common and most are noncancerous (benign). A single polyp may appear or polyps may grow in clusters. Polyps usually range in color from reddish purple to cherry red.

Understanding the Problem. Cervical polyps are diagnosed during a pelvic examination. Even though these polyps are rarely cancerous, you may choose to have them removed because they are prone to bleeding, usually after intercourse and between menstrual periods. Your health-care provider will also have the tissue analyzed to make sure the polyps are not malignant.

Treatment Options. Most polyps can be removed in a simple office procedure. Because the cervix is not particularly sensitive to pain, the procedure can be done without an anesthetic. Your health-care provider will insert a special instrument into the vagina. The polyp is then twisted until it is detached. It is then sent to a laboratory for analysis.

If abnormal bleeding continues after the polyp is removed, your provider may recommend an endometrial biopsy, hysteroscopy (see page 542), or a dilation and curettage (D & C), a minor procedure in which the lining of the uterus is scraped and the tissue analyzed (see page 539).

CERVICAL DYSPLASIA

Cervical dysplasia, also known as cervical intraepithelial neoplasia, does not produce any noticeable symptoms. Rather, abnormal cervical cells are detected during a Pap test. Changes in cervical cells can range from mild to severe; if left untreated, though, the most severe cases can eventually progress to invasive cervical cancer.

Dysplasia is a progressive disorder. With mild dysplasia, the abnormal cells develop little over time and pose no danger. With moderate and severe dysplasia, however, the condition is regarded as precancerous and, if left untreated, can progress to cancer. Dysplasia is found primarily in premenopausal women, usually in their twenties and thirties but sometimes even younger.

Women who have a sexual history that involves multiple partners seem to be at highest risk for this disorder. However, not all cases of cervical dysplasia are related to sexual activity. Cigarette smokers, those with impaired immune systems, and women who have had previous dysplasia or cervical cancer are at increased risk for cervical dysplasia. You also are at a higher risk of development of cervical dysplasia if you have had certain types of human papillomavirus (HPV), a sexually transmitted viral infection (see page 457).

Understanding the Problem. If your Pap smear result shows dysplastic cells, your health-care provider may order other diagnostic tests, including a colposcopy and possibly a biopsy, to determine the extent of the problem. For a colposcopy, your clinician will insert a speculum into your vagina to hold the vaginal walls open, and, using a special magnification instrument called a colposcope, he or she will check the cervix. During this office procedure, you should feel no more pain than during a routine pelvic examination.

If a lesion is found on your cervix, a small sample of tissue will be removed for analysis by a laboratory. Some women report that this biopsy feels like a sharp pinch.

After these initial tests, a surgical procedure called a cone biopsy may be necessary if the entire lesion cannot be seen with the colposcope. A cone biopsy is also a form of treatment used when severe dysplasia has been diagnosed. In this procedure, a cone-shaped sample of the cervix is removed and analyzed for signs of disease. General, spinal, local, or epidural anesthesia may be used, and the procedure may be performed in a hospital or outpatient surgery unit. You will need to rest at home afterward for a day or two, and you will probably have a bloody vaginal discharge for a couple of weeks after the procedure. Many practitioners, however, now use an office procedure called a *loop electrosurgical excision procedure* (LEEP) (see page 531).

Sometimes mild cervical dysplasia simply disappears. In some cases, the biopsy itself removes all abnormal cells. Some women with cervical dysplasia, however, require further treatment to halt the progression of these abnormal cells. Studies suggest that moderate and severe cervical dysplasia slowly progresses over a period of years. The women at greatest risk of eventual development of invasive cervical cancer are those who have persistent dysplasia despite treatment. In one study of such women, 22 percent went on to have invasive carcinoma.

Treatment Options. The goal of treatment is to destroy the abnormal tissue, a task that sometimes can be accomplished in the health professional's office. Mild forms of dysplasia are often treated with cauterization, cryosurgery, or laser surgery.

Cauterization destroys tissue with heat, electricity, or chemicals; cryosurgery uses freezing to kill diseased tissue; and laser surgery involves the use of a high-energy beam of light that vaporizes the abnormal cells. For many precancerous changes, laser surgery seems the most effective while causing the least damage to surrounding tissue.

In the event your dysplasia is more severe, your health-care professional may recommend conization (cone biopsy), as mentioned earlier, or LEEP. Women with severe cervical dysplasia are usually cured by conization, although the procedure may weaken the cervix (see *Incompetent Cervix*, page 302).

LEEP, the loop electrosurgical procedure, involves drawing a thin wire through the tissue of the cervix to remove a thin slice. Because the procedure is done in the office under local anesthesia, it is less expensive and more convenient than a conventional cone biopsy. LEEP is performed under magnification with a colposcope, allowing for precise removal of just the surface cervical layers.

If you have severe or recurrent dysplasia, your clinician may recommend a hysterectomy, the removal of your uterus, especially if childbearing is not an issue for you.

No matter what treatment you and your health-care provider choose, cervical dysplasia requires frequent follow-up care because new lesions can develop on the cervix or even in the vagina. Many doctors recommend a Pap smear every three months for the first year and then every six to twelve months.

THE PAP TEST

The Pap test or Pap smear is a simple procedure that most women take for granted as part of their annual pelvic examination. Despite its simplicity, few screening tools have been as effective in cutting cancer deaths.

The Pap smear has been used since 1943, when George N. Papanicolaou established its value as a simple method of screening for premalignant changes in cervical cells. Since that time, the death rate from cervical cancer has dropped 70 percent, largely because the Pap test, performed during routine annual pelvic exams, can detect very early malignancies while they are still highly curable. Moreover, the test can detect changes in cervical cells before they progress to cancer. Early treatment of precancerous conditions has reduced the incidence of invasive cervical cancer by 50 percent. The test has been so successful that today cervical cancer is highly unusual in women who have regular Pap smears.

The Pap smear itself is a painless procedure, typically done during a regular pelvic examination. Using a wooden spatula, brush, or cotton swab, your health-care provider scrapes the surface of your cervix and inside the cervical canal. A sample of cells is then sent to a laboratory, where it is analyzed under a microscope for the presence of abnormalities.

Within a few days or weeks, your health professional learns the results of the test. A negative result means your cervix is probably normal, although there is a 10 to 20 percent chance of error.

If abnormal cells are present, a colposcopy may be ordered: A magnifying instru-

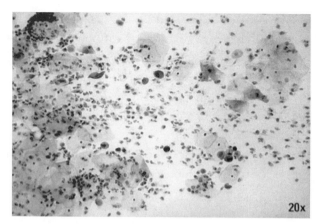

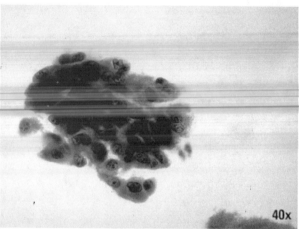

In conducting a Pap smear, your health-care provider will gather sample cells from the cervix. Those cells are then examined under a microscope. In the top photograph is a Pap smear within normal limits (a "negative" result). In the other, magnified twice the size of the normal Pap smear, is a positive Pap test, in which a squamous cell carcinoma is apparent.

ment is inserted into the vagina, allowing the clinician to see the cervix and take a sample of the abnormal tissue (see page 548).

The American College of Obstetricians and Gynecologists recommends that all women have annual Pap smears once they are over the age of eighteen. Annual Pap smears are recommended for even younger women if they are sexually active since cervical cancer occurs most often in women who have been sexually active. However, to cut costs, some health management programs recommend Pap smears every third year. One recent study showed that although there was no increased risk to women tested every two years, the incidence of cervical cancer increased 3.9 times in those who went three years between Pap tests and 12.3 times in women who waited a decade between tests.

CERVICAL CANCER

The most common symptom of cervical cancer is vaginal bleeding, usually after intercourse, between periods, or after menopause. There may be a watery, brownish discharge that is foul-smelling. In its advanced stage, after the cancer has spread beyond the cervix, there may be back and leg pain and swelling, loss of appetite, weight loss, and intestinal obstruction.

As a result of widespread screening with the Pap test, cancer of the cervix has steadily decreased over the past few decades; even so, an estimated 13,500 new cases are diagnosed in American women every year, making this the third most common malignancy of the female reproductive tract. Six thousand women in the United States die each year from this disease.

The vast majority of cervical malignancies are squamous cell carcinomas; 10 to 15 percent are adenocarcinomas. Squamous cell cervical cancer appears to be associated with early and frequent sexual activity and cervical viral infections with certain types of human papillomavirus (HPV).

Most women who have cervical cancer have not had a Pap smear for several years. Cancer of the cervix most often occurs in women between the ages of forty and seventy, with the median age fifty-four. Black women have a higher incidence of this disease than other groups.

Although cervical cancer occurs in women who have no risk factors, it is more likely to occur in women who had sexual intercourse before the age of eighteen, have had multiple sexual partners, gave birth at an early age, and have had certain types of human papillomavirus.

Understanding the Problem. If your Pap smear result and symptoms suggest a malignancy, your health-care provider will do a cervical biopsy to obtain a sample of the tissue, a procedure that usually can be done in the office.

If the biopsy reveals cancer, the clinician will determine whether the cancer has spread to the uterus by scraping the uterine lining for tissue samples, a procedure called dilation and curettage (D & C) (see page 539). The extent of the disease (the stage of the cancer) determines the most effective treatment. This pretreatment evaluation may also include routine blood studies, an electrocardiogram, a chest X ray, computed tomography (CT) scan, an intravenous pyelogram (IVP), and a barium enema test.

The prognosis depends upon how early the cancer is diagnosed and treated. When cervical squamous cell carcinoma is detected in its early stages—that is, when the tumor is relatively small and has not spread beyond the cervix into other organs—it is almost always curable: Ninety percent of women are alive five years after diagnosis and treatment. In its most advanced stage, when the cancer has spread to distant organs, the five-year survival rate is only about 7 percent. The majority of cervical cancers, however, are diagnosed in earlier stages when the outcome is promising—primarily because they are found during routine Pap tests.

The outcome for adenocarcinoma of the cervix, however, is generally poorer, because it is typically diagnosed at a later stage.

An estimated one third of women with cervical cancer have a recurrence of disease six or more months after treatment. When this cancer metastasizes or spreads, it is most likely first to invade the pelvis and, in some cases, the abdomen, liver, lung, and bone.

Treatment Options. Treatment approaches for cervical cancer vary; they include surgical intervention and radiation.

SURGERY. An option for small, early-stage cancers is a cone biopsy (see page 535). This procedure, performed in the hospital under anesthesia, involves the removal of a cone-shaped piece of the cervix, including the malignant area. If the borders of the cone are free of disease and the cancer has invaded only minimally below the surface of the cervix, it is likely that all the cancerous tissue was removed. Conization is generally reserved for women who wish to have children, because the recurrence rate is higher than after hysterectomy.

When the cancer involves a large part of the cervix or extends into the uterus, a radical hysterectomy is the primary surgical option. During this procedure, your surgeon will remove your uterus, upper vagina, and surrounding tissue and lymph nodes. The ovaries may be left to maintain natural estrogen levels.

A radical hysterectomy has advantages when compared to radiation, the other treatment sometimes used for this type of cancer. The operation allows your surgeon to explore the pelvis and abdomen for signs that the cancer has spread. And women who have a hysterectomy often are able to function better sexually than those who have radiation, which may scar vaginal tissue, impairing its elasticity and lubrication capabilities. When this occurs, intercourse can be extremely painful or even physically impossible. Moreover, some women who are treated with radiation may suffer injury to the bowel, which in some cases may necessitate a colostomy, a surgery in which the colon is connected to an artificial opening in the skin of the abdomen so that feces can be eliminated. With modern radiation therapy, however, those complication are rare. The disadvantages of radical hysterectomy include short-term complications such as infection, which occur in under 2 percent of cases, and more serious injuries to the urinary tract or bowel.

If your cancer has spread to your lymph nodes, your health professional may advise radiation therapy after surgery.

RADIATION. The cure rates for radical hysterectomy and radiation therapy are nearly the same for early cancers and those that have just begun to spread to the vagina.

Radiation therapy may involve both external and internal radiation. External therapy is delivered by a machine, whereas in internal radiation, radioactive material is implanted within your cervix and the upper part of your vagina while you are under anesthesia. This type of treatment requires that you remain hospitalized for several days while the implantation irradiates the cancerous tissue.

Complications associated with radiation seem to be related to the radiation dosage, the size of the area treated, and the sensitivity of your tissues to this type of treatment. However, radiation equipment and techniques have improved significantly in recent years, reducing tissue damage and other adverse side effects. Even with improvements, though, some women still have diarrhea, rectal bleeding, and fatigue after radiation therapy, but these generally end once treatment is completed. Scarring in the irradiated area may lead to a narrowing and shortening of the vagina. Vaginal or rectal ulcers and bowel problems such as severe pain during bowel movements sometimes occur as a result of radiation therapy, typically a year or more after the treatment ends.

CHEMOTHERAPY. Cancer-fighting drugs, either alone or in combination, have not been very successful in treating cervical cancer and are usually prescribed for recurrent cervical cancer or disease that is advanced. Chemotherapy may prolong life if the cancer recurs but does not cure the disease. Chemotherapy is also being increasingly used in conjunction with radiation for some more advanced tumors.

Because chemotherapy kills normal cells as well as cancerous ones, there are often severe side effects. Temporary hair loss, extreme fatigue, mouth sores, dry mouth, nausea, vomiting, diarrhea, bleeding, and a susceptibility to infection are all common among chemotherapy patients.

FOLLOW-UP CARE. As with other malignancies, once you have had cervical cancer, you will need to see your clinician more often than the average person, even in the absence of symptoms. During your checkups you can expect to have a complete physical and pelvic examination as well as a Pap test.

CONE BIOPSY

During a cone biopsy, also called conization, *a cone-shaped slice of the cervix is removed and analyzed for the presence of cancer or premalignant cells. The method is a way of both diagnosing and treating cervical dysplasia (abnormal changes in the cervix that in some women progress to become cervical cancer) and sometimes the earliest stage of cervical cancer.*

As a diagnostic tool, conization of the cervix is used when the gynecologist is unable to do an adequate exam with the colposcope (a magnifying instrument that views the cervix); when a biopsy sample of the cervix shows cancer or premalignant cells; or when the biopsy specimen shows only a slight cell abnormality whereas the Pap smear result suggests a more substantial problem (indicating that diseased tissue was not included in the sample). Conization also is used as a treatment for the most advanced precancerous lesion of the cervix, also known as carcinoma in situ, *when a severe dysplasia has not yet infiltrated deeper tissue.*

If your health-care provider recommends conization, the procedure will be done in the hospital with anesthesia. The gynecologist uses a scalpel, electrocautery, or laser to remove a piece of the cervix, including the suspect tissue. The tissue is then analyzed for disease. If the margin of the tissue sample is free of premalignant cells, this may be all the treatment you need, although you will have to be followed closely because new lesions may appear. In one study of women who had conizations and the margins were free of disease, 98 percent showed no sign of recurrence five years later. When the margins contained premalignant cells, the rate fell to 70 percent.

Some health professionals recommend a hysterectomy when the conization edges contain premalignant cells. This can be a difficult call because not all women in this situation have a recurrence of the disease. In one study of twenty-one women whose conization margins showed dysplasia, only four had a recurrence, in some cases as much as six years later. The rest remained disease-free up to fifteen years. Reconization is a less radical option.

After conization you may be advised to take it easy for a day or two, although many women feel well enough to return to their normal activities the next day. The major short-term complication of this procedure is a bloody discharge that usually lasts for about two weeks. Once the discharge has stopped—a sign your cervix is healed—you can resume intercourse.

Conization may increase the risk of incompetent cervix (see page 302). An alternative procedure known as LEEP (see page 531) may present less of a risk but is less effective than conization for very severe dysplasia or early cervical cancers.

CERVICITIS

The most common symptom of cervicitis, or cervical inflammation, is a grayish or yellow vaginal discharge. Pain during and bleeding after intercourse are also common. Even without these symptoms, however, you may have cervicitis. More than 60 percent of women with this problem have no indication that there is anything wrong.

Cervicitis is an inflammation of the cervix. In most women with cervicitis, the culprit is a sexually transmitted infection, usually chlamydia. In one study done by a team in Seattle, chlamydia organisms were found in the cervical specimens of half of forty women with cervicitis, yet in only two of sixty women without cervical inflammation. *Neisseria gonorrhoeae*, the bacterium that causes gonorrhea infection; trichomonas; and viral agents such as herpes simplex and human papillomavirus can also cause cervicitis.

Any woman can have cervicitis. However, most cases are caused by sexually transmitted infections. An estimated 30 to 40 percent of women who visit clinics that treat sexually transmitted diseases have cervicitis, and 8 to 10 percent of college women who visit student health clinics have this ailment.

Understanding the Problem. If you have the symptoms of cervicitis, your health-care provider will attempt to determine the organism responsible for the inflammation. During a pelvic examination, he or she will obtain a sample of your cervical secretions that will be sent to a laboratory for analysis. To rule out the possibility of cancer or premalignancy (dysplasia), the clinician also may do a Pap test.

Treatment Options. The usual treatment is an antibiotic effective against the specific organisms responsible for your cervicitis. If the cause is a sexually transmitted disease, your sexual partner also should be treated to prevent you from becoming reinfected.

A follow-up culture of your cervical secretions may be done after the antibiotic therapy has been completed to make sure the infection is gone.

Cervicitis usually resolves after the appropriate antibiotic is prescribed, although some strains of gonorrhea may be resistant to certain drugs. The primary danger of cervicitis is that the infection, if left untreated, can migrate to the upper genital tract, scarring the fallopian tubes and ultimately impairing fertility. Prompt and proper treatment is essential.

Nabothian Cyst

Nabothian cysts are fluid-filled lumps on the cervix. If you are one of the many women who have a nabothian cyst, you will have no symptoms.

A nabothian cyst occurs when a mucus gland on the cervix becomes blocked; the obstruction commonly occurs when new tissue grows over the gland. Named for Martin Naboth, a German anatomist, nabothian cysts occur singly or in multiples. These cysts are commonly found in adult women and are not a sign of disease. Nabothian cysts are usually discovered by a health professional during a pelvic examination. They generally do not cause any symptoms or problems.

Treatment Options. No treatment is necessary.

Uterine Disorders

Your uterus or womb is a hollow, muscular cavity lined with moist, pink, velvety tissue, called *endometrium*. Under normal conditions, the uterus is no more than three inches long and holds barely a teaspoonful of fluid. The walls are made of smooth, highly elastic muscles. During pregnancy, the uterus is able to expand up to forty times its normal size to house and nourish a developing fetus. A relatively short time after childbirth, the uterus not only stops stretching, but also returns to its original size—or pretty close to it.

Like any organ, the uterus is subject to various diseases, most of which are not lifethreatening. The exception is uterine cancer. Fortunately, this cancer is usually curable when it is caught in its early stages.

In this section we will explore some of the most frequently seen problems that occur in the uterus.

UTERINE RETROVERSION

Women with uterine retroversion (a tipped or tilted uterus) usually have no symptoms. Rarely, a woman with uterine retroversion will find intercourse painful, particularly when her partner thrusts deeply. In general, however, the discomfort is not due to the position of the uterus but to endometriosis (see page 545), which may be the cause of the retroversion.

If you have uterine retroversion or retroflexion, your uterus is tipped, tilting backward instead of lying in the more common forward position, with the closed end nearer to the front of the body. In the past, retroversion was considered a cause of discomfort or infertility, but it is now recognized to be a normal variation.

About 20 percent of all women have a tipped uterus. If you have uterine retroversion, your clinician will be able to feel it during a pelvic examination.

Uterine retroversion is not a disease and does not require any treatment. During pregnancy, the supports around the uterus may be weakened or stretched, causing the uterus to rest slightly lower in the vaginal canal. However, there is no increased risk for miscarriage or infertility as a result of a tilted uterus.

If intercourse is uncomfortable, try assuming the top position. In this position, your partner's penis is less likely to touch your ovaries, which most often are the source of the sensitivity.

Your health-care provider should also determine whether you have endometriosis or something else that is causing your pain (see *Endometriosis and Adenomyosis*, page 545).

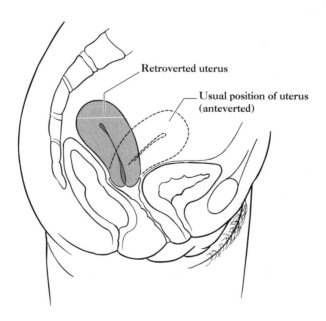

*The uterus in about one in every five women is tipped backward (*retroverted*).*
This is a normal variation.

DILATION AND CURETTAGE

Dilation and curettage, also known as "D & C," is a minor surgical procedure in which the clinician dilates the normally tight cervix and uses a thin, spoon-shaped instrument called a curette *to scrape the lining of the uterus.*

Most D & Cs today are done on an outpatient basis—either during an office visit or in the hospital—with a local anesthetic or a light general anesthetic. A D & C has value in both diagnosing and treating certain conditions.

If you are having problems with your period—especially if you are menstruating too often or your flow is unusually heavy—the health professional may be able to determine the cause by examining samples of your uterine lining under a microscope. If an office biopsy of the endometrium (uterine lining) suggests a precancerous problem or polyp, a D & C may then be necessary.

As a method of treatment, the D & C may be used to remove endometrial polyps. Although fibroid tumors can be scraped during the procedure, in most cases these benign tumors require hysteroscopy (see page 542) or major surgery for removal.

Some women who miscarry do not expel all the products of conception. When this occurs, a D & C can be used to empty out the uterus.

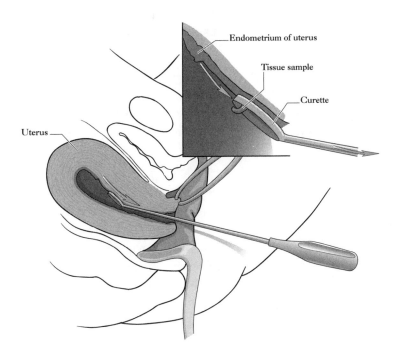

A dilation and curettage is a minor surgical procedure. To perform a "D and C," the clinician uses a thin instrument called a curette to remove a tissue sample from the lining of the uterus.

If your clinician recommends that you have a D & C, you may have some vaginal bleeding for a few days after the procedure, as well as some cramping and back pain. If the procedure is done in the hospital, you can generally go home the same day. Once home, however, you should abstain from intercourse or tampon use for as long as your clinician recommends, generally until the bleeding stops.

Dilation and curettage can also be used to abort an embryo; for a discussion of that use of the procedure and the broader context of the abortion debate, see page 127.

UTERINE CANCER

The primary symptom of uterine cancer is abnormal bleeding. In women who have already gone through menopause, vaginal bleeding will inexplicably recur. Women who have this disease and are still menstruating will have bleeding between periods. A pink, watery vaginal discharge also is common.

Uterine cancer is the most common malignancy of the female reproductive organs. An estimated 33,000 new cases of uterine cancer are diagnosed each year in the United States, three times the number of cervical malignancies and 1.5 times that of ovarian cancer. The most prevalent form of uterine cancer, called *endometrial cancer* or *adenocarcinoma*, originates in the uterine lining,

An estimated one in one hundred women will eventually have uterine cancer. Most of these cancers occur around or after menopause. This does not mean that young women are immune to this disease: An estimated 5 percent of uterine cancer occurs in women under the age of forty.

There are many risk factors associated with this type of cancer. White women have nearly twice the incidence of this disease that black women do. It used to be that women who took estrogen replacement therapy were at increased risk because the high doses of estrogen stimulated the uterine lining, causing it to proliferate. But the current practice of combining progestin with estrogen prevents the uterine lining from building up and seems to eliminate the higher risk of uterine cancer.

Women with polycystic ovary syndrome, ovarian tumors, and other conditions that stimulate estrogen production over a long period also are at increased risk. As a group, women who have never had children are twice as likely to have uterine cancer as women who have. Because many of these women do not ovulate, the uterus is not exposed to sufficient levels of progesterone to counteract the effects of estrogen. Women who have a late menopause (after the age of fifty-two) are 2.4 times as likely to experience uterine cancer as those who stop menstruating before the age of forty-nine—again, because of exposure to excess estrogen.

Overweight women have an increased risk of this disease because fat tissue produces excess estrogen. If you are twenty to fifty pounds overweight, your risk of uterine cancer is increased threefold; the multiple is times ten if you carry more than fifty extra pounds.

Understanding the Problem. Uterine cancer is not noticeable during a pelvic examination. Routine Pap smears do not examine interior uterine cells and only detect this malignancy about half the time.

If your symptoms suggest cancer of the uterus, your health-care provider will need to obtain a sampling of the uterine lining. The biopsy is a procedure that usually can be done in the office without anesthesia, although some health-care professionals use a mild anesthetic on the cervix. A slender tube with a piston and a hole at the end is put into the uterus. The clinician pulls back on the piston and draws a piece of the endometrium into the tube.

After the tissue is removed, your uterus will cramp for a few seconds, but you should feel well enough to go about your normal activities afterward. If there is any question as to the biopsy result's accuracy, a D & C (see page 539) can be done to confirm the finding.

When cancer is found, a series of diagnostic tests will be done to determine whether the disease has spread to other organs.

However frightening a diagnosis of uterine cancer may be, it is responsible for fewer deaths each year than either ovarian or cervical cancer. The outlook for this relatively slow-growing malignancy depends upon the tumor type and the stage at which it is diagnosed. Generally, younger women with uterine cancer have a better prognosis than their older counterparts. The overall five-year survival rate for most early-stage tumors is 72 percent. Rarely, the tumor is a faster-growing type, which radically lowers a woman's chance of survival.

Treatment Options. The most commonly recommended treatment for uterine cancer is a hysterectomy. Usually both fallopian tubes and ovaries are also removed not only to block estrogen production, but to prevent the malignancy from infiltrating those organs as well. Some lymph nodes also may be removed and analyzed for the presence of cancer cells.

RADIATION. Radiation is sometimes used in combination with surgery or alone when a woman is unable to tolerate surgery. Depending upon the severity of the cancer, the radiation may be confined to the pelvis or, in more extensive disease, may include the entire abdomen.

MEDICATIONS. When uterine cancer has spread outside the pelvis or when it recurs in the same area years after the initial diagnosis and treatment, antiestrogen hormones such as a progestin may be prescribed. The combination of cancer-fighting drugs (chemotherapy) and hormonal therapy may also be effective.

FOLLOW-UP. Once you have been treated for cancer of the uterus, you will have to adhere to a regular schedule of clinical visits. Although 90 percent of recurrences occur within five years of the diagnosis, 10 percent appear more than five years later, demonstrating the need for long-term follow-up.

HYSTEROSCOPY

When Jillian told her gynecologist about the abnormal bleeding that had plagued her for months, she assumed the doctor would schedule a dilation and curettage (D & C), a procedure she had had years before to investigate a similar complaint. Instead, the doctor suggested she have hysteroscopy, a relatively new but increasingly popular procedure that allows her gynecologist to see the inside of the uterus.

A week later Jillian was admitted to the hospital for same-day surgery. Although some women are awake during the procedure, Jillian and her gynecologist had decided that because the examination can be uncomfortable, she would be better off with a general anesthetic.

After Jillian was asleep, her gynecologist inserted a special lighted instrument called a hysteroscope *into her uterus through the vagina. The doctor then introduced a gas substance that distended Jillian's uterine cavity, making it easier to see and to operate on, if necessary.*

This procedure, which usually can be accomplished in twenty minutes, currently is being used to diagnose a variety of uterine ailments, including congenital abnormalities, abnormal bleeding, infertility, repeated miscarriages, and to locate an intrauterine device that is broken or out of position.

If surgery is necessary, surgical instruments can be introduced through the hysteroscope. Uterine polyps, some fibroid tumors, and damaged intrauterine devices can be removed during hysteroscopy. A laser can be introduced into the uterus through the hysteroscope to destroy abnormal tissue. Some practitioners are experimenting with sterilization techniques using the hysteroscope. Various methods can also be used to destroy the uterine lining in women who have severe menstrual abnormalities as an alternative to hysterectomy.

In the course of the hysteroscopic examination, Jillian's doctor discovered the problem: a large uterine polyp, which she removed. Within a few hours, Jillian was back home. She had cramping and minor bleeding that day but felt well enough the next morning to return to work.

Like almost any medical procedure, hysteroscopy is not without risks, although the complication rate is less than 2 percent. The most common complications include perforation of the uterus, pelvic infection, and excessive bleeding. If after a hysteroscopy you experience severe pain, fever, or chills or are bleeding more than you would during your period, call your doctor.

Although hysteroscopy is a valuable diagnostic tool, you should be aware that there are some conditions that make this procedure dangerous to some women. If you are pregnant you should not have a hysteroscopy. Nor should a woman with a pelvic infection have this procedure because the gas or liquid that is used to expand the uterus flows out the fallopian tubes and can carry the infection throughout the reproductive organs.

FIBROIDS

Many women with fibroids, benign tumors of the uterine wall, have no symptoms. Those who do have symptoms generally complain of heavy or prolonged menstrual periods, abnormal bleeding, and pain or pressure in the lower abdomen. Some women with fibroids have difficulty in getting pregnant or problems during the pregnancy.

Fibroids, also called *leiomyomas* or simply *myomas*, are the most frequently seen tumors of the pelvis; an estimated 40 percent of all women have fibroids. They are virtually always found in the uterus, but fibroids may occasionally be found nearby in the abdomen. It is possible to have only one fibroid, but most women with this problem have several tumors. The size of a fibroid typically ranges from the size of a pea to that of a grapefruit.

Researchers have not established what causes fibroids, but it appears that estrogen is necessary for their growth. Although they are normally slow-growing tumors, fibroids are likely to increase substantially when the estrogen level is high, specifically during pregnancy. However, most pregnancies are not adversely affected. Fibroids usually do not increase in size with oral contraceptives or during hormone replacement therapy after menopause. However, women with fibroids are more likely to have abnormal bleeding when put on hormone replacement therapy.

One in three women with fibroids has pelvic pain. Women who have never had children are more likely to have fibroids and be bothered by symptoms than the rest of the population.

Understanding the Problem. Most fibroids can be felt by your health-care provider during a pelvic examination. Fibroids often are found during an ultrasound examination for an unrelated problem.

Most fibroids never become malignant or cause serious problems. If you do have fibroids, however, you will need to see your health professional on a regular basis for monitoring. Some women with heavy bleeding may have iron-deficiency anemia, a condition that can be corrected by taking an iron supplement. Most fibroids shrink or disappear altogether after menopause even if you take estrogen replacement therapy.

Treatment Options. If your fibroids are causing pain or producing other symptoms, surgery may be recommended. The two surgical options available are hysterectomy—the removal of your uterus—and a myomectomy, a procedure in which the tumor alone is removed. Whether you want children will help determine which surgery is right for you. About one in four women who opt for a myomectomy do end up eventually having a hysterectomy, mainly because the fibroids recur. The complication rate for myomectomy is also higher than that of hysterectomy. Discuss the options with your health-care provider and make the decision together.

Recently developed treatments use medications to control symptoms from fibroids. How well these medications work and for how long are still being studied.

ENDOMETRIAL POLYPS

Most endometrial polyps produce no symptoms. When these soft, small growths of the uterine lining do cause problems, you are most likely to notice spotting between periods or, if you are post-menopausal, staining. Some women also have pelvic cramps and heavy, unusually long periods. Sometimes a polyp will protrude into the vagina, causing cramping as it expands the opening of the cervix.

Endometrial polyps, growths that are attached to a stalk, appear singly or in multiples. Some are very small; others are so large that they fill the uterine cavity. The cause is unknown, although some researchers suspect estrogen may be involved.

Endometrial polyps occur in women of all ages, although the peak incidence is found between the ages of forty and forty-nine. Endometrial polyps are noted in an estimated 10 percent of women whose uterus is examined at autopsy, so the problem is thought to be relatively common.

Understanding the Problem. Because most endometrial polyps do not cause symptoms, the majority are discovered when the uterus is examined after a hysterectomy that is done for other reasons. These polyps also are sometimes discovered during the diagnostic tests hysteroscopy (see page 632) and hysterosalpingogram (page 630).

If a polyp protrudes into your vagina, your health-care provider will be able to see it during a pelvic examination. When you have symptoms but the polyp cannot be seen, your clinician may do a hysteroscopy, a minor procedure in which the uterine lining is inspected.

Endometrial polyps are not dangerous, although a very small percentage are malignant. Most malignant polyps, however, are in an early stage of malignancy and as a result are highly curable.

Treatment Options. Endometrial polyps can be surgically removed with dilation and curettage (see page 539) or via the hysteroscope (see *Hysteroscopy*, page 632). After removal, the polyp will be analyzed for signs of malignancy. In some cases, polyps may recur.

ENDOMETRIAL HYPERPLASIA

Endometrial hyperplasia is an overly thick uterine lining. The predominant symptom is abnormal vaginal bleeding that occurs between periods, or irregular periods. However, some women with this condition have no symptoms.

Endometrial hyperplasia occurs when the uterine lining becomes too thick, often as a result of irregular ovulation that in turn makes menstruation irregular.

Although this disorder can occur at any time during the reproductive years, it is more common just prior to menopause, when periods tend to be erratic. Endometrial hyperplasia also occurs frequently in menopausal women who take estrogen replacement therapy. When estrogen is taken without a progestin component, the uterine lining builds up excessively.

Understanding the Problem. If endometrial hyperplasia is suspected, a small sample of your uterine lining will be removed for analysis through a slender tube inserted into your uterus. This procedure, called a biopsy, can be done in your health professional's office. You will feel cramping for a few seconds but afterward should be able to go about your normal activities.

Most endometrial hyperplasia is not dangerous and resolves without treatment. A small percentage, however, contain cells that have the potential to become malignant. Women who have this type of hyperplasia—called *atypical*—have a greater risk of development of cancer of the endometrium than do women with other types of hyperplasia. The danger sign that doctors watch for is "lawless bleeding," that is, bleeding that does not show any pattern.

Treatment Options. The recommended treatment will depend upon the severity of your hyperplasia. If there are no signs of malignancy, your health-care provider may recommend progestin or birth control pills for a few months to halt the rapid growth of the uterine lining.

If you are postmenopausal or have atypical hyperplasia—the kind that may eventually progress to a malignancy—your clinician may advise a hysterectomy. For younger women who want to preserve their childbearing potential, high doses of progestin may be adequate therapy, but close follow-up is necessary.

ENDOMETRIOSIS AND ADENOMYOSIS

Endometriosis, in which bits of uterine tissue travel from the uterus and become implanted on surrounding organs, causes pain, especially on the first two days of menstruation, that typically continues for the duration of your period. Other symptoms include infertility, a sharp pain deep in the pelvis during intercourse, and pain during bowel movements. Some women have no symptoms.

Adenomyosis, in which endometrial tissue grows in the muscular walls of the uterus, often causes menstrual cramps that last throughout your period, worsening as you age. You also may have prolonged and excessive bleeding during your period. Like some women with endometriosis, many with adenomyosis are asymptomatic.

Endometriosis is a chronic and often progressive condition in which pieces of uterine tissue escape the uterus and become attached to the outside of other pelvic organs. The most common sites invaded by endometrial tissue are the ovaries, but the tissue can embed itself inside the fallopian tubes and on the outer surface of the uterus, the broad ligament, and the bowel. On rare occasions, endometriosis causes tissue to be present in a woman's bladder, kidney, lung, arms, or legs.

Adenomyosis—also called *endometriosis internal*—occurs when endometrial tissue begins to grow in the muscular walls of the uterus itself. Some women have both endometriosis and adenomyosis.

As a woman's hormones prepare her body for menstruation, the wayward tissue—just like the endometrial lining of her uterus—thickens and then begins to bleed as her period starts. But unlike menstrual flow, which escapes through the vagina, the blood from the implanted tissue has no place to go. Bleeding into the pelvic cavity causes pain and irritates surrounding tissue. Scar tissue forms and thick bands of adhesions can bind organs together.

The severity of symptoms does not always correlate with the degree of disease. Some women with extensive endometriosis may have no symptoms at all, and others with minimal disease may experience severe pain.

Researchers don't know what causes this uterine tissue to stray from its proper place. It is known that in all women some menstrual flow backs up into the fallopian tube and spills out into the pelvis. And yet all women do not experience endometriosis. Whether this tissue successfully implants may depend on a faulty immune system. Some evidence indicates a possible genetic predisposition to endometriosis.

Experts estimate that as many as 15 percent of American women of childbearing age have endometriosis, although the problem is often minor and many women are unaware of it.

The typical endometriosis patient is in her thirties and has never had a child. Teenage girls, too, can have endometriosis. If your mother or sister has severe endometriosis, your risk is enhanced. One in ten women with severe disease has a mother or sister who also has endometriosis. Those with a family history are more likely to have the disease earlier and have more severe endometriosis than other women.

An estimated 30 to 45 percent of infertile women have endometriosis. And yet, many women with the disease have no difficulty getting pregnant. However, there is a causal relationship between severe endometriosis and infertility. Because the disease is often progressive, some women may have children and later become infertile as the condition worsens.

Understanding the Problem. Most health-care providers will be able to feel scarring suggestive of endometriosis during a pelvic exam, but the only way to be completely sure the disease is present is to do a laparoscopy, a minor surgical procedure that allows the health-care provider to examine the reproductive organs through a lighted instrument inserted into the abdomen (see page 554). Frequently endometriosis is diagnosed incidentally during a laparoscopy for other problems.

If your clinician suspects you have adenomyosis, he or she will do a pelvic examination to see whether your uterus is swollen, a characteristic associated with this disease. The uterus in a woman with adenomyosis is sometimes two or three times the normal size. Uterine size alone is not sufficient to make a diagnosis, however, and adenomyosis is more reliably diagnosed by using MRI (see page 636). Although adenomyosis can be painful, this condition is usually harmless. Severe anemia can occur, though, if menstrual blood loss is too heavy.

Endometriosis often worsens with time and spreads to sites throughout the pelvis and occasionally beyond. Yet treatment often improves the symptoms. However, the only real cure is menopause or removal of the uterus and ovaries.

Treatment Options. If you are diagnosed with early-stage endometriosis and want to have children, your health-care provider may recommend that you not postpone pregnancy because the condition may worsen and cause infertility. Pregnancy may also improve the condition, possibly because the high level of progesterone of pregnancy or the lack of menstrual bleeding allows the organs to heal.

MEDICATION. If you want to postpone pregnancy for at least a few years, your health-care practitioner will prescribe hormonal medication to stop menstruation. Some medications may have a direct effect on the implants, causing them to shrink. Oral contraceptives are sometimes used, although some women quit this therapy because of discouraging side effects such as weight gain, nausea, increased appetite, irritability, and depression.

Danazol, a derivative of testosterone, was frequently prescribed at one time. However, this medication is usually associated with bloating and sometimes with acne and mood changes. Although three out of four women who use danazol notice significant improvement, about 40 percent will have a recurrence of endometriosis and adenomyosis years after discontinuing the medication.

At present, the most popular medications for endometriosis and adenomyosis are called *gonadotropin-releasing hormone (GnRH) agonists*, which temporarily simulate menopause. Side effects, chiefly hot flashes, are less troubling than those associated with danazol and can be controlled with small doses of estrogen. About 60 percent of women who try this therapy are able to become pregnant afterward.

SURGERY. When immediate pregnancy is desired, surgery may be used to destroy all the visible implants. Increasingly, surgeons are opting for laparoscopic surgery in the treatment of endometriosis, using either a laser or electrocautery to destroy or excise the diseased tissue. Although symptoms usually abate after surgery, recurrences are common. This is in part due to the fact that some microscopic-sized implants may be missed during surgery.

For women who have advanced endometriosis or adenomyosis that produces severe symptoms and who do not wish to become pregnant, a hysterectomy with bilateral salpinoophosectomy (the removal of the uterus and ovaries) may be recommended.

DES-RELATED DISORDERS

Beginning in the late 1940s, as many as three million women were given the oral estrogen diethylstilbestrol (DES) to prevent miscarriage or premature birth. It is now known that DES is not an effective treatment for miscarriage or premature birth, but that is not the worst of it: Female children born to mothers who took DES during pregnancy have an increased risk of a rare cancer of the vagina and cervix, as well as a host of congenital reproductive abnormalities. In the early 1970s, the use of DES during pregnancy was abandoned.

The following examines the most common health problems encountered by women exposed to DES during their fetal development:

Clear Cell Adenocarcinoma of the Vagina and Cervix. This rare and fast-growing tumor appears mainly to strike women whose mother took DES during pregnancy. In 1971 a special registry was established to trace this disease among women who were born after 1940. As of 1990, 555 women with this tumor had been reported; 65 percent of them definitely had been exposed to DES in the womb. Another 10 percent may have been exposed.

Clear cell adenocarcinoma is rare even among DES daughters, affecting only one of one thousand women exposed to DES. This cancer has struck females as young as seven and as old as thirty-seven, with the average age in the late teens.

Vaginal Adenosis and Other Vaginal Abnormalities. Girls born to DES mothers frequently have a birth defect in which a glandular tissue normally found in the cervix is incorporated into the vaginal walls. An estimated 30 to 40 percent of women whose mother took this drug are thought to have this condition, which is called *vaginal adenosis.* Structural abnormalities of the vagina also are common, but these usually do not interfere with pregnancy.

Tissue and structural abnormalities change over the years and sometimes disappear.

Uterine Abnormalities. Irregularities in the size and shape of the uterus occur in more than half of DES daughters.

Pregnancy Outcome. Women exposed to DES in the womb occasionally experience difficulty during pregnancy. It is estimated that premature births, ectopic (tubal) pregnancy, and miscarriage occur in half of DES-exposed women. Even so, more than 80 percent of DES daughters who want to have a baby are able to do so eventually.

YOUR HEALTH CARE. If you are a DES daughter, it is important that you have regular checkups so your health-care provider can check for any changes in your cervical and vaginal tissue that might indicate cancer.

During pregnancy your health-care provider may advise an early ultrasound to be sure the embryo has implanted properly in the uterus. Later in the pregnancy you will be carefully observed for any signs that your cervix is dilating early, an indication that your baby might be born prematurely.

COLPOSCOPY

If you have an abnormal Pap smear result or suspicious vaginal lesions, or you are one of the many women whose mother took diethylstilbestrol during pregnancy, your clinician may want to do a colposcopic examination.

The colposcope is a magnifying instrument that allows your health-care provider to look for signs of abnormality on the surface of your cervix and vagina.

This examination can be done during an office visit and takes about fifteen min-

utes. As with any pelvic exam, you will be asked to put on a gown, lie on the examining table, and place your feet in stirrups. The clinician will then insert a speculum into your vagina to hold the vaginal walls open. He or she then will place the colposcope between your legs; the instrument does not touch you. Since one purpose of this test is to determine why a Pap smear finding was abnormal, your health professional may use a small instrument to take a sample of tissue (biopsy) that can be evaluated for the presence of cancer or a premalignant condition. Although most women do not find the examination any more uncomfortable than a routine pelvic exam, you may feel a pinching sensation if your doctor removes a sample of tissue for biopsy. Some women also have minor bleeding, but your clinician will make sure the bleeding has stopped before he or she removes the colposcope. After the examination, you should have no problem going about your normal activities.

OVARIAN AND FALLOPIAN TUBE DISORDERS

You are born with all the eggs you will ever have—an estimated one to two million—stored in your two ovaries, those walnut-sized organs located four to five inches below your waist.

The ovaries have two important jobs. From the time you reach puberty until menopause, each month one ovum (egg) ripens and is sent on its way up the fallopian tube. If the ovum is met by sperm, it may be fertilized. The other important task of the ovaries is to produce female sex hormones, estrogens and progesterone, which regulate the menstrual cycle and produce your feminine characteristics.

Most of the time a woman's ovaries and fallopian tubes are healthy. But like other organs, the ovaries and fallopian tubes can become diseased. Sexually transmitted infections can settle in the fallopian tubes, causing scarring that results in infertility, a condition known as pelvic inflammatory disease (see Chapter 19, *Sexually Transmitted Diseases and Other Infections*, page 440). However, the most common problems are benign cysts and tumors, some of which resolve without treatment.

In this section we will look at the most commonly diagnosed disorders of the ovary as well as cancer of the fallopian tubes, a rare but often deadly malignancy.

OVARIAN CYSTS AND SOLID TUMORS

Most ovarian cysts and benign tumors produce no symptoms. However, symptoms that may occur include a dull ache in your abdomen, a sensation of abdominal fullness, pain during intercourse, abnormal periods, or an abrupt sharp pain in your lower abdomen. Emergency symptoms are fever and sometimes vomiting, associated with sudden and severe abdominal pain and/or cold, clammy skin, and rapid breathing, indicating that the cyst has ruptured, or that the ovary has twisted, cutting off its blood supply.

A cyst is a fluid-filled sac. A tumor is simply a growth, which can be either cystic or solid, benign or malignant—although some tumors have both solid and cystic matter. There are several types of cysts and solid tumors. Most cysts disappear eventually, requiring no treatment. Some, however, may be ovarian cancer.

Since many tumors do not cause pain, they are often discovered during a routine pelvic examination.

A number of different types of tumors affect women of various ages. The least common cyst, thecalutein, is often associated with pregnancy. The most common ovarian cyst is called *a follicular cyst*. The most common benign solid ovarian tumors, *fibromas*, are generally seen in women who are near or past menopause. Another benign ovarian tumor is the *teratoma*; these rarely occur in young girls before puberty, are less rare in teenagers, and are relatively common in women between the ages of twenty-five and fifty. Teratomas usually have cystic and solid components.

Understanding the Problem. If during a pelvic exam your clinician feels something suspicious on your ovary or if you have symptoms indicative of a cyst, he or she may recommend an ultrasound (see page 637). Sometimes a laparoscopy (see page 554) is done to confirm the diagnosis. During this procedure, a thin, lighted instrument is inserted into a tiny incision near your navel, allowing the surgeon to see your ovaries.

Most cysts and solid tumors are not cancerous. Many disappear without treatment. For example, in nearly all cases, a follicular cyst will either rupture or shrink on its own within a few weeks. However, when a cyst does not go away on its own, surgical removal is necessary to resolve the problem and rule out the possibility that it is malignant. Solid tumors always require removal for resolution. Tumors that have cystic areas as well as solid components are more difficult to diagnose.

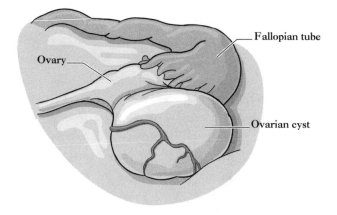

A fluid-filled sac called a cyst *can develop on the ovary. Some are large, some small, and, while most require no treatment, some may result in ovarian cancer.*

Treatment Options. If you are still menstruating, your health-care provider may recommend watching the cyst without treatment for a month or two because it will probably go away on its own. Oral contraceptives, used by some practitioners, have not been shown to be more effective than a watch-and-wait approach. However, if you are nearing or have already completed menopause, your doctor may suggest surgery because of the increased risk of ovarian cancer in this age group.

Surgery. Solid tumors that do not resolve on their own require surgery, which may be carried out through a laparoscope or by an opening in the pelvic cavity. If a cyst or solid tumor is large, the entire ovary may have to be removed. In a postmenopausal woman with a solid tumor or cyst, a hysterectomy with removal of both ovaries may be considered as a safety precaution against cancer in these organs. Some women feel that this is an extreme approach, though many doctors will argue that it is wise treatment because the ovaries are no longer producing estrogen and ovarian cancer is a deadly disease that primarily strikes postmenopausal women. Discuss the options with your provider before making a decision.

POLYCYSTIC OVARIES

If you have polycystic ovarian syndrome—also called Stein–Leventhal syndrome *after the doctors who first described the disease—you will have unpredictable periods because women with polycystic ovaries ovulate infrequently, if at all. Infertility is also a symptom. Approximately 70 percent of women with this syndrome have hirsutism (excessive hair growth), typically on the upper lip, chin, cheeks, chest, abdomen, inner thighs, and back. Many women also are overweight.*

Polycystic ovarian syndrome is an endocrine disorder that begins around puberty, when the body produces excess amounts of androgens (male sex hormones) and inappropriate levels of gonadotropins (hormones that stimulate the ovaries). The ovaries of women with this disorder are enlarged. For reasons that are not completely understood, the ovarian follicles in the ovary form cysts instead of developing and releasing eggs. Both ovaries may be filled with cysts.

Understanding the Problem. If you have the symptoms of polycystic ovaries, your clinician will first do a pelvic exam during which he or she will be able to feel whether your ovaries are enlarged. Blood tests to measure the hormone level confirm the diagnosis.

Polycystic ovaries are not life-threatening but without treatment may lead to other problems. For example, extremely irregular periods cause the uterine lining to build up, a condition called *endometrial hyperplasia*, which in some cases may become malignant (see page 544).

Infertility due to polycystic ovaries can nearly always be treated successfully.

Treatment Options. If you are not trying to become pregnant, your health professional may prescribe oral contraceptives or progestins to regulate your period. If you want to con-

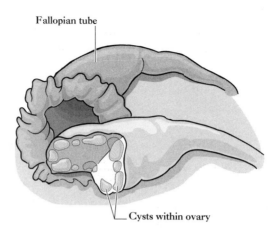

Fallopian tube

Cysts within ovary

In women with polycystic ovaries, multiple cysts develop within the ovaries and can interfere with ovulation and lead to other complications.

ceive, you will be given a fertility drug such as clomiphene to stimulate ovulation. This drug is successful in inducing ovulation most of the time, although only half of the women who take it actually become pregnant, presumably because hormone levels are not completely normalized. Women who do become pregnant while taking this drug are about 5 to 10 percent more likely to give birth to twins.

When clomiphene does not work, drugs called *menopausal gonadotropins* may be successful. This drug regimen, however, is more complicated, expensive, and time-consuming. The incidence of side effects as well as multiple pregnancy is also higher.

SURGERY. Your physician may perform a laparoscopy, during which he or she will cauterize the cysts on your ovaries. This procedure can reduce the androgen level and induce ovulation in most women. Because it works only temporarily and may cause scar tissues to form around the ovaries, this operation is not frequently used.

OVARIAN CANCER

Ovarian cancer is insidious because in its early stages most women have no symptoms. Later, as the disease progresses, discomfort in the abdomen is so mild that it is easy to ignore. By the time the abdomen becomes swollen enough to prompt a woman to seek professional help, the disease has often entered its late stage.

Cancer of the ovaries is the second most common malignancy of the female reproductive system (uterine cancer is more common), but it is the leading killer. An estimated 20,500 new cases of ovarian cancer are diagnosed each year in the United States, and the disease claims 12,500 lives. Not surprisingly, the high death rate is related to the difficulty in detecting this disease, which produces so little early warning.

Despite many studies, we still don't know what causes ovarian cancer.

Most women with ovarian cancer are between the ages of fifty and seventy, although this malignancy can also strike younger women.

Certain risk factors are associated with this disease. If you started menstruating earlier than the average and had a late menopause, your risk may be higher. Women who have had infertility problems or who have never given birth to a child also are at increased risk. Women whose mother had ovarian cancer are at somewhat higher risk of the disease than the rest of the population. Women with two affected relations are at substantially higher risk. White women have a higher incidence of ovarian cancer than black women. In contrast, oral contraceptive use seems to offer substantial protection from ovarian cancer.

The use of talcum powder on the genitals as well as a mumps infection prior to starting menstruation have both been suggested as risk factors but have not been confirmed.

Understanding the Problem. Most ovarian cancers are detected during routine pelvic examinations when the health-care provider feels a mass on the ovary. If you are under the age of forty-five, there is only a small chance that the tumor will be malignant; even in women over forty-five, 67 percent of ovarian masses are benign.

To determine whether your tumor is benign or malignant, your doctor will order a series of tests that may include ultrasound studies. If you have a solid tumor rather than a cyst, it will be removed and examined for malignancy.

Like that of all cancers, the outcome of ovarian cancer depends upon how early it is diagnosed. When ovarian cancer is caught early, the five-year survival rate is between 60 and 80 percent. However, the overall five-year survival rate for all stages of this disease is only 30 to 40 percent.

Treatment Options. If you plan to give birth in the future and if your tumor is a particularly low-grade cancer confined to one ovary, your surgeon may remove only the cancerous ovary to preserve your childbearing ability. Most ovarian cancers, though, have the potential to spread to the other pelvic organs; for this reason, both ovaries as well as the uterus, lymph nodes, and omentum, a fatty apron that drapes over the intestine, are usually removed.

RADIATION. Radiation therapy seldom helps and is not used for most ovarian cancers.

CHEMOTHERAPY. Cancer-fighting agents are frequently used following surgery to treat ovarian cancer. Two drugs, cytoxan and cisplatin, used in combination, seem fairly effective, and more recent regimens include the use of taxol, a substance derived from the bark of the Western yew, and other drugs.

Chemotherapy alone is usually effective in shrinking a tumor, but generally, after twelve to eighteen months, the malignancy begins to grow again.

CANCER OF THE FALLOPIAN TUBE

Many women who have cancer of the fallopian tube do not have symptoms. About half of those who have this rare malignancy notice abnormal or excessive vaginal bleeding or a watery discharge. Some women complain of abdominal pain.

Cancer that originates in the fallopian tube is the rarest of the gynecological malignancies; only about one thousand cases of primary fallopian tube cancer have been reported. The fallopian tube is, however, frequently the site of cancers that have spread from other organs, usually the ovary and uterus. The cause of this disease is unknown.

Cancer of the fallopian tube is more likely to occur in women in their fifties, but the reported age range is from eighteen to eighty years of age.

Understanding the Problem. This type of cancer is difficult to diagnose because most women do not have symptoms. If symptoms are present, laparoscopy (below), a minor surgical procedure, and ultrasound may be used to make the diagnosis.

The prognosis for this rare cancer depends upon the stage of the disease at diagnosis. If the disease is confined to the tube itself, the five-year survival rate is 70 to 80 percent. Overall, the five-year survival rate for all stages of fallopian tube carcinoma is 40 percent.

Treatment Options. If you have cancer of the fallopian tubes, you will need to have a total hysterectomy, and that includes the removal of your ovaries, fallopian tubes, and uterus. When the cancer is caught early, this may be all the therapy you need.

RADIATION. Radiation therapy is not useful for this cancer.

CHEMOTHERAPY. For most tubal cancers, you will be treated with cancer-fighting agents. Cisplatin, in combination with other drugs, has been successful in prolonging life in some women with advanced fallopian tube cancer. Tubal cancer is treated similarly to ovarian cancer.

Overall five-year survival rate for all stages of this disease is 30 to 40 percent.

LAPAROSCOPY

Laparoscopy can be credited with changing the practice of gynecology in recent years. This outpatient surgical technique has made it possible to diagnose and treat many conditions that once would have required a costly hospital stay and major surgery.

The laparoscope is a long, slender tube with a tiny light on one end. It is inserted through a small incision in the abdomen, enabling the gynecologist to see clearly the reproductive organs. A general anesthetic is most commonly used for this procedure because the abdomen is inflated with gas (carbon dioxide), which provides more space for the gynecologist to work yet makes it more difficult for you to breathe on your own.

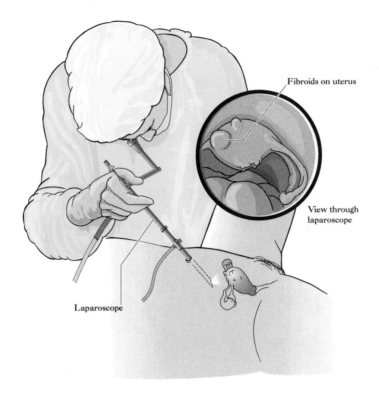

Fibroids on uterus

View through
laparoscope

Laparoscope

*Laparoscopy will enable your clinician to literally see into your abdomen in order to
identify abnormalities and, in some cases, to correct them surgically.*

In some cases, a laparoscopy may be used simply to diagnose a problem. Often, however, surgery to correct the problem can be performed during the laparoscopy. By
inserting surgical instruments through the laparoscope, or through additional small
incisions, the surgeon avoids making larger incisions that can necessitate longer stays
in the hospital and extended recuperation time.

　　There are many conditions for which laparoscopy is used in gynecology. Probably
the most common is sterilization. The technique also is used to remove an intrauterine
device that has perforated the uterus, to treat ectopic pregnancy, to cut adhesions, and
to diagnose and treat endometriosis.

　　If you are having problems becoming pregnant, your health-care professional may
recommend laparoscopy, for both diagnosis and treatment. The procedure also is used
to evaluate women who have severe pelvic pain and to diagnose congenital defects.

　　Your recovery after a laparoscopy should be relatively easy. Your abdomen may
be a bit distended for a day or two, and you may feel a little discomfort but most
women have no significant problems. In most cases, a woman is allowed to go home
within a few hours after the procedure.

❧

CHAPTER 24

The Cardiovascular System and Related Conditions

CONTENTS

For years heart disease was regarded as a male concern by both the medical community and the public. Most studies on heart conditions used only men until 1993. However, questions raised and research conducted recently indicate that seeing heart disease as a male concern is a serious misconception.

In one of the first studies that followed women over an extended period, the Framingham Heart Study, researchers discovered that, of women who were diagnosed as having had heart attacks, 45 percent died within one year. This figure stood in stunning contrast to 10 percent of symptomatic men who died within the first year.

Even though the health community as a whole has reconsidered its understanding of women and heart disease in the last decade, and the media have reflected this shift in the last few years, there is, nevertheless, a prevalent notion that the number-one killer of women is cancer. It is startling to realize, though, that heart disease, not cancer, is the leading cause of death in women over the age of fifty. It is responsible for more women's deaths than *all* cancers—including breast, uterine, and ovarian—combined.

The consequences of these misconceptions are many. Today heart disease remains alarmingly underrecognized and undertreated in women. The general understanding of symptoms, for example, reflects common male complaints. Take, for example, the story of Johanna (see page 560).

Men often complain of chest pressure—"an elephant sitting on my chest." A woman suffering from heart problems, on the other hand, typically describes a burning sensation in the chest or upper abdomen. Usually these sensations are coupled with nausea, sweating, and light-headedness, thus differentiating heart problems from indigestion. Nevertheless, women tend to disregard the signs because they do not correspond closely enough to the descriptions of male symptoms they have read.

Too often women delay seeking treatment. As a whole, women seek treatment significantly later than men with similar heart-related symptoms, increasing the likelihood that a woman's heart attack will be fatal or be associated with more complications like heart failure and stroke.

When women do consult health-care professionals, their complaints are less likely to be recognized as potential heart problems. When Shawntel described her symptoms, for example, her health-care professional told her that she had indigestion and gave her an antacid. Marilyn was told that in all likelihood her symptoms were stress-related, and a sedative was prescribed. Had they been men describing the same symptoms, statistics tell us that, at the very least, diagnostic tests would have been ordered, including an electrocardiogram (ECG), which records variations in the heart's electrical activity in order to diagnose abnormal cardiac rhythm and heart damage.

When a woman's heart condition is properly diagnosed, conventional pharmaceutical remedies are more likely to be prescribed than the more aggressive interventions—angioplasty, thrombolytic therapy, or bypass surgery—commonly offered to men (see page 572).

The bottom line? Women are more likely to die of heart attacks than men; this is especially true within the first week of experiencing symptoms. Women are roughly twice as likely to have repeat heart attacks within a year of their first, even when the first attack has been diagnosed correctly. Furthermore, women have twice as many strokes as men—and the death rate from stroke for black women is 43 percent higher than for white women.

Finally, because so much emphasis in heart treatment rests on prevention and life-style moderation, the fact that heart disease in women is so dramatically underrated means that women have less opportunity to make the same informed choices in terms of nutrition, cardiovascular fitness, and overall health. However, by painting a more accurate picture of a woman's risk for heart disease, by increasing her awareness of the symptoms of heart problems, a woman can make the appropriate adjustments in her diet and in her life-style as well as more accurate assessments of any heart-related pain and discomfort.

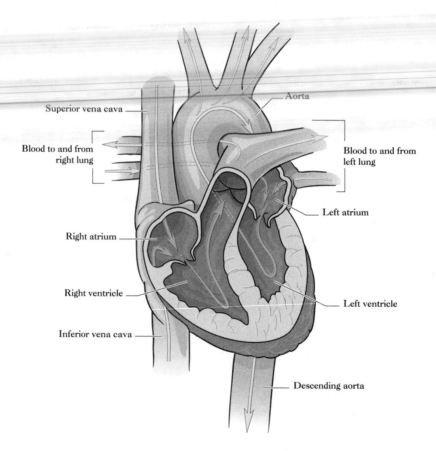

In the deceptively complex workings of the heart—which is essentially the pumping mechanism that delivers blood to the body—the blood flows from the upper and lower halves of the body through the superior vena cava and inferior vena cava, respectively. It collects in the right atrium, then flows into the right ventricle, which pumps blood to both lungs to pick up oxygen. The oxygen-rich blood returns from the lung to the left atrium before moving on to the left ventricle, which pumps blood to the aorta and descending aorta and on to the entire body.

In this chapter, we will look at how the healthy heart works, at the factors that put a woman at greater risk for heart disease, at specific heart diseases and disorders, and at those symptoms that should sound an alarm for heart problems.

THE HEALTHY HEART

At the center of the cardiovascular system is the heart, the body's pump. It moves blood through an intricate network of blood vessels, delivering nutrients and oxygen throughout the body. The regular and rhythmic muscular contractions of the heart muscle work the pump.

The heart is a four-chambered organ, divided into right and left sides, lower and upper

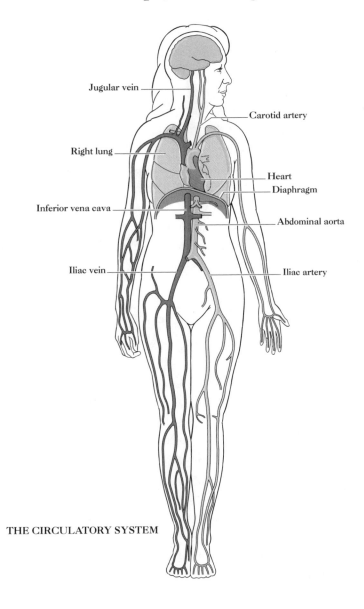

Jugular vein

Carotid artery

Right lung

Heart

Diaphragm

Inferior vena cava

Abdominal aorta

Iliac vein

Iliac artery

THE CIRCULATORY SYSTEM

chambers. The upper chambers are called the *right atrium* and *left atrium*; the lower are called the *right* and *left ventricles*; the atria and ventricles are connected by valves that regulate the rhythm of blood flow between the chambers.

Blood vessels called veins deliver blood from the tissues to the right atrium. This blood, depleted of oxygen during its journey through the body, is high in carbon dioxide that it has absorbed from the body's tissues. The blood then passes down into the right ventricle, which pumps it into the lungs, where carbon dioxide is eliminated and oxygen is absorbed. From the lungs, the bright red oxygenated blood travels through the left atrium to the left ventricle and is then pumped out through the aorta to all tissues of the body.

The typical heart rate—the pace at which the heart pumps—is 60 to 90 beats per minute, which amounts to about 100,000 beats a day. However, heart rates vary from person to person and according to activity. The heart will naturally pump more slowly when you are at rest. When you exercise, contractions increase to provide additional oxygen to the body's muscles and tissues. At each beat, two to three ounces of blood is pumped throughout the circulatory system.

The vascular system consists of an intricate web of blood vessels, which become smaller as they stretch away from the heart and larger as they near the heart. The aorta, the principal artery leading away from the left ventricle, subdivides into large arteries that, in turn, branch into smaller vessels called *arterioles*. These small vessels supply blood to tiny capillaries, which provide oxygen to the tissues. The capillaries absorb carbon dioxide. The blood then returns to the heart by way of veins.

More than the veins, which by the very nature of their task need to be less muscular and elastic, the arterial network works harder and is subject to greater pressure as it receives blood directly from the heart. The whole system is a complex one, subject to various ailments and the deteriorating effects of aging.

JOHANNA'S STORY

For several days, Johanna experienced a burning sensation in the upper part of her abdomen. She dismissed it as heartburn.

Yet the discomfort was tenacious. What was more, she felt nauseated and lightheaded. She'd break out in a cold sweat, even though she hadn't engaged in any activity that was particularly strenuous.

She discounted these symptoms as menopausal. When the discomfort refused to abate and became more acute, she called her doctor. But because she was tentative over the phone about the seriousness of the symptoms, she was not given an appointment for another week. As it turned out, the appointment was a week too late. Later that night, Johanna's husband drove her to the hospital emergency room, where it was found that she had suffered a heart attack.

Earlier, a friend had urged Johanna to take her symptoms seriously, suggesting that they might signal heart disease. Why would Johanna—who is sophisticated and thoughtful in most other areas—ignore these sensations for so long? She just couldn't reconcile her experience with what she knew about heart attacks. But actually what she understood and what most people understand to be heart-related symptoms are based on a man's experiences.

Johanna received excellent treatment once her heart problem had been correctly diagnosed, and she survived the experience. But she sustained heart tissue damage she might not have, if treatment been more immediate.

CARDIOVASCULAR DISEASE AND DISORDERS

The term *cardiovascular disease* is popularly associated with heart attack. In fact, cardiovascular disease involves the entire cardiovascular system. In the case of a heart attack, the symptoms are severe, acute, and centered within the heart muscle, whereas other kinds of cardiovascular problems, such as heart failure, stroke, and aneurysm, involve the arteries, veins, lungs, or brain. Wherever heart disease manifests itself, however, at issue are the health and functioning of the entire system.

Many problems of the cardiovascular system arise from a condition called *atherosclerosis*, in which deposits of fatty tissue called *plaque* can cause the arteries to narrow and harden. When this happens, blood flow is restricted and tissues are deprived of the nutrients and oxygen they need to function.

For too many years, it has been an accepted belief that women were not subject to heart and coronary artery disease in any meaningful numbers. Although younger women are less likely than men to have atherosclerosis and other heart-related illnesses, the incidence of cardiovascular disease rises rapidly after menopause. At any age, women who smoke and are diabetic are at particular risk.

Premenopausal women are protected by the estrogen produced by their ovaries. Although the direct relationship between this female hormone and heart disease is not completely understood, estrogen offers substantial protection from atherosclerotic disease. However, after menopause when estrogen production stops, the frequency of heart disease in women rises to equal that of men. Estrogen replacement therapy after menopause can reduce this rise by about 50 percent (see page 90 for a discussion of estrogen replacement therapy). The U.S. Food and Drug Administration (FDA) has approved use of the medication raloxifene (Evista) for osteoporosis. When used by women after menopause, raloxifene mimics the beneficial effects of estrogen on bone density (thereby offering protection against osteoporosis) and on blood fats (thus protecting against coronary artery disease). An additional advantage is that the use of raloxifene has not been found to increase the risk of uterine and breast cancer.

It is important for a woman's good health and longevity to adapt to any number of changes in her life, but making appropriate dietary and other adjustments to minimize the risks of heart disease is essential during and after menopause. Stopping smoking is the single most important way to reduce risk and should be a priority for women at any age (see *High Risk Factors*, page 565).

ANGINA

Also called angina pectoris, *angina is marked by a tight, crushing, often suffocating band of pressure centered beneath the sternum (breastbone). The sensation of tightness may spread to the throat or arm. It generally occurs during strenuous exercise or emotional stress and may bring with it feelings of anxiety or a fear of impending death.*

Frequently a warning sign of serious heart disease, angina is usually brought on by physical exertion such as heavy lifting, rigorous exercise, or sexual activity; by extreme cold; by indigestion after a large meal; or by emotional stress. The sensation of severe constriction or pressure typically lasts for a minute or two, although it may last as long as fifteen minutes. Discomfort may be severe and often radiates into the left shoulder, back, neck, or arm. There may be sensations of heaviness and burning as well.

Angina occurs whenever the amount of blood reaching the heart muscle is insufficient. During exercise, for example, the heart muscle needs more oxygen as the heart increases its pace. However, if the coronary arteries (which provide the heart's blood supply) are narrowed and unable to accommodate the increase in blood flow, chest pain results. Angina, therefore, is a warning sign of coronary artery disease, in which arteries become blocked by fatty accumulations called *plaque*.

When the discomfort occurs frequently, occurs at rest, or increases in severity, it may signal an impending heart attack (see page 573). Angina is actually quite common, occurring in men after the age of thirty, in women after menopause.

Angina attacks should be taken seriously and a medical practitioner consulted.

Understanding the Problem. Many women experience occasional chest pains after strenuous exertion. Although most of these sensations last at most a few minutes, they may signal coronary artery disease and, as such, should be discussed with a health-care clinician.

Your clinician may recommend an *electrocardiogram* or blood tests to rule out possible heart muscle damage, especially if the chest pain has lasted longer than ten minutes. To test for coronary artery disease and angina, one or several tests may be done, including the use of a *Holter monitor*, in which a twenty-four-hour ECG records heart activity for evaluation; an *echocardiogram*, which uses ultrasound to examine heart structure and function; an *exercise stress test*, which determines, through graded exercise, any compromise in the heart's functioning and capacity; *radionuclear imaging* or *thallium scanning*, which uses a short-lived radioactive substance injected into a vein to create a computer image of the blood supply to the heart muscle; and a *coronary angiogram*, in which an X-ray dye is injected through a catheter to create an image of the heart arteries. In addition, your health-care provider may order blood tests to check blood sugar, cholesterol, triglyceride, and thyroid hormone levels and blood count (see *Blood Tests*, page 625).

Treatment Options. If you experience chest pains, stop any activity that may have brought on the pain so that you ease the strain on your heart and reduce its need for oxygen. This should relieve the discomfort. Then contact your clinician. If the discomfort does not diminish within a few minutes, or if the frequency or severity of the attacks increases, seek immediate medical attention.

LIFE-STYLE CHANGES. There is no question that heart disease is addressed most effectively through preventative measures. Discomfort such as angina can often be alleviated by making adjustments in your health habits.

Smoking, obesity, and a diet rich in fat and processed foods all diminish your heart's efficiency. Besides, quitting smoking, losing weight, and eating a healthy, low-fat diet may actually eliminate symptoms of angina by addressing the underlying problem of atherosclerosis.

A responsible exercise routine, specifically an aerobic program that includes regular, rhythmic movement, will improve the heart's capacity. Anyone with angina should develop an exercise program with the approval and guidance of her health-care practitioner.

MEDICATION. The most common pharmacological treatment for acute attacks of angina is the prescription drug *nitroglycerin*, which works to dilate (open) the arteries, thereby increasing blood flow. Nitroglycerin pills are usually dissolved under the tongue, or nitroglycerin spray is administered under the tongue. Nitroglycerin works in a remarkably short time—usually in less than a minute—to lessen discomfort. It can cause headaches in some people, though this side effect is usually mild.

Some health-care providers will prescribe *calcium-channel blockers* or *beta-adrenergic blockers* for angina. Calcium channel blockers increase blood flow by interrupting the normal flow of calcium through heart channels and dilating arteries. Beta-adrenergic blockers decrease the heart rate and blood pressure, and that, in turn, may reduce symptoms of angina. Recent research also suggests that women over fifty taking one to six aspirin per week had a 25 percent decreased risk of heart attack. For younger women, no such benefit has been found.

SURGERY. If neither life-style changes nor medication eases chest pain or if the symptoms occur with greater intensity or frequency, your clinician may recommend *angioplasty*, a catheterization technique that clears plaque formations from the arteries, or *coronary artery bypass surgery*, in which surgically implanted veins or arteries divert blood flow from the aorta past the obstruction.

ATHEROSCLEROSIS
Commonly referred to as "hardening of the arteries," atherosclerosis describes a condition in which fatty deposits accumulate with the lining of the artery wall, thus obstructing blood flow. Atheroscle-

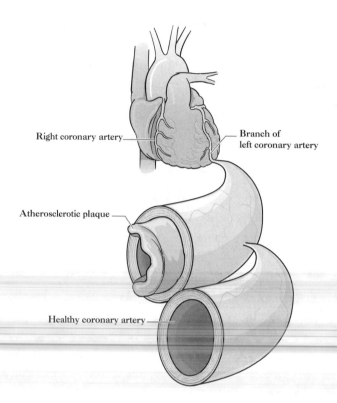

*Fatty deposits of atherosclerotic plaque can accumulate in the linings of the arteries, increasing
the risk of heart attack and stroke.*

*rosis can mean problems in circulation and increased vulnerability to heart attack, aneurysm,
stroke, and other cardiovascular diseases.*

Atherosclerosis is a disease in which plaque, or deposits of fat and calcium, accumulates
over time within the walls of the arteries. The arterial channels become encrusted, narrowed and rigid, and, as a result, blood flow is impeded.

Atherosclerosis is the starting point for much of cardiovascular disease. The impact of
atherosclerosis is felt in those areas to which blood flow has been reduced. A partial blockage to the heart, for example, can cause angina, or sensations of pain or constriction around
the heart that frequently radiate to the left shoulder and down the left arm. Total coronary
blockage can result in a heart attack (see page 573). Strokes occur when there is a blockage
of blood flow to the brain (see page 577). Atherosclerosis of the aorta or arteries to the leg
can produce muscle pain as you exercise, a condition called *claudication.*

In addition, pieces of the fatty deposits may break off and travel some distance through
the vascular system before they block blood flow to an organ, a complication called *embolism.*

Understanding the Problem. A woman may experience very few overt symptoms of atherosclerosis as it develops. A health-care professional might suspect atherosclerosis if, dur-

ing a routine stethoscopic examination, there is a blowing or rushing sound from the neck, abdomen, or groin area. He or she may be alerted by a decrease in pulsations in the arteries around the wrist, leg, or foot.

Your clinician may order a CT scan of the abdomen (see page 635) to look for weakened and enlarged areas of the aorta called an *aneurysm*, which frequently results from atherosclerosis. Often, a clinician will recommend arteriography, in which a dye is injected into an artery in the groin and X rays are taken to identify areas of blockage. Too often atherosclerosis remains undetected until an artery is completely blocked and the condition has been signaled by a heart attack or stroke.

Treatment Options. One of the most effective ways of preventing atherosclerosis is by adjusting your life-style. Because hypertension increases the susceptibility of blood vessels to accumulated plaque, it is important to keep blood pressure under control by limiting salt and fat intake and, in some cases, treating high blood pressure and elevated cholesterol with medication (see page 568). Smoking promotes the development of atherosclerosis and is the single most important risk factor.

Weight control, too, is a key element in preventing coronary heart disease. Women who are overweight, especially those whose excess body fat centers around the midsection of the body, are at higher risk. Women with diabetes have a five times greater risk of development of heart disease, so that minimizing the likelihood of serious heart disease means managing blood sugar level.

Finally, a regular exercise routine not only enhances the heart muscle's tone, endurance, and efficiency, it also lowers blood pressure, decreases levels of fats in the blood, and keeps weight down. Aerobic exercises, such as swimming, walking, and running, which involve continuous, rhythmic activity, are considered the best for the health of your heart.

HIGH RISK FACTORS

Almost any man who has a routine medical examination will be warned, Keep your blood pressure low, quit smoking, watch your weight and diet, get plenty of exercise. *As he gets older, his health-care professional will likely urge upon him, with greater vehemence, an understanding of risk factors and the importance of managing his life in ways that minimize these factors.*

Only within the last few years, however, have women been urged to assume a more health-conscious approach to diet and exercise. Although women are subject to the same risk factors as men, they face the additional concern of increased heart disease associated with loss of estrogen after menopause. At the same time, a woman is less likely to understand the relationship between life-style and heart disease, though in fact her risk is not considerably lower than a man's. In fact, by the time she is sixty, a woman's chance of dying from heart attack or stroke equals a man's.

There are a number of factors that seem to contribute to heart disease—some can be controlled and some lie outside a woman's control.

Smoking. *There is no question that smoking increases a woman's risk of heart disease. Smoking damages the linings of the arteries, making them more susceptible to plaque accumulation. Nicotine overstimulates the heart by signaling the adrenal gland. Smoking reduces oxygen in the blood through the toxic effects of carbon monoxide, a process that decreases oxygen carried to the heart muscle as well as other tissues. And, of course, smoking damages the respiratory system, which plays an essential role in the circulatory process.*

Once a woman quits smoking, regardless of how long she has smoked, her risk for heart disease diminishes significantly. Studies show that within ten years of quitting, a woman actually returns to a nonsmoker's risk level.

Hypertension. *Also called* high blood pressure, *hypertension means simply that the blood in the circulatory system is being maintained at an exaggeratedly high pressure. This puts pressure on the heart, arteries, and veins, contributing to heart disease by weakening and stiffening the blood vessels. As a result, they become more vulnerable to plaque accumulation. Hypertension can be controlled through diet—specifically through lessening salt and sodium consumption—and in some cases through antihypertensive medications (see page 569).*

Diet. *The way in which a woman eats contributes significantly to the way her heart functions. Because salt increases fluid retention and blood volume, for example, the heart must work harder. Cutting down on the amount of salt we shake over our food as well as the salt we consume in processed foods, therefore, may increase the efficiency of the heart. Salt poses another threat to the heart since it counters the effect of diuretics that are often used for hypertension (see page 569).*

The kinds and amount of fat our bodies must process also affect the way the heart functions. By altering our diet, we can replace saturated fats with unsaturated fats; eating fewer foods high in cholesterol can also reduce the risk of atherosclerosis (see page 563).

Empty-calorie foods, that is, heavily processed foods or those that derive most of their calories from simple sugars, should be replaced with foods high in nutritional value in order to prevent obesity. Diets that center on grains, pastas, poultry, fish, fruits, vegetables, and very lean meat are healthier than those that rely on fatty or fried foods. Fish in particular is thought to contribute to a healthy heart; not only is fish low in unhealthy cholesterol (see page 570), but some fish contain fats that appear actually to combat the detrimental effects of cholesterol.

Limit consumption of butter, shortening, and eggs. Although calcium is an essential part of a healthy diet, especially for women, since it works to guard against hypertension and osteoporosis, low-fat milk and cheeses are better choices than whole milk or cheese (see Understanding Cholesterol, *page 570).*

Obesity. *Health-care professionals use the term* obesity *when actual weight is 20 percent greater than ideal weight. Obesity is associated with heart disease because there is often a correlation between overweight and high levels of cholesterol in the blood (see page 570). Obesity is often accompanied by high blood pressure or diabetes. Developing a sensible diet and exercise regimen can reduce the risk for heart disease substantially (see* Nutrition, *page 45).*

Exercise. *Women who get little regular exercise tend to be at greater risk for heart problems. Exercise, especially aerobic exercise that is characterized by repetitive, rhythmic movement, strengthens the heart muscle, builds muscle, keeps weight down, and lowers blood pressure. If, however, you have had heart problems in the past, it is important to consult your medical practitioner as you develop an exercise program.*

Diabetes. *As troubling as diabetes is in itself, its complications, including heart disease and stroke, can be even more disabling and life-threatening. A chronic condition in which the pancreas does not produce adequate amounts of insulin, diabetes results in the body's inability to process dietary sugars. When insulin production is insufficient, glucose builds up in the bloodstream rather than entering the cells. This invites the concentration of blood fat along the arterial walls and impedes blood flow.*

Diabetes poses a major health threat, especially to women over forty, who as a group are more likely than men to have the disease in adulthood. Adult-onset diabetes often occurs in women who are at highest risk for heart disease—those who have high blood pressure, who lead a sedentary life, who are obese, and who do not monitor their diet. Diabetes can be successfully managed through regular use of insulin (see page 463). In light of the condition's impact on the heart, it is essential that diabetic women get their blood sugar level under control.

Heredity. *Genes and family health habits in relation to smoking, eating, and exercise make family history an important factor in heart disease. Clearly, if heart disease runs in your family, you would do well to take preventative measures.*

Stress. *The relationship between emotional stress and cardiovascular health has not been clearly established. However, the Framingham Study, which looked at women and heart disease, indicated that women who work outside the home are less likely to suffer heart attacks than those who do not. At the same time, those who have children; stressful, unsatisfying jobs; and unsupportive husbands and bosses suffer more heart attacks.*

There have been much talk and disagreement about personality styles in relation to stress management and heart disease. Although there is no clear conclusion, what does seem clear is that finding a balance between activity and leisure enhances both a healthy and a satisfying life.

Hormones. *Both estrogen and progesterone seem to play a part in the body's processing of cholesterol (see page 570). Heart disease increases for women around menopause because the body's production of estrogen that provides earlier protection drops during menopause. Heart disease also increases in younger women who have had their ovaries surgically removed unless they are given estrogen replacement therapy.*

Research shows that replacement estrogen reduces the risk of coronary heart disease after menopause by about 50 percent. A similar reduction in stroke has been noted by some studies.

HYPERTENSION

Everyone's blood pressure goes up when they are frightened, running, or worried. But blood pressure should return to normal levels once the stress is over. In some people, the blood pressure stays up all the time. Hypertension, or high blood pressure, is a condition in which blood travels consistently through the arterial channels at elevated pressure, the force of which damages the circulatory system. Although high blood pressure produces few evident symptoms, its long-term effect can be seen in heart, cardiovascular, and kidney damage. Unless managed, hypertension can lead to early death.

Hypertension is commonly referred to as "the silent killer." Although some people with high blood pressure may experience headaches, dizziness, fainting spells, nosebleeds, and ringing in the ears, most individuals do not have any symptoms at all. It is estimated that some sixty million Americans have high blood pressure, yet only half are aware of it. Meanwhile, it does its damage silently and methodically over a period of years. Fortunately, it is easy to diagnose, and treatment in the form of life-style changes and medication is very effective.

Blood pressure is determined by the interaction of the brain, the kidneys, and the blood vessels in response to a variety of stimuli. There may be identifiable medical reasons for high blood pressure, among them Cushing's syndrome (see page 437), adrenal gland tumors, and kidney problems. For some women, high blood pressure occurs during pregnancy or, rarely, stems from oral contraceptive use. The most common type of hypertension—called *essential hypertension*—has no known cause.

We know that blood pressure has a tendency to rise significantly with age and menopause. It is estimated that about 50 percent of women over sixty-five have high blood pressure. African-American women experience hypertension in greater numbers than white women, and at a younger age. For black women, the condition tends to be more severe and serious, resulting more often in death, specifically from strokes. Although the reason for this increased severity is not completely understood, many conjecture that a genetic adaptation in blood pressure evolved to accommodate the African climate. Others point to such factors as the stress inherent to poverty, diets high in salt and fats, obesity, and limited access to health care that many African-American women face.

Untreated high blood pressure creates an environment ripe for heart attack, stroke, kidney damage, and loss of vision, as well as other complications. The heart must work harder to pump the same amount of blood, and the pressure with which it is pumped increases. When blood vessels are subjected to high blood pressure for extended periods, they thicken and lose their elasticity. If, simultaneously, excessive fats are present in the blood, a hard fatty substance called *plaque* builds up inside the linings of the arteries. Blood flow to the heart, brain, and kidneys, as well as to other body tissues and organs, becomes obstructed. The resulting condition, *atherosclerosis*, is a primary factor in heart attack, coronary artery disease, congestive heart failure, and stroke (see *Atherosclerosis*, page 563).

The kidneys are particularly vulnerable and responsive to variations in blood flow that result from high blood pressure and its complications. When blood flow through narrowed arteries decreases, kidney function is compromised. A hormone called *renin* is then released, prompting the vessels to constrict and further accelerating blood pressure. The kidneys lose their ability to process impurities in the blood. Toxic waste products may accumulate in the blood as a result of end-stage kidney failure.

Understanding the Problem. Your health-care professional will routinely check your blood pressure during most visits using an instrument called a *sphygmomanometer*, or blood-pressure cuff. Healthy blood pressure varies widely but averages around 120/80 millimeters of mercury (mmHg). The first number (120, for example) indicates the pressure while the heart is pumping blood into the arteries *(systolic pressure)*; the second number corresponds to pressure as the heart is resting as it fills with blood for the next beat *(diastolic pressure)*. High blood pressure is generally identified when it consistently reads higher than 140/90 mm. When the second number is high, the heart is under pressure even when it should be resting. Since blood pressure naturally varies according to time of day, activity, and emotional stress levels, a diagnosis of high blood pressure should be based on a series of readings taken days or weeks apart rather than on only one reading,

Treatment Options. Life-style changes, often in conjunction with oral medication, can successfully return blood pressure to a normal range for most people and prevent life-threatening damage to major organs.

Life-style. The first priority if you are a smoker is to quit. Next, limit the amount of salt you consume—the more salt you have in your body, the more water you retain. This adds to the amount of fluid being pumped, and the amount of work your heart must do, which translates into higher blood pressure. Therefore, reducing salt intake will reduce blood pressure.

Third, make other dietary changes to control your weight; extra pounds also demand extra effort from your heart. Fourth, exercise to strengthen the heart, to reduce the amount of fats in your blood, and to lessen stress.

Medications. Many years ago, the drug of choice in treating hypertension was almost universally a *diuretic*. Sometimes called water pills, diuretics increase the rate at which urine and salts are eliminated from the body, thereby reducing the amount of total fluid in the body.

Over-the-counter water pills are not effective against hypertension. Prescription diuretics are more potent, but their use must be supervised by your health-care professional because they can cause dehydration, urinary problems, elevated uric acid and blood glucose levels, fatigue, muscle weakness, and leg cramps. Diuretics can drain the body of potassium, so people who take them should, as a rule, eat such potassium-rich foods as bananas, apricots, avocados, broccoli, and beans.

Although diuretics are still a part of many antihypertension regimens, several newer drugs are now available to lower blood pressure. These include beta-blockers, calcium-channel blockers, angiotensin-converting enzyme (ACE) inhibitors, and vasodilators. Beta-blockers (beta-adrenergic blockers) reduce the heart's demand for blood by inhibiting the stimulating effects of adrenaline. They are not recommended for the elderly, or for people with a history of asthma or severe heart failure. In some cases, they may cause fatigue and depression. They also may lessen sexual desire. If the dosage is too high, dizziness and fainting spells may result.

Calcium-channel blockers curb calcium absorption in the cell that would otherwise narrow the smaller arteries. Angiotensin-converting enzyme (ACE) inhibitors interfere with the body's natural chemical processes that constrict blood vessels. Vasodilators relax the blood vessel walls, allowing more blood to flow through. Some women who take vasodilators complain of headaches, swelling around the eyes, palpitations, shortness of breath, or dizziness.

UNDERSTANDING CHOLESTEROL

The concept of blood lipids may seem confusing at first. Yet a fundamental understanding can reduce some of the confusion and help you sort through much of the contradictory information on your way to establishing a sensible way of eating.

Cholesterol is one of several fats, or lipids, present in the blood. The body manufactures 8 percent of its own cholesterol in the liver and uses it to make cell walls and hormones. Our bodies also derive cholesterol from the food we eat.

Lipids bind with proteins, forming lipoproteins, which then carry the fat in the blood. High-density lipoprotein (HDL) is instrumental in transporting fat away from body cells to the liver, where it is broken down. HDL helps to prevent the concentration of cholesterol and fats within the artery walls. It is called the "good cholesterol." In general, women tend to have a higher HDL level than men. Exercise raises HDL level; smoking lowers it.

Low-density lipoprotein (LDL), known as "bad cholesterol," contains the largest proportion of cholesterol of any of the lipoproteins. LDL causes accumulation of fatty materials within the artery walls, a significant factor in the risk of heart attack and stroke.

A third type of blood lipids is triglycerides. High levels of triglycerides generally are thought to promote atherosclerosis, although their role is not completely under-

stood. In fact, some health professionals believe that triglycerides contribute very little to the development of coronary heart disease.

Blood cholesterol levels generally increase with age, particularly among women after menopause. Estrogen helps maintain the beneficial ratio of HDLs to LDLs. When estrogen levels decline at menopause, women's total cholesterol readings tend to rise. Replacement estrogen taken orally reestablishes a healthier balance and prevents much of the increase in heart risk that otherwise accompanies menopause. In contrast, estrogen replacement therapy may also raise the body's level of triglycerides, which some researchers suggest raise heart disease risk. Some progestins, which are often taken in conjunction with estrogen, may counteract some of the benefits of estrogen, although the decrease in cardiovascular risk may be retained.

An estimated fifteen million American women have a high blood cholesterol level that puts them at risk for heart disease. These women show levels of at least 260 milligrams (mg), whereas the American Heart Association (AHA) recommends a level of 220 mg. In addition, the average American consumes 400 to 700 milligrams of cholesterol a day; the AHA suggests an upper limit of 300 milligrams a day.

There is no question that lowering cholesterol level in the bloodstream reduces the risk of heart attacks and heart attack deaths. For every 1 percent drop in cholesterol level, adults lower their chance of having a heart attack by 2 percent. Although women have not been included in most past studies, one recent study shows that the benefit of low-cholesterol diets is greater for women than for men.

How is a woman to translate information about cholesterol into healthy eating habits? The answer is simply, Eat sensibly. Decrease total fat consumption. Whenever possible, make complex carbohydrates—grains, beans, and legumes—the center of your meals. Foods that come from animals—meats, eggs, dairy—tend to be higher in cholesterol. Choose fish and poultry over red meat. When you want meat, select very lean cuts. Low-fat and nonfat milk, cheese, and yogurt provide the calcium women need without adding significantly to blood cholesterol levels. Emerging research suggests that a low-fat diet is not just a healthy choice but that it can reduce the atherosclerotic process and help clear out plaque from arterial vessels. Just because people have eaten poorly does not mean it is too late to start on a healthy diet. The American Heart Association recommends several heart-healthy diets, rich in fruits and vegetables, that will help women regain their health.

Switch from saturated or hydrogenated oils such as butter and margarine to olive oil and canola oil. Read labels of processed foods to avoid oils and fats.

Not all products derived from vegetables have a low fat content. Palm and coconut oils, for example, have no cholesterol, but are very high in saturated fats. The process of hydrogenating, used to harden oils and blend peanut butter, converts some harmless unsaturated fats into saturated fats. Therefore, the label "no cholesterol" by itself does not mean that a food is certifiably heart-healthy.

In short, when it comes to keeping blood cholesterol level within a healthy range, less fat, no smoking, and more exercise are the keys.

TILDA IS WORRIED

Almost every time Tilda opens a newspaper or popular magazine, she finds another article on cholesterol and its effects on heart disease. She recognizes the importance of this information and feels that she needs to understand the relationship between cholesterol and health. She'd like to be able to apply what she reads to her dietary and exercise habits.

Yet every article seems to offer information and advice that conflicts with the previous one she read. No sooner does an article admonish the reader to give up eggs or substitute margarine for butter than another article appears praising the egg for delivering a high-quality, highly digestible form of protein. And a third accuses margarine of containing "transfatty" acids that may also contribute to heart disease. She saw on the television show 60 Minutes *that it might be a smart strategy to drink a glass of red wine each day as the French do; subsequently, she read that wine may actually increase the incidence of breast cancer in women.*

Tilda's so confused that at her last checkup she got a little impatient with her doctor. "I'm just trying to do the right thing, and all these researchers can't seem to make up their mind. What do I do?" She told him she had virtually given up trying to adjust her eating habits in the hope of controlling her cholesterol level but feels all the more anxious as a result.

Tilda's doctor offered her some sound advice. She is basically healthy, with no known heart disease or diabetes or other chronic health problems. She is approaching menopause, and she's conscious of the fact that her father died of a heart attack, and her mother had a mild stroke a few years ago.

Tilda's doctor advised her to change her diet right away. She is to avoid fats, of course, and to eat less meat. Foods high in cholesterol are also to be avoided. And don't eat too too many sweets, he advised her. On the other hand, she doesn't have to abandon everything she likes in favor of nothing but nuts and berries. A little wine? A glass a day may even be beneficial.

He had some more advice about wading through the health information the media offered her.

"You're a person who's curious about the world, Tilda," he observed. "But you don't believe everything you read, do you, when it comes to politics or the news of the world? The same should be true of research findings."

He explained that most scientific studies examine a small population of people, which allows researchers to control the number of variables in any given study. That makes for good science, of course, but it also tends to narrow the applicability of the findings to the population at large, not to mention to an individual, like Tilda, with her own set of habits and genetic inheritance.

"Use your good sense," her physician advised; "when you sit down to dinner, eat sensibly. When you read the paper, remember that research findings—like yesterday's newspapers—shortly become yesterday's news. Sometimes they get refined and recycled into healthy dietary practice; sometimes they end up on the rubbish heap."

HEART ATTACK

Frequently unprovoked by physical activity or emotional stress, a heart attack is usually signaled by intense chest pain or prolonged, heavy pressure. The sensation may radiate to the left shoulder and arm, the back, and even the teeth and jaw. Often, women who are suffering heart attacks will experience burning sensations in the upper abdomen or midsternum. These symptoms are often accompanied by shortness of breath, sweating, nausea, vomiting, fainting, and light-headedness. But women may never have any chest discomfort, experiencing back or shoulder pain instead.

When a blood clot (thrombus) or narrowed artery (caused by atherosclerosis) interferes with the supply of blood to the heart, the heart is deprived of oxygen and nutrients. As a result, part of the heart muscle dies. This is a heart attack, or *myocardial infarction* (MI).

Although the experience of pain and discomfort may be similar in heart attack and angina, there is an important difference: With angina, the interruption to the blood flow is temporary and the pain soon subsides; with a heart attack, the blood supply to a portion of the heart is completely shut off, causing that part of the heart muscle to die. The pain of a heart attack does not abate when physical or emotional stress subsides. Nor will it respond to nitroglycerin (see *Angina*, page 562).

Without exception, a heart attack is a grave medical emergency. If you experience any of these symptoms, stay calm but seek help immediately. Early treatment is essential. Go to your local emergency room or call your area's emergency medical number. A new recommended strategy is to take one 600 mg aspirin tablet if you believe you are experiencing heart attack symptoms. The antiplatelet action of aspirin may help decrease the clot formation.

Understanding the Problem. Because of the seriousness of the condition, treatment and assessment procedures will commence almost immediately, whether in the hospital emergency room or in an emergency vehicle. Blood pressure will be taken and an electrocardiogram will record heart rhythms (see page 557). Typically a person who has had a heart attack will be advised to stay in the hospital, where other tests may be ordered, including blood tests to detect enzymes that are produced as a by-product of damaged heart tissue. In addition to the ECG, a number of other tests will aid in the diagnostic process. For example, a *coronary angiography*, an X-ray procedure in which dye is injected into the artery to illustrate blockage. An angiogram can help confirm any suspicion of heart damage.

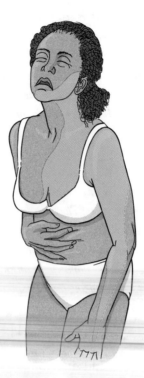

The pain or burning sensation of a heart attack may be felt not only in the chest around the heart but also in the left shoulder, neck, and arm.

Treatment Options. After a heart attack patient's condition has been stabilized, a team of health-care professionals will begin to work out a treatment plan based on the patient's history and condition.

MEDICATION. A wide range of medications is available to dissolve blood clots and to facilitate blood flow. Thrombolytic agents such as *streptokinase* or *tissue plasminogen activator*, delivered through a catheter or injected into a vein, help dissolve clots. These drugs work best when used within a few hours of the heart attack but they are not recommended for anyone who has recently had surgery or a stroke or anyone who has an ulcer or a bleeding disorder.

Nitrates, often injected into the vein during or immediately after a heart attack, work to dilate blood vessels and increase the oxygen supply to the heart. Nitrates also may be prescribed to manage the condition over the long run. They are most commonly administered under the tongue, applied to the skin as an ointment or patch, or prescribed in long-acting tablets. *Beta-adrenergic blockers* inhibit the stimulating effects of adrenaline on the heart, resulting in slower heartbeat, lower blood pressure, and a reduction in the amount of oxygen needed.

Another, more familiar medication, *aspirin*, may be beneficial after a heart attack because it decreases the accumulation of platelets and in so doing impairs the formation of a clot. Many health-care professionals recommend that women who have coronary artery disease or who are recovering from bypass surgery take aspirin daily. However, if there is a history of stroke or high blood pressure, bleeding disorders, ulcers, or impaired liver or kidney function, aspirin would not be recommended.

ACE inhibitors are often prescribed after heart attack to lower blood pressure and limit the extent of heart muscle damage.

If a woman continues to experience pain after a heart attack, a doctor may prescribe an analgesic drug, such as morphine.

Balloon angioplasty is a procedure sometimes used to clear a blocked artery. A relatively uncomplicated procedure performed usually under local anesthesia, angioplasty involves inserting a small inflated balloon at the site of the arterial obstruction.

Bypass Surgery. In those cases in which a blocked artery cannot be cleared with either medication or angioplasty, *cardiac bypass surgery* may be performed. Surgeons construct a *shunt*, or detour around the obstructed artery, using a section from another artery or a vein, usually taken from the chest or the leg. During this procedure, the chest is opened and a heart/lung machine sustains circulation as the new segment is attached to the heart. Many women who undergo bypass surgery or angioplasty experience direct relief and are able to resume their active life; the procedures also decrease the risk of angina and sudden death. However, in light of the considerable expense of the surgery as well as the physical scarring left by the procedure, it is important to explore other treatments, including medication and life-style modification, before turning to bypass surgery.

CONGESTIVE HEART FAILURE

Congestive heart failure is the condition created when the heart is unable to pump out adequate blood to the tissues. Symptoms include breathlessness, weakness, fatigue, and swelling in the ankles.

Almost always serious and frequently life-threatening, congestive heart failure occurs when the heart's efficiency diminishes. The failing heart cannot push adequate blood out to tissues throughout the body. Congestion develops in the veins as the blood returning to the heart backs up.

Often this condition develops after the heart has been working at an accelerated pace for a prolonged period, as with hypertension (see page 568) or when the heart muscle doesn't receive enough oxygen because of blockage in the coronary arteries or rapid arrhythmias.

If the heart weakens on its right side, blood backs up into the veins of the legs and liver, causing *edema*, or swelling, in the lower legs and ankles. If there is failure on the left side, the lungs become congested with fluid. This condition is called *pulmonary edema* and causes difficulties in breathing. In many cases, both sides of the heart fail.

In addition to fluid retention, swelling, and shortness of breath, congestive heart failure causes physical fatigue and reduced endurance since the blood supply to the muscles is drastically curtailed.

Congestive heart failure may stem from conditions created by earlier heart attacks—specifically, by weakened heart muscle tissue.

Understanding the Problem. Early signs of congestive heart failure may go unnoticed, but they usually become worse over time. Swollen ankles, especially after standing for some time; feelings of weakness and breathlessness after routine activities; and shortness of breath even during sleep are typical. Women who suffer from congestive heart failure often report feelings of dread and anxiety with these episodes of constricted breathing.

During a routine physical examination, a health-care professional might hear sounds in the heart or lungs that suggest congestive heart disease. If there are swollen neck veins, signs of an enlarged liver, and edema of the feet, blood and urine tests may be ordered to check kidney function. Other tests that may be indicated include an *electrocardiogram* to monitor heart rhythms and detect signs of damage from previous heart attacks, chest X rays to explore the possibility of enlarged heart and congested lungs, and an *echocardiogram*, which uses ultrasound to detect heart muscle or valve problems.

Treatment Options. If congestive heart failure is diagnosed, your clinician will help you make the kind of life-style changes that suit your needs and your condition. There should be a balance between rest—to conserve energy and to prevent taxing your heart even more—and movement, to maximize healthy circulation. Your diet should be altered so that you consume less salt and fat and are able to reach and maintain a healthy weight.

MEDICATION. Angiotensin-converting enzyme (ACE) inhibitors are likely to be the mainstay of treatment for congestive heart failure. These drugs dilate arteries and improve blood flow, thus lowering blood pressure and reducing strain on the heart.

Diuretics may also be prescribed to aid the body in ridding itself of salt and fluid. This decreases swelling throughout the body and helps eliminate fluid in the air spaces of the lungs. By their very nature, diuretics bring about more frequent urination. You may also need to compensate for the resultant loss of potassium by adjusting your dietary consumption of the mineral with bananas and orange juice.

Digitalis can help increase the strength of the heart's pumping action, and *vasodilators* expand the arteries to ease blood flow and lessen the demand on the heart. Medications that help return the heart's rhythm to normal may be prescribed if the cause of the heart failure was related to an arrhythmia.

SURGERY. In some cases, congestive heart failure has been caused or exacerbated by a weak heart valve. An artificial valve can be surgically implanted to replace the defective one. Where a leak between heart chambers or damaged cardiac tissue interferes with the heart's efficiency, surgery to repair heart tissues may be advised. *Bypass surgery* or *angioplasty* may be required if there are blockages in coronary arteries.

JUDY'S SEX LIFE

As frightening as the experience had been, Judy felt grateful that she had survived her heart attack and had come through the bypass surgery so well. As her doctor advised, she made adjustments in terms of her diet, her weight, and her exercise habits. So three months after the ordeal, she was feeling better than she had for years. She was back to her normal activities with only slight modification.

One lingering concern was about sex. Was what she had always heard in reference to men—that once you've had a heart attack, you can say good-bye to your sex life— true for her as well?

Judy was smart. Instead of worrying and wondering, she asked. Her health-care practitioner explained: Any notion that a person—man or woman—must forgo sexual activity after a heart attack, stroke, or heart surgery is simply a myth. After a reasonable time to allow for recovery and with a little common sense and awareness of her body's responses to exertion, there should be no reason that she cannot return to a satisfying and active sex life.

STROKES AND TIAs

A stroke results when the blood supply to the brain is disrupted. Among the signs that a stroke has occurred or warnings that one is about to occur are a deterioration of speech, vision, or sensation; a sudden weakness or numbness in the face, arm, or leg on one side of the body; a severe and persistent headache; dizziness or unsteadiness; and sudden memory loss. Emergency symptoms include any of the signs described that comes on with startling abruptness, a sudden loss of consciousness, or complete or partial paralysis that is not related to an injury.

The term *stroke* actually describes a series or variety of events that occur when the blood supply to a part of the brain is interrupted. The most common form of stroke is a *cerebral thrombosis*, which happens when a clot develops in an artery narrowed by atherosclerosis.

A second type, *cerebral embolism*, is caused when a piece of the plaque or a blood clot attached to the lining of a blood vessel breaks free and travels through the bloodstream to lodge in one of the arteries leading to the brain.

A third form, *cerebral hemorrhage*, occurs when an artery bursts, flooding brain tissue with blood, causing both pressure on brain tissue and loss of blood flow to the brain. Usually a cerebral hemorrhage is caused by an injury to the head or an *aneurysm*, a blood-filled sac that has ballooned out from a weak spot in the artery wall.

Once they begin, stroke-related symptoms may progress or fluctuate over a period of days. Typically, when the stroke is caused by an embolism, a clot of undissolved matter, that travels through the bloodstream and wedges in the artery to the brain, the symptoms are rapid and serious. When it is caused by a thrombus (a clot that develops within an artery), the symptoms develop more slowly and over a longer period.

Transient ischemic attacks (TIAs) occur when blood loss to the brain is temporary. In this case, symptoms, including sensations of weakness, tingling or numbness, blind spots or blurred vision, loss of balance and poor coordination, usually last only a few minutes. Frequently due to atherosclerosis (see page 563), TIAs can be a warning sign that a major stroke is imminent; these ministrokes often precede a serious stroke by days, weeks, or months. TIAs, then, are like angina. They signal that tissues need oxygen but do not represent the tissue death seen in stroke.

Although young women in general are at low risk for stroke, women who smoke face a significantly greater risk at any age. The chances of stroke also seem to rise slightly among women who take oral contraceptives. Long-term, untreated hypertension also increases the likelihood of strokes. Diabetic women, especially those who have hypertension, are highly vulnerable to stroke and should take special care to keep their blood pressure within a normal range. Also, the chances of having a stroke naturally increase with age.

Understanding the Problem. A stroke is invariably a serious medical emergency. If you experience any stroke-related symptoms, contact a health-care professional immediately.

Before determining treatment, a clinician will try to identify the type and location of the stroke. Other factors, such as tumors, that could have precipitated the attack must be assessed. An *angiogram* (an X ray that permits the clinician to trace blood circulation) and *computed tomography* (CT) or *magnetic resonance imaging* (MRI) (both of which use computerized scanning equipment to create diagnostic images; see page 636) will likely be ordered for these purposes.

Treatment Options. When a stroke causes prolonged loss of consciousness, treatment will include hospitalization and, in many cases, intensive care. A woman who has experienced a severe stroke may need life-support equipment to provide oxygen, nutrients, and medication as well as catheterization to handle bladder functions.

MEDICATION. Once a stroke has occurred, medications cannot correct the damage. However, some doctors will prescribe anticoagulants, or blood thinners, to prevent further damage to brain tissue and to counteract the blood's exaggerated tendency to clot. These medications require close monitoring since they present an increased danger for women with high blood pressure and can enhance the possibility of hemorrhage.

If it appears that a woman suffers from TIAs, aspirin may be suggested. Because it inhibits the way blood platelets clump together, aspirin reduces the body's tendency to clot. In addition, a woman with symptoms of TIAs will be urged to monitor and control blood pressure.

SURGERY. In cases of cerebral hemorrhage in which blood has leaked into the tissues, surgery may be indicated. The decision to operate is usually determined by the location and progress of the hemorrhage. Surgery may also be advised to remove an aneurysm or a malformation in specified arteries.

SMOKING. Whether you have had a stroke, have experienced TIAs, or are simply worried about the risk of them, quit smoking. Smoking is a significant risk factor for strokes and TIAs and increases your risk of many other disorders.

PERIPHERAL VASCULAR DISORDERS

Any condition that disrupts the circulatory system and creates problems in the body's extremities and organs is called a peripheral vascular disorder. Blood clots, including arterial embolism and thrombosis, can produce pain and numbness, as well as sensations of cold in the hands and feet. Aortic aneurysm, *an abnormal swelling within the artery, can result in pain in the abdomen or back.* Phlebitis *is clotting and inflammation within a vein, often leading to tenderness, pain, redness, and swelling of the affected limb.* Varicose veins *are enlarged, twisted veins that function poorly and predispose the vein to the clots of* phlebitis.

The vascular system relies on clear passage and vessel elasticity to move blood, which contains nutrients and oxygen, to the body's tissues. However, a number of conditions can disrupt blood flow in a significant way.

A blood clot, for one, can develop in a specific site along the arterial wall, obstructing the flow of blood. A blood clot developing in a vessel is called a *thrombus* and is often a consequence of the rupture of an atherosclerotic plaque accumulation. A woman may then experience intermittent leg cramps and cold, painful sensations in her hands or feet. Under some circumstances, this condition can bring about gangrene, a serious condition in which tissue in the arm or leg has actually died.

Similar symptoms may be experienced when an *embolus* forms. Unlike a thrombus, which is a blood clot that remains stationary, an embolus is a piece of atherosclerotic plaque or blood clot that has broken free from the artery wall and is carried through the circulatory system until it becomes lodged. When an embolus or a group of emboli wedges in the artery of a leg or arm, blood flow is blocked, and pain, pallor, and numbness can result. If the condition is not monitored and promptly treated, arm or leg tissue below the obstruction can die.

An *aneurysm* is a weakness of an artery wall that results in a ballooning of the blood vessel. It is not uncommon for a clot to form in the aneurysm, increasing the risk of embolism. The greatest risk is that the weakened wall will rupture, allowing blood to flow into surrounding tissue. This can produce shock, loss of consciousness, or stroke (see page 577). Although an aneurysm can form in any of the blood vessels, it occurs most commonly in the aorta, the main blood vessel leading away from the heart and brain blood vessels. High blood pressure and atherosclerosis increase the likelihood of aneurysm.

Phlebitis refers to a condition that develops when a clot occurs in a vein, resulting in swelling and inflamation. Phlebitis appears most commonly in the leg, producing considerable pain, tenderness, redness, and swelling. It may arise with pregnancy, bed rest, paralysis, a malignancy, long trips on planes or cars, and, rarely, oral contraceptives. Superficial clotting is usually visible under the skin. Clotting deep within the vein is often detected with ultrasound or an X-ray examination.

Varicose veins are primarily a cosmetic concern that becomes more apparent with age. The dilated blue veins residing close to the surface of the skin result from a malfunction of the valves in the veins. There is often a familial pattern and varicose veins are ten times more common in women than in men. During pregnancy, a woman's veins naturally stretch with the increased volume of blood that passes through them. The veins and valves weaken. As a result, rather than working efficiently to propel blood directly up to the heart, some valves may fail to close properly, allowing blood to pool at certain sites. The veins then become enlarged. Previous phlebitis and obesity contribute to the development of varicose veins. "Spider-burst veins" are actually arteriole growths in which purple blood vessel patterns can be seen through the skin. These growths are harmless and present little more than a cosmetic concern (see *Sclerotherapy*, page 181).

Understanding the Problem. Although many of the symptoms of peripheral vascular disorders may seem merely troublesome, it is important to discuss them with your medical practitioner. Once the nature and location of the discomfort are described, he or she will measure blood pressure and feel for pulsations, especially around the affected area.

With phlebitis and varicose veins, careful observation is often enough to make an accurate assessment of the problem. If a blood clot or aneurysm is suspected, an angiogram (a method of X ray that uses dye injected into the affected area), ultrasound (a method of computer imaging that uses sound waves), or CT (a method of computer scanning using X rays; see page 635) may be recommended to confirm its existence. Accurate diagnosis is important because an embolism can result if the blood clot is in a vein and is not treated with blood thinners.

Treatment Options. Some peripheral vascular conditions—depending upon the diagnosis—need only to be monitored or can be addressed through slight life-style modifications. Others require immediate medical intervention.

VARICOSE VEINS. Often, the discomfort and progression of varicose veins can be checked with self-help measures. Avoid standing or sitting for any length of time. Engage in regular exercise such as swimming, walking, and biking, to improve circulatory flow and decrease pressure on the veins. Some women find that support hose and stockings help relieve pressure as well. When the skin around the varicose veins becomes itchy or ulcerated, some health practitioners may recommend surgery to strip or remove the veins and tributaries. This kind of surgery is done primarily to improve the appearance of the area.

PHLEBITIS. Treatment of phlebitis may involve applying heat to the affected area, elevating the arm or leg, or using anti-inflammatory medications. Usually anticoagulants are recommended. A woman may need to be hospitalized for heparin therapy before oral anticoagulants are started. She will need to have frequent follow-up blood tests to keep the blood clotting within a prescribed range. If administered intravenously, these drugs will prevent new clots from forming as the body dissolves the old clot. In some instances of phlebitis, it may be necessary to insert a filter or tie off a vein to prevent the clot from breaking loose and traveling to the lung.

ANEURYSM. Blood pressure medications are sometimes used in the early treatment of aneurysm. If symptoms are minor and the aneurysm is small, your health-care professional may simply follow the condition over time, perhaps recommending periodic scanning through ultrasound or CT (see page 635) to watch for any changes in size. Surgical removal or replacement of the damaged area of artery may be recommended if there seems to be a risk of rupture.

EMBOLISM. When an embolism occurs, blood flow must be restored within a few hours to prevent permanent damage to the affected limb. Typically, a clot-dissolving drug injected directly into the affected artery will break up the embolism. If the health of the limb is at immediate risk, surgery may be performed using a balloon-tipped catheter to withdraw the clot directly from the artery. In either case, anticoagulant medication may be prescribed to guard against the development of future clots.

CHAPTER 25

Oral Disorders

CONTENTS

As a child, you may have been marched to the dentist twice a year. Your mouth was inspected for cavities and you were handed a shiny new toothbrush for being so cooperative. In those days your biggest concern was that the dentist would find a cavity and you'd have to endure a shot of novocaine.

Now that you're past the years when you are most cavity-prone, you may think you're out of the woods. You may be tempted to pay little attention to your oral health. In truth, oral health is as important during adulthood as it was when you were a child. Your mouth, like the rest of you, has grown up, and now your biggest oral health risk is no longer decay but periodontal disease. Both can lead to tooth loss.

In this chapter we will explore the most pressing oral health problems encountered by women.

PERIODONTAL DISEASE

People with periodontal disease have swollen, soft, red gums that bleed easily, often after brushing. As the disease progresses, the gums recede. You may notice an unpleasant taste in your mouth or have chronic bad breath. Some people have pain in a tooth when eating hot, cold, or sweet foods. Eventually, teeth loosen and fall out.

Periodontal disease is a major dental concern for people over the age of thirty-five and in mild forms often is found in even younger people. This usually painless disease occurs in the gums, ligaments, tooth sockets, and jawbones, the structures that hold the teeth in place.

There are two common forms of periodontal disease, gingivitis and periodontitis. Gingivitis, or inflammation of the gums, is caused when plaque, a sticky film that forms on the

THE HEALTHY TOOTH

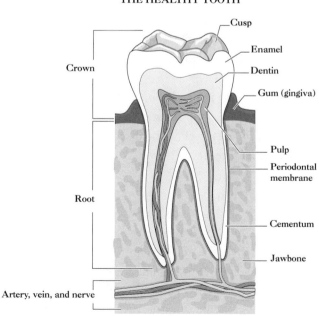

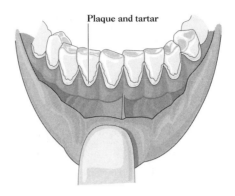

Plaque and tartar are most likely to develop at the gum line and can result in periodontal disease.

teeth, accumulates around the gum line. Mild gingivitis is common among adults. If gingivitis is left untreated, the disease can progress to become periodontitis, a condition in which not only the gums, periodontal ligaments, and tooth sockets become inflamed, but abscesses and erosion of the jawbone can also occur. Plaque-filled pockets form between the teeth and gums, trapping more plaque. The result is increased inflammation, which, over time, causes the gums to detach from the teeth. Sometimes the invading bacteria cause infection and pus oozes from around the teeth. Eventually, the socket that holds the tooth in place can't help but erode. When this happens, the tooth loosens and may fall out. Bacteria and infection can spread to other areas of the body, including the heart.

Understanding the Problem. Periodontal disease in either form can be diagnosed during a routine dental exam. Most healthy gums are pale pink and firm and will not bleed easily. During an examination, the dentist will examine your gums for signs of inflammation and plaque deposits.

The course of periodontal disease depends upon when it is diagnosed. If you have gingivitis, a strict program of oral hygiene and regular visits to your dentist can probably get your teeth back on the right track. If, however, the disease has progressed to periodontitis, surgery may be needed to save your teeth.

Treatment Options. The first step in the treatment of periodontal disease is to remove the plaque and tartar (plaque after it has hardened) from the teeth. This thorough cleaning is called a *scaling* and is done by either your dentist or a dental hygienist in the dental office. Even in a healthy mouth, a scaling can be uncomfortable because of the sharp tools used to scrape the tartar from around the teeth. If your gums are already inflamed, this process may be more uncomfortable but is necessary to make your mouth healthy.

After a cleaning, you will need to follow a strict program of oral hygiene. This includes brushing your teeth after eating (at least twice a day) and flossing daily. Regular professional cleanings are also fundamental to the maintenance of a healthy mouth.

If you have periodontitis, scaling and proper hygiene may not be enough. There are surgical procedures that may be used to treat periodontitis. One gives unexposed areas a thorough cleaning and involves lifting the gum tissue and scrubbing the area around the teeth and bone. The gum is then sutured back into place. Another procedure is called a *gingivectomy*. The gums are trimmed to decrease the depth of pockets and then the gum line is covered with a puttylike packing, which allows the gums to heal. Damage to bone can often be corrected with a procedure that involves replacing the diseased bone with healthy bone or a bone substitute.

In some cases, orthodontia may be recommended to straighten crooked or overcrowded teeth. Although overcrowding does not cause periodontal disease, it does make it more difficult to clean your teeth properly and, as a result, can make you more susceptible to periodontal disease.

KELLY'S STORY

The dental hygienist tipped the chair back, instructed Kelly to open her mouth, and then began to pick her way gently around Kelly's teeth and gums. Kelly felt as if she were waiting for a grade that would be posted, after a particularly difficult exam back in college.

A moment later she felt a wave of relief wash over her. "Looking good," the hygienist said, continuing to probe.

Three months before, the scenario in the dental chair had been different. With the carefree air of a person with few dental problems in her past, Kelly had plopped down in the chair thinking she might even doze a little, when suddenly she felt an unexpected pain. The metallic taste of blood in her mouth brought her to the realization this was no routine dental visit.

The news had been that she had gingivitis, the early stage of periodontal disease. When the dentist asked whether she flossed, Kelly felt defensive. Of course she flossed. How often? the dentist wanted to know. Well—Kelly couldn't remember the last time. Maybe once a week or so, she finally admitted, a little sheepishly.

After showing Kelly a few pictures of people with severe periodontal disease, the dentist laid out a stringent program of oral hygiene that included brushing three times a day and flossing after breakfast and dinner. She demonstrated proper brushing techniques, showing Kelly how to brush gently around the gum line to remove plaque, and also recommended that she use special toothpicks or stimulators to remove plaque from the gum line and between the teeth.

After three months of this stepped-up oral hygiene regimen, Kelly got the good news: Her gums were pink and firm. On this dental visit, her mouth was healthy. But she would have to work to keep it that way.

DENTURES

Good teeth just seemed to run in Martha's family. Both her parents were in their eighties, their natural teeth still in fine working order. Maybe that's why Martha had never been concerned about her own teeth. They were straight and they did the job, even if they didn't look great.

As she approached sixty, Martha noticed pain when she chewed certain foods. When she looked at her gums, she saw that they were red and puffy. When one of her teeth seemed loose, Martha made an appointment with a dentist.

The news wasn't good. Martha had severe periodontal disease and decay. The dentist recommended extracting all the teeth and replacing them with dentures. Martha hesitated before choosing such a drastic option, but after learning more about dentures, she decided that they were the best solution.

Dentures are artificial teeth that are made and fitted by a dentist called a prosthodontist. *A full set of dentures consists of an upper and a lower set of teeth that fit over the gums. The dentures are removed at night and stored in a cleaning solution. Although a person who wears dentures often has trouble eating certain foods such as corn on the cob and whole apples and may lose some sensation in eating because the roof of the mouth is covered by the upper denture, most people eventually adjust to the change. However, complete dentures have only 20 percent of the chewing efficiency of natural teeth.*

A month after Martha got her dentures, they still felt a little strange, but friends commented on how natural they looked. And Martha agreed. She liked the way she looked when she smiled.

TOOTH DECAY

If you have a decayed tooth or cavity, your first symptom may be pain or oversensitivity in the tooth after eating something sweet or particularly hot or cold. Many people with cavities, however, have no early symptoms.

Cavities, also called *dental caries*, occur when your mouth's natural bacteria convert the sugars and other carbohydrates you eat into acid. Together, the bacteria and acid form the sticky substance we know as plaque. This plaque, which is also host to minute food particles, lies on the teeth, especially in the pits and fissures of molars and around the gum line. If it is not removed, the acid then wages war against tooth enamel, causing tiny openings or cavities in the enamel.

Tooth decay does not happen overnight. It typically takes a year or two for a cavity to form in an adult tooth, less in a primary tooth.

Children and young adults are more likely to have cavities, although some people are prone throughout their lives. A more prevalent problem for adults than surface cavities are root caries, decay in the root of the tooth.

Understanding the Problem. Since there are often no symptoms of early cavities, most are found during routine dental examinations. Others are diagnosed when a raging toothache drives the sufferer to seek out the services of a dentist. Long-standing cavities that go untreated can penetrate the dentin beneath the tooth enamel, allowing bacteria access to the core of the tooth. When this happens, the blood vessels in the tooth swell, pressing on the nerves, and you may have severe pain. Sometimes the nerves and blood vessels die.

Most cavities can be treated easily and the tooth saved. If an abscess develops, however, a root canal may be necessary to save the tooth. Even after such treatment, some teeth may be too damaged to survive and may need to be pulled.

Treatment Options. The treatment requires the decay be removed and the cavity then filled. If the filling will be visible, a tooth-colored filling that matches the color of the teeth will be used; a filling of silver amalgam is the usual choice when the cavity is in the back teeth. Sometimes gold, a stronger restorative, is used in back teeth, but this is significantly more expensive. Typically, the small prick of a local anesthetic being injected into the gum is the most uncomfortable part of having a tooth filled. The dentist then drills out the decay and fills the hole. If the cavity is so large that the tooth cannot support a filling, a porcelain jacket or metal crown may be necessary.

If decay has penetrated to the core of a tooth, you will need a *root canal.* This procedure is also required to save a tooth that has been traumatically injured. A dental specialist called an *endodontist* typically performs this procedure, which is usually done in several stages in the dental office.

If severe infection is present, the doctor prescribes antibiotics first, to reduce the bacteria and allow the anesthesia to work better. After injections of a local anesthetic, the dentist gently removes the diseased nerve tissues (pulp) of the tooth. All traces of diseased nerve tissue and bacteria are then removed by flushing the root canal with a sterile solution. Medication is inserted into the root canal to clear up any infection, then the root is packed with a sealer and a temporary filling to close up the tooth. A few weeks later after the tooth has healed, a permanent filling or crown is put in place to complete the process.

TOOTH LOSS

A tooth or teeth may be knocked out or loosened as a result of an accident, but in adults, tooth loss is usually the result of disease, most commonly untreated tooth decay and periodontal disease.

A century ago, a middle-aged person with all his or her own teeth was a relatively rare sight. Today, however, thanks to vast improvements in oral hygiene and dental techniques for treating tooth diseases, fewer people lose their teeth.

Understanding the Problem. Should you lose a tooth in an accident, call your dentist immediately (if you can't reach the dentist, go to the nearest emergency room); the tooth—

if you have it—may be able to be reimplanted. Whether or not the tooth can be reimplanted depends upon how quickly you get help and how the tooth is handled. If a tooth is knocked out, the following guidelines should be followed:

1. Successful reimplantation depends upon the tooth's being reimplanted no more than two hours after it was knocked out and preferably within thirty minutes.
2. Handle the tooth by the crown only.
3. Clean the tooth in tap water but not under the faucet; do not scrape dirt off the tooth.
4. Try to insert the tooth into your empty gum socket and then bite down gently on gauze or a wet tea bag to keep it in place while you are en route to the dentist.
5. If you can't get the tooth into its socket, place it in a cup of milk, your own saliva, or mild salt water.

If you lose teeth to disease, they can only be replaced with artificial teeth. Once you lose a tooth, it is important to have it quickly replaced. If not, other teeth may drift toward the empty space, eventually altering your bite.

Treatment Options. The treatment for accidental tooth loss is reimplantation whenever possible.

In the event that the reimplantation is unsuccessful or teeth are lost as a result of dental disease, the treatment is to replace the missing teeth.

If all your teeth need to be removed, you will need a full set of dentures (see page 586). Often, however, your tooth loss may involve no more than a few teeth or even one tooth. Then your dentist may make a partial denture or bridge that can be fixed permanently into your mouth or removed for cleaning, depending upon the location of the missing teeth and the condition of your remaining teeth.

Another approach is to anchor artificial teeth directly to the upper or lower jaw in a manner resembling the way real teeth are held in place. Implants are artificial roots that are placed into the jawbone to replace missing teeth. For most people, the procedure can be done in a dental office with local anesthesia. The implants are made of biocompatible metal and are small anchors shaped like screws, cylinders, or blades. Bone cells in the jaw will require three to six months to attach to the implant to give it maximum strength. Replacement teeth are then attached to the part of the implant that projects through the gums.

Dental implants can provide support for a fixed bridge, a single tooth, or an entire denture. Not everyone is an ideal implant candidate, so discuss this option with your dentist. Tooth implants can be more expensive and time-consuming to make and fit than traditional dentures but may offer a more permanent solution.

DRY MOUTH

Some people, particularly those taking certain prescription drugs (including some antidepressants, antihistamines, anti-inflammatories, muscle relaxants, antihypertensives, decongestants, and certain diuretics), experience the sensation known as dry mouth. Quite literally, the mouth feels uncomfortably dry. Although older women are more likely to experience dry mouth, the cause is less a consequence of aging than a result of hormonal changes, radiation therapy, and certain systemic diseases.

The medical explanation is simple: Too little saliva is secreted to maintain the usual moistness in the mouth. This results in plaque buildup, especially under the gum line, which can lead to inflamed gums and root decay. In severe cases, the bacteria destroy the tooth's support structure, causing the tooth to become loose and fall out. Or, the root decay eats through the root and the tooth breaks at the gum line.

If you experience dry mouth, try decreasing your intake of caffeine or nicotine. Drink water when the parched feeling is bothersome. If the discomfort continues, consult your health-care provider. He or she may recommend you use a dry-mouth gum to help moisten the mouth. Fortunately there is help available to the millions of people with this condition. There are many products that can help alleviate the problems of dry mouth, and they are available at most drugstores or through your dentist. Special toothpastes, chewing gum, gels, and sprays function as artificial saliva to help protect the teeth. Artificial saliva products include MouthKote, Optimoist, and Glandosane.

For the prevention of loss of minerals from the teeth as a direct result of dry mouth, fluoride is also important. Estrogen is also advocated as a prophylactic measure for treating osteoporosis, which affects the jawbone, especially in women who have had teeth removed. Further research will be necessary to determine how effective hormone replacement therapy is in alleviating dry mouth in aging women.

PREVENTION STRATEGIES

Your teeth were designed to last a lifetime. Whether they do or not depends upon how you take care of them.

As we've seen in this chapter, the main threats to tooth longevity are decay and periodontal disease, both of which begin with the sticky substance we know as dental plaque. You should try to keep your teeth as plaque-free as possible. Another contributing factor to tooth decay is the acid that forms in your mouth when you eat sugars and other carbohydrates, so diet is also a factor in the war against cavities.

The following suggestions will help you to keep your teeth healthy:

1. To help prevent tooth decay, watch your diet. We now know that sugar is not the only culprit in tooth decay; other carbohydrates also are converted into acid on the teeth, which then can eat through the enamel, forming a cavity. Yet a balanced diet is dependent upon a certain percentage of carbohydrates in your daily intake.

The solution is not to eliminate carbohydrates but to know the proper time to eat them. First, it is better to eat sweets or carbohydrates with a meal rather than between meals. Limit consumption of sweet or sticky foods. Moreover, whenever possible, brush your teeth within twenty minutes of eating these foods. If you can't brush, at least try to rinse your mouth with water.

2.   Brush your teeth at least twice a day (more often if you are cavity-prone or your dentist has advised that you tend to have heavy plaque deposits). Use a fluoride toothpaste, which will help prevent cavities.

3.   Dental floss should be a normal part of your everyday dental care. Dentists recommend flossing at least once a day prior to brushing.

4.   If you find that plaque accumulates around your gum line, try using special toothpicks or stimulators to help remove plaque buildup from around the gums and between the teeth.

5.   See your dentist twice a year for a checkup and thorough cleaning to remove any hardened plaque or tartar that has formed on the teeth.

CHAPTER 26

Musculoskeletal Disorders

CONTENTS

If there was ever a miracle of mechanics, it is the human musculoskeletal system. This system encompasses the entire body, from the top of your head to the tip of your toes. It consists of 206 bones, 650 muscles, and assorted joints that allow you to run a race, whack a tennis ball, swim laps at your local pool, and, quite simply, get out of bed in the morning. Moreover, the system assumes the role of bodyguard, protecting more delicate components like the heart, lungs, and brain.

Stripped to its basics, the body begins with the bones that make up the skeleton. Bone, a living and constantly evolving substance, is made up of proteins, minerals, and cells. Your skeletal system is, in essence, the body's foundation, supporting it as well as functioning as a depository for important minerals such as calcium and phosphate.

Bones are interconnected at junctions known as joints, which function as hinges, allowing the bones to move within certain limits. Each joint is cushioned by cartilage that acts as a shock absorber. Bands of fibrous tissue, the ligaments, bind the parts of each joint together.

Muscles are attached to two or more bones and are made of elastic fibers that allow them to expand and contract, thus producing movement at the joints. When a muscle contracts, the bones attached to it move. Virtually all the muscles in the human body work with a partner. If, for instance, you contract the biceps muscle in your arm, the arm will flex; if you contract the opposing triceps muscle, your arm will extend.

Most of us have little reason to think about our muscles and bones until something happens to remind us that they are there and vulnerable. Often that not-so-gentle reminder is in the form of trauma that results in a broken bone or sprain. Or, it may be a nagging backache that makes life miserable. Women in particular have the threat of osteoporosis hanging over their head as they age. This potentially crippling bone disorder typically strikes after menopause and is silent until the calcium-depleted bones begin to fracture.

Many of the disorders we will discuss in this chapter are not serious problems. Most backaches, for example, though uncomfortable, do not pose a threat to your health. This is not to say that you can or should dismiss these minor complaints. On the contrary, musculoskeletal complaints account for nearly 10 percent of all doctor visits in this country and are the leading cause of disability and absenteeism from work.

ABDOMINAL AND INGUINAL HERNIAS

If you suffer from an abdominal hernia, you may have pain or discomfort when bending or lifting. There may be a tender lump in your groin. Emergency symptoms are nausea and vomiting.

A hernia occurs when any part of an organ (usually the intestines) protrudes through a weak spot or tear in the muscular wall that holds the abdominal organs in place. Sometimes the blood supply to the herniated area is cut off. When this happens, the hernia is said to be strangulated, a condition that requires immediate surgery.

The two primary types of hernias are inguinal and paraumbilical.

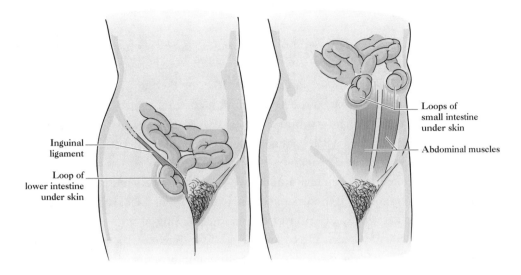

Inguinal ligament

Loop of lower intestine under skin

Loops of small intestine under skin

Abdominal muscles

Hernias occur when portions of the intestine protrude through weak spots or tears in the abdominal wall. When a hernia occurs at the groin near the vaginal opening, it is termed an inguinal hernia; when in the vicinity of the navel, a paraumbilical hernia.

INGUINAL HERNIA. This hernia in women develops in the groin near where the round ligament exits from the abdomen to join with the tissue surrounding the vaginal opening. Inguinal hernias are more common in men, in whom they develop in the groin near the area where the cord that suspends the testes passes from the scrotum into the abdomen.

PARAUMBILICAL HERNIA. This hernia, more common in women than in men, occurs when a weakness develops in the abdominal wall muscles that surround the navel.

Understanding the Problem. Your health-care provider should be able to feel the bulge of a hernia during an examination. When a strangulated hernia goes untreated, the trapped tissue dies because of a lack of blood. This condition, called *gangrene*, is life-threatening.

Treatment Options. Surgery is the recommended treatment for large hernias or those that are producing symptoms. After a local, spinal, or general anesthetic is administered, the surgeon makes a small incision and pushes the protruding tissue back into its proper place. The weakened muscle or tissue is then repaired to prevent the same thing from happening again. The procedure typically takes an hour or less.

If the hernia is strangulated and gangrenous, the affected section of the intestine is removed and the healthy ends sutured together.

After the surgery, you will be encouraged to get on your feet as soon as possible (usually within a day) to help your recovery. You will be instructed to call your clinician at the first sign of redness or pain around the incision site. You should also avoid heavy lifting. Most people are able to resume exercise or other strenuous activities within a month.

BACKACHE

The symptoms of backache are pain and stiffness that may occur during exertion or even when your body is at rest.

One of the oldest and most common ailments afflicting the human race is backache, a problem that can occur anywhere on the back but most commonly affects the lower back.

Sometimes a backache can be attributed to a serious spinal problem such as a prolapsed disk or arthritis. However, the backache that plagues most of us from time to time is called "nonspecific" because there is no apparent cause.

Perhaps you're like Paula, a college student who wakes up every morning stiff and sore but by midmorning is fit enough to work out at the gym. Or, your backache may have more in common with Kelly's; Kelly, a computer analyst, after sitting in front of a computer all day, is bothered by aches and pains all evening. Kim, a first-time mother, spends a good part of her day lugging around her well-fed toddler, carrying him upstairs when he's too tired to walk, bending awkwardly to put him into his car seat. Lately, she's been feeling pain and pressure every time she hoists her child onto her hip.

In most cases, nonspecific back pain is due to a strained ligament or muscle spasms. Emotional stress also can cause back pain in some people. Whatever the cause, back pain is one of the most common causes of missed work due to illness.

Understanding the Problem. If your backache persists or the pain is severe, see your health-care provider. He or she will question you about the pain and perform a physical examination. To rule out a serious underlying cause like a disk problem, the clinician may recommend a diagnostic test such as an X ray.

Although a backache can make going about your daily activities tantamount to conquering Mount Everest, most backache will subside with time and rest. Unfortunately, however, many back pain sufferers have recurrences.

Treatment Options. If a serious problem with a disk is found, special therapies or surgery may be necessary. However, the recommended treatment for most nonspecific backache is rest and the application of alternating heat and cold on the affected area. You also can take an analgesic such as aspirin for the pain.

PREVENTION. The following are ways to help prevent the back strain that can cause backache:

1. When you lift, bend your knees, not your back.
2. Extra pounds put extra stress on your skeletal system. If you are overweight, start a diet and exercise program.
3. Consult your health-care provider regarding a stretching and exercise regimen. Some simple daily exercises—including sit-ups and leg lifts—will strengthen the muscles involved and may help prevent recurrences.

CARPAL TUNNEL SYNDROME

If you have carpal tunnel syndrome, you may feel numbness or a tingling in the fingers. Pain from the wrist may shoot up your forearm or down into the palm of your hand. For many, the pain is worse at night and may actually awaken them from sleep. Shaking the hand may relieve the pain.

The carpal tunnel is a narrow byway through your wrist that protects the median nerve, which provides sensation to some of your fingers. When the tissues around this passageway become swollen or inflamed, the nerve is compressed, producing numbness and pain.

Carpal tunnel syndrome, which may affect one or both wrists, is most common in middle-aged women. Workers employed in jobs that subject the wrist to repetitive motion, like typists, people who work at computers all day, meat cutters, carpenters, violinists, and mechanics, are at higher risk for this disease because of the physical demands of their occupation.

In some cases, carpal tunnel syndrome is found in tandem with other medical problems such as diabetes and rheumatoid arthritis. Pregnancy also can cause the syndrome, but the problem usually disappears after the baby is born.

Understanding the Problem. If you have the symptoms of carpal tunnel syndrome, your health-care provider may order a test called an *electromyogram*. This hour-long outpatient

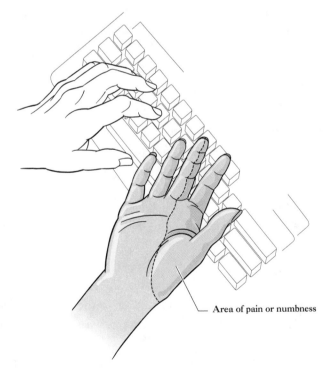

— Area of pain or numbness

When the structures of the wrist put pressure on the median nerve where it passes through the carpal tunnel, an ailment called carpal tunnel syndrome results, producing pain or numbness as indicated.

procedure involves placing a thin needle electrode into each muscle being studied. You will feel a brief, sharp pain each time the needle is inserted. A fine wire leads from the needle to an electrical instrument that detects the muscle's electrical currents, indicating whether these impulses are stalled in the carpal tunnel, a sign that the nerve is compressed.

Carpal tunnel syndrome is painful and in some cases makes it impossible for a sufferer to do his or her job. With proper treatment, however, the pain can be relieved and permanent damage to the hand and wrist prevented.

Treatment Options. Your clinician may prescribe a wrist splint that immobilizes the wrist, yet allows the hand to function almost normally. If this fails to eliminate the pain, cortisone injections may be used to reduce swelling and inflammation.

If the pain persists after these measures have been tried, surgery to relieve pressure on the nerve is recommended. This involves widening the carpal tunnel to lessen the pressure on the median nerve. The surgery has become quite routine, and most people regain full use of their wrist and hand within a few weeks.

FOOT PROBLEMS

If you have a foot problem, you are probably reminded every time you put on a pair of tight shoes or spend more time than usual on your feet: You experience pain or discomfort that makes getting about painful.

Foot problems run the gamut. The cause may be simple corns and calluses that, although unsightly and uncomfortable, are no threat to your health; more serious problems are foot ulcers, a common problem among diabetics. If left untreated, foot ulcers can lead to amputation of the infected foot. Fortunately, most foot problems are less serious and more easily treated.

Judging from the pointed toes and stiletto heels that women force their feet into, it isn't surprising that foot problems are more commonly found in women. In many cases, the problems can be prevented by simply wearing better-fitting shoes.

The following briefly describes the most common foot problems.

CORNS AND CALLUSES. These are hard, thick layers of skin, often between the toes or on the heels, that are caused by constant pressure or repeated friction on the skin. Poorly fitted shoes are the most common cause.

BUNIONS. A bunion is a painful bony protrusion that develops at the base of the big toe when the toe overlaps the next one. The bunion protrudes from the normal profile of the foot. Many people have a genetic predisposition to bunions; in many cases, the cause is not known.

HAMMERTOE. A hammertoe is the condition in which any toe, most often the second one, becomes bent and painful. The toe develops a clawlike appearance. This condition may occur in diabetics as a long-term consequence of the disease.

INGROWN TOENAIL. If you have an ingrown toenail, the sharp end of the nail has grown into the skin surrounding the nail. The tissue around the nail may become red and swollen, causing pain. An ingrown toenail can be caused by poorly fitting shoes, by toenails that are unusually curved, or by the improper cutting of the nails.

FOOT ULCERS. An ulcer on the foot is an open sore surrounded by inflamed tissue. If the sore is infected, pus may leak. This ailment is more likely to occur in diabetics who have blood vessel or nerve deterioration in their extremities.

Understanding the Problem. Many foot problems can be treated at home, often by simply opting to wear better-fitting shoes. If your problem persists, however, see your health-care provider or a podiatrist, a licensed professional who, although not a medical doctor, is trained in the diagnosis and treatment of foot disorders.

If you have a bunion, the health-care provider may take an X ray to confirm his or her visual diagnosis. In the event of a foot ulcer, the clinician may order an ultrasound to check for any arterial blockage in your leg.

Most foot problems are not dangerous. The exception is a foot ulcer in a diabetic, which can eventually lead to infection and even death of the affected tissue.

Treatment Options. Many foot problems can be relieved by wearing more comfortable shoes. To prevent ingrown nails, cut the nails straight across. If you have corns and calluses, try soaking your feet and then using a pumice stone to abrade gently the thickened skin, and layers of it will, over time, slough off. If you have an infection, your clinician will prescribe warm soaks and a topical antibiotic. In severe cases of hammertoe, your provider may recommend an appliance inserted into the shoe to help straighten the toe.

For foot ulcers caused by poor circulation, your health practitioner may recommend you wear support hose to aid your circulation and prevent future ulcers. Elevating the feet periodically also may help. Sometimes surgery on the arteries is necessary to increase blood flow to the foot.

OSTEOARTHRITIS

If you have osteoarthritis, you will notice pain in a joint during or after use. The joints may become swollen and difficult to bend. If the joints on your fingers are affected, bony lumps may develop at the end joint (Heberden's nodes).

Jean, a grandmother who will soon celebrate her seventieth birthday, loves to do needlepoint in her spare time. But lately the joints of her fingers have been so swollen that her needlework has been relegated to the sewing basket in the back of a closet. Some days she has to grit her teeth to manage the simple task of buttoning a button or zipping a zipper. Jean, who suffers from osteoarthritis in her fingers, is in good company. Although this very common disease does sometimes occur in younger people, most, like Jean, are in their later years. Although the precise mechanisms that cause this disease are unknown, the wear and tear to which the joints are subjected are a major factor.

If you have osteoarthritis, the cartilage cushioning the impact on the joint gradually wears away. Over time, the normally smooth surface becomes rough and unable to protect the joint. Eventually the ends of the bones produce painful and disfiguring lumps.

Osteoarthritis commonly occurs in the neck, back, knee, hip, or fingers. In most cases, the disease is limited to one or a few joints.

Understanding the Problem. Your health-care provider may be able to diagnose osteoarthritis on the basis of your symptoms and a physical examination. He or she may order an X ray of the affected joint to see whether you have a bone spur, an indicator of osteoarthritis. If the problem is more generalized, your health-care provide may order further tests to exclude rheumatoid arthritis (see page 475).

Osteoarthritis can be very painful, although often the pain recedes within a year of its appearance. Over time, other joints may also be affected, but the good news is that this ailment is rarely crippling.

Treatment Options. The goal of treatment is to decrease pain and maintain or improve joint function. This is done in the following ways:

MEDICATION. Jean's pain usually can be controlled with over-the-counter analgesics. For more severe cases of osteoarthritis, corticosteroid drugs are often used to reduce pain and swelling; these are especially helpful when the arthritis affects weight-bearing joints such as the knee or ankle.

EXERCISE. If you have osteoarthritis, you should consult your clinician or physical therapist about an exercise program to improve your range of motion. Isometric exercises, for example, do not put stress on the joint yet strengthen the surrounding muscles, thereby protecting the vulnerable joint. Jean, for example, performs a series of finger exercises every day to help prevent stiffening in her fingers.

Excessive weight on an arthritic joint will worsen the problem, so if you are carrying extra pounds, consider dieting, especially if you have arthritis in your back, hip, or knee.

SURGERY. When joint deterioration is severe, surgery to replace the diseased joint may be recommended. Hip replacement (see page 601), hand surgeries, and even knee replacements are becoming increasingly commonplace.

OSTEOPOROSIS

Osteoporosis is a condition of decreased bone mass or low bone density, which is found in one in four women over the age of forty-five. A first sign often is vertebral fractures, signaled by low back pain, and, as the disease progresses, sometimes with a loss of height and development of stooped posture. Osteoporosis, however, produces no back pain or other overt symptoms until weak bones begin to fracture.

Osteoporosis occurs when too much bone is lost, too little bone is formed, or both occur, generally after the onset of menopause. The more bone tissue that is lost, the more porous the bones become, making them subject to fracture.

Although men also can experience osteoporosis, this disease is more common in women. White and Asian women are at the highest risk. Other risk factors include being underweight, smoking, and consuming a diet that is low in calcium.

Understanding the Problem. For many women, the first sign of osteoporosis is a broken bone, typically a wrist or hip. The break is often the result of a minor accident, one that would not damage a healthy bone. Upon examining an X ray of the break, your health-care provider may be able to distinguish that the bone appears less dense than a healthy bone would.

If your X-ray result indicates osteoporosis, your clinician may also order blood and urine tests to see whether your porous bones are due to other causes. A bone density test may also be ordered to measure the amount of bone in different parts of your skeleton and predict your risk of future fractures.

The principal consequence of osteoporosis is bone fracture. Three areas of the skeleton prone to osteoporosis-related fractures are the radius, or the lower arm bone; the vertebrae in the spine; and the hip.

COLLES FRACTURE. A stumble or fall may result in a fractured wrist as a person attempts to break the fall with a hand, and the wrist absorbs much of the shock. Typically it is the outer bone in the lower arm, the radius, that breaks, having been weakened by bone demineralization.

Recovery is usually complete after proper treatment. However, a wrist fracture may be an early indication of osteoporosis—and a signal you should discuss the best strategies for preventing further bone loss with your health-care provider.

VERTEBRAL FRACTURES. The twenty-two bones in the back—the vertebrae—are especially subject to the demineralizing effects of osteoporosis. The result can be fractures that result from falls, or heavy lifting or even occur spontaneously without apparent connection to any physical action.

Often the first outward sign of a vertebral fracture is a dull, nagging pain. Over time, however, a series of such fractures will result in a loss of body height and a bent-over posture. Commonly known as dowager's hump (*kyphosis*) and associated with very old and frail women, this condition can be painful as well as disfiguring.

HIP FRACTURES. Literally hundreds of thousands of women a year sustain broken hips; in fact, this injury is the most serious result of the bone loss that results from osteoporosis. The head and neck of the upper leg bone, the portions near the hip joint, are especially subject to demineralization, weakening them. In some cases, women fall and fracture their hips; in others, the bone break occurs *before* the fall, caused by a normal motion or even a simple shifting of weight.

In severe cases, osteoporosis can be a debilitating disease. It can also kill. Forty thousand deaths occur annually as a result of osteoporosis, mainly after hip fractures and complications like pneumonia and blood clots that result from extended immobility.

Treatment Options. The best way to battle this disease is to take steps early to prevent it. Although some clinicians argue that a woman prone to osteoporosis will eventually have some signs of the disease regardless of her life-style, most agree that the greater peak bone density a woman acquires, the better her skeletal system will fare. (*Peak bone density* occurs at age thirty; 98 percent of bone density is achieved by age twenty.)

The National Institutes of Health recommend that women consume 1,200 milligrams (mg) of calcium per day at ages eleven to twenty-four; 1,000 mg for adult women; 1,200 mg for pregnant or lactating women; and 1,500 mg for postmenopausal women not taking estrogen and all women over sixty-five. Foods rich in calcium include dairy products, beans, nuts, whole-grain cereals, and leafy green vegetables. Calcium supplements also are available if you don't think the food you eat is giving you the calcium you need.

Exercise that uses a combination of motion and weight on the limbs is great for strengthening the body. Bicycling, dancing, jogging, weight training, and just plain walking are excellent both for young women who want to prevent osteoporosis and for elderly women who have the disease but want to prevent it from worsening.

MEDICATION. Studies have shown that hormone replacement therapy at the time of menopause will help prevent osteoporosis. Concern about an increased risk of cancer is a common reason for not using therapy. New nonhormonal medications that build bones now being used include alendronate, calcitonin, and raloxifene (see also *Hormone Replacement Therapy*, page 90).

SURGERY. If you suffer a fracture, you may require surgery to set the bone. In the case of a hip fracture, screws or metal pins may be inserted. If the bones are badly deteriorated, hip replacement surgery may be necessary (see page 601). Hip operations of all sorts are major surgeries that often require extended hospital stays and rehabilitation thereafter. Only about half of the women who suffer hip fractures regain normal function in their hips, so appropriate physical and occupational therapies are essential.

HIP REPLACEMENT

When Leslie remembered her life the way it once was, the thing she missed most was the dancing. Years of ballet during her formative years had taught her to hold her body ramrod straight and move with grace.

That was before arthritis had hit early with a vengeance, chewing up her right hip joint until a mere walk across the room was an exercise in torture.

When she was forty-two, having endured three years of using a cane, Leslie was advised by her doctor to consider having a hip replacement.

Today surgeons are able to re-form knees, fingers, and, most commonly, hips, using artificial replacement parts. In a typical year, there are more than 100,000 hip replacement surgeries in the United States alone.

When you consider that the average person takes about a million steps annually, it isn't surprising that some once-serviceable hips go on the blink. To get an idea of how your hip joint works, make a fist with your right hand and twist it into the cupped palm of the left. The fist represents the top of the thigh bone and the cupped palm the hipbone. Every time you take a step, the ball of the leg bone turns inside the socket of the hipbone. This socket starts out well cushioned but often that cushioning begins to

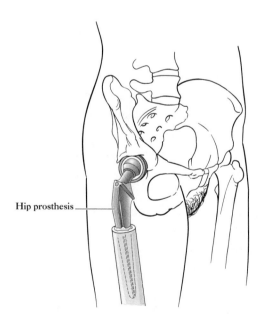

Hip prosthesis ————

In a hip replacement or hip arthroplasty, the joint between the pelvis and upper leg is replaced by a man-made ball-and-socket prosthesis, as indicated here in this cutaway drawing.

wear thin, sometimes simply as a result of age, often as a result of disease. When this happens, the pain can be excruciating.

Although other joints are commonly replaced, by far the most successful and most common joint replacement is that of the hip, the procedure that Leslie elected to have. This surgery involves removing the top of the thigh bone and inserting a steel ball on a stem. The socket of the hipbone is replaced with a polyethylene cup. Depending upon the materials used, the implants are fastened with acrylic cement or positioned so the bone actually grows into the porous surface of the implant, locking it in place.

Although a hip replacement is major surgery and, like any major operation, carries risk, more than 90 percent of these operations do what they are intended to—allow the person to walk without pain. Leslie is one of those success stories. It's only been a few weeks since the surgery and she is still undergoing physical therapy and will be for a while. No, she hasn't resumed ballet. But she feels like a new person. She is getting ready to throw away the cane. And for the first time in years, a long walk in the park doesn't seem an insurmountable task.

SCOLIOSIS

Scoliosis is an abnormal sideways curvature of the spine. The spine typically develops two curves, the first to one side of the body and the other to compensate for the first. People with scoliosis usually have an asymmetrical rib cage and one protruding shoulder blade.

Carly, a twelve-year-old, came home with a note from the school nurse after the sixth grade had been screened for scoliosis. The examining doctor had detected a curve in Carly's back. Alarmed, Carly's parents took her to the pediatrician, who had the girl bend forward so that she could examine her spine. And there it was: a very slight curve near the top of Carly's back, which made her right shoulder blade appear slightly larger than the left.

Stunned, the parents wanted to know how this could happen. They'd always been diligent about taking their daughter for her yearly checkups. They encouraged Carly's interest in sports as a way of keeping her body strong. Perhaps this growth spurt that had rendered her a head taller than most of the boys in her class and had made her feel uncomfortable was responsible? Yes, her mother reported, come to think of it, she had noticed Carly slumping.

The pediatrician explained that it was unlikely that her slumping had anything to do with her spine's curvature. She explained that in the majority of cases, scoliosis can be traced to genetic factors. Although the curvature may begin early in life, it is often undiscovered until adolescence. Girls are more commonly affected than boys.

Understanding the Problem. Scoliosis usually can be detected during a physical examination of the spine. The pediatric examination should include a careful look at the back, both when the child is standing straight and when she is bending forward.

When scoliosis is found, an X ray is often taken to determine the degree of the curvature.

The outcome of scoliosis is highly variable. The curvature may progress as the child grows, even into adulthood, especially with pregnancy and excessive weight gain.

When left untreated, a severe curvature will cause the vertebrae to rotate, separating the ribs on one side of the body and narrowing them on the other. In addition to causing much pain, this can make it difficult for the heart and lungs to function properly and ultimately can shorten life.

Treatment Options. The goal of treatment is to prevent the curvature from increasing. How this is done depends upon the severity of the scoliosis when it is diagnosed.

Luckily for Carly, her curvature was relatively minor, about fifteen degrees. So her doctor recommended a program of daily exercises to strengthen the muscles of the spine and improve her posture. Had the curvature been worse (usually between twenty and forty degrees), Carly would have been fitted with a spinal brace, which she would wear all day for a period of years to prevent further curvature.

In cases in which the curvature is more than forty degrees, spinal surgery that involves the insertion of a metal rod is usually recommended to correct the deformity.

SPINAL STENOSIS

If you have spinal stenosis, also known as lumbar stenosis, *you may have pain in your buttock, thigh, and calf, usually when you walk or stand. Typically, the pain stops when you sit down or bend forward.*

Spinal stenosis can be the result of changes that occur with arthritis or of a congenital narrowing of the spine that causes compression at the lower end of the spinal canal.

Understanding the Problem. If you have these symptoms, your health-care provider will conduct a physical examination and may order a computed tomography (CT) scan to determine whether the spinal canal is narrowed.

Treatment Options. When pain is persistent and severe, spinal surgery to relieve the pain and pressure may be necessary.

FIBROMYALGIA

The symptoms of this disease are widespread aches, pains, and stiffness; fatigue, often in conjunction with insomnia and disturbed sleep pattern; headaches; and a tingling sensation in the muscles.

If you have fibromyalgia (also called *fibromyositis* and *fibrositis*), you may think you have the flu but without an accompanying fever. The cause of this poorly understood disorder isn't known, although emotional stress may increase its risk, and deep-sleep (stage IV sleep) disturbances or interruptions may cause a flare-up. Underused muscles may also be a contributing factor. Typically, the stiffness is worse with inactivity.

Fibromyalgia is most common in women between twenty and fifty, although it can strike men as well and at any age.

Understanding the Problem. No one test can confirm or exclude fibromyalgia, so your physician will need to do a thorough history, examination, and even laboratory tests to exclude other diseases before making this diagnosis.

Although a chronic condition, fibromyalgia is neither progressive nor a serious health threat.

Treatment Options. Treatment involves changes in life-style. Sometimes it may be as simple as taking aspirin for the pain and buying a firmer mattress. Daily exercise, hot baths, and elimination of stress whenever possible also may be helpful. Antidepressant drugs such as amitriptyline, which increase stage IV sleep, may be prescribed. (Regular sleeping pills, on the other hand, interrupt deep sleep, worsening fibromyalgia.)

Skin Problems

CONTENTS

If the pictures Janet and the rest of us see in magazines are to be believed, American women have no shortage of perfect complexions. Whether peaches and cream or burnished ebony, the skin that is held up to us as ideal is poreless and pimple-free, as empty of lines and creases as a fresh sheet of fine stationery. Never mind that the women who possess such skin are almost as rare as winter roses in a backyard garden.

A more common scenario is the one Janet sees every time she looks in the mirror. In her midthirties, Janet, with her fair complexion, is already beginning to see the effects of too much sun. In the last couple of years, imperceptible lines have evolved into deep crinkles around her eyes. The skin on her cheeks is dry and slightly rough, especially during the winter. And around her period, her chin erupts with pimples that seem much worse than the ones she remembers from her teenaged years. Although Janet's skin is not as terrible as she sometimes thinks, it's a long way from where she'd like it to be.

It wasn't always like that. In childhood, a woman's skin, the organ that protects the body's vital organs and serves as a heat regulator, is close to perfection. Most young children have healthy, beautiful skin that is neither dry nor oily. Unfortunately, those days are over for most of us with the advent of the hormonal roller coaster we know as puberty. As a result of increased oil production, three out of four teenagers have some degree of acne. Interestingly, acne also is a common problem among women in their thirties and forties, many of whom did not have pimples during their teenaged years. Add to the equation years of sun exposure—a skin's worst enemy—and the natural aging process during which skin loses its elasticity and begins to sag, and you can see what skin is up against.

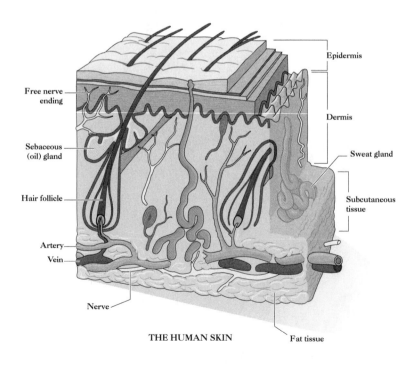

THE HUMAN SKIN

Not that your skin isn't prepared for some amount of abuse. Skin is a remarkably resilient material. It has to be to stand up to the rigors of day-to-day life.

Skin is composed of three layers: the visible layer, called the *epidermis*, which lies along the *dermis*, and the *subcutaneous tissue* beneath. Every square inch of skin contains millions of cells, nerve endings, oil and sweat glands, and hair follicles, as well as a complex network of blood vessels that provide nourishment.

The outer layer of your skin is constantly being replenished. Every month new skin cells move upward to the skin's outer surface, where they become smaller and change into a protein called *keratin*. When you wash your face, these cells flake off, revealing fresher-looking skin, and the process begins again. The skin's middle layer, the dermis, is a dense bed of strong fibers that give strength and elasticity to the skin. With age, the dermis becomes thinner and the skin more transparent.

The deepest skin layer, the subcutaneous tissue, is composed mainly of fat through which blood vessels and nerves run. The source of your skin's oil and sweat glands is found in this layer. Like the dermis, this component of the skin also thins as the body ages.

The appearance of the skin is to a large degree influenced by heredity. Some people are simply genetically programmed to have clear, beautiful skin, just as others inherit shapely legs or perfect teeth. If you have an olive or dark complexion, for example, chances are your skin will not show the ill effects of sun exposure as readily as the fair skin of a woman like Janet. Conversely, if acne runs in your family, you too may have a tendency to have this skin condition.

If you feel shortchanged by heredity, take heart. Although it isn't possible for a middle-aged skin to look the way it did before adolescence, great strides have been made in the treatment of skin disorders that detract from appearance; cosmetic surgery (see page 162) also offers a variety of skin treatments, should you feel more extreme measures are needed.

In this chapter we will explore some common skin problems and ways in which the conditions can be treated to improve the appearance and health of the skin. Most of these problems, although unsightly and uncomfortable, do not pose a real risk to your overall health. The exception is skin cancer, which we also will discuss. Since proper care is a crucial element in both keeping your skin safe from skin cancer and preventing premature aging, we will address ways to protect yourself from the sun's damaging rays.

ACNE

If you have acne, you will see blackheads on your face, neck, shoulders, and/or back. You will have pimples on the surface of the skin or boil-like cysts under the skin.

Acne is an unsightly and often stubborn ailment that affects three out of four teenagers and many women in their thirties and forties. Although acne typically occurs in people with oily skin, some women with dry skin will have pimples, sometimes the result of using too much moisturizer or oily cosmetics on the skin.

The specific cause of acne is unknown, although we know it can be influenced by increased sebaceous (oil) gland activity, which in turn may be influenced by stress, hormonal changes, increased sweating, genetic factors, and, in rare instances, diet.

Understanding the Problem. In normal skin, oil or sebum is secreted by sebaceous glands contained in the skin's hair follicles. The oil then travels to the surface of the skin. In a person with acne, the sebum, along with dead skin cells, clogs the pores. When this occurs, the oil solidifies and forms a white plug. If this blockage occurs deep beneath the surface of the skin, the pore is closed off and a whitehead forms. When it is near the surface, the top of the plug becomes dark, hence the name *blackhead*.

Pimples occur when the oil in the pores reacts with bacteria. Pimples can occur near the surface or deep down below, where larger cysts or lumps can form. These sometimes lead to scarring.

The course of acne varies. Some people are plagued from early adolescence well into adulthood, and others may only have a problem for a short time. Many girls and women notice an acne flare-up prior to their period but are not bothered the rest of the month. Others may have constant breakouts.

With the exception of cystic acne, most pimples will not leave permanent scars on the skin. Acne can, however, damage self-esteem and confidence, especially in young people.

Treatment Options. If your acne is mild, you may want to try treating it at home before you see a doctor. The first step is finding the right soap or cleanser, one that removes dirt and oil without overdrying the skin. Use only moisturizers or cosmetics which are labeled oil-free or noncomedogenic; in order to prevent secondary infection or scarring, do not pick or squeeze pimples. Avoid abrasive scrubs that can cause inflammation and worsen acne.

You might want to try benzoyl peroxide, an over-the-counter cream or lotion that kills the bacteria inside the pores and peels the skin's surface, thus helping to open clogged pores. In the past, many women have been discouraged with this treatment because they found it dried out the skin, leaving it chapped and red. Rather than the 5 to 10 percent concentrations that are most commonly found, a 2.5 percent dose of benzoyl peroxide is now available and may be preferable. Moreover, do not apply the solution immediately after washing your face, when the pores are open and your skin is especially vulnerable to irritation. Wait twenty minutes or so before applying benzoyl peroxide.

If this treatment is going to be successful, you should notice improvement after three weeks of morning and evening application. You can then graduate to a higher-strength product if your skin is not irritated.

MEDICATION. Although the previously mentioned treatments are often successful in improving mild acne, many people have a more persistent or severe acne problem that requires the expertise of a dermatologist.

For the treatment of acne, dermatologists may prescribe an oral antibiotic such as tetracycline or minocycline in order to reduce the number of bacteria in the skin. The antibiotics have anti-inflammatory effects that also can help reduce acne. Unfortunately, some women experience vaginal yeast infections or stomach pains while using oral antibiotics.

Topical antibiotics in the form of swabs or lotions also are often used. Available by prescription only, topical medicines such as erythromycin kill the bacteria in the skin's hair follicles and are usually used twice a day. The use of combination benzoyl peroxide and erythromycin may reduce the bacterial resistance to erythromycin, which often occurs with topical antibiotics used alone.

Another medication frequently used in recent years is Retin-A, the vitamin A derivative that has enjoyed widespread publicity as a possible treatment for lines and wrinkles caused by too much sun exposure.

Retin-A works by forcing the follicles to empty their oil and accumulated cells and debris and avoid the formation of blackheads. If your doctor suggests Retin-A, you will be instructed to use a pea-sized amount after you wash your face at night. Retin-A can, however, be very irritating and drying to the skin in the first weeks of treatment, making it extremely important that you use small amounts (a pea-sized quantity will do your entire face). Also, use a gentle nondrying cleanser or soap on your skin. Your acne will probably worsen initially because Retin-A will bring debris to the surface that was deep in the pores. Women who use Retin-A will also be extremely sun sensitive, so they should always wear a powerful sunscreen and a hat outdoors while using the preparation to prevent sun damage to their skin.

The final drug in the arsenal against acne is Accutane, an oral medication derived from vitamin A. This powerful drug works by essentially shutting down the oil glands. Although it is effective in the treatment of all forms of acne, because of its side effects most doctors prescribe Accutane only in very severe cases such as cystic acne or when other treatments have failed.

Before you consider using Accutane, you should know that studies have shown that as little as one dose of the drug can cause birth defects such as heart disorders and ear and facial abnormalities if used during pregnancy. Thus, most doctors insist their patient have a pregnancy test prior to starting treatment and to be diligent about birth control during the time the drug is taken. There is no evidence, however, that a child conceived after its mother discontinues Accutane is at a greater risk than normal for birth defects. Wait at least one month after discontinuing use of Accutane to attempt pregnancy.

In some cases Accutane users have reported such serious side effects as liver malfunction and blurred vision, although these problems were reversed after the drug was discontinued. More common complaints include extremely dry skin, cracked lips, itching, increased sun sensitivity, peeling of the palms and soles of the feet, and generalized body aches.

Despite its drawbacks, Accutane is amazingly effective against acne. If your doctor recommends this treatment, you will take the drug once or twice a day for up to twenty weeks.

In 60 percent of cases, the acne then disappears for good; 30 percent of Accutane users have marked improvement if not total cure and the remaining 10 percent need another twenty-week course of treatment.

SURGERY. If you have cystic acne, your doctor may have to make a small incision in the skin so the cyst can drain, a procedure that is done in the office, usually without anesthetic. Or, your dermatologist may inject cortisone directly into a cyst to reduce the inflammation and expedite the healing process.

When acne has caused noticeable facial scars, cosmetic surgery is an option. One technique involves the injection of collagen under scars caused by cysts that have destroyed normal tissue. Another is called *dermabrasion*. This procedure uses a motorized wire brush to remove the skin's top layer. A third option is a new technique of laser resurfacing, which also removes layers of skin to improve the appearance of acne scars. Deep "ice-pick" scars may require punch incisions, in which a small hole is made in the skin and dermabrasion or resurfacing is done thereafter.

ACNE AT MIDLIFE

Unlike most of her friends, Roni never had a pimple as a teenager. But now at the age of forty, while most of her peers are lamenting lines and crinkles, Roni has a full-blown case of acne.

"Crow's feet I can handle," Roni says as she sits in her dermatologist's office, "but not this," she says, pointing to her face. "Not zits on top of the wrinkles."

For the first few weeks she tried to ignore the new crop of pimples that blossomed on her chin and forehead. She told herself that it was occurring because she was getting her period or that her job as a securities analyst was unusually stressful that month. But her period came and went, her work slowed down, and although some pimples cleared up, they were soon replaced by the next generation.

She found herself avoiding mirrors, canceling appointments. Finally, she decided the problem wasn't going to go away by itself so she made an appointment to see the dermatologist.

Roni left the doctor's office feeling that maybe her skin wasn't hopeless after all. The doctor, a woman about her own age, reassured her that acne during midlife—probably caused by the body's changing hormones—was a common and very treatable problem among women. She prescribed four medications: a daily dose of the oral antibiotic minocycline, plus a topical antibiotic that Roni uses on her skin twice a day, a mild solution of benzoyl peroxide to use at bedtime, and Retin-A.

A month later when she returned to the doctor, Roni's skin still had a few break-outs—but it had noticeably improved and she was feeling the situation was under control.

BIRTHMARKS

Birthmarks are skin markings that appear before or shortly after birth.

There are many different kinds of birthmarks. Milia, for example, are small white bumps that resemble whiteheads on a newborn's face. Salmon patches or stork bites are collections of blood vessels that appear as flat pink spots on the eyelids, upper lip, and back of the neck in roughly half of all newborns. Hemangiomas are noncancerous tumors made of newly formed blood vessels and may be bright red protrusions that can appear anywhere on the body but often disappear spontaneously. However, purple flat patches, called port-wine stains, are present at birth and are usually permanent.

Treatment Options. Milia, stork bites, and most hemangiomas eventually disappear spontaneously and treatment usually is not necessary. Laser therapy is often used to treat a port-wine stain, preferably in infancy or childhood. They may become deeper as the person ages.

DERMATITIS

A person with dermatitis may have red and itching skin. Blisters may form on the surface of the skin and may weep. You may notice a thickening of the skin, particularly in the folds of the elbows, on the backs of the knees, or around the ankles. Greasy-looking scales may appear on the skin. You may have stubborn dandruff.

Dermatitis is a term used to describe a wide variety of inflammations of the skin. These bothersome and common skin conditions have a variety of causes; the cause determines the symptom.

The following are the most common types of dermatitis:

CONTACT DERMATITIS. This common form of dermatitis is caused by contact with a substance to which you are sensitive. One irritating substance that causes contact dermatitis in almost anyone is poison ivy. But many other substances cause reactions only in highly sensitive people. For example, you may have a skin rash every time you use makeup on your skin. The most common causes are fragrances and preservatives.

NEURODERMATITIS. This skin condition is caused by repeated scratching at a site that becomes thickened and extremely itchy as a result of the constant rubbing. It is characterized by red patches that are thickened from constant scratching.

ATOPIC DERMATITIS. Atopic dermatitis, also called *infantile eczema*, typically begins in infancy as scaling and redness, usually within body folds, that produces an intense itching sensation. Atopic dermatitis frequently runs in families. Most children tend to outgrow it as they move through adolescence, but it can persist into adulthood. People with this skin problem often have allergies such as asthma, nasal congestion, and hives.

STASIS DERMATITIS. People with varicose veins or other vascular conditions that reduce the blood supply to parts of the body may experience statis dermatitis. This problem most often occurs in the legs, especially around the ankles, where fluid can accumulate and weaken tissue. When this occurs, the skin can become inflamed, causing itching. In addition, sores, ulcers, and pigmentation (darkening) may form.

SEBORRHEIC DERMATITIS. Greasy scaling, especially in the folds at the sides of the nose, above the bridge of the nose, and over the breastbone, is characteristic of seborrheic dermatitis, a chronic condition that can be controlled but not cured.

Understanding the Problem. Some types of dermatitis can be readily diagnosed during an examination of your skin. However, if your doctor suspects contact dermatitis, he or she will want to determine the source. This can be done with patch testing, during which small amounts of various substances are applied to your skin (typically on your back) and covered with an adhesive. Forty-eight hours later the area is uncovered and examined for signs of a reaction.

Common substances that are often the culprits in contact dermatitis are mild chemicals such as hexachlorophene in soap, acetone in nail-polish remover, and thimerosal in contact lens solution. Antihistamines, antibiotics, plants, rubber, metals, and cosmetics also can cause a skin reaction, even after years of use with no problem.

Dermatitis is not a dangerous condition, but it can be annoying, unsightly, and itchy.

Treatment Options. Treatment will depend upon the cause. For instance, if you have contact dermatitis and tests show that you are allergic to an ingredient in an over-the-counter product, you should simply stop using the product containing the irritant.

In other types of dermatitis, the first step may be to stop the scratching so the skin can heal. Your doctor may recommend a cortisone preparation to reduce the inflammation and itching. Some of these products are sold over the counter; higher-strength formulas can be obtained only with a prescription. For severe itching, an antihistamine also may be prescribed. Frequent shampooing with a medicated shampoo also may be recommended for a person with seborrheic dermatitis.

People with stasis dermatitis may find that using support hose and elevating the legs while at rest improve their symptoms. In severe cases, surgery may be required to resolve sores, ulcers, and underlying vascular problems.

EXCESSIVE HAIR

Excessive hair *refers not to a shining crown of beautiful tresses but to an abnormal amount of facial or body hair. If you have excessive facial or body hair, also called* hirsutism, *you may notice a definite mustache above your upper lip; coarse, dark hair on your chin or cheeks; or an excessive amount of hair on your chest.*

Medical Disorders and Diseases of Women 613

A twenty-seven-year-old store manager, Trudy first experienced hirsutism during puberty, the time when androgen hormones produce a host of physical changes in a girl's body, including the development of pubic and armpit hair. With the same thick black hair and olive pit eyes as her Greek grandparents on her mother's side, Trudy is typical of most women with this problem. Hirsutism tends to be more common among women of Southern European or Middle Eastern extraction, though many women may notice a slight increase in body and facial hair as they age.

Trudy thinks the light growth of hair on her upper lip is unattractive. Yet she, like most women with hair that is considered in excess of our societal norm, is basically healthy and has no chronic hormone imbalance. However, hirsutism can be a symptom of an underlying problem, especially if it occurs suddenly. Adrenal and ovarian tumors or a condition called polycystic ovaries (see page 551) are sometimes responsible for the growth of excessive hair. Drugs such as the antiseizure medication Dilantin, some medications used to treat hypertension, and various medications containing testosterone also can cause a significant increase in body and facial hair.

Understanding the Problem. If you have a sudden increase in your body or facial hair, your doctor will want to rule out a medical problem such as a tumor. The vast majority of women with hirsutism, however, have what is known as idiopathic hirsutism, that is, excessive hair growth due to an unknown cause. Idiopathic hirsutism occurs when the activity of male hormones that are naturally present in women is increased, though the cause of this sudden increase in activity is unknown. Women with idiopathic hirsutism have normal menstrual cycles, healthy reproductive organs, and no signs of tumors or other problems. For them, hirsutism is a cosmetic problem rather than a medical one.

Treatment Options. The treatment of hirsutism depends upon your doctor's findings. If you have a tumor, you may need surgery. In some cases, the problem may be solved by discontinuing a certain medication.

Sometimes drugs are used to treat idiopathic hirsutism. Oral contraceptives may be used to suppress male hormone levels. Oral contraceptives can be dangerous when used by smokers over the age of thirty-five, but the solution is to stop the cigarettes, not the pills.

Oral contraceptives are the preferred method of decreasing the growth of new hair, but do not affect existing hair. Depending upon the location of the unwanted hair, popular methods for removal include plucking, shaving, bleaching, waxing, and electrolysis, the most permanent method of hair removal. Laser removal of hair is becoming a more popular form of treatment of excessive body hair.

HAIR LOSS
Signs of hair loss include small bald batches on the scalp, a general thinning of the hair, a loss of eyebrow and eyelash hair, and sometimes, a complete loss of all body hair.

There are two types of temporary hair loss: the more common gradual hair loss and alopecia areata (patchy hair loss). Permanent hair loss due to a genetic predisposition toward baldness occurs in women as well as men, although female-pattern baldness is rarely as severe as that found in men.

As she ages, every woman notices some hair loss, which is due to hormonal changes that occur as she reaches menopause. Simple wear and tear also plays a role, especially for women who bleach or perm their hair. Illness, poor diet, stress, and use of certain medicines can take their toll on your hair.

For about 2 percent of the population, hair loss is abrupt. These people may have alopecia areata, a condition in which large smooth and painless bald spots (up to three inches across) appear on the scalp. The causes have not been established, but suspected causes are a familial predisposition to hair loss and autoimmune reactions within the body.

Treatment Options. The diagnosis of alopecia areata is easily made because of its unique appearance. Ninety percent of those who lose hair because of alopecia areata have regrowth within two years, but if regrowth does not occur spontaneously, cortisone injections will usually stimulate regrowth.

When female-pattern hair loss is not severe, a change of hairstyle may be enough to give the appearance of more hair. With substantial thinning or bald patches, some doctors may recommend the use of topical minoxidil, which may slow progression of hair loss.

Another option for moderately severe hair loss is hair transplantation, an expensive procedure in which a specialist implants tiny plugs of hair follicles into the bald areas of the scalp. Although the transplanted hair usually falls out within a few weeks, new hair soon grows in to take its place. Several transplantation sessions may be necessary to achieve the results you want.

MOLES

Moles are spots on the skin that can vary in color from flesh-toned to blue or black. Some are smooth, others raised or wrinkled.

Almost everyone has benign skin spots called *moles*, which are actually nests of pigment cells. A small percentage of moles produce malignant melanoma, a deadly form of skin cancer (see page 617), but most are harmless.

Understanding the Problem. It is a good idea to examine periodically your moles for any change in color, size, or shape. If you suspect a mole is changing or if it begins to itch, hurt, or bleed, see your health-care provider. If he or she suspects malignant melanoma, a skin biopsy—a procedure in which a part of the mole is removed after a local anesthetic is injected into the area—will be performed and the tissue analyzed.

The vast majority of moles are harmless and never require removal unless for cosmetic reasons.

Treatment Options. If a mole is being irritated by contact with your clothing or the appearance is objectionable, you can have it surgically removed. This procedure is done in your doctor's office after a local anesthetic is injected into the site.

ROSACEA

Rosacea appears as an inflammation on your cheeks, nose, forehead, and chin. Pimplelike pustules may appear in the reddened areas. Your nose may be red and bulbous.

Rosacea, chronic inflammation of the face, most frequently is found in fair-skinned individuals who blush easily. Women have this condition more often than men, although men are more likely to have a red, bulbous nose. Rosacea can occur at any age. Its cause is unknown, although the symptoms are the result of the enlargement of blood vessels just below the skin's surface.

This ailment is sometimes mistaken for acne and was once called *acne rosacea* because in many cases pimplelike pustules appear in the reddened areas. The pimples associated with rosacea, however, do not stem from blackheads and whiteheads as they do in skin with true acne.

Understanding the Problem. Rosacea can be diagnosed by your health-care provider during a close examination of your skin. Although it does not pose a threat to your physical health, it can damage your self-esteem if not treated.

Treatment Options. Some people have noticeable improvement if they avoid hot or spicy foods, hot drinks, and alcohol, all of which tend to dilate the blood vessels.

Your doctor may prescribe both oral and topical antibiotics to decrease the number of pimples. Gradually, the dose of antibiotic is reduced until it is eventually discontinued without the return of pimples. Laser therapy also is often used to eliminate prominent superficial vessels in order to diminish the red component of the condition.

PSORIASIS

The symptoms of this skin disorder include dry, red, raised often painful bumps with silvery, flaking scales, usually on the scalp, elbows, knees, and buttocks. Other symptoms are itching, cracked skin; bleeding from the scales; loosened and discolored nails; and joint pain and stiffness.

Although the cause of this common, persistent skin disorder is unknown, it appears to have a genetic component.

Normally, new skin cells take about a month to travel from the lowest skin layer to the top layer (the epidermis), where they die and are shed. But when psoriasis is present, the process takes only three or four days; as a result, dead skin cells pile up and form thick scales.

Attacks vary in severity. Some people may have only a few spots on isolated areas; others may be covered with cracked skin, scales, and pustules.

If you have psoriasis, expect your condition to wax and wane. A flare-up may be triggered by a seemingly insignificant skin injury like an insect bite or a minor cut or scrape. Attacks are also triggered by viral or bacterial infections, excessive alcohol consumption, certain medications, stress, a bad sunburn, or cold temperatures. After an attack, many people have periods of remission. Some medications, including some antihypertensives and anti-inflammatories, may worsen symptoms, so check with your health-care provider.

An estimated three million Americans have psoriasis; 100,000 have severe symptoms. The onset of this disease is generally gradual and occurs most often between the ages of ten and thirty-five.

Understanding the Problem. Your clinician will be able to make the diagnosis simply by looking at your skin. A skin biopsy will confirm the diagnosis.

The outlook for people with this disease depends on its severity. There's no cure for psoriasis, and though the symptoms can be treated, it may be painful and hard to live with.

In one in ten people with psoriasis arthritis develops. Another risk is secondary infection during a flare-up. In rare instances psoriasis will cover the entire skin surface; this is a medical emergency requiring immediate treatment.

Treatment Options. Avoid being overweight since psoriasis is aggravated when it occurs in skin folds. Controlled exposure to sunlight may be helpful. Don't scratch, pick, or rub the patches, to prevent thickening them and increasing your risk of secondary infection.

MEDICATION. If you have a mild case of psoriasis, over-the-counter moisturizing creams will prevent dryness, and ointments containing cortisone will relieve symptoms. Bathe with mineral salts or oatmeal to soothe skin. If your scalp is involved, you may need to use a phenol and sodium chloride lotion.

For severe psoriasis, physicians now prescribe the anticancer drug methotrexate to slow the production of skin cells.

PHOTOTHERAPY. When psoriasis is severe, phototherapy at a hospital or clinic may be recommended. This treatment, usually lasting for three weeks, involves sensitizing the skin with a coal-tar ointment and then exposing it to ultraviolet light. Another treatment—PUVA therapy—combines oral medications with ultraviolet A light irradiation.

SKIN CANCER

Molly noticed the tiny white bump on the side of her nose when it began to bleed one morning after she had just washed her face. She at first shrugged off the incident, thinking that she had just been a little rough with her washcloth. The next day one of her third-graders interrupted her lesson on nouns and verbs to tell her that her face was bleeding. When Molly looked in the mirror, she saw the tiny pearly protrusion crusted over with blood.

A week later she sat, stunned, while her dermatologist told her it looked like skin cancer, although he couldn't be sure until the growth was removed and analyzed. A few days later the report came back: Molly did indeed have a "basal cell carcinoma."

All across the country, men and women like Molly are hearing this diagnosis at an unprecedented rate; more than 500,000 new cases are diagnosed each year. The reason? A society that glories in that bronze glow that comes from basking in the sun. Those most at risk are fair-skinned, blue-eyed, blond, or redheaded; people with dark skin have the least chance of development of a skin cancer.

When Molly first was told she had a skin cancer, her thoughts went back to a dear friend who years before had died after a struggle with a virulent form of skin cancer, malignant melanoma. But her doctor quickly reassured her that there are three different basic forms of skin cancer, the most highly curable of which is basal cell, the type that Molly had. The following briefly describes the skin cancers—basal cell, squamous cell, and malignant melanoma—and their treatment and prognosis.

Basal Cell. *This highly curable form of skin cancer accounts for 75 percent of all malignancies and most commonly affects people who, like Molly, are over forty. Basal cell carcinoma occurs in the epidermis, the outer layer of the skin, and is generally found in areas exposed to sunlight.*

This is a slow-growing cancer that rarely spreads to other parts of the body. If neglected, however, it can invade nearby tissues. Basal cell cancer can be cruelly disfiguring if not promptly treated.

Treatment usually involves the removal of the growth, which is done under a local anesthetic in the doctor's office. When treated early, basal cell cancer is 95 percent curable, although those who have this form of cancer may have another lesion at some time or have a recurrence in the area from which the growth was removed.

Squamous Cell. *This cancer develops in the midportion of the epidermis. It may appear as a firm, red nodule or flat lesion with a scaly or crusted surface. Squamous cell cancer may arise from a precancerous tumor called* actinic *or* solar keratosis, *a flat, wartlike lesion caused by the sun. Like basal cell cancer, this form of skin cancer most frequently is found in areas of the body that are exposed to sunlight. It usually occurs after the age of fifty and is more likely to be found in light-skinned people. Squamous cell cancer is more aggressive than basal cell carcinoma and can invade the lymph nodes and internal organs if not treated promptly.*

If you have a squamous cell cancer, the lesion and the surrounding tissue must be removed. Sometimes radiation is used after surgery to prevent the spread of the malignancy. When it is treated early, the cure rate of this disease is about 95 percent.

Malignant Melanoma. *This is the most deadly form of skin cancer, beginning painlessly from cells that produce the skin's pigmentation. An estimated 70 percent of malignant melanoma appears on normal skin; 30 percent arises from an existing mole that has recently undergone changes. Thus, if you have moles, you should have them periodically examined by a health-care professional for signs of color changes, irregular borders, irritation, or growth.*

The incidence of malignant melanoma has doubled in this country in the past twenty years. Again, those most at risk have fair skin that sunburns easily. An important risk factor is a history of blistering sunburns that occurred during childhood or adolescence.

The cure rate of this disease depends upon when it is diagnosed. If caught before it has infiltrated deep within the skin, the cure rate is 85 percent. Once the tumor has spread to the lymph nodes or to other organs, however, the five-year survival rate is only 30 percent.

Doctors say the best way to prevent skin cancer is to protect yourself from the sun. Since her bout with basal cell cancer, Molly, an avid biker and skier, is a convert to that philosophy. These days she won't leave her house without applying a strong sunscreen to her face and other exposed parts of her body. Molly is doing everything she can to prevent another skin cancer.

PROTECTING YOUR SKIN

However wonderful the warm glow of the sun makes you feel, it is your skin's worst enemy. Too much sun exposure will age you prematurely and, worse, increase your risk of eventual development of skin cancer.

Sunlight is made up of different kinds of rays, the most dangerous of which are ultraviolet (UV) rays, which alter the physical and chemical composition of the skin after exposure. There are two main types of UV rays: The more damaging, UV B rays, disrupt certain light-sensitive proteins, setting off a chemical reaction in the blood vessels, which produces sunburn and swells the skin. Moreover, collagen, the substance that gives youthful skin its flexibility and firmness, is damaged, although the effects aren't seen for years. UV B rays are responsible for many of the changes that cause aging and skin cancer. The other culprit, UV A rays, stimulates the production of melanin, the brown color or tan that occurs with sun exposure. This is the skin's way, in fact, of trying to shield itself from the sun. These darker cells travel to the upper layers of the epidermis, the skin's top layer, drying and flaking off. Skin cell growth after sun exposure is sped up in an effort to provide protection, giving the skin a leathery, dry look.

Short of becoming nocturnal, there is no way to achieve 100 percent protection from the sun. Nor would you want to, as the sun also has some health-giving benefits in moderate exposures. The following should allow you to enjoy the outdoors and keep your skin safe.

1. Wear a sunscreen every day, year-round. Some people make the mistake of thinking a sunscreen is only necessary for days when they are basking at the beach. Although it is true that the summer sun's rays are stronger and thus more damaging, your skin is still exposed to damage on a winter afternoon spent playing in the snow or taking a walk.

2. Select the best sunscreen for your needs. Sunscreens work by absorbing the harmful rays. They are rated with a sun protection factor number (SPF). Most doctors recommend that everyone use a sunscreen with at least an SPF of 15. This is a means of comparing sunscreens. An average person using SPF 15 could be in the sun about three hours without burning. Sunscreen must be applied twenty minutes before exposure and reapplied often. Use a generous amount of sunscreen for each application. Keep in mind that most sunscreens need to be reapplied often if you are perspiring or after swimming if they are not waterproof. In addition to the SPF, also read the label carefully to make sure the product blocks both UV B and UV A rays. Some are effective against UV B rays only.

3. Wear a large hat when you are in the sun. Beach umbrellas, clothing, and shade also help protect your skin.

4. If you feel you must sunbathe, try to do it before 10:00 a.m. or after 2:00 p.m., when the sun's rays are the least dangerous.

5. Be aware that some medications increase your sun sensitivity, making it more important than ever that you take steps to protect yourself. Some sleeping pills, pills for high blood pressure, oral contraceptives, antibiotics, and Retin-A make your skin especially vulnerable to sun damage.

Medical Tests

CONTENTS

It is difficult to imagine the practice of modern medicine without the plethora of diagnostic tests that have helped take some of the guesswork out of diagnosing disease.

Years ago, a cancer might have been growing in a woman's breast for years before even the experienced fingers of her health-care practitioner could detect it. Today, mammography is saving lives by identifying tiny tumors years before they can be felt by the most practiced of hands.

The major incision required for some pelvic surgeries has been replaced to a large degree by a wound small enough to be covered by a Band-Aid. Thanks to laparoscopy, a procedure that uses a fiber-optic instrument inserted into the abdomen through a small incision, gynecologists now can clearly see the pelvic organs, search out disease, and even carry out some surgeries.

And modern-day scanning technology such as computed tomography and magnetic resonance imaging has moved giant steps beyond the capacities of the ordinary X ray.

In this section, we will discuss the various type of diagnostic tests health-care practitioners use to help identify and locate problems. Some, such as routine blood tests and Pap smears, are done in the absence of symptoms, simply as a precaution. Others—biopsies, X-ray scans, and tests on the reproductive system—are usually reserved for women with symptoms or when other tests indicate a possible problem.

Some of the tests we will describe are invasive, requiring that the interior of your body be penetrated by an instrument. Invasive tests are necessary when your clinician must see the organ or when a biopsy—the removal of a piece of tissue—is necessary. Noninvasive tests produce an indirect view of the inside of your body. An ultrasound, for example, is noninvasive.

Keep in mind that some diagnostic tests carry the possibility of side effects, although most don't pose a serious threat. As with all elements of health care, you, with the guidance of your provider, must weigh the potential benefit of any procedure against its potential risk.

BIOPSIES

A biopsy is the removal of a sample of tissue, which is then sent to a laboratory and analyzed for the presence of disease.

Most biopsies are done using a needle, a scalpel, or a special tool inserted through fiber-optic instruments used to examine the windpipe, lungs, gastrointestinal tract, or other organs.

After tissue samples are extracted, most are chemically treated and sliced into thin sections, which are then placed on glass slides and stained to provide contrast.

Breast Biopsy. If you have a lump in your breast or an abnormal mammogram finding, your health-care provider will recommend a breast biopsy, the definitive step in determining whether you have breast cancer.

A mammogram is taken prior to the biopsy to help identify any suspicious areas in the breasts. Then the biopsy is usually performed under a local anesthetic on an outpatient basis. A wedge of breast tissue is removed and then examined by a pathologist for cancer cells. Some clinicians use a needle to withdraw cells from the tissue instead of making an incision in the breast, although the findings of this method may be inconclusive.

If your health-care provider recommends a breast biopsy, do not automatically assume the worst. Of all fifty-year-old women who have biopsies, only about one woman in five has breast cancer.

Cone Biopsy. A cone biopsy, also called *conization*, is a surgical procedure in which a cone-shaped section of the cervix is removed for diagnosis or treatment.

A cone biopsy would probably be recommended if, for example, you have abnormal areas on your cervix that cannot be adequately examined by your practitioner during a colposcopy (see page 548). Conization also is used diagnostically to determine whether a precancerous cervical change (see below) has spread beyond the surface of the cervix, if a small sample of tissue taken from the cervix is normal yet a woman's Pap smear result contains abnormal cells, or if a standard biopsy sample of the cervix contains abnormal cells.

As a treatment, conization is often used to eradicate cervical intraepithelial neoplasia (CIN), a condition in which premalignant changes occur in the cervical lining. If you are of childbearing age and have a cervical cancer that has only superficially infiltrated the underlying tissue, conization rather than a hysterectomy could be used to remove the cancer, and you would retain the ability to have a child. Women who opt for conization for the treatment of early cancers, however, must have frequent follow-up examinations.

Conization is performed with a scalpel, laser, or electrocautery instrument that both cuts and cauterizes blood vessels.

Conization is usually done as an outpatient procedure in the hospital with anesthetic; some practitioners prefer a light general anesthetic, and others anesthetize only the pelvic region. After the anesthetic takes effect, a colposcope—an instrument that allows the clinician to see the cervix under magnification—is placed in front of the vagina. The practitioner then removes a cone-shaped section of the cervix that includes the abnormal area. The section will be analyzed and the extent of disease determined. Occasionally, absorbable sutures are sewn into the cervix to reduce blood loss.

Many women experience minor bleeding after a cone biopsy that may last several days or even a week or two. After this procedure, you may want to take it easy for a couple of days, although many women feel well enough to return to work the next day. As for long-term risks, in some women who have this procedure an incompetent cervix develops, making it difficult to support a pregnancy to term.

Endometrial Biopsy. Endometrial biopsy involves removing a sample of the uterine lining, the endometrium.

Several situations might require this test. If, for example, you and your partner are unable to conceive a child, an endometrial biopsy can help determine whether you are indeed ovulating. Another indication for this procedure is abnormal bleeding that cannot be explained. An endometrial biopsy may also be done to confirm a chronic uterine infection.

An endometrial biopsy is often done in an office setting, usually without an anesthetic, although some clinicians will give you a local injection to prevent pain. The test, although not intensely painful, will cause your uterus to cramp for a couple of minutes while the instrument is in place. A small sample of tissue is then suctioned by a syringe or portable pump.

Most women have no complications after an endometrial biopsy. The major problem associated with this procedure is a perforated uterus, which occurs in about one or two women out of every thousand who have the biopsy.

Endometrial biopsy is more than 90 percent accurate in diagnosing cancer of the endometrium. However, if you continue to have unexplained bleeding after an endometrial biopsy, your clinician may recommend a dilation and curettage (D & C) and/or hysteroscopy (see pages 539 and 542) to identify the source. In some instances, hysterectomy is required to stop the bleeding.

Bone Marrow Aspiration and Biopsy. During a bone marrow aspiration, a teaspoon of marrow—the spongy material that serves as the production site of most of your body's blood cells—is withdrawn through a slender sleeve of metal. A bone marrow biopsy involves the removal of a small, solid core of intact marrow. The procedures are often done at the same time.

Examination of the marrow sample obtained through either procedure will determine whether you have a blood disorder such as leukemia.

A bone marrow aspiration or biopsy can be done in an office, laboratory, or hospital. Prior to the procedures, a local anesthetic is injected into the area from which the marrow will be removed, typically from the back of the pelvic bone.

During the test, you will feel pressure when the needle punctures your skin. As the marrow is being removed, most people feel a deep pain in the bone, but this ends in a matter of seconds. The procedure itself takes only a few minutes. After the needle is withdrawn, the wound is covered with a bandage. The area may be tender and bruised for several days; in rare instances, bleeding after the procedure may also occur.

Liver Biopsy. A liver biopsy is done when your symptoms suggest that you may have a liver disease such as cirrhosis, hepatitis, or cancer.

Prior to a liver biopsy, you will be instructed not to eat or drink for several hours. The test, which is usually done in the hospital as an outpatient procedure, is performed after the area of your lowest right rib is sterilized and anesthetized with a local injection. While you lie on the examining table, you will be asked to take a deep breath and hold it. The clinician then inserts the needle into your liver. Once the needle reaches its target, it is rotated and withdrawn a few seconds later with a sample of liver tissue. The tissue is then sent to a laboratory for analysis.

After a dressing is placed on the wound, you will be put to bed for three or four hours and your vital signs monitored periodically. If during this time you feel light-headed, tell your health-care provider. This could be a sign of internal bleeding. Some people feel some discomfort from the procedure and may require a mild analgesic. However, most people have no complications and are able to go home within a few hours.

Lung Biopsy. In this procedure, a fiber-optic flexible tube called a *bronchoscope* enables your health-care provider to search your airways for tumors, foreign objects, or other abnormalities. The practitioner can then use the instrument to remove a sample of lung tissue for analysis.

You will be told not to eat or drink for at least six to twelve hours prior to the bronchoscopy. Typically, fiber-optic bronchoscopy is performed in the hospital on an outpatient basis. Most clinicians administer a local anesthetic through the nostrils or mouth to depress your cough and swallow reflexes. Many providers also give a sedative to help you relax.

After you are relaxed, the bronchoscope is inserted through either your nose or your mouth. As the tube is inserted, the provider watches on a small television screen as the tube progresses down the windpipe and into the smaller airways. After the airways have been thoroughly examined and a sample of tissue taken, the bronchoscope is withdrawn.

Most people report no pain with fiber-optic bronchoscopy, and there are rarely complications after this procedure. However, to prevent choking you should not eat or drink until the anesthetic wears off and you regain normal swallowing and cough reflexes.

Biopsy of the Colon. The best way of examining the colon or large intestine is with a colonoscope, a thin fiber-optic tube that can be threaded up the five-foot intestine, sometimes even into the lower length of the small intestine.

Colonoscopy may be recommended if you have blood in your stool, pain during bowel movements, bloody diarrhea, altered bowel habits, or abdominal pain or simply to rule out cancer, especially if you have a family history of colon cancer. In some cases, a colonoscopy is done after an X-ray result indicates an abnormality.

During the colonoscopy, your provider is looking for polyps, ulcerations, or abscesses that may indicate ulcerative colitis, or signs of cancer. In the course of the procedure, the health-care practitioner will remove tissue samples for analysis. In some cases, the problem itself can be treated during the colonoscopy. For instance, if your clinician finds polyps, he or she can remove them.

Prior to having this procedure, you will be given dietary instructions and a laxative to take the night before so that your intestine will be empty for the exam. Before the test begins, you will be given a sedative to relax you during the somewhat uncomfortable procedure. The procedure requires only a matter of minutes to complete.

Although hemorrhage and perforation of the colon can occur during colonoscopy, these complications are rare.

BLOOD TESTS

Of all the tests that health-care practitioners use to rule out or help diagnose disease, blood tests are the most common and certainly the easiest from most patients' standpoint.

A small amount of blood contains a remarkable number of indicators of a person's state of health. By studying the results of your blood work, your health-care provider can gain valuable insight. Depending upon the particular test ordered, blood can indicate whether or not your kidneys are functioning properly, whether your liver is diseased, whether an infection is brewing somewhere in your body, whether there is a dangerous level of fats in your blood, whether a woman who seems unable to become pregnant is indeed ovulating, and much more.

Blood samples are usually taken during a routine physical examination or when there are specific symptoms. Some tests such as the one that measures the blood level of fats require an overnight fast, but most need no advance preparation. Blood samples may be analyzed in your provider's office or in a medical laboratory.

Blood can be drawn from several spots. If only a drop or two is needed, it is usually squeezed from your finger after the skin is stuck with a tiny sharp instrument. Many tests, however, require at least a full syringe of blood, which is taken from a vein, typically one in your forearm. After the nurse or technician selects the vein, he or she cleans the area with alcohol and then inserts the needle. Blood passes through the needle and into an attached tube. If several blood tests are ordered, additional tubes are subsequently attached to the needle, so it isn't necessary to repeat the puncture.

There are hundreds of tests that can be performed on your blood. The following are some of the most common.

Complete Blood Count. An important part of any complete checkup is the complete blood count (CBC), a test that counts each type of blood cell in a given volume of your blood and looks for any abnormalities in the size and shape of your blood cells.

This blood test measures the amount of hemoglobin (the substance that ferries oxygen throughout the bloodstream), the percentage of red blood cells, the number and kinds of white blood cells, and the number of platelets.

An abnormal CBC result is often the first clue that a person has a health problem such as anemia, an infection, or leukemia.

Blood Chemistry Group. This test, which may be used in various combinations, includes an analysis of electrolytes, blood sugar (glucose), a series of liver function tests, tests for kidney function, and a measurement of albumin, a protein in the blood.

Lipids. To determine whether you may be at risk for coronary artery disease, your health-care provider may test the lipids or fats in your blood. A lipid test provides measurements for cholesterol, high-density lipoprotein (HDL) cholesterol, and triglycerides. If your measurements are higher than normal, your clinician may recommend a low-fat diet, more exercise, or certain medications to help bring the numbers into the normal range.

Erythrocyte Sedimentation Rate. In diagnosing certain illnesses, sometimes it is necessary to know the rate at which red blood cells settle to the bottom of a container. In such instances, an *erythrocyte sedimentation rate*, also called a sed rate or ESR, will be performed on your blood sample.

If the cells settle faster than is considered normal, your health-care provider will want to investigate further to determine whether you have an infection, inflammation, anemia, rheumatoid arthritis, rheumatic fever, or even malignancy.

Maternal Serum Screening. If you are pregnant, your state of health has an impact not only on you, but on your developing fetus. Thus, it is important from the onset for both you and your health-care provider to know whether you have any problems that could adversely affect the outcome of your pregnancy.

One way to determine whether you have a preexisting condition that could cause a problem or that calls for special measures during your pregnancy is the maternal serum screening, a blood test that is usually given at the first or second prenatal visit.

The maternal serum screening provides your provider with key information. Blood type, an Rh factor profile (see page 301), blood count, antibodies in the blood, and presence of a sexually transmitted disease are just some of the information gleaned from this important test.

From this information, your clinician can tailor your prenatal care to fit your special health needs. For example, if the test shows you to be Rh-negative, meaning you lack the Rh component in your blood, you need to have regular blood tests throughout your pregnancy to ensure that your body is not producing antibodies that might harm your developing fetus.

Thyroid Studies. If you have symptoms suggestive of a thyroid problem, your health-care practitioner will order tests that measure blood levels of certain hormones such as thyroxine and thyroid-stimulating hormone.

Enzyme Tests. An enzyme test determines whether you have abnormal levels of particular enzymes in your blood that indicate damage to the liver, pancreas, heart, or another organ.

When these organs are functioning properly, enzymes are found only in minute quantities in the blood. However, when an organ is damaged by disease, enzymes can leak out into the blood. The result is an abnormally high enzyme level, which will help your provider pinpoint the source of your problem.

PRENATAL TESTING, MONITORING, AND OTHER PROCEDURES

A generation ago, a pregnant woman could do little more than wait—and wonder whether she would give birth to a healthy baby. Today, prenatal testing has taken some of the guesswork out of pregnancy. You'll still have to wait and see whether your child inherited your red hair or your partner's dimples. But if you have a family or personal history of certain diseases, or you have reached the age when your risk of bearing a child with a genetic abnormality is higher, you may want to consider some prenatal tests.

Amniocentesis. As many women delay pregnancy well into their thirties and even forties, prenatal testing has become an important component of obstetrics because of the increased risk of chromosome problems in babies born to older mothers.

A test that can provide valuable information on fetal development is amniocentesis, a procedure that many health-care providers offer pregnant women, particularly those over the age of thirty-five and those who have a family history of Down's syndrome or spina bifida. Amniocentesis can also be done in the last trimester of pregnancy to determine whether the baby's lungs have sufficiently developed to allow for early delivery in the event of a pregnancy complication.

The developing fetus floats in a pool of fluid that contains valuable clues to health. The fluid contains fetal cells, as well as protein, fats, enzymes, carbohydrates, hormones, and fetal urine, which make it an ideal testing fluid. Amniocentesis involves removing a small amount of the fluid from the amniotic sac. Cells in the fluid are then grown in a laboratory and examined for abnormalities. Amniocentesis is most often used to detect Down's syndrome, but more than a hundred different tests can be carried out on the fluid samples, each for a different birth defect. Examination of the cells also reveals the baby's sex, which is important if you have a family history of disorders such as hemophilia or muscular dystrophy.

If you and your partner decide on amniocentesis, the test typically will be scheduled between your fifteenth and eighteenth weeks of pregnancy, though the procedure can be done as early as twelve weeks. Less than one woman in two hundred has a miscarriage as a result of the procedure.

The test is usually performed in the hospital or doctor's office on an outpatient basis. The first step after you arrive is an ultrasound so that your health-care provider has a road map to guide him or her in placing the needle. The clinician then inserts the needle, which is about the diameter of a needle used to draw blood from your arm but much longer since it has a greater distance to travel to reach its target. After the fluid is drawn and the needle removed, the small wound is covered with a bandage and you are free to leave.

The procedure takes only ten to fifteen minutes to perform and is not painful. Some women notice that their abdomen is tender around the needle site for a day or two after the procedure.

What is more difficult for most women than the procedure itself is waiting to learn the results, which are not available for up to four weeks. The vast majority of women get good news. But if there is something wrong, you and your partner then are faced with deciding whether to continue with the pregnancy or abort the fetus.

Alpha-fetoprotein Analysis. Alpha-fetoprotein (AFP) is a protein produced by the baby's liver which passes into the mother's blood via the placenta. When a woman is about sixteen weeks pregnant, her physician can take a routine blood sample and measure the amount of AFP in her blood.

The physician expects to find a certain level of AFP in the sample, a sign that the fetus is developing normally. However, a high level suggests a number of possibilities. A miscarriage may be imminent, or the mother may be carrying twins. Very high levels of AFP suggest the possibility of neural tube defects such as spina bifida, a condition in which the vertebrae do not fuse, leaving the spine open. An unusually low amount of the protein may indicate the possibility of Down's syndrome or another chromosomal abnormality.

Many health-care practitioners recommend their patients have the test. However, the test results are not absolute but are expressed as statistical probabilities. Thus, some couples prefer to avoid the anxiety that certain results might produce. If an AFP blood test comes back with a reading that suggests a low risk of neural tube disorder, for example, your infant in all likelihood will not have one. On the other hand, an abnormal AFP concentration does not necessarily mean that there is something wrong with your child. The first thing to remember is that these disorders are relatively rare; neural tube defects occur in only one or two babies out of one thousand. Yet fifty out of every one thousand women tested appear to be at higher risk. This sometimes is due to the fact that the pregnancy is more advanced than was initially suspected, or the woman is carrying twins (multiple births automatically raise the AFP level).

If the AFP level is high, the test will have to be repeated. If the result of a test conducted on another blood sample is also abnormal, your provider will order an ultrasound examination to see whether a defect can be found. If there is still no evidence of a problem, he or she will offer you amniocentesis. For a low AFP level, repeating the test is of no benefit, but an amniocentesis may be recommended to evaluate for chromosomal abnormalities.

Chorionic Villus Sampling. Chorionic villus sampling, like amniocentesis, is a prenatal test used to determine whether the fetus has certain genetic abnormalities. This test, however, has the advantage of being done in the early weeks of pregnancy.

During the first trimester of pregnancy, the products of conception do not fill the uterine cavity as they will later. The embryo is establishing its home inside the sac of membranes, while the outer membrane, the chorion, is branching in treelike structures throughout the uterine cavity. In later weeks, these villi will form the placenta. Although the membrane is not part of the fetus, it does contain fetal tissue, so analyzing it can divulge a wealth of information. The test gives the same information as amniocentesis, including the gender of the fetus, and appears to offer the same degree of accuracy.

Chorionic villus sampling involves the removal of a small amount of this villus material, which can be studied and the cells examined for evidence of chromosomal abnormalities.

As with amniocentesis, the most likely candidate for this procedure is a woman over the age of thirty-five or one with a family history of Down's syndrome or other genetic abnormalities.

During this procedure, the clinician uses an ultrasound to enable him or her to guide a catheter or small tube into your cervix or a needle through the abdomen. Villi are located and a syringe is used to suck material into the catheter.

The main advantage of this procedure over amniocentesis is that it can be done earlier in pregnancy. Then, if there is a problem with the fetus, abortion at this stage of pregnancy is generally much safer and less traumatic.

However, chorionic villus sampling is not as effective as amniocentesis in detecting some disorders. And, in some cases, a clinician will recommend a woman have amniocentesis if the findings of a chorionic villus sampling are questionable, so you may end up having two tests instead of one.

As for the safety of this invasive prenatal test, women who have chorionic villus sampling have a small risk of miscarriage, but the risk is somewhat greater than for those who opt for amniocentesis.

Fetoscopy. During fetoscopy, the health-care practitioner uses a long, thin scope inserted into the abdomen to view the fetus. A fetoscopy allows the clinician to look for abnormalities, obtain samples of fetal blood and skin for analysis, perform liver biopsies, and even do some corrective surgical procedures.

The technique used for this test is similar to that of amniocentesis, except that the fetoscopy needle is thicker. After the needle is passed through the abdomen and into the amniotic cavity, the scope is inserted through the needle. Miniature surgical instruments also can be manipulated within the fetoscope.

This procedure, although useful in detecting some defects, is not perfect. Sometimes the amniotic fluid is so cloudy that it is difficult to see the fetus. Then, too, the field of view is limited, so that the clinician can see only small parts of the fetus at any given time.

Fetoscopy is not without its risks. About 5 percent of women who have fetoscopy miscarry after the test. Moreover, there is a risk of infection.

In recent years, improvements in sonography and deoxyribonucleic acid (DNA) analysis have substantially reduced the need for fetoscopy. Thus, most providers do not recommend this test unless there is a good chance that a fetus has a congenital problem that cannot be diagnosed through other means.

REPRODUCTIVE AND UROLOGICAL TESTS

A multitude of diagnostic tests are available to help health-care practitioners see and, in some cases, correct defects in the reproductive and urological organs. Many of the following tests have become routine in both the diagnosis and treatment of infertility.

Hysterosalpingogram. If you are having difficulty getting pregnant or carrying a pregnancy to term, a hysterosalpingogram (HSG) may be part of your diagnostic workup.

The hysterosalpingogram is an X-ray technique that involves the injection of contrast material through the cervical canal. Problems such as fallopian tubes blocked by scar tissue and uterine malformations are likely to be uncovered with this examination. You should not have this procedure, however, if you have a pelvic infection or vaginal bleeding, are pregnant, or are allergic to iodine.

Although HSG is not new technology—the test was first described in 1914—recent refinements have both reduced radiation exposure and allowed for more precise imaging. A hysterosalpingogram can be performed in a radiology laboratory, hospital, or office setting.

If your health-care provider recommends a hysterosalpingogram, you will be asked to lie on an examining table and place your feet in stirrups, just as you would during a routine pelvic examination. A speculum is then inserted into your vagina and an instrument is attached to your cervix. The health-care practitioner then injects a contrast material (liquid dye) through a small tube into the uterus and fallopian tubes, after which X rays are taken. During the test, you will be able to see your reproductive system on a television screen as the contrast dye highlights your organs. If, for example, your tubes are blocked, the obstruction will be visible because the dye will not be able to continue up the tube.

This test is typically uncomfortable as the dye infiltrates your uterus. After the procedure, some women have cramps, nausea, dizziness, and/or a bloody vaginal discharge, but these symptoms generally pass quickly. Complications, though rare, can be serious and include pelvic infections, uterine perforation, and allergic reactions to the contrast material.

Colposcopy. When a Pap smear finding indicates premalignant cells on the cervix, the next step is often a test called a *colposcopy.*

During this office procedure, the gynecologist uses a magnifying instrument to examine the cervix carefully for signs of premalignant cells or an actual cancer of the cervix. This test also may be used in the evaluation of women whose mother took the female hormone diethylstilbestrol (DES) during pregnancy, because these DES daughters are at an increased risk for developing vaginal and cervical cancers.

A colposcopy is performed while you are lying on the examining table with your feet in stirrups. A speculum is inserted into the vagina to hold open the vaginal walls; the colposcope is then placed in front of your vagina. Using this magnifying instrument, the clinician is able to view clearly the surface of the cervix for signs of disease. He or she then will remove tissue from suspicious areas. This biopsied tissue is examined in a laboratory to determine the extent of disease and ultimately the recommended treatment.

During this procedure, you may have some minor bleeding, but that will be stopped before the instrument is removed.

Cystourethroscopy. Cystourethroscopy, which allows the heath-care provider to see inside your bladder and urethra, is used to evaluate bladder control problems, recurring urinary tract infections, painful urination, chronic inflammation, and symptoms that indicate a possible bladder cancer.

Cystourethroscopy is a relatively simple procedure that can be performed in your clinician's office. You will remain awake during it, although your provider may inject a local anesthetic into the urethra to make you more comfortable. A tiny tube, the cystourethroscope, is then threaded up your urethra and into the bladder. On the end of the tube are a special lens and fiber-optic lighting system that allow the examiner to see clearly the structures through which the cystourethroscope passes.

Through the lens on this device your clinician may observe that a structural abnormality in the bladder itself, for example, is contributing to your high incidence of infection. Or the cystourethroscope may reveal a bladder stone.

In some cases, the provider may remove a sample of tissue during the procedure for biopsy to aid in the diagnosis of your problem.

Hysteroscopy. Hysteroscopy was reportedly first used in 1869 to remove a polyp from the lining of a woman's uterus. Today, this relatively simple method of visualizing the inside of the uterus has become increasingly used in both the diagnosis and treatment of disease.

The procedure involves the insertion of a long, hollow-tubed instrument into the vagina and up into the cervix. The hysteroscope has a fiber-optic light and a channel for inserting various surgical instruments.

If you have recurrent abnormal bleeding or a history of miscarriage, are having difficulty getting pregnant, or have had an abnormal hysterosalpingogram finding, you may be a candidate for this procedure.

When hysteroscopy is used as a diagnostic tool, it is usually performed in the health-care provider's office or in the hospital. After you have undressed and put on a gown, you will be given an injection to numb your cervix or a mild general anesthetic. The hysteroscope is then inserted into the cervix. A gas or liquid is pumped through the instrument to distend the uterine cavity, to allow the clinician to do a more thorough examination of the uterus.

Hysteroscopy also is used in the surgical treatment of uterine disorders. Using the hysteroscope as a guide, the clinician can remove intrauterine devices, endometrial polyps, and benign tumors. Lasers can be directed through the hysteroscope to vaporize abnormal uterine tissue.

Most women who have a hysteroscopy have no complications after the procedure. However, potential problems include abnormal bleeding, pelvic infection, and uterine perforation. If you are pregnant or have a pelvic infection, you should not have this test.

Laparoscopy. In the past twenty-five years, few things have had as profound an effect on the practice of gynecology as laparoscopy, the outpatient surgical technique that allows clinicians to view the female reproductive organs through a small incision in the abdomen.

Prior to the 1970s, when this technique came into increasing use, most gynecological surgery had to be performed through a major surgical incision in the abdomen (laparotomy), requiring a significant hospital stay and recuperation period. Today, many of those same conditions can be both diagnosed and treated with laparoscopy, which usually requires only a brief hospital stay and minimal recuperation time.

Laparoscopy may be recommended to evaluate chronic pelvic inflammatory disease or endometriosis, two conditions that could cause infertility. Women who have pelvic pain for which no obvious cause can be found also often undergo this procedure.

Laparoscopy can be used to perform sterilization; to remove ectopic (tubal) pregnancies, adhesions, cysts, and benign tumors; to recover lost intrauterine devices; to take a biopsy sample of abnormal tissue; and to treat endometriosis.

If your health-care provider recommends that you have a laparoscopy, the procedure may be done in the hospital or in an outpatient surgical center. You will be instructed not to eat or drink for the eight hours prior to the procedure. Your anesthetic will depend upon the surgeon, but most practitioners prefer a general anesthetic.

After the anesthetic takes effect, the gynecologist will make a small incision in your abdomen. Although techniques vary, often a needle is then inserted and your abdominal cavity inflated with carbon dioxide. The laparoscope, a long metal tube with a lens and light, is then inserted, allowing the clinician a direct view of your reproductive organs. When surgery is indicated, the surgical instruments can be manipulated through additional small incisions.

After the procedure, your vital signs will be checked for several hours before you will be allowed to go home. You may have some pain and discomfort, but in most cases that should disappear within a couple of days. Most women who have diagnostic laparoscopy are able to return to work in one or two days; those who have surgery with the laparoscope may require a longer recuperation, depending upon the specific problem. However, recovery time is significantly shorter than it is with the traditional laparotomy.

As in any surgery, there can be complications with laparoscopy, although they are relatively rare. Lacerated blood vessels, injuries to the intestines, or cardiovascular problems that stem from inflating the abdomen with gas sometimes occur.

Dilation and Curettage. In this minor gynecological procedure, the cervix is dilated and an instrument is inserted to scrape or vacuum the lining from the uterus. A D & C is commonly performed when a woman has unexplained heavy bleeding. It is also a useful tool in diagnosing uterine and cervical cancers.

A D & C also may be used to treat certain problems. Some uterine polyps, for example, can be removed by this procedure. If your health-care practitioner suspects you have endometrial hyperplasia, a condition that occurs when the uterine lining grows too thick and that in some cases has the potential eventually to become cancerous, he or she may scrape your endometrial lining, to establish clearly the diagnosis.

This technique is also commonly used after a miscarriage to remove any leftover products of conception from the uterus.

If you have a problem that warrants a D & C, the procedure may be done in your gynecologist's office with a local anesthetic. Some clinicians, however, prefer to hospitalize their D & C patients and use a general anesthetic so that the pelvic muscles are completely relaxed, allowing for a more complete examination.

After the anesthetic takes effect, the gynecologist begins gradually to dilate the opening to your cervix, using a series of tapering rods, each one thicker than the last. After the opening is sufficiently enlarged, the provider may insert into the cervix a long, thin, spoon-shaped instrument called a *curette* to scrape the uterus; alternatively, a low-pressure vacuum aspiration device can be used to aspirate the endometrial tissue.

After a D & C, expect to have some bleeding from the vagina for a few days. Many women also have cramps or lower back pain. Most, however, feel fine within a couple of days.

Although you can resume your normal activities as soon as you feel well enough, you should not have intercourse or use tampons until cleared to do so by your clinician.

The Pap Smear. Perhaps one of the easiest medical tests a woman can and should have is the Pap smear, a simple scrape of your cervical cells taken during the annual gynecological checkup.

Few people will argue that the Pap smear has played a major role in the fight against invasive cervical cancer. Since the early 1940s, when this test became widely used as a screening tool, the death rate from cervical cancer has dropped 70 percent because the Pap smear can detect precancerous changes at a stage when they are almost always curable.

A Pap smear is typically done during the annual pelvic examination. During the examination, the clinician uses a wooden spatula, brush, or cotton swab gently to scrape cells from the surface of your cervix and from the cervical canal itself. The cells are then sent to a laboratory for analysis.

A negative result means that the cells are normal; an abnormal test result may not mean anything definite. Do not be alarmed should your health-care practitioner's office call you to report an abnormal Pap smear finding. This does not necessarily mean you have cervical cancer or even a precancerous condition. In some cases, all that may be necessary is a follow-up Pap smear. Or your provider may recommend a biopsy or a procedure called a *colposcopy* (see page 548).

You should be aware also that the Pap smear is not infallible. There is a low percentage of false-positive and false-negative results.

Who should have this test and how often? Clinicians recommend that women begin having Pap smears after they become sexually active or by the age of eighteen.

How often you should have a Pap smear depends upon whom you talk to. Annual Pap smears used to be recommended; however, concern over the cost-effectiveness of widespread screening programs has led some medical groups to modify their recommendations. The National Cancer Institute (NCI), for example, now recommends a Pap smear every one to three years for low-risk women between the ages of thirty-six and sixty. For women over the age of sixty who have had two consecutive negative Pap smear results, the NCI suggests there is no further need for testing. The American Cancer Society's recommendation for women under the age of sixty is similar, except that it endorses annual Pap smears for women thought to be at high risk for cervical cancer. These include women who had intercourse before the age of eighteen and those who have had many sexual partners.

Discuss with your health-care practitioner your Pap smear schedule. Because the test is relatively inexpensive, virtually painless, and potentially lifesaving, many clinicians still recommend yearly Pap smears for their patients.

Pregnancy Testing. Your period is late and you've been feeling a little funny. Could you be pregnant?

The best way to know for sure is to have a pregnancy test. Long before your provider can diagnose pregnancy with a physical examination, a simple test of your urine can detect the presence of human chorionic gonadotropin (hCG), a hormone the fertilized egg begins to secrete when it is four days old. The hormone spreads in body fluid to tissue throughout your body. Initially it is at its highest level in the blood, but within a few days it also can be detected in the urine.

Most women these days have a urine test to determine pregnancy, either at the clinician's office or with a home pregnancy test. These tests depend upon a reaction between the hCG and an anti-hCG antibody. A second reaction then takes place to determine whether the first reaction has occurred. This usually involves a color change.

Home pregnancy test kits have become increasingly popular in recent years. They have been simplified so that they are relatively easy to use. They also allow a women to find out within minutes in the privacy of her own home whether or not she is pregnant. It is important when using a home pregnancy test, however, to follow the instructions to the letter. Moreover, to increase your chances of getting an accurate reading, be sure to "catch" your first urine of the day because it is more highly concentrated than subsequent voiding.

What kind of track record do urine tests have in predicting pregnancy? The earlier the pregnancy, the greater the risk of a false-negative result from a urine test. If, for example, your period is four to seven days late, about three fourths of the time a urine test done in your health-care provider's office will detect pregnancy. Two weeks after a missed period, the detection rate rises to close to 100 percent. Home pregnancy tests have about a 95 percent accuracy rate ten days after a missed period.

Most pregnancies are diagnosed with a urine test because a blood pregnancy test is more expensive and takes longer. There are, however, times when the more accurate blood test is necessary. For instance, if a woman is being monitored for a miscarriage or tubal pregnancy, her hCG level may increase more slowly than normal. Only the blood test will measure the absolute level and permit comparisons to be made over time.

SCANS AND X RAYS

Although basic X rays have long been in use, newer scanning techniques are allowing clinicians to delve deeper into the body's mysteries without so much as lifting a scalpel, pinpointing areas of disease that in another time would have been missed. Moreover, this noninvasive procedure often eliminates the need for riskier invasive procedures.

Computed Tomography. Computed tomography, better known as CT scanning, provides detailed pictures of soft body tissues. Many times more sensitive than a conventional X ray, the CT equipment produces an ultrathin X-ray beam that shoots through the body from various angles. Different tissues absorb varying amounts of the beam. The intensity of the beam that emerges from your body is then measured by an X-ray detector. A computer then receives and analyzes the information, measuring the beam's penetration and using the data to produce a three-dimensional composite in which body tissues appear in varying shades of gray. Bone, for example, appears white on the image; air shows as black.

Using this composite, the radiologist can create individual cross sections or slices of tissue to be displayed on a screen for examination or in photographic images. These cross sections of tissue reveal significantly more information than does a standard X ray.

CT scanning has revolutionized the diagnosis of central nervous system disorders. In gynecology, a CT scan might be used to detect a suspected pituitary gland tumor and to determine the extent of a malignant tumor in the pelvis. Sometimes it can also help distinguish benign from malignant tumors.

CT scans can be done in the hospital or in an outpatient radiology center. Before the scan, a contrast medium or dye may be injected into your vein or given orally or rectally. Because some dyes contain iodine, you will be asked before the test whether you are allergic.

You will lie on a movable table, which is guided into the center of the CT scanner, a machine shaped like a doughnut. While you remain still, the machine rotates and X rays are beamed through the designated segments of your body. After this painless procedure, you will be able to go home and return to your normal activities.

Magnetic Resonance Imaging. Magnetic resonance imaging (MRI) uses magnetism and radio waves to produce a similar image to that of the CT scan.

This safe and painless procedure relies on the creation of a magnetic field after the patient is put into the MRI machine. Within the tunnel-shaped machine, the switching on and off of the magnetic field causes the nuclei of atoms to produce energy. The response depends upon the type of body tissue and its water content. An energy detector then measures the responses of the atoms, and the data are analyzed by a computer, which creates a photograph that can be broken down, slice by slice, by the examining radiologist.

MRI is especially useful for producing images in the brain, where soft and hard tissue meet; in the spinal cord; and in parts of the body affected by stroke. Because the MRI clearly delineates the brain's white and gray matter, it is often used to diagnose nerve fiber diseases such as multiple sclerosis. In gynecology, MRI is frequently used to identify malignant tissue and certain congenital reproductive defects and to evaluate the anatomical characteristics of the vagina. Magnetic resonance imaging is more accurate than CT scans in evaluating the spread of uterine and cervical malignancies.

MRIs can be done on an outpatient basis, either in the hospital or in a radiology center. This test, like the CT scan, sometimes includes the injection of a contrast material. After you have undressed and put on a gown, you will be asked to lie on a movable bed, which then passes into the access tube, an enclosed area where the test is done. The procedure may take as long as an hour.

Although this is a totally painless and noninvasive test, many patients complain of feeling claustrophobic inside the enclosure. However, the inside of the tube is well lit and you can hear and speak to the technician during the test.

Mammogram. The mammogram is a special breast X ray that can detect early cancers of the breast, in many cases years before they will ever be felt.

Who should have mammograms and how often? Because breast cancer is rare in women under the age of thirty-five, most providers do not recommend mammograms for their patients before that age unless they have a family history of the disease.

Around the time you turn forty, your clinician may recommend a baseline mammogram, an X ray to be kept on file for comparison purposes in the future. Most women in their forties are advised to have a mammogram every year or two. Beyond the age of fifty, providers recommend an annual test because the risk of developing this disease increases as you age.

Your mammogram will be done as an outpatient procedure, either in the hospital or in a radiology center. After you have disrobed and put on a gown, you will be asked to stand in front of a special X-ray machine. The technician will then help you place your breast on a shelf that projects from the machine. Another shelflike projection is then lowered on top to compress the breast; compression is important because dense areas of breast tissue must be spread apart so that any hidden cancers can be found. X rays are then made and the procedure is repeated on the other side. In most centers, you will learn the results within a few days after the test.

You may be concerned about your radiation exposure during the procedure. Improvements made in recent years in the equipment have enabled radiologists to decrease substantially the amount of radiation during a mammogram and few experts will disagree that the benefits of this test greatly exceed the risks of radiation exposure. Improvements in imaging techniques have also made the test more accurate than ever, although a mammogram is not infallible; occasionally the test will miss a tumor or indicate a problem where none exists.

A mammogram can be uncomfortable because of the breast compression. To help minimize discomfort, do not schedule your test just before or during your period, when your breasts may be more tender.

Ultrasonography. Another common imaging technique is ultrasound, which uses acoustic waves to create an image of internal organs.

Studies have shown this diagnostic method to be safe for both mothers and their developing infants, and as a result this painless and noninvasive technique has had a major impact on the practice of obstetrics. Today, an ultrasound—also called a *sonogram*—is commonly used to evaluate the gestational age, size, position, and growth rate of the fetus.

An ultrasound also is useful in detecting abnormalities in the unborn and in identifying a multiple pregnancy. If there is a question about whether the fetus might be growing in your fallopian tube instead of the uterus, your clinician may recommend an ultrasound. This simple procedure also is frequently used to investigate unexplained vaginal bleeding, lack of menstrual flow, and abdominal pain and can locate a misplaced intrauterine device and differentiate between solid tumors and cysts. Ultrasonography also is a valuable tool in infertility studies.

Ultrasonography uses a wandlike device called a *transducer* to produce and receive high-frequency sound waves. These sound waves, too high for you to hear, pass into your tissue and then are reflected. The reflected waves are interpreted by a computer and are then displayed as images on a video screen. To the untrained eye, these images may bear little resemblance to body organs. Photographs are then made so that the images can be studied by the radiologist.

If your health-care provider recommends an ultrasound, you will be given instructions on how to prepare for the examination, which will vary, depending upon what part of your body is being studied. If, for example, you need an abdominal ultrasound, you may be told not to eat or drink for twelve hours prior to the test, whereas a pelvic ultrasound sometimes requires that your bladder be full to elevate the uterus and ovaries and provide an acoustic window for the sound waves.

During the brief exam, which may be done in a clinician's office, radiology center, or hospital outpatient department, you will lie on a table, where a technician will apply a gel-like substance over the area to be studied. The transducer is then passed back and forth across the lubricated area and the pictures made.

After the test, you will be able to go home and resume your normal activities.

Glossary

Abdominoplasty. Plastic surgery performed on the abdomen. Also known as a "tummy tuck."

Abortion. The termination of a pregnancy before the fetus becomes viable, by extraction or natural expulsion.

Abscess. A localized collection of pus.

Adenomyosis. Invasive but benign growth of the *endometrium* (the inner surface lining of the uterus) into the muscle wall of the uterus.

Adenosis. The disease of a gland. See also *Vaginal adenosis.*

Adhesion. Abnormal tissue that binds organs together. Also the meeting and knitting of two tissue surfaces, as in wound healing.

Adoption. The legal assumption of responsibility for rearing a child who is not one's own.

Adjuvant. A substance that enhances or hastens the action of another ingredient in a medicine or a second therapy designed to increase the effectiveness of the first.

Adrenal glands. The pair of glands found over each kidney that produce a variety of hormones including epinephrine, norepinephrine, and the corticosteroid hormones.

Aerobic. That which requires oxygen to live. Aerobic exercise does not exceed the body's ability to the tissues being exercised.

Afterbirth. The placenta and membranes used to nourish and contain a fetus during gestation, which are expelled from the uterus very shortly after childbirth.

Agoraphobia. Overwhelming anxiety about being in public places.

AIDS. Acquired immunodeficiency syndrome. The series of infections that occur as the last stage of infection by the human immunodeficiency virus (HIV).

Alcoholism. The uncontrollable need to drink alcohol on a regular basis.

Alopecia areata. Loss of hair in patches, usually on the scalp.

Amenorrhea. The absence or cessation of menstruation. This occurs normally as a result of pregnancy, lactation, or menopause; and abnormally as a result of surgery or problems of the reproductive tract, systemic diseases, emotional disorders, endocrine disorders, or hormonal imbalances.

Amniocentesis. A test to determine fetal maturity and some abnormalities. A sample of amniotic fluid is extracted from the amniotic sac, using a long needle inserted through the abdomen, for later laboratory analysis.

Amniotic fluid. The liquid that surrounds and protects a developing fetus in the womb.

Amniotomy. Rupture of the fetal membranes to induce or expedite labor.

Anaerobic. That which does not require oxygen to live, such as certain bacteria. In exercising, vigorous bursts of activity that exceed the oxygen supply and thereby create a growing oxygen deficit are termed *anaerobic.*

Anemia. A decrease in circulating red blood cells.

Anesthesia. Partial or total loss of sensation and sometimes consciousness, usually caused by the administration of an anesthetic agent. In some cases the agent can be administered to a localized area either topically or by injection, causing loss of sensation to only that area. In general anesthesia, the entire body is anesthetized using injected and/or inhaled drugs.

Aneurysm. The localized swelling or bulging or a blood vessel, usually an artery, which forms a sac.

Angina pectoris. Chest pain and feeling of constriction about the heart caused by a temporary loss of oxygen, via the blood supply, to the heart.

Angioma. A benign tumor formed principally of blood vessels or lymph vessels.

Angioplasty. The altering of a blood vessel either by surgery or the insertion of a balloon inside the artery.

Anorexia. Loss of appetite.

Anorexia nervosa. A psychiatric disorder characterized by severely restricted caloric intake. Usually found in girls twelve to twenty-one years old but can occur in older women and men. The condition can result in severe weight loss and even death.

Anovulation. Lack of ovulation.

Antibiotics. A broad group of medicines that inhibit or destroy bacterial microorganisms.

Antibody. A protein of the immune system that destroys or controls foreign substances (*antigens*) and thus protects against common infections.

Antigen. A substance foreign to the body that triggers the production of antibodies.

Antihistamine. Any of a number of drugs that oppose the action of histamine in the body.

Anxiety. A feeling of uneasiness, apprehension, worry, or dread.

Aorta. The principal artery in the body; it carries blood from the heart and distributes it to a series of smaller arteries that carry the blood on to other parts of the body.

Apgar score. A system of scoring an infant's physical condition one and five minutes after birth. The tests, named for the anesthesiologist Virginia Apgar, assign points for heart rate, muscle tone, respiration, response to stimuli, and color. The Apgar score is used to determine whether an infant needs immediate medical intervention such as help in breathing (ventilation). The score does not predict future health or intellect.

Areola. The pigmented area surrounding the nipple of the breast.

Arousal. Alertness; also the state of sexual excitement.

Arrhythmia. Irregular heartbeat.

Arterioles. Small arteries that carry blood from larger arteries to capillaries.

Arteriosclerosis. The term, now infrequently used, for various conditions in which the walls of arteries become thickened, hard, and less elastic, often making them less able to circulate blood freely.

Artery. Major blood vessel that carries blood from the heart to other tissues of the body.

Arthroplasty. The surgical repair or replacement of a damaged or diseased joint.

Artificial insemination. The placement of semen into the vagina or cervix by means other than intercourse.

Aspiration. The withdrawing of fluids or objects by suction from the nose, throat, or lungs; also the breathing of fluids or objects into the nose, throat, or lungs.

Asthma. A condition of airway constriction characterized by coughing, wheezing, and difficult breathing. Usually a consequence of inhaled allergens or infection of the respiratory tract.

Asymptomatic. Without symptoms.

Atherosclerosis. The accumulation of fatty plaques on the walls of arteries; the usual cause of arteriosclerosis. See also *Arteriosclerosis*.

Atrophic vaginitis. Vaginal inflammation due to low estrogen level, often after menopause.

Atrophic vulvar dystrophy. Ailment now more generally known as *lichen sclerosis*, a chronic skin disorder characterized by itchy flat white areas found in the genital and anal area.

Atrophy. Wasting of tissue, often caused by disease or lack of use.

Autoimmune response. The immune system's reaction to a perceived foreign substance, the result of which is production of antibodies against one or some of the body's own tissues.

Bacteria. Any of a class of microscopic organisms, some of which are beneficial to biological processes, and some of which cause disease.

Bacterial vaginosis. Inflammation of the vagina associated with overgrowth of several different kinds of bacteria.

Barbiturates. A group of drugs used as sedatives that depress the nervous and respiratory systems.

Bartholin's gland. A small mucus gland located near the vaginal opening.

Basal cell carcinoma. A skin malignancy that rarely spreads.

B cell. Lymphocyte found in the bone marrow that produces antibodies to fight infection.

Benign. Harmless.

Biopsy. A testing procedure involving the removal of a small piece of tissue for microscopic examination.

Bipolar disorders. Psychiatric disorders, the most common example of which is manic-depressive illness, in which a person suffers wild mood swings from euphoria to deep despair.

Blepharoplasty. Plastic surgery performed on the eyelid.

Blood pressure. The pressure placed on the walls of the arteries.

Bloody show. Release of the mucus plug at the opening to the vagina, often before the onset of labor.

Boil. A skin abscess.

Bone marrow. The soft material that fills bones and that is the site for blood cell formation.

Braxton Hicks contractions. Intermittent painless uterine contractions that occur in pregnancy. Often misunderstood as signs of labor.

Breech position. A fetus presenting bottom down instead of head down.

Bulimia nervosa. A psychiatric disorder characterized by binge eating, followed by purging through self-induced vomiting and diarrhea, excessive exercise, strict dieting or fasting, and an abnormal concern about weight and body shape.

Bypass surgery. A procedure to circumvent an obstructed artery by installing an alternate route for blood.

Cancer. The broad term for various diseases characterized by uncontrolled growth of tissues to form tumors. In some forms the tumors are self-contained; in others they can spread to various other parts of the body.

Carbohydrates. A group of chemical compounds including sugars and starches found in cereals, grains (and thus breads and pastas), fruits, and vegetables.

Carcinogen. A cancer-causing substance.

Cardiac. Relating to the heart.

Cardiopulmonary. Relating to the heart and lung.

Cardiovascular. Relating to the heart and blood vessels.

Carpal tunnel syndrome. A condition of the hand and wrist characterized by a sensation of pain, numbness, tingling, or prickling of the thumb, index finger, ring finger, and palm of the hand and into the arm, caused by pressure on a nerve.

Cerebral. Relating to the brain.

Cervical cap. Contraceptive device of flexible material that serves to cover the uterine cervix, the neck of the uterus.

Cervicitis. Inflammation of the uterine cervix.

Cervix. The neck of an organ, such as the uterus.

Cesarean birth. Also known as *cesarean section*; a procedure in which a baby is surgically removed from the womb through an abdominal incision.

Chancre. A hard ulcer that can be the first sign of syphilis. May appear almost anywhere on the body. See *Syphilis.*

Chancroid. A nonsyphilitic but highly infectious venereal ulcer.

Chemotherapy. Treatment of disease using chemicals that have a direct effect on the diseased cells or on the disease-causing organism. Commonly used in treating cancer.

Child abuse. Neglect or inadequate physical care and supervision of children (including lack of food, clothing, or supervision; inadequate medical care; and psychological remoteness from children); may also involve physical, emotional, and sexual abuse.

Chlamydia. A group of bacteria that cause a variety of illnesses, including venereal infections passed between men and women. These infections, if left untreated, can cause infertility in women. See *Pelvic inflammatory disease.*

Cholesterol. Fatlike substance formed in the liver and found in foods of animal origin. Cholesterol is distributed to the blood, brain, and liver and can be deposited on the walls of arteries as a result of being carried in the blood. It is important in the formation of sex hormones. Some forms of cholesterol contribute to heart disease when large amounts are consumed over a long period.

Chorionic villus sampling (CVS). An early test to determine the chromosome count of a fetus in which a sample of cells of the outer portion of the membranes surrounding the fetus is removed using a catheter inserted into the cervix or a needle in the abdomen.

Chronic fatigue syndrome. An illness of unknown origin characterized by severe, prolonged exhaustion. Symptoms include mild fever, sore throat, unexplained muscle weakness or pain, generalized fatigue for at least a day after normal exertion, headache, and certain neuropsychological symptoms including depression, forgetfulness, intolerance of light, severe irritability, inability to concentrate, and sleep disturbance.

Claudication. Cramping of the calf muscles during exercise, caused by inadequate blood flow.

Climacteric. The gradual ending of a woman's reproductive ability at the conclusion of which, over several years, a woman no longer menstruates.

Clitoris. The highly sensitive erectile organ of a woman's genitals.

Coitus. Sexual intercourse between a woman and man in which the man inserts his penis into the woman's vagina.

Coitus interruptus. Coitus in which the penis is removed before ejaculation. An ineffective contraceptive method.

Collagen. A fibrous protein found in connective tissues of the skin, cartilage, bone, and ligaments.

Colles fracture. A fracture of the forearm just above the wrist, displacing the hand backward and outward. Common in patients with osteoporosis.

Colon. The large intestine. It connects the small intestine to the anus and completes the digestive processes begun in the small intestine, extracts water from undigested food, and stores waste for excretion.

Colostrum. The liquid produced by a new mother's breasts for the first few days after childbirth, before true lactation begins. It contains quantities of protein, calories, antibodies, and lymphocytes, all beneficial to a baby.

Colposcopy. The direct examination of vaginal and cervical tissues for abnormal growth using a colposcope, a device with a magnifying lens.

Condom. A thin sheath worn over the penis during sexual intercourse to prevent pregnancy and the spread of venereal disease.

Cone biopsy. A surgical procedure to test for disease in the cervix, in which a cone-shaped slice of the cervix is removed and analyzed. The procedure is done in a hospital with the patient under anesthesia.

Congestive heart failure. A disease characterized by edema and shortness of breath caused by the heart's inability to pump efficiently.

Contraception. The prevention of pregnancy.

Contraindication. The presence of a circumstance that makes a form of treatment unacceptable.

Coronary. Pertaining to the blood vessels that supply the heart.

Coronary artery disease (CAD). A narrowing of the arteries that supply blood to the

heart, creating an inadequate supply to the myocardium. Usually caused by atherosclerosis.

Corpus luteum. Body formed from the follicle once ovulation has occurred; it secretes estrogen and progesterone.

Cryotherapy. Use of cold in treatment of disease.

Curette. A spoon-shaped device used for removing tissue from the uterus, such as polyps, and specimens for diagnosis.

Cushing's syndrome. A disease caused by the extra production of certain adrenal hormones.

Cyst. A closed sac or pouch that contains fluid.

Cystitis. Inflammation of the bladder.

Cystocele. Bulging of the bladder against the roof of the vagina, sometimes causing incontinence; often a consequence of childbirth.

Cystourethroscopy. Examination of the bladder and urethra using a cystoscope, a device inserted through the urethra into the bladder.

Cytology. The study of cells.

D & C. See *Dilation and curettage.*

DTs. See *Delirium tremens.*

Delirium. A state of mental confusion characterized by disorientation, hallucination, and often disordered speech.

Delirium tremens. Also known as acute alcohol withdrawal, this disorder is a complication of alcoholism and is characterized by some or all of the following: restlessness, irritability, confusion, trembling, convulsions, hallucinations, and constant and nonsensical talking. The autonomic nervous system can become overactivated, producing fever, heart arrhythmia, and profuse sweating.

Depression. Illness characterized by altered mood that produces sadness, hopelessness, and loss of interest in the normal pleasures of life such as food, sex, friends, hobbies, work, or entertainment. Symptoms include changes in eating and sleeping patterns, fatigue, feeling of being unable to think or concentrate, feeling of worthlessness, excessive or inappropriate guilt, and frequent thoughts of death or attempted suicide.

Dermabrasion. A surgical procedure of abrading the skin using sandpaper or other mechanical implements. Used for removing acne scars, birthmarks, tattoos, or fine wrinkles of the skin.

Dermatitis. Inflammation of the skin.

Dermis. The second layer of skin. See *Epidermis.*

Diabetes mellitus. A chronic disorder characterized by an excess of glucose in the blood. The two major forms of the disorder are known as type 1 (insulin-dependent), in which a person secretes little or no insulin, and type 2 (non-insulin-dependent), in which insulin is produced, but it cannot be properly used by the body. Type 1 requires the daily injection of insulin; type 2 may be controlled through diet and other means.

Diaphragm. A cup-shaped contraceptive device made of plastic or rubber that fits over the cervix.

Dilate. To expand an organ or orifice.

Dilation and curettage. A surgical procedure in which the cervix is expanded (dilated) and then the uterine wall is scraped.

Dilation and extraction. A surgical procedure in which the cervix is expanded and a fetus and its surrounding membranes are removed.

Dilator. Any of a number of mechanical devices used to stretch an organ such as the cervix.

Domestic abuse. Physical attacks, verbal abuse, threats, humiliation and intimidation, withholding of support and care, destruction of personal property, and psychological and emotional abuse by a partner.

Donovanosis. A venereal disease characterized by tumors or growths, initially painless, in the genital area. Also known as *Granuloma inguinale.*

Dysfunction. Abnormal or impaired function.

Dysmenorrhea. Pain associated with menstruation.

Dyspareunia. Painful sexual intercourse.

Dysplasia. The abnormal growth of tissue.

Dysthymia. Chronic mild form of depression.

Dysuria. Painful urination.

Eclampsia. A life-threatening condition that can occur from the twentieth week of pregnancy through the first week after delivery, the symptoms of which include hypertension; protein in the urine; swelling of the legs, feet, and face; severe headaches; spots before the eyes; stomach pain; nausea; convulsive seizures; and coma. Usually the result of untreated preeclampsia. See *Preeclampsia*.

Ectopic pregnancy. A misplaced fertilized egg, often in a fallopian tube.

Edema. A swelling of body tissues.

Effacement. The thinning of the cervix during labor to allow dilatation for passage of the baby.

Ejaculation. The discharge of semen during male orgasm.

Electrocautery. The destruction of tissue by heat from an electric source.

Embolism. Obstruction of a blood vessel, usually by a blood clot, but can also be caused by an air bubble, fat, collection of tissue, or other foreign entity.

Embryo. The stage of human development between conception through the tenth week after fertilization.

Endocarditis. Inflammation of the endocardium, the inner lining of the heart.

Endometriosis. Formation of endometrium at a site other than the lining of the uterus.

Endometrium. The tissue that lines the uterus, which is shed each cycle and which serves as the nesting place for a fertilized egg.

Enterocele. A protrusion of small intestine through the wall of the vagina.

Enzyme-linked immunosorbent assay (ELISA). A test for determining the presence of certain antigens, antibodies, or hormones in the body. Often used in testing for HIV antibody.

Epidermis. Superficial layer of skin.

Epidural anesthesia. A procedure often used during labor in which a local anesthetic is injected into the space that surrounds the spinal cord (the epidural space), thus numbing the body below the waist.

Epilepsy. A recurrent disorder in which brain neurons suddenly discharge abnormally, altering consciousness and often producing convulsions.

Episiotomy. An incision made in the tissues around the vaginal opening (perineum) toward the end of labor to prevent them from tearing and to enlarge the opening and ease delivery.

Estrogen. Female sex hormone responsible for development of secondary sex characteristics and cyclic changes such as menstruation and pregnancy. Men produce a small amount of the hormone.

Fallopian tubes. The two ducts, one on each side of the uterus, that convey the eggs from the ovaries to the uterus.

False labor. Irregular uterine pains and contractions that mimic labor, but that do not dilate the cervix.

Family practitioner. A physician who provides comprehensive medical care for each member of a family.

Fats. A group of compounds composed of fatty acids that serve as sources of stored energy for the body, insulation of tissue, protection of certain organs, and help in normal growth and development. Fats also make food taste and smell good, thus leading to overeating, causing a variety of increased risks for cancers and cardiovascular disease.

Fertility. The state of being able to reproduce or conceive a child.

Fertilization. The process of union in which the ovum and sperm meet to conceive an embryo.

Fetal alcohol syndrome (FAS). Birth defects due to a mother's alcoholism during pregnancy. May include slowed growth and mental deficiency.

Fetoscopy. A procedure for examining a fetus in the womb using a fiber-optic device inserted in the womb.

Fetus. The developing infant from the third month of gestation to birth. See also *Embryo*.

Fibrocystic breasts. A common condition of the breast characterized by lumps that fluctuate in size and tenderness with the menstrual cycle.

Fibroid. The colloquial term for *leiomyoma*, a common benign tumor found in the uterus.

Flooding. A method of treating an anxiety disorder by repeatedly exposing a person to an especially feared object or situation until it no longer produces anxiety.

Follicle. A small secretory sac or gland of the ovary, hair, skin, and intestine. Ovarian follicles produce the hormone estrogen.

Fontanel. Either of the two soft spots on an infant's head where the skull bones have left a gap.

Forceps. A surgical instrument used for grasping.

Foreplay. A couple's fondling of one another for sexual stimulation immediately before intercourse.

FSH. Follicle-stimulating hormone. Hormone secreted by the pituitary gland during the menstrual cycle that causes the development of ovarian follicles, which in turn release an egg.

G-spot. Possible spot on the vaginal wall that, when stimulated, produces a fluid from the urethra at the time of orgasm. The term comes from the initial of the last name of the first researcher who worked on a study in the 1980s.

Galactorrhea. Milk flow from the breast unrelated to nursing an infant.

Gamete intrafallopian transfer (GIFT). A surgical procedure in which an ovum is extracted from a follicle, examined, and paired with sperm; then both are placed in the fallopian tube, where they can unite naturally.

Genitals. The female and male reproductive organs.

German measles. See *Rubella*.

Gestation. The time between conception and birth, in humans an average of forty weeks.

Gestational diabetes. Diabetes that develops in about 2 percent of pregnant women who previously had no diabetes. It usually can be controlled by diet, often disappears at delivery (although it may dispose a woman to later development of diabetes), and poses little risk to a fetus when properly managed.

Gingivectomy. The removal of gum tissue.

Gingivitis. Inflammation and tenderness of the gums, most often caused by poor dental hygiene.

Gland. An organ that secretes substances to be used elsewhere in the body.

GnRH. Gonadotropin-releasing hormone. A hormone that induces release of FSH and LH.

Gonorrhea. A contagious venereal disease caused by the bacterium *Neisseria gonorrhoeae* and characterized by painful urination; urethral, vaginal, or penile discharge; and abdominal tenderness. Many women have no symptoms or symptoms that are very mild. Disease can be treated with antibiotics and prevented by the use of condoms.

Gout. Hereditary form of acute arthritis usually marked by inflammation and pain in the knee or foot (usually the great toe), that is caused by excessive uric acid level in the blood.

Granuloma inguinale. A venereal disease characterized by granular tumors felt as painless nodules in the genital area. Can be treated with antibiotics.

Group practice. A collection of physicians of one or more specialties who share office space and billing.

Gynecology. The study of the diseases related to women's reproductive organs, more generally the study of women's reproductive health.

Hammertoe. The condition in which any toe but most often the second one becomes bent and painful. The toe assumes a clawlike appearance.

Harassment. Continual annoyance and intimidation by someone that impede normal functioning of another person.

Heart attack. The common term for myocardial infarction: the interruption of blood to a part of the heart caused by a blockage of one of the coronary arteries. Myocardial infarctions are painful and sometimes fatal.

Heberden's nodes. Hard nodules on the joints of the fingers; one of the visible manifestations of arthritis of the fingers.

hCG. Human chorionic gonadotropin. A hormone secreted by a fertilized human egg, which can be found in urine; in pregnancy tests, this hormone is often the first sign of conception.

Hematoma. A collection of blood under the skin or in an organ caused by a broken blood vessel.

Hemorrhage. Severe or abnormal internal or external bleeding.

Hemorrhoid. Mass of swollen veins in and around the anus that can cause discomfort from itching, pain, and bleeding.

Hepatitis. Inflammation of the liver, caused by viral or bacterial infection, or physical or chemical agents. Symptoms include fever, jaundice, and enlarged liver.

Hepatitis B. Inflammation of the liver caused by the hepatitis B virus. Today, children are routinely inoculated against this form of hepatitis.

Hernia. The protrusion of an organ into surrounding tissue.

Herpes. The common name for an infection by the virus herpes simplex which takes the form of sores. When found in and around the mouth they are known as fever blisters or cold sores. Herpes simplex can be transmitted sexually and is then known as genital herpes and is characterized by development of painful sores in the genital area.

Hirsutism. The excessive or unusual growth of body or facial hair, most often in women; caused by abnormal production of or sensitivity to male hormones.

Histamine. A chemical substance found in body tissue that is responsible for allergic reactions; also stimulates gastric juices. Histamine is released when cells appear threatened by an invader. The site swells and becomes congested, creating hives on the skin, sneezing, running nose, itching eyes, or asthma.

Hormones. Chemical substances produced by glands that are transported through the blood to other parts of the body, where they stimulate and regulate various body functions. See also *Estrogen, FSH, hCG, LH,* and *Progesterone.*

Hormone replacement therapy (HRT). Estrogen and/or progestin given orally, vaginally, transdermally (using a patch), or by injection to lessen the effects of menopause.

Human immunodeficiency virus. Known as HIV, the virus that causes acquired immunodeficiency syndrome (AIDS).

Human papillomavirus. Known as HPV; the virus that causes genital warts.

Hymen. A membrane that partially covers the vaginal opening.

Hyperemesis. Excessive vomiting.

Hyperplasia. Excessive growth of tissue.

Hypersomnia. Excessive sleep.

Hypertension. Known also as high blood pressure, a condition in which blood is pumped through the body under higher than normal pressure.

Hyperthyroidism. Condition in which the thyroid gland overproduces thyroid hormone, causing the metabolic rate to increase.

Hypochondriasis. Excessive concern about one's health.

Hypomania. A mild manic episode.

Hypomenorrhea. Menstrual flow that is scanty but regular.

Hypopituitarism. A condition caused by inadequate pituitary hormones.

Hypothyroidism. Condition in which the thyroid gland underproduces thyroid hormone, resulting in a slowing of the body's functioning.

Hysterectomy. The surgical removal of the uterus.

Hysterosalpingogram. A test to determine the presence of obstructions, tumors, or adhesions in the uterus or fallopian tubes that could impair fertility. A liquid contrast medium is injected through a small tube into the uterus and fallopian tubes, and then X rays are taken.

Hysteroscopy. Inspection of the uterus with a scope passed through the cervix.

Immune system. All of the tissues, organs, and physiological processes that protect the body from abnormal or foreign proteins and thus protect it from *infection*.

Implants. See *Mammoplasty*.

Impotence. A man's inability to achieve or maintain an erection through sexual intercourse.

Incest. Sexual abuse by family members.

Incompetent cervix. A disorder that appears during pregnancy when the cervix opens prematurely without contractions.

Incontinence. The inability to control the release of urine or feces.

Infection. The condition in which the body or a part of it is invaded by a virus, bacterium, or other microorganism.

Infertility. Inability to conceive a child.

Inflammation. The body's reaction to injury, whether from a physical blow, irritation, or infection; characterized by swelling, pain, heat, and redness.

Inguinal hernia. The most common form of hernia or protrusion, which develops in the groin.

Intercourse, sexual. The insertion of a man's penis into a woman's vagina.

Interstitial cystitis. A condition of unknown origin in which a woman's bladder is inflamed and irritated.

Intraductal papilloma. A benign tumor of the breast that occurs in the milk ducts.

Intrauterine. Within the uterus.

Intravenous. Into or within a vein.

In vitro fertilization (IVF). A method of conception that occurs outside the body; eggs are harvested from the ovaries, fertilized by harvested sperm, then placed back in the uterus.

Irritable bladder. See *Unstable bladder*.

Kegel exercises. Exercises to strengthen the pelvic floor that involve the tightening of the perineal muscles and the anal sphincter.

Keratin. The tough protein found in hair, nails, and skin.

Kidneys. Pair of bean-shaped organs located at the back of the abdomen, one on each side of the spine. They excrete urine and help regulate the body's water, electrolyte, and acid–base content.

Labia. Four liplike folds of tissue surrounding the vagina consisting of the outer labia majora and the inner labia minora.

Lamaze classes. Classes which prepare parents for childbirth by practicing breathing techniques that lessen the need for anesthesia. The techniques teach how to relax using rhythmic breathing during the involuntary contractions of labor. Named for the French obstetrician Fernand Lamaze, who developed the techniques.

Laparoscopy. Interior examination of the abdomen using a device called a laparoscope, a lighted telescope.

Lawless bleeding. Bleeding that does not show any pattern.

Learned helplessness. A pattern of behavior marked by passivity and fatalism based on the feeling that one is helpless. Often seen among the elderly experiencing chronic illness, loss of family and friends, and increasing loss of control of their life.

Lesbianism. Sexual preference of women for other women.

Lesion. An area of tissue damaged by disease process or injury.

LH. Luteinizing hormone. Substance secreted by the pituitary gland that stimulates ovulation and the development of the corpus luteum.

Libido. Sexual drive.

Lichen sclerosis. Chronic skin disease consisting of itchy white areas in the genital and anal areas.

Ligaments. Strong fibrous bands or sheets of tissue that connect bones or organs to one another.

Liposuction. A surgical method of removing fat beneath the skin using a suction device.

Lumpectomy. The surgical removal of a tumor from the breast without removing the entire breast or any lymph nodes. Also known as a *Tylectomy.*

Lymph nodes. Small round organs that act as filters preventing bacteria and other invaders from entering the bloodstream. They are found superficially in groups at three primary sites: the neck, armpit, and groin.

Lymphocytes. Disease-fighting white blood cells produced in the lymph nodes that circulate throughout the body to protect against microbial invasion.

Malaise. General discomfort, feeling of illness, and uneasiness that often signal an infection.

Malignant. Harmful. Usually used in reference to cancer.

Mammogram. A breast X ray to screen for cancer.

Mammoplasty. Plastic surgery of the breast.

Mammary gland. The gland in the breast that secretes milk.

Manic-depressive. Common type of bipolar psychiatric disorder, in which a person experiences wild mood swings from euphoria to despair.

Mastectomy. Surgical removal of a breast, usually to stop the spread of cancer.

Mastopexy. Surgical support of a large breast.

Mastitis. Inflammation of the breast, usually caused by bacteria. Nursing women are most susceptible.

Masturbation. Sexual stimulation by oneself.

Maternal alpha-fetoprotein analysis. A blood test done between the fifteenth and eighteenth weeks of pregnancy to determine the level of the protein alpha-fetoprotein, which when present at high levels signals increased risk of neural tube defects or at low levels of Down's syndrome or other chromosome abnormalities.

Meconium. The stool of a newborn for about the first three days, composed of salts, amniotic fluid, mucus, bile, and epithelial cells. It is usually dark green in color, tarry in consistency, and odorless.

Melancholia. Obsolete term for depression.

Melanoma. A dark, irregularly formed malignant skin tumor, usually caused by sun exposure. The most dangerous form of skin cancer.

Menarche. The onset of menstruation, usually between the ages of nine and sixteen, the average being twelve to thirteen.

Meningitis. Inflammation of the membranes surrounding the spinal cord or brain.

Menopause. The ending of menstrual periods. See also *Climacteric.*

Menorrhagia. Excessive menstrual bleeding.

Menstruation. The monthly shedding of endometrial tissues when no pregnancy has occurred.

Metabolism. The process by which the body changes all food into energy and tissues, then breaks down these substances into waste products.

Metastatic. Pertaining to the moving of cells from a cancer in one part of the body to another, often through the lymph system, bloodstream, or spinal fluid.

Metastasize. To spread disease by the moving of cells from one part of the body to another.

Midwifery. The art of assisting in delivering babies, usually referring to the work done by midwives, people trained specifically in the delivery of babies, usually nurses in the United States.

Miscarriage. The spontaneous termination of pregnancy before twenty-four weeks.

Missed abortion. A miscarriage in which the embryo or fetus dies in utero, but neither it nor the placenta is expelled naturally.

Mite. Tiny member of the spider family, some of which are responsible for the onset of asthma; others are parasites and cause the communicable skin disease scabies in humans and mange in animals.

Mittelschmerz. Abdominal pain during the middle of the menstrual cycle, at the time of ovulation.

Molluscum contagiosum. A mildly contagious viral skin disease of children and young adults characterized by small waxy tumors of the skin filled with white cheesy matter.

Morning sickness. Nausea and vomiting many women experience in the early stages of pregnancy, usually from around the fifth or sixth week to around the twelfth week; may be accompanied by headache, dizziness, and exhaustion.

Myocardial infarction. Heart attack; the partial or complete blocking of one or more arteries to the heart, causing blood flow to diminish or stop and heart tissue to die. Symptoms include a feeling of heavy pressure or squeezing pain in the chest, which may extend to the shoulder, neck, and arm, to the back, teeth, or jaw. Symptoms may also include nausea and vomiting, shortness of breath, and sweating.

Narcolepsy. A chronic disorder characterized by overwhelming drowsiness and the desire to sleep during the day at inappropriate times, such as during conversation, while standing, or when eating.

Natal. Referring to birth.

Natural family planning. A method of contraception in which a couple refrain from sexual intercourse around ovulation, which is determined by a woman's keeping a record of her basal temperature and evaluating her vaginal secretions. Can also be used to achieve conception.

Neonatal. Concerning a newborn infant from birth to four weeks old.

Nodule. A small clump of cells forming a knob, knot, or swelling.

Obesity. Abnormal amount of body fat; usually defined as weight 20 percent above normal for bone structure, height, and age.

Obstetrics. The practice of medicine relating to care of women during pregnancy, childbirth, and the six weeks or so following childbirth.

Occiput posterior position. Unusual fetal position in labor or at delivery in which the infant's head is face up toward the mother's front, causing the position sometimes to be called "sunny-side up."

Oligomenorrhea. Infrequent or scanty menstrual flow.

Oral. Pertaining to the mouth.

Orgasm. Sexual climax of either intercourse or stimulation. Signaled in a woman by contractions of the muscles around the vagina, in a man by the ejaculation of semen.

Osteoarthritis. Common degenerative disease of the joints, characterized by destruction of cartilage, overgrowth of bone with spur formation, and decreased function. Also known as wear-and-tear arthritis.

Osteomalacia. Disease of the bones characterized by deficient calcification of bone matrix. Osteomalacia can be caused by vitamin D and calcium deficiency, in which the bones become soft and brittle and a person experiences pain in the limbs, spine, pelvis, and chest. The adult form of rickets.

Osteoporosis. Reduction in bone mass that increases the risk of fracture. It may be due to a variety of conditions and diseases but usually occurs in older people (especially women) as a result of decreased sex hormone level.

Otoplasty. Plastic surgery of the ear.

Ovary. One of two glands located in a woman's lower abdomen, beside the uterus, that produce the ovum and the hormones estrogen and progesterone.

Ovulation. The monthly release of an ovum (egg) from an ovary. This happens about fourteen days before the beginning of the next menstrual flow. Once the ovum is released, it travels through the fallopian tube, where it may become fertilized by a sperm. If it does become fertilized, it becomes attached to the wall of the uterus, which has been prepared; if not, it is passed out of the body with the menstrual flow (the membranes lining the uterus made ready for a fertilized ovum).

Oxytocin. A hormone that stimulates the muscle cells in the breast to eject milk. Also simulates the uterus to contract, thus inducing or speeding up labor.

Pap smear. Named for George Nicholas Papanicolaou, the scientist who developed a test for the early detection of cervical cancer, by which a small sample of shed tissue cells are taken from the vagina or cervix, stained, and then studied microscopically.

Parasite. An organism that lives on or within another organism, or at the expense of the other organism, known as the host, without contributing to the survival of the host.

Paraumbilical hernia. This hernia, more common in women than men, occurs when a weakness develops in the abdominal wall muscles that surround the navel.

Passive smoking. Breathing the smoke of others; known to be a health hazard.

Pathogens. Microorganisms that can produce disease.

Pediculosis pubis. Infestation of the genital region with crab lice. Also known as crabs.

Pelvic inflammatory disease. Often abbreviated PID, infection of the uterus and fallopian tubes. It can cause infertility. Often caused by infection with gonorrhea or chlamydia. See *Gonorrhea* and *Chlamydia*.

Pelvis. The basin-shaped bone structure that connects the spine with the lower limbs.

Penis. The male organ used for urination and sexual intercourse.

Percutaneous umbilical cord sampling. A prenatal test performed to obtain fetal blood. A needle is inserted through the abdomen and uterus to the umbilical vein, from which a blood sample is taken. Usually done during the third trimester, in the evaluation of Rh disease.

Perimenopausal. The time around menopause.

Periodontitis. Inflammation, infection, and often degeneration of the supporting structure of the teeth, including gums and bones, as a result of chronic gingivitis, poor dental hygiene, or systemic disease, causing tooth loss.

Peyronie's disease. A disease which causes hardening of the penis into a distorted, curved shape, especially when erect.

Pharynx. Back of the mouth to the upper portion of the throat; the passageway from the nose to the larynx and from the mouth to the esophagus.

Phlebitis. Inflammation of a vein, most often of the leg, causing tenderness, pain, and acute swelling.

Placenta. The spongy structure that develops in the uterus during gestation and serves to nourish the fetus. Once the infant is delivered, it is shed.

Placental abruption. Premature separation of the placenta from the uterus.

Placenta previa. Placenta that is implanted over the cervix; can cause bleeding during the third trimester.

Plaque. A deposit. Dental plaque is composed of a gummy mass of bacteria and other material beginning on the surface of a tooth and spreading to the roots; it is the cause of cavities as well as gum disease. Cardiovascular plaque is fat deposits on the walls of arteries, which over time restrict blood flow.

Pleura. The membrane that surrounds the lungs and chest cavity.

Polycystic. Made up of many cysts.

Polycystic ovarian syndrome. An endocrine disturbance causing the ovaries to grow multiple cysts and prevent ovulation.

Polyps. Benign tumors attached by a stem; usually found in the uterus, colon, and nose.

Postpartum. Occurring after delivery of a baby.

Preeclampsia. Serious complication of pregnancy signaled by hypertension, swelling, and protein in the urine.

Premature birth. Delivery of a baby before thirty-seven weeks of gestation (normal gestation is forty weeks).

Prenatal. Before birth.

Pregnancy. The carrying of a developing embryo and fetus.

Premenstrual syndrome (PMS). Discomfort some women feel during the few days before menstruation begins. Symptoms include irritability, mood changes, anxiety, emotional tension headache, breast tenderness, and swelling.

Priapism. A painful disorder in men characterized by continuous erection, usually without sexual desire.

Primary ovarian failure. Undeveloped or absent ovaries, often due to chromosomal abnormalities, which prevent a girl from ovulating and reaching full puberty.

Prodrome. A symptom that signals the onset of a disease.

Progesterone. A female hormone responsible for the changes of the endometrium that prepare the uterus for implantation of a fertilized egg. Also important in the development of the mammary glands once an embryo has been conceived.

Prolactin. A hormone produced by the pituitary gland that signals the breast to produce milk.

Prolactinoma. A tumor of the pituitary gland that causes excess prolactin to be produced.

Prolapse. A dropping or falling of an organ, such as the uterus.

Prophylactic. Any routine or device that prevents disease and infection, such as good oral hygiene for the teeth or the use of a condom during sexual intercourse.

Prostaglandins. A wide-ranging group of substances found throughout the body that affect or regulate a variety of organs and tissues.

Proteins. Nitrogen compounds found in animal and plant foods that provide amino acids necessary for the growth and repair of tissue.

Pruritus vulvae. Itching of the female genitals.

Puberty. The period during which the secondary sex characteristics of boys and girls mature.

Pulmonary. Concerning the lungs.

Pulmonary edema. Fluid in the lungs.

Quickening. The first movements of the fetus a woman feels, usually between the eighteenth and twentieth weeks of pregnancy.

Radiation therapy. The use of X rays or radionuclides (such as radium) to treat disease, especially cancer.

Recommended dietary allowances (RDAs). The amounts of vitamins and minerals thought necessary to prevent nutritional deficiencies, based on age and sex groupings. Determined by the Food and Nutrition Board of the Nutrition Research Council, a part of the National Academy of Sciences.

Rectocele. A bulging of the rectum against the back wall of the vagina, causing a sensation as of something about to fall from the vagina.

Rectum. The lower portion of the large intestine closest to the anus.

Relapse. The return of a disease or symptoms after apparent recovery.

REM sleep. Rapid eye movement sleep. A state of sleep during which the eyes move rapidly and during which most dreaming occurs. REM sleep is the state from which a person most easily wakes. REM and non-REM sleep alternate during the course of a sleep period.

Remission. The lessening or disappearance of a disease.

Renal. Concerning the kidneys.

Resection. Removal of an organ or tissue.

Retrograde ejaculation. Ejaculation of fluid into the bladder rather than through the urethra. Sometimes a result of prostate surgery.

Retroversion. Tipping back of an organ, especially of the uterus.

Rh blood group. A blood group that some people have and that when present is referred to as *Rh-positive.* When the Rh factor is absent, the blood type is Rh-negative. Rh-negative

mothers' bodies sometimes produce antibodies against Rh-positive fetuses. See *Rh incompatibility.*

Rheumatoid arthritis. A chronic systemic disease most often affecting the hands, knees, and hips and characterized by inflammation, stiffness, swelling, and pain.

Rh incompatibility. An incompatibility of blood types between a mother and fetus requiring medical supervision during pregnancy and, in most cases, a blood transfusion for the fetus after delivery.

Rhinoplasty. Plastic surgery of the nose.

Rosacea. A chronic skin disease of the nose and face characterized by pimples and extra growth of skin cells.

Rubella. Also known as *German measles,* an acute infectious viral disease causing a slight itchy rash, drowsiness, slight fever, and sore throat. In pregnant women may cause fetal abnormalities.

Sacrum. The triangular pelvic bone at the base of the spine just above the coccyx or tailbone. Formed of five fused vertebrae, it constitutes the base of the vertebral column.

Scabies. Highly communicable skin disease caused by tiny mites that burrow into the skin and lay eggs, causing intense itching and rash to the infected areas: hands, between fingers, wrists, armpits, genitals, under the breasts, and inner thighs.

Scaling. Dental procedure in which *plaque* and *tartar* are mechanically removed from the teeth by scraping.

Sclerosis. Hardening or thickening of tissue.

Sclerotherapy. Treatment using an agent to harden or thicken, such as the weak vein of a hemorrhoid.

Scoliosis. Sideways curvature of the spine.

Scrotum. A pouch beneath the penis that holds the testicles.

Seasonal affective disorder. A mood disorder characterized by depression, drowsiness, fatigue, and difficulty in concentrating. SAD occurs more often during the winter months and is often treated with bright lights, especially during the morning.

Sebaceous glands. Oil-producing skin glands found all over the body, most of which open into hair follicles.

Sebum. Fatty secretion of the sebaceous glands.

Secretion. Glandular process of producing a substance; also the substance produced.

Separation anxiety. The distress a young child feels on being separated from a parent.

Septum. A partition that divides a cavity such as the nose.

Sex therapy. Counseling or psychotherapy to treat sexual dysfunction.

Sexual harassment. Unsolicited and unwanted sexual advances, especially from an employer to an employee.

Sheehan's syndrome. A condition caused by damage to a pituitary gland that causes a decrease in pituitary hormone secretions, which control many of the body's functions.

Sickle-cell anemia. A hereditary, chronic, and serious blood disorder characterized by severe anemia, susceptibility to infection, improper development in infants and children, and a host of other problems.

Side effects. Unwanted actions caused by a treatment used for a specific illness.

Sleep apnea. The symptom of a variety of sleep disorders characterized by a stoppage of breathing during sleep, lasting more than ten seconds and happening at least thirty times during a seven-hour period of sleep.

Spasm. Involuntary movement or muscle contraction.

Sperm. Male sex cells. Short for *spermatozoa*.

Spermatozoon. A mature male sex cell, which when united with a female ovum produces an embryo. Plural is *Spermatozoa*.

Spermicide. Chemical birth control agent that kills *spermatozoa*.

Sphygmomanometer. A blood pressure gauge; a cuff is applied to the upper arm, inflated, then slowly deflated while the pulse is heard with a stethoscope.

Spina bifida. Congenital defect of the spinal column in which the spinal cord or its membranes are pushed through the vertebrae.

Spinal column. The vertebrae that enclose the spinal cord.

Spinal cord. The column of nerve tissue running from the neck to the coccyx that links the nerves of the trunk and limbs to the brain.

Spinal stenosis. Constriction of the spinal canal.

Spirochete bacterium. A group of bacterial microorganisms responsible for a variety of diseases including Lyme disease and syphilis.

Spontaneous abortion. The ending of a pregnancy without outside intervention. Also known as a miscarriage.

Squamous cell carcinoma. A form of skin cancer involving flat, scaly cells.

Staging. The process of classifying cancerous tumors with regard to their spread.

Stein–Leventhal syndrome. See *Polycystic ovarian syndrome.*

Stenosis. Narrowing of a passageway or opening.

STDs. Abbreviation for *sexually transmitted diseases.*

Sterility. The inability of a woman or man to conceive a child.

Sterilization. The process of killing microorganisms on surfaces (such as surgical instruments) using heat, chemicals, radiation, or certain filtering techniques. Also the process of making a man or woman unable to conceive a child, including *tubal ligation* for a woman or *vasectomy* for a man.

Stillborn. A baby dead at delivery.

Stroke. Medical emergency often involving loss of consciousness followed by paralysis, due to blockage of an artery or vein or sudden bleeding in the brain. Symptoms can include complete or partial paralysis of one side of the body and loss of speech.

Subcutaneous tissue. The fatty layer underneath the skin.

Substance abuse. Overuse of drugs (prescription, illegal, alcohol) that cause physical and mental impairment.

Surrogate parenting. A method of parenting when a woman is infertile, in which the spouse's sperm is artificially inseminated into another woman. If the surrogate becomes pregnant, she carries the fetus to term and agrees to give up all rights to the child.

Syphilis. A chronic communicable venereal disease caused by a spirochete bacterium.

Tartar. Hardened dental plaque.

Tay–Sachs syndrome. An inherited disease caused by an enzyme deficiency and characterized by serious developmental problems. Affected children do not usually live beyond four years.

T cells. Lymph cells that are an important part of the immune system.

Thalidomide. Sedative and sleeping pill used widely in Europe in the early 1960s. Discontinued when it was found to cause severe birth defects. Now in use for the treatment of some immunologically mediated diseases.

Therapeutic abortion. Abortion performed when the health of the mother is at risk if the pregnancy continues, or if the fetus is known to be severely damaged or unlikely to live. Term often used synonymously with *voluntary abortion.*

Thoracic. Concerning the chest or thorax.

Threatened abortion. The onset of symptoms of possible loss of a fetus, including vaginal bleeding with or without pain as the first sign.

Thrombosis. The formation or existence of a blood clot in a blood vessel that can block the blood supply from reaching its destination.

Thrombus. A blood clot that blocks the flow of blood in a blood vessel.

Thyroid gland. An endocrine gland found at the base of the neck that secretes an iodine-containing hormone that affects the metabolism, growth, and development.

Tissue. A collection of similar cells that work together and thus form a structure.

Topical. Applied to the surface.

Toxic shock syndrome (TSS). A serious disease caused by the bacterium *Staphylococcus aureus* that can cause a high fever, bodywide rash, lowered blood pressure, fainting, vomiting or diarrhea, severe muscle pain; can involve the kidneys, liver, blood, and nervous system. The disease has been associated with the use of tampons by menstruating young women, but it can also occur in men, menstruating women not using tampons, and nonmenstruating women. It has also been found in people with streptococcal infections.

Transient ischemic attacks (TIAs). Temporary stoppages of blood flow to the brain, causing sudden dizziness, or a feeling of light-headedness; can also cause blindness in one eye, paralysis of one side of the body, loss of speech, loss of touch sensation, difficulty swallowing, staggering, and numbness, depending on what part of the brain is affected. TIAs are usually caused by atherosclerosis of blood vessels to the brain.

Transverse lie. A fetus that is positioned crosswise in the uterus instead of head down.

Trichomoniasis. Infections caused by a type of protozoan parasite. Found fairly commonly in the vagina, where it causes discharge, itching, and burning. Can be transmitted through sexual intercourse, requiring that both partners be treated. Also found in the intestines, where it can cause diarrhea.

Tubal ligation. A permanent form of birth control, in which a woman's fallopian tubes are blocked from releasing eggs by using a ring or clip or through electrocautery.

Tumor. A growth of extra tissue. Tumors may be benign, causing no inherent harm, or malignant (cancerous) and can spread.

Tylectomy. See *Lumpectomy.*

Ulcer. An open sore.

Ultrasonography. The practice of using inaudible sound waves to produce an image of an organ or tissue. When the waves penetrate tissue, they change velocity, depending on the density of the material encountered, and send echoes that can be recorded electronically or photographically. Used diagnostically and during pregnancy to measure the growth of a fetus.

United States Recommended Dietary Allowances (USRDAs). See *RDAs.*

Unstable bladder. Involuntary contraction of bladder muscles causing the sudden, urgent, and sometimes uncontrollable need to urinate. Also called *Irritable bladder* or *Urge incontinence.*

Urethra. The canal from which urine is discharged; in men it also delivers semen.

Urethritis. Inflammation of the urethra, causing painful urination.

Urinary tract. The organs and ducts that collect and eliminate urine, including the bladder and urethra.

Urinary tract infection (UTI). Bacterial infection of the urinary tract, causing painful urination. Risk factors for sexually active women for UTI include use of a contraceptive diaphragm, failure to urinate after intercourse, and prolonged intercourse or cunnilingus.

Uterine. Concerning the uterus.

Uterus. The pear-shaped muscular reproductive organ of the lower abdomen that contains and nourishes an embryo from implantation through delivery. Also known as the *womb.*

Vacuum abortion. The ending of a pregnancy by use of a device that sucks the fetus and other membranes from the uterus.

Vagina. The passageway that connects a woman's uterus and external genitalia, through which the menstrual flow passes, an infant is delivered, and into which a man's penis is inserted and semen delivered.

Vaginal adenosis. A birth defect in which a glandular tissue normally found in the cervix is incorporated into the vaginal walls.

Vaginal sponge. A birth control device in which a sponge soaked with spermicide is inserted into the vagina before intercourse.

Vaginismus. Painful spasm of the vaginal muscles due to anatomical abnormality or, more often, fear of penetration.

Vaginitis. Vaginal inflammation due to infection or irritation, causing discharge, itching, and sometimes painful urination.

Varicose veins. Swollen veins, seen most often on the legs and causing pain in the feet and ankles.

Vascular. Concerning blood vessels, such as veins and arteries.

Vas deferens. The duct that carries a man's sperm from the testes to the urethra.

Vasectomy. A surgical birth control method in which a portion of the vas deferens is tied, making a man's ejaculate sterile.

Venereal disease. Any disease, bacterial or viral, transmitted through sexual intercourse, heterosexual or homosexual. Also known as *Sexually transmitted disease,* or *STD.*

Venereal warts (HPV). Warts around the anus and genitals, caused by a sexually transmitted virus.

Vernix. A white sebaceous covering that protects the developing skin of a fetus.

Virus. Any of a large group of submicroscopic organisms that can cause a variety of diseases ranging from the common cold to AIDS.

Vitamins. A group of organic substances found in food that are vital for normal metabolism, growth, development, and maintenance of the body.

Vulva. A woman's genitals, including the clitoris and labia.

Vulvitis. Inflammation of the female external genitals.

Vulvar cysts. Cysts found in the vulva, as a result of blocked glands, childbirth trauma, or surgery.

Weight-bearing exercise. Exercises such as walking, jogging, and weight training that serve to strengthen muscles and bones.

Western blot. A test used for analyzing protein antigens, especially in determining the presence of HIV.

Zygote. Fertilized egg.

Zygote intrafallopian transfer (ZIFT). A method of conception in which eggs are harvested from a woman, fertilized in a laboratory, and then placed back into the woman's fallopian tubes.

Index

Index **675**